HANDBOOK OF

PHASE I/II CLINICAL DRUG TRIALS

HANDBOOK OF PHASE I/II CLINICAL DRUG TRIALS

EDITED BY

JOHN O'GRADY, M.D., F.R.C.P., F.F.P.M.
European Medical Director
Daiichi Pharmaceuticals U.K. Ltd.
London, England

PIETER H. JOUBERT, M.D., F.C.P. (S.A.)
Head, Clinical Pharmacology Science
F. Hoffmann — La Roche Ltd.
Basel, Switzerland

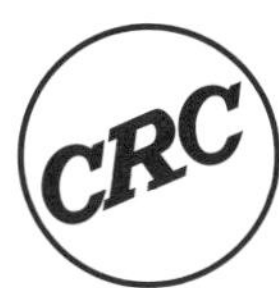

CRC Press
Boca Raton New York London Tokyo

Acquiring Editor: David Grist
Project Editor: Renee Taub
Marketing Manager: Susie Carlisle
Direct Direct Manager: Becky McEldowney
Cover design: Dawn Boyd
PrePress: Carlos Esser
Manufacturing: Sheri Schwartz

RM 301.27
.E37
1997

Library of Congress Cataloging-in-Publication Data

Handbook of phase I/II clinical drug trials / edited by John O'Grady,
Pieter H. Joubert.
p. cm.
Rev. ed. of : Early phase drug evaluation in man. 1990.
Includes bibliographical references and index.
ISBN 0-8493-9230-6 (alk. paper)
1. Drugs--Testing. 2. Clinical trials. I. O'Grady, John.
II. Joubert, Pieter H. III. Early phase drug evaluation in man.
[DNLM: 1. Drug Evaluation. 2. Clinical Trials, Phase I.
3. Clinical Trials, Phase II. QV 771 H2367 1997]
RM301.27.E37 1997
615'.7'0287—dc20
DNLM/DLC
for Library of Congress 96-23811
CIP

This book contains information obtained from authentic and highly regarded sources. Reprinted material is quoted with permission, and sources are indicated. A wide variety of references are listed. Reasonable efforts have been made to publish reliable data and information, but the author and the publisher cannot assume responsibility for the validity of all materials or for the consequences of their use.

Neither this book nor any part may be reproduced or transmitted in any form or by any means, electronic or mechanical, including photocopying, microfilming, and recording, or by any information storage or retrieval system, without prior permission in writing from the publisher.

All rights reserved. Authorization to photocopy items for internal or personal use, or the personal or internal use of specific clients, may be granted by CRC Press, Inc., provided that $.50 per page photocopied is paid directly to Copyright Clearance Center, 27 Congress Street, Salem, MA 01970 USA. The fee code for users of the Transactional Reporting Service is ISBN 0-8493-9230-6/97/$0.00+$.50. The fee is subject to change without notice. For organizations that have been granted a photocopy license by the CCC, a separate system of payment has been arranged.

The consent of CRC Press does not extend to copying for general distribution, for promotion, for creating new works, or for resale. Specific permission must be obtained in writing from CRC Press for such copying.

Direct all inquiries to CRC Press, Inc., 2000 Corporate Blvd., N.W., Boca Raton, Florida 33431.

© 1997 by CRC Press, Inc.

No claim to original U.S. Government works
International Standard Book Number 0-8493-9230-6
Library of Congress Card Number 96-23811
Printed in the United States of America 1 2 3 4 5 6 7 8 9 0
Printed on acid-free paper

FOREWORD

This book is a new edition of *Early Phase Drug Evaluation in Man*, published in 1990. In the Foreword to that edition, I wrote that regrettably there was ample evidence that the time taken for the development of a drug from marketing to discovery was lengthening. Ten to twelve years was then quoted as the norm, but I was aware of at least one instance where it had taken more than seventeen years. In part, this disappointing trend was attributable to an increased demand for information on the safety and efficacy of the compound before it could be registered for sale. Clearly there is a need, long perceived by basic scientists, to conduct the early evaluation of drugs in humans more effectively and more rapidly. The management of the industry has often not appreciated sufficiently that there is a great deal of difference between the approach needed for the investigative first testing of a new chemical entity in humans and that needed to organize large-scale Phase III clinical trial programs. There is now a much greater appreciation of these factors. In part this has been brought about by the ever-increasing cost and time constraints within the pharmaceutical industry.

This book is particularly valuable in continuing to concentrate on the initial investigations of the properties of new drugs in humans. I am most impressed by the list of contributors, who are all recognized experts in their field. The international nature of these experts from industry and academia is also noteworthy. As with the earlier edition, this volume will have served its purpose well if it encourages the clinical scientist to use the most appropriate methods in an expeditious way to provide information necessary for decision making in drug development. Despite progress in recent years, this is still an area where months, if not years, and considerable cost could be saved by more imaginative management.

I am pleased to see the comprehensive approach that John O'Grady and Pieter Joubert have continued for this book. Not only does it describe in detail the essential animal tests needed before investigating a drug in humans, but it also discusses legal and ethical considerations. However, the major part of the book deals with the assessment of drug activity in humans, and has drawn on the experience of many internationally recognized clinical pharmacologists. These contributions are of particular importance because of the detailed practical guidance given for the early assessment of new drugs in most major therapeutic areas and in some particularly important indications.

I have no doubt that the expertise provided in this comprehensive book will continue to enable the early phases of drug testing in humans to be speeded up. Thereafter, one hopes that the clinical scientists responsible for Phase III studies might be pursuaded to pick up the ball and run with it as fast as their colleagues in the early stages of drug discovery.

Sir John Vane
London, October 1996

APR 28

PREFACE

The first edition of *Early Phase Drug Evaluation in Man* was so well received that the editors were convinced that a second edition was warranted. Scientific advances and increasing competitiveness in drug development have underlined the importance of fast, targeted, early drug development and quick go/no go decisions. With a never-ending flood of literature to deal with, it is a daunting task to get information together to plan a drug development program or to design a key study. With the growing limitations on time and resources in the pharmaceutical industry and in academia, a readily available practical information source is indispensable. With this in mind we have enhanced the practical nature of the book, and this is reflected in the new title, *Handbook of Phase I/II Clinical Drug Trials*, which reflects the philosophy of providing practical guidance for cost-effective early drug development in humans.

This edition contains a wealth of new material, and almost all chapters have been rewritten or extensively revised. The general layout of the earlier edition has been maintained. The first four sections deal with the preliminaries to studying drugs in humans, as well as considerations common to early drug trials in humans. Subsequent chapters deal with specific therapeutic areas and indications.

Several new chapters have been added. Studying *in vitro* metabolism in human hepatocytes (Chapter 3) is an area of growing importance, particularly in anticipating potential drug interactions. Genetic engineering has opened up a complex area of drug development and biotechnology products (Chapter 8) such as cytokines or their inhibitors pose special problems in terms of production, indication finding, and safety. In terms of specific indications, chapters on Alzheimer's disease and Parkinsonism have been added. We are confident that all of the key areas in early drug development have been addressed and that the indication areas cover a wide range of important topics.

The two overriding considerations in putting the chapters together has been the focus on practical guidance and decision making based on sound science and high ethical standards. We are confident that this book will be a valuable aid to both pharmaceutical industry sponsors and investigators (be they academic or CRO based) in asking the right questions and designing the right studies to maintain a competitive edge in the face of financial and time restrictions.

We are sorry that Otto Linet, who co-edited the first edition, was not able to contribute to this edition. We would like to thank all the contributing authors for their efforts to enable us to put together so much valuable information and expertise in a single volume. We would also like to thank David Grist at CRC Press for his guidance and assistance, as well as Hazel Gunn and Amy Pawelzik for secretarial support.

John O'Grady
Pieter Joubert
Basel and London, October 1996

THE EDITORS

John O'Grady, M.D., F.R.C.P., F.F.P.M., after graduating in medicine, trained in General Medicine and also in Clinical Pharmacology and Therapeutics to achieve specialist registration. Subsequently, he held medical appointments at the Radcliffe Infirmary in Oxford, Royal Postgraduate Medical School, Hammersmith Hospital, Hospital for Nervous Diseases, Queen's Square, London, and St. Bartholomew's Hospital, London.

Formerly Head of the Clinical Pharmacology Section at Wellcome Research Laboratories, he was then made Medical Director at Rhone-Poulenc and visiting Professor at the University of Cape Town, South Africa.

Currently, he is Medical Director for Europe, Daiichi Pharmaceuticals U.K. Ltd., Director of Imperial Cancer Research Technology Limited, and visiting Professor of Clinical Pharmacology and Therapeutics at the University of Vienna, Austria.

Dr. O'Grady is a member of the Board of Management, Faculty of Pharmaceutical Medicine as well as Examiner to the Royal College of Physicians and External Examiner at the University of Guildford, Surrey. He is a Fellow of the Royal Statistical Society, member of the British Pharmacological Society, and various other learned bodies.

He has published widely in the field of medicine and in clinical pharmacology and therapeutics. He has been editor of several books dealing with drug effects in man, including a standard textbook of *Pharmaceutical Medicine.*

Pieter Joubert, M.D., F.C.P. (S.A.), obtained his Bachelor's degree in Physiology and Biochemistry, then graduated in medicine with postgraduate qualifications in Pharmacology and Internal Medicine. Subsequently, he held clinical appointments at the University of the Orange Free State before joining the Department of Clinical Pharmacology. He was awarded a Merck International Fellowship in Clinical Pharmacology and trained in that area under Professor Louis Lasagna at the University of Rochester.

Dr. Joubert was founding Professor and Head of the Department of Clinical Pharmacology and Therapeutics at the Medical University of Southern Africa. During this period he was Deputy Dean of the Faculty of Medicine and Member of the University Council. He also served as a member of the South African Medicines Control Council as well as of The South African Medical Research Council. Dr. Joubert has served on the Editorial Boards of several South African publications, including the Monthly Index of Medical Specialties (MIMS).

Dr. Joubert joined Hoffmann-La Roche, Basel, as Head of Pharmacodynamics and is currently global Head of Clinical Pharmacology within the Clinical Science Group.

Currently Honorary Professor of Pharmacology and Therapeutics at the Medical University of Southern Africa and Fellow of the American College of Clinical Pharmacology, he is a member of the ICH/EPPIA Efficacy Topic Group and is on the teaching faculty of the European Diploma in Pharmaceutical Medicine.

Dr. Joubert has published widely on various aspects of Clinical Pharmacology, Clinical Toxicology, and Therapeutics.

CONTRIBUTORS

Dr. Wade J. Adams
Drug Metabolism Research
Pharmacia & Upjohn, Inc.
7000 Portage Rd.
Kalamazoo, MI 49001
U.S.

Dr. Karl-Heinz Antonin
MDK Bayern
Gabelsbergerstrasse 2a
97080 Würzburg
Germany

Professor Jill F. Belch
Department of Medicine
University of Dundee
Medical School
Ninewells Hospital
Dundee DD1 9SY
Scotland

Professor Gustav G. Belz
Centre for Cardiovascular Pharmacology
Alwinenstr. 16
65189 Wiesbaden
Germany

Professor Peter R. Bieck
Department of Chemical Dependency
VA Medical Center 116A
1310 24th Ave. South
Nashville, TN 37212-2637
U.S.

Dr. Martin Birkhofer
Bristol-Myers Squibb Co.
Rte. 206 & Provinceline Rd.
Princeton, NJ 08543
U.S.

Professor Olivier Blin
Laboratoire de Pharmacologie Médicale et Clinique
CHU Timone Faculté de Médecine
27 Blvd. Jean Moulin
13385 Marseille
France

Dr. J. Raymond Bratty
Clinical Pharmacology and Diabetes Clinical Research
Pennyfoot St. Knoll Pharmaceuticals
Nottingham NG1 1GF
England

Dr. Colin Broom
Clinical Research Development and Medical Affairs
SmithKline Beecham Pharmaceuticals
King of Prussia, PA
U.S.

Dr. André Bryskier
Clinical Pharmacology, Antiinfectives
Roussel Uclaf
102 Rte. de Noisy
F-93230 Romainville
France

Dr. Stephen Carter
Bristol-Myers Squibb Co.
Rte. 206 and Provinceline Rd.
Princeton, NJ 08543
U.S.

Dr. Anne Dawnay
Department of Clinical Biochemistry
St. Bartholomew's Hospital
London EC1A 7BE
England

Dr. Jasper Dingemanse
Clin-Pharma Research Ltd.
Haupstrasse 56
CH-4127 Birsfelden
Switzerland

Ian C. Dodds-Smith
McKenna and Co.
Mitre House
160 Aldersgate St.
London EC1A 4DD
England

Dr. K. M. Donaldson
Brighton Pharmacia & Upjohn Clinical Research Unit
Brighton General Hospital
Elm Grove
Brighton BN2 3EW
England

Dr. Carlos A. Dujovne
Department of Medicine
University of Kansas Medical Center
3901 Rainbow Blvd.
Kansas City, KS 66160
U.S.

Dr. Alan M. Edwards
Regional Medical Director,
Asia-Pacific Region
Fisons Pharmaceuticals
12 Derby Rd.
Loughborough
Leics LE11 0BB
England

Dr. P. M. Farr
Department of Dermatology
University of Newcastle-upon-Tyne
Framlington Place
Newcastle-Upon-Tyne NE2 4BW
England

Dr. R. M. Ferris
Division of Pharmacology
Burroughs Wellcome Co.
Cornwallis Rd.
Research Triangle Park, NC 27709
U.S.

Professor Peter I. Folb
Department of Pharmacology
University of Cape Town Medical
School
Observatory 7925
South Africa

Dr. John R. Gibson
Pharmaceutical Development
Allergan, Inc.
2525 Dupont Drive
Irvine, CA 92713-9534
U.S.

Dr. Peter A. Harris
Medical Director
Therexsys Ltd.
University of Keele Science Park
Keele
Staffordshire ST5 5SP
England

Dr. W. S. Harris
Department of Medicine
University of Kansas Medical Center
39th St. and Rainbow Blvd.
Kansas City, KS 66103
U.S.

Dr. J. D. Harry
Director, Clinical Pharmacology
Pharmacia & Upjohn, Inc.
Fleming Way
Crawley
West Sussex RH10 2LZ
England

S. J. Held
Professional Nutrition Systems
1900 W. 47th Pl.
Westwood, KS 66205
U.S.

Dr. Susan Hellmann
Clinical Cancer Research
Bristol-Myers Squibb Co.
5 Research Parkway
Wallingford, CT 06492-7660
U.S.

Dr. Robert L. Holland
Director, Clinical R&D — Europe
Upjohn Laboratories Europe
2780 Puurs
Belgium

Dr. Gwilym Hosking
Department of Clinical Neurology and Psychiatry
The Wellcome Foundation
Langley Court
Beckenham
Kent BR3 3BS
England

Dr. Mark Hovde
Director
DataEdge, Inc.
501 Office Center Drive
Fort Washington, PA 19034
U.S.

Dr. Christopher G. Jones
Zeneca Pharmaceuticals
Alderley Park
MacClesfield
Cheshire SK10 4TJ
England

Dr. Finian Kelly
Knoll Pharmaceuticals
Nottingham NG1 1GF
England

P. E. Krehbiel
Department of Medicine
University of Kansas Medical Center
3901 Rainbow Blvd.
Kansas City, KS 66160
U.S.

Dr. J. J. E. Kusmierek
Director of Development
Sanofi Recherche
9 Rue du President S. Allende
F-94256 Gentilly
France

Dr. C. M. Lawrence
Department of Dermatology
University of Newcastle-upon-Tyne
Framlington Place
Newcastle-Upon-Tyne NE2 4BW
England

Dr. Christopher G. G. Link
Zeneca Pharmaceuticals
Alderley Park
MacClesfield
Cheshire SK10 4TJ
England

Dr. Vasant K. Manna
Skin Department
Royal London Hospital
Whitechapel
London E1 1BB
England

Dr. Pran K. Marrott
Director, Cardiovascular Medicine
Berlex Laboratories, Inc.
300 Fairfield Rd.
Wayne, NJ 07470-7358
U.S.

Dr. Graham R. McClelland
Head, Clinical Pharmacology Operations
Roche Products Ltd
P.O. Box 8
Welwyn Garden City
Herts AL7 3AY
England

Dr. John McEwen
Department of Clinical Pharmacology
Ninewells Hospital and Medical School
Dundee DD1 9SY
Scotland

Dr. Joe Mercer
CNS Clinical Pharmacology
Division of Clinical Pharmacology
Glaxo Wellcome Research and Development
Greenford
Middlesex UB6 OHE
England

Professor Jean-Louis Montastruc
Service de Pharmacologie Clinique
Faculté de Médecine
37 allées Jules Guesde
31073 Toulouse
France

Dr. Kevin P. J. O'Kane
Department of Medicine
University of Edinburgh
Western General Hospital
Crewe Rd.
Edinburgh EH4 2XU
Scotland

Dr. Nicole Onetto
Clinical Cancer Research
Bristol-Myers Squibb Co.
5 Research Parkway
Wallingford, CT 06492-7660
U.S.

Dr. Nancy Pauly
Central Research and Development
Rhône Poulenc Rorer
20 Ave. Raymond Aron
92165 Antony
France

Professor O. Rascol
Service de Pharmacologie Clinique
Faculté de Médecine
37 allées Jules Guesde
31073 Toulouse
France

Dr. Stots B. Reele
Zeneca Pharmaceuticals
1800 Concord Pike
P.O. Box 15437
Wilmington, DE 19850-5437
U.S.

Dr. Paul E. Rolan
Medical Director
Medeval Ltd.
Manchester Science Park
Lloyd St. North
Manchester M15 6SH
England

Dr. Edmond Roland
Central Research and Development
Rhône Poulenc Rorer
20 Ave. Raymond Aron
92165 Antony
France

Dr. Marcel Rozencweig
Clinical Cancer Research
Bristol-Myers Squibb Co.
5 Research Parkway
Wallingford, CT 06492-7660
U.S.

Dr. J. A. Salmon
Department of Pharmacology
Wellcome Foundation Ltd.
Langley Court
Beckenham
Kent BR3 3BS
England

Dr. Lee P. Schacter
Yale Cancer Center
333 Cedar St.
New Haven, CT 06520-8028
U.S.

Professor J. M. Senard
Service de Pharmacologie Clinique
Faculté de Médecine
37 allées Jules Guesde
31073 Toulouse
France

Professor Sam Shuster
Department of Dermatology
University of Newcastle-upon-Tyne
Framlington Place
Newcastle-Upon-Tyne NE2 4BW
England

Dr. Wolfgang Söhngen
Grünenthal GMBH
0-52220 Stolberg
Germany

Dr. Whaijen Soo
Vice-President
Clinical Science
Hoffmann-La Roche Inc.
340 Kingsland St.
Nutley, NJ 07110-1199
U.S.

Dr. C. Thalamas
Centre d'Investigation Clinique
CHU Toulouse Purpan
31059 Toulouse
France

Dr. Malcolm Thomas
Clinical Pharmacology Division
Glaxo Wellcome Research and
Development
Greenford Rd.
Greenford
Middlesex UB6 0HE
England

Professor G. T. Tucker
Department of Medicine and
Pharmacology
University of Sheffield
Royal Hallamshire Hospital
Glossop Rd.
Sheffield S10 2JF
England

Dr. Shri C. Valvani
Director, Pharmaceutics and Drug Delivery
Systems Research
The Upjohn Company
301 Henrietta St.
Kalamazoo, MI 49007
U.S.

Dr. Steven J. Warrington
16 The Knoll
Beckenham
Kent BR3 2JW
England

Dr. David J. Webb
Department of Medicine
University of Edinburgh
Western General Hospital
Crewe Rd.
Edinburgh EH4 2XU
Scotland

Dr. Catherine Weil
Bristol-Myers Squibb
Chaussée de la Hulpe 154
1170 Brussels
Belgium

Dr. Frank Wells (retired)
The Brick House
3 The Granaries
Tudderham St. Martin
Ipswich, Suffolk 1P6 9BW
England

Dr. Keith A. Wesnes
Chief Executive
Cognitive Drug Research Ltd.
Beech Hill
Reading RG7 2BJ
England

Dr. B. J. R. Whittle
Department of Pharmacology
Wellcome Foundation Ltd.
Langley Court
Beckenham
Kent BR3 3BS
England

Dr. Benjamin Winograd
Bristol-Myers Squibb
Chaussée de la Hulpe 154
1170 Brussels
Belgium

D. Wood
Department of Pharmacology
University of Cape Town Medical School
Observatory 7925
South Africa

CONTENTS

PART I. PRELIMINARIES TO TESTING IN HUMANS

1. The Pharmaceutical Background, *S.C. Valvani* 3
2. The Pharmacological Background, *B.J.R. Whittle, J.A. Salmon, and R.M. Ferris* 15
3. The Metabolic Background, *W.J. Adams* 23
4. Animal Tests as Predictors of Human Response, *D. Wood and P.I. Folb* 35
5. The *In Vitro* Assessment of Human Hepatic Drug Metabolism, *G.T. Tucker* 51

PART II. ORGANIZATION AND DECISION MAKING

6. Decision Points in Human Drug Development, *S.B. Reele* 67
7. Principles in Costing and Administration, *M. Hovde* 81
8. Biotechnology, *P. Harris* 93

PART III. ETHICAL AND LEGAL CONSIDERATIONS

9. Ethical Aspects of Research in Healthy Volunteers, *S.J. Warrington* 103
10. Bioethics and Industry: Ethical Aspects of Research in Patients, *F. Wells* 111
11. Legal Liabilities in Clinical Trials, *I.C. Dodds-Smith* 123

PART IV. MEASURING DRUG ACTIVITY IN HUMANS

12. Study Design and Assessment of Wanted and Unwanted Drug Effects in Phase I/II Trials, *M. Thomas* 157
13. The Assessment of Pharmacokinetics in Early Phase Drug Evaluation, *P.E. Rolan* 169

PART V. ASSESSMENT OF DRUG EFFECTS ON THE CARDIOVASCULAR SYSTEM

14. Noninvasive Measurement of Cardiovascular Response, *K.M. Donaldson and J.D. Harry* 179
15. Antianginal Drugs, *N. Pauly and E. Roland* 197
16. Antiarrhythmic Agents, *P.K. Marrott* 213
17. Antihypertensive Drugs, *K.P.J. O'Kane and D.J. Webb* 217
18. Drugs for Heart Failure, *G.G. Belz and P.H. Joubert* 237
19. Peripheral Arterial Disease, *J.J.F. Belch and W. Söhngen* 249

PART VI. ASSESSMENT OF DRUG EFFECTS ON THE RESPIRATORY SYSTEM

20. Anti-Asthmatic Drugs, *A.M. Edwards* 281

PART VII. ASSESSMENT OF DRUG EFFECTS ON THE CNS

21. Measurement of CNS Effects, *F. Kelly and J.R. Bratty* 295
22. Antiepileptic Drugs, *J. Mercer and G. Hosking* 305
23. Anxiolytics and Hypnotics, *G.R. McClelland* 317
24. Antidepressants, *J. Dingemanse* 329
25. Antipsychotic Agents, *C.G.G. Link and C.G. Jones* 347
26. Alzheimer's Disease and Other Dementias, *R.L. Holland and K.A. Wesnes* 355
27. Antiparkinsonian Agents, *J.L. Montastruc, O. Rascol, J.M. Senard, O. Blin, and C. Thalamas* 373

PART VIII. ASSESSMENT OF DRUG EFFECTS ON THE GASTROINTESTINAL SYSTEM

28. Gastrointestinal Effects, *K.H. Antonin and P.R. Bieck* 385
29. Anti-Ulcer Drugs, *C. Broom* 401

PART IX. ASSESSMENT OF DRUG EFFECTS ON THE GENITO-URINARY SYSTEM

30. Diuretics, *J. McMurray and J. McEwen* 415
31. Renal Side Effects, *A. Dawnay* 425

PART X. ASSESSMENT OF DRUG ACTIVITY IN THE SKIN

32. Measurement of Skin Response to Drugs, *S. Shuster, P.M. Farr, and C.M. Lawrence* 437
33. Drugs for Eczema, *J.R. Gibson and V.K. Manna* 447

PART XI. ASSESSMENT OF DRUGS USED FOR THE TREATMENT OF METABOLIC DISORDERS

34. Phase II Trials with Lipid-Acting Drugs, *C.A. Dujovne, P.E. Krehbiel, W.S. Harris, and S.J. Held* 463
35. Development of Antidiabetic Therapy Phases I and II, *J.R. Bratty and F. Kelly* 475

PART XII. ASSESSMENT OF THE EFFECTS OF CHEMOTHERAPEUTIC AGENTS

36. Antibiotic Development, *A. Bryskier* 485
37. Antiviral Drugs, *W. Soo* 511
38. Anticancer Drugs, *L.P. Schachter, M. Birkhofer, S. Carter, R. Canetta, S. Hellmann, N. Onetto, C. Weil, B. Winograd, and M. Rozencweig* 523

PART XIII. ASSESSMENT OF DRUGS AFFECTING THE INFLAMMATORY PROCESS AND PAIN

39. Analgesics, *R.L. Holland* 537

Index 547

Part I. Preliminaries to Testing in Humans

Chapter 1

The Pharmaceutical Background

Shri C. Valvani

CONTENTS

1 Introduction 3
2 Background 3
3 Preformulation Considerations 4
4 Dosage Form Considerations 6
5 Biological Considerations 7
6 Physicochemical Considerations 9
7 Summary 11
References 11

1 INTRODUCTION

The primary goal of most research-based pharmaceutical organizations around the world is to discover, develop, and procure necessary regulatory approvals for marketing new drugs for the treatment or prevention of diseases in humans and animals. This chapter deals primarily with pharmaceutical considerations for the development of new chemical entities. A comprehensive discussion of all pharmaceutical considerations in the design and development of all types of dosage forms or drug delivery systems for various routes of administration is beyond the scope of this chapter, rather it focuses on pharmaceutical considerations for dosage forms generally developed for preclinical safety assessment and early human testing.

Over the last several years, the amount of data required for early testing and registration of new products has significantly increased. Global consolidation of the pharmaceutical industry with strategic mergers and acquisitions continues to exert pressures for accelerating drug development. It is generally recognized that the requirements for registration from many countries have differed not only in content but also in how the data is formatted for regulatory reviews. This has culminated in the desire to harmonize registration requirements. The International Commission on Harmonization of Technical Requirements for Registration of Pharmaceuticals for Human Use (ICH) has undertaken an ambitious goal to reduce or eliminate redundant technical requirements for testing and registration of products. While ICH does not cover the entire world, it is focused toward development of unified standards for new drug registrations in the regions with the three largest consumers of pharmaceutical products, the U.S., the European Community, and Japan. The ICH is co-sponsored by the regulatory agencies, compendial groups, and major industrial organizations from these three regions. Major topics covering quality, safety, and efficacy of new products in different stages of harmonization include stability testing, impurities, validation, light stability, and stability of biotechnology products.

2 BACKGROUND

The discovery phase of new chemical or molecular entities usually involves chemical synthesis or isolation from natural sources. With the advent of genetic and protein engineering, a new generation of drugs, protein or polypeptide molecules, is beginning to be introduced. During the past ten years, many new drugs derived from biotechnology sources, such as cytokines, erythropoietins, plasminogen activators, blood-plasma factors, hormones, growth factors, insulin, monoclonal antibodies, and rDNA vaccines have appeared in global markets and numerous products are under development. Because most protein drugs and large peptides cannot be synthesized, they are produced via genetic engineering or recombinant DNA techniques, fermentation or cell culture, isolation, and purification steps. A decision to develop new drugs often depends on the results of early "screening" which involves testing of new drug molecules

0-8493-9230-6/97/$0.00+$.50
© 1997 by CRC Press, Inc.

using whole animals or *in vitro* techniques to determine the pharmacological response which reflects potential therapeutic benefit(s) or unmet medical needs.

Once the new drug has been shown to possess the desirable therapeutic or pharmacological promise during initial screening, it must undergo determination of purity, potency, stability, and other properties leading to development of early dosage forms for extensive evaluation of preclinical safety and pharmacokinetics or biopharmaceutics testing before early testing in humans can begin. The requirements for clinical trials of new drugs vary considerably depending on the regulations within each country. Initial testing of new drugs in humans requires a comprehensive dossier of information for the regulatory review and approval process. Specific guidelines for the format and content and submission of regulatory documents for pharmaceutical and other sections must be followed before studies in humans can be undertaken. The use of sound scientific principles, adherence to regulatory guidelines, and rational science-based approaches is critical to successful testing and development of new drugs.

When the decision is made to develop a new compound, usually the first step is to prepare a sufficient quantity of active drug substance so that the multidisciplinary approach to early investigation and development can begin. Synthesis of bulk drug substance at this early stage is often carried out on a small laboratory scale from several tens of grams to a few kilograms depending on the expected dosage and toxicology testing protocol needs.

New drugs for preclinical safety assessment, usually in two different animal species (e.g., rodents and non-rodents), must be formulated in a dosage form or a delivery system which will deliver the drug in a way that maximizes the "availability" of drug for thorough evaluation of drug related toxicity. Drug formulation development for toxicological evaluation needs to be optimized to conveniently deliver the drug to the animal species in question and also to minimize any non-drug related concerns. The development of early dosage forms for preclinical testing and eventually for early testing in humans requires an interplay of physicochemical, biological, and dosage form considerations.

For new drugs, preclinical studies are expected to provide data that should help understand the dose/activity relationship, the dose/toxicity relationship, the relationship of route and dose frequency to activity/toxicity, and the potential risk for clinical toxicity. The determination of no-effect or toxic levels in animals should involve not just maximizing the dosage administered, but achieving the highest systemic level of exposure with the lowest dosage administered. Therefore, the toxicology formulation development phase may require the design and development of several drug formulations of varying compositions (e.g., vehicle, additives, pH, etc.). The goal is to identify a formulation which will achieve the highest exposure with the lowest dosage and yet is tolerated by the animal species involved for the duration of toxicity studies. Sometimes high enough exposure for toxic levels may not be achievable because of limitations imposed by the physicochemical properties of the drug.

3 PREFORMULATION CONSIDERATIONS

The development process usually begins with the preformulation characterization of drug substance. Preformulation is the study of critical physicochemical properties which could affect the drug's biological performance, processing, design, and the development of an efficacious dosage form. Critical physicochemical properties of a compound include solubility, lipophilicity, stability, diffusivity, particle size, pKa, and crystal form. Table 1 lists these and additional parameters which may be evaluated during the preformulation investigation stage. Most of these are molecular properties of the drug and provide a sort of "fingerprint" of the drug molecule. A thorough understanding of these characteristics is important for successful formulation design and development.

Some of the preformulation parameters may be affected by processing, e.g., rate of dissolution, specific surface area, and/or flow properties of the drug may be affected by particle size reduction via micronization, milling, or by manipulation of crystallization procedures. Development of formulations for toxicology testing, early human evaluation, or for eventual marketing may not require extensive in-depth evaluation of all of these parameters. It largely depends on the type of drug, dosage form, or the route of administration. For example, for solid dosage forms, stability of the drug in the solid state to various environmental factors such as temperature, moisture, and light, etc. should be investigated in greater detail, while solution formulations (parenteral or oral), degradation mechanisms, and kinetics of solution stability may require critical evaluation. Likewise, for aerosol delivery systems for inhalation, particle size, shape and surface characterization, and solubility and compatibility with vehicle and propellants are some of the important considerations. For proteins and polypeptide macromolecular drugs, biological activity is often dictated by molecular conformation and, thus, is largely governed by

Table 1 Preformulation Characterization of Bulk Drug Substances

- Chemical structure and molecular weight
- Organoleptic properties
  - Color, odor, taste
- Chemical purity and identity
  - Level and identification of impurities
  - Spectral properties (infrared, ultraviolet)
- Physical properties
  - Particle size, shape, and frequency distribution
  - Bulk density
  - Microscopic characterization
  - Surface area
  - Surface activity
  - Effect of milling/micronization
- Aqueous solubility
  - pH solubility profile
  - Effect of temperature
  - Effect of solubilizing agents
  - Effect of buffers, ionic strength
- Non-aqueous solubility
  - Pure solvents
  - Mixed cosolvents
  - Effect of pH
- *In vitro* dissolution or drug release rate
  - Bulk drug and pure drug compact
  - Effect of particle size, surface area
  - Partition coefficient
  - Octanol/water systems
  - Alkane/water systems
- Ionization constants (pKa)
  - Aqueous and non-aqueous systems
- Biopharmaceutics properties
  - *In vitro* absorption/transport properties
- Crystalline properties
  - Melting point
  - Polymorphism (effect on bioavailability)
  - Thermal analysis (DSC, TGA, etc.)
  - Isomerism
- Mechanical properties
  - Viscoelastic properties
  - Compressibility
  - Flowability
- Solution stability
  - pH rate profile
  - Degradation rate and mechanism
  - Effect of temperature
  - Photolytic degradation
  - Oxidation/hydrolysis
  - Presence of metals
  - Non-aqueous solution stability
  - Ionic strength
  - Effect of additives
- Solid state stability
  - Effect of temperature
  - Effect of humidity
  - Effect of light
  - Effect of oxygen/nitrogen
  - Effect of additives

non-covalent forces. Therefore, conformational stability, including denaturation and aggregation, and an assessment of biological activity must be addressed during formulation development of proteinaceous drugs. For targeted or site specific drug delivery systems, for example, monoclonal antibodies, consideration of biochemical and transcellular events at the cellular level is important.

Preformulation investigation usually commences with complete analytical characterization of the drug substance with regard to chemical purity, including the level and nature of impurities. For proteins, peptides, and other biologicals, evaluation of trace contaminants, such as viral, nucleic acid, endotoxin, antigen, foreign protein, and microbial contamination, may be carried out as part of the initial characterization in addition to several other specific tests for purity and identity. For conventional organic drug molecules, early chemical synthesis often is directed toward maximizing chemical purity of the drug, while minimizing the impurities and residual organic volatile solvents.

Isolation and identification of impurities, which may be present in the drug substance beyond a certain level, are required by most regulatory agencies worldwide. In this regard, under ICH guidelines on impurities in new drug substances, applications for marketing new drugs would need to demonstrate that all impurities above a certain level (e.g., 0.1%) have been identified.[1,2] Specific guidelines on testing and qualification of process and drug-related organic impurities, inorganic impurities, and residual solvents are discussed in the guidelines. The ICH guidelines emphasize the importance of specification limits for purity of the drug substance. A scientific rationale for impurities specification based on safety considerations needs to be provided. It clearly states that the limits for impurities should be set no higher than the level which can be justified by the safety data and no lower than the level which can be achieved by the manufacturing process and analytical capability.

Early evaluation of chemical purity and impurity characterization is critical for ensuring that drugs with no additional or higher level of impurities, as compared with what has been used for toxicology assessment in animals, will be used in the formulations for early human testing. Generally, the process involves finding impurities, quantitation of impurities, and isolation and identification of impurities above a threshold level. For new drug molecules with one or more assymetric (chiral) centers, where two or more enantiomers are possible, characterization of stereoisomeric composition as well as preclinical evaluation of enantiomers is required.[3] Specific stability indicating assay methodology, which will resolve impurities, as well as degradation products, needs to be developed and validated for bulk drug substance and also for formulations for animal and human testing.

In addition to analytical characterization, determination of important physicochemical properties, such as melting point or boiling point, ionization constant(s) for electrolyte drugs, partition coefficients, isoelectric point for protein drugs, spectroscopic properties (e.g., infrared), and polymorphic characterization is critical to establishing identity and purity of the drug molecule.

From a physical standpoint, the goal of the pharmaceutical scientist is to design and develop a dosage form for marketing that is stable (at least for a period required for successful marketing — usually two years), elegant, contains the precise amount of drug, will deliver the drug in the most available form, and can be consistently manufactured on a large production scale in an economic manner to meet market needs after regulatory approvals. Because formulations and processes intended for large-scale marketing may often be different from those used for early testing in humans, a link between the pivotal clinical batches and commercial process need to be established, usually by demonstration of their bioequivalence.

4 DOSAGE FORM CONSIDERATIONS

A review of pharmaceutical dosage forms available in global markets would indicate that tablets and capsules are by far the most widely used dosage form, primarily because of advances in the technology of manufacture, flexibility in dosing, stability, elegance, and ease of ingestion, etc. Table 2 provides a list of the major pharmaceutical dosage forms and drug delivery systems in use today. A detailed listing of different types of tablet dosage forms appears in the table. Similar listings can be constructed for each of the other dosage forms; however, for brevity, other dosage forms are listed in their simplest form. Because the goal of toxicology testing is to define the toxicity/activity/safety relationship, administration of very high concentrations or doses of formulations for preclinical safety testing in animals is usually required during early stages. This leads to the development of solution or suspension formulations of drug for toxicological testing.

For early metabolic or bioavailability studies in animals and/or humans, a parenteral solution, for intravenous administration, is often required in order to assess drug disposition and clinical pharmacology. Other dosage forms, such as tablets, capsules, liquids, semisolids, and other delivery systems may

Table 2 Dosasge Form or Drug Delivery System Considerations

Tablets
Compressed
Layered
Sugar coated
Film coated
Enteric coated
Chewable
Delayed release
Extended release
Sublingual
Buccal
Effervescent
Hard filled capsules
Soft gelatin capsules
Suppositories
Emulsions
Microemulsions
Gels/creams/ointments
Oral solutions
Parenteral solutions
Ophthalmic solutions
Aerosols
Suspensions
Lyophilized powders
Ready-to-use injections
Liposomes
Transdermals
Biodegradable polymer systems
Bioerodible polymer systems
Microspheres
Nanoparticles
Surgical foams
Edible foams
Softgels/hydrogels
Micellar solutions
Monoclonal antibodies
Implants/pumps
Microsponges

also be used for toxicology testing and for early human studies. One of the key requirements for these formulations is that they must present the drug in the most bioavailable form in order to achieve the highest *in vivo* exposure (usually denoted by maximum concentration and area under the curve), and they must be stable for the duration of investigational studies. Isotonicity and physiological pH are important considerations for parenteral formulations for toxicology testing. Suspensions must possess good homogeneity to deliver uniform dosing and should demonstrate acceptable physical stability, especially minimal settling tendency with good resuspendibility. The U.S. regulations require that the formulations for toxicology testing must be manufactured in accordance with Good Laboratory Practice (GLP). Similar regulatory requirements are generally recommended in other parts of the world for the conduct of toxicology studies and clinical studies.[4,5]

5 BIOLOGICAL CONSIDERATIONS

The ultimate goal in the drug design and development process is to improve or optimize the biological performance of drugs. Biological performance can be regarded as the most efficient delivery of drug substance to the site at which it is needed the most and at such a rate of delivery that it elicits the most beneficial therapeutic response while minimizing undesirable side effects.

It is generally recognized that physical chemical properties of the drug and pharmaceutical considerations with regard to route of administration play an important role in governing the overall biological performance of drugs. Some of the important parameters influencing the biological performance are the absorption and transport processes across biological barriers. The nature of these biological barriers and enzymatic, metabolic, or biochemical events associated with these barriers generally depend on the route of administration. For example, endothelial barriers are important for target specific delivery to liver, lungs, or reticular endothelial system; cellular barriers for targeting to tumor and other specific cells; and epithelial barriers are dominant for oral, topical, transdermal delivery, etc. Because a majority of the drugs are administered by the oral route, we will critically examine the factors influencing the gastrointestinal process for drug absorption and transport. This requires consideration of biological and physicochemical factors.

Table 3 shows some of the important biological factors which govern gastrointestinal absorption. The absorption process depends on the complex interplay of some or most of these factors. Drug absorption, whether it is through gastrointestinal tract, nasal cavity, buccal mucosa, or other barriers requires that the drug must be transported in a molecular form across the barrier membrane. Biological membranes are composed of small amphipathic molecules, phospholipids, and cholesterol, the association of which creates lipoidal bilayers in an aqueous environment. Embedded in the matrix of lipid molecules are proteins which are generally hydrophobic in nature. It is generally thought that most lipid-soluble drugs can pass by passive diffusion through the lipid membrane from regions of high concentration to regions of low concentration. A few drugs can pass through active transport, often by carrier-mediated transport or through specific transporters.

Table 3 Biological Considerations for Oral Drug Delivery

Membrane transport mechanism
Active transport
Passive diffusion
Facilitated diffusion
Gastrointestinal pH
Stomach
Duodenum
Jejunum
Ileum
Colon
Surface and bulk pH
Stomach emptying and gastrointestinal motility
Fasting
Non-fasting
Hydrodynamics
Type of food
Enzymes of the gastrointestinal tract
Lumenal
Surface bounds
Intercellular
Specificity and distribution of
Bile acid secretions
Intestinal flora
Malabsorption due to disease state
Pharmacological drug effects

Similarly, the pH of the intestinal contents in various segments, the presence of biliary salts, enzymes, the type and nature of food, the intestinal flora, and the disease state will all influence the drug absorption process. It is generally thought that the presence of enzymes, e.g., proteolytic enzymes and other specific enzymes, inhibits or limits the absorption of the large peptide or protein drugs. In addition, the extent of absorption in the gastrointestinal tract for drugs is largely influenced by the gastric emptying time as well as the transit time through the small intestine.[6] In this regard, gamma scintigraphy and other techniques have been extensively used for evaluation of food effects and other variables such as stress, exercise, density, etc. Interactions with other concomitantly administered drugs, protein binding, and disease state can also significantly affect the absorption process. The pharmaceutical scientist must consider these factors in the design of formulations for animal and human studies.[7-9]

Most solid dosage forms for oral administration (tablets, capsules, and powders) must first undergo disintegration followed by dissolution of drug particles and transport of drug molecules into the gut. Extended or delayed release solid dosage forms may release the drug by surface erosion, biodegradation, osmotic pressure, or other mechanisms. Active drug molecules then diffuse across the gut mucosa into the systemic circulation either by active transport or by passive diffusion process. The drug may undergo a variety of enzymatic and/or metabolic conversions, transport and deposition into several organs, possible biotransformation, and finally excretion by one or more specific routes. A small fraction or most of the drug entity may eventually reach the receptor site where the desired therapeutic response is achieved.

6 PHYSICOCHEMICAL CONSIDERATIONS

Table 4 shows some of the physicochemical properties involved in drug absorption and transport processes. Lipophilicity of the drug or the membrane-water partition coefficient and solubility are two of the most important properties of the drug molecule which have profound influence on these processes.

Table 4 Physicochemical Considerations for Drug Delivery

Drug molecular properties
Lipophilicity
Molecular weight/size
pKa of the weak acid/base
Chemical stability
Enzymatic stability
Solubility
Crystal form
Coprecipitates
Particles size
Dissolution
Micellar solubilization
Cosolvent solubilization
Polymer complexation
In vitro precipitation
Hemolysis
Molecular interactions
Drug-drug complexation
Drug-drug interactions
Drug-mucoid polysaccharides
Drug-heavy metal ions
Protein binding
Adsorption

The parameters listed in Table 4 are extremely important in formulation design and development for preclinical testing or for evaluation in humans. For example, for parenteral administration via the intravenous route, drugs must be formulated in the solution form. Solubility of the drug in a particular aqueous system or a mixed organic cosolvent system will determine the limitation within which the drug may be formulated. Often, during the preclinical investigation phase, high concentrations or doses of drugs must be administered to determine the toxicological response. This creates a challenge for the pharmaceutical scientist, who must develop a formulation which not only will be in the solution form, but must remain so without precipitation at the site of injection and in the body tissues and fluids. Furthermore, the drug or the formulation intended for the intravenous route should not cause significant hemolysis, local irritation, or incompatibility with blood components. *In vitro* and *in vivo* techniques for studying precipitation potential upon injection and hemolysis potential have been reported and are employed in drug development.[10-16]

In whatever form the drug is administered, it must be available in the solution form, often after dissolution of solid dosage forms, before absorption across biological barriers can occur. Even when solutions with limited aqueous solubility are given via the oral route, they may precipitate in the stomach or intestinal region, because of either pH changes or solubility limitation, and then they must redissolve before absorption can occur. Drugs with low solubility may dissolve slowly in the gastrointestinal tract. The rate of dissolution may be the rate-determining step in the absorption process.[17] Development of a method for *in vitro* dissolution rate for solid dosage forms is of vital importance in the characterization of bioavailability since the rate of dissolution determines the rate and extent to which the substance is absorbed. Drugs with poor or low aqueous solubility often present the greatest challenge for pharmaceutical scientists and frequently may be associated with bioavailability problems. For example, digitoxin, griseofulvin, some steroids, indomethacin, chlorpropamide, and other drugs with low solubility are considered to have large variation in biological availability. These types of drugs present significant challenges to demonstrate bioequivalence to link early formulations with those developed for commercial use.

Because of limitations in aqueous solubility, various solubilization techniques may be investigated to increase the apparent solubility to achieve the desired formulation goal. Solubilization techniques, including the use of surface-active agents, e.g., polysorbates, sorbitan esters, quaternary ammonium compounds, and sodium lauryl sulfates, have been successfully used for formulations of pharmaceutical compounds.[18-20] However, the use of surface active agents often present toxicology problems and cannot be used for certain routes of administration.

Cosolvents, such as polyethylene glycols, propylene glycol, glycerin, alcohol, and others are often employed to improve the solubility behavior of drugs with low solubility or poor stability in aqueous solutions. The solubility of a drug increases exponentially as a function of cosolvent concentration. In general, the lower the aqueous solubility, the greater the solubilizing capacity by these cosolvents. Of course, some of these and other cosolvents have toxicological implications and constraints on the route of administration. Several drugs, such as digoxin, phenytoin sodium, diazepam, chlordiazepoxide, etc. are formulated in a variety of cosolvent systems.[21-26] Such drugs are often injected slowly to avoid precipitation or pain on injection.[27-29] They may also cause muscle damage after intramuscular injection of cosolvent mixtures.[30]

For drugs with weak ionizable groups, an improvement in solubility for drug formulation can be achieved by controlling the pH within reasonable bounds, depending on the ionization constant (pKa) of the drug molecule. Alternatively, an improvement in solubility can be accomplished by formation of a salt by chemical modification, complexation, coprecipitate formation, and a variety of other techniques.[31-35]

While low aqueous solubility may be a problem or limitation for the above situations, it is often desirable for the development of most controlled- or sustained-release delivery systems.[36] Often prodrugs or other chemical modification efforts are undertaken to reduce the solubility or improve solution stability.[37-39] The taste of organic drug molecules has been shown to be a function of aqueous solubility. For example, increasing the chain length of clindamycin esters, thus reducing the aqueous solubility, dramatically improves the taste.[40]

For poorly absorbed drugs which do not undergo significant degradation or first-pass metabolism, membrane permeability and the dose-to-solubility ratio are the key parameters controlling drug absorption.[41] The membrane permeability for drugs absorbed by passive diffusion depends on the membrane-water or oil-water partition coefficient (a measure of lipophilicity). While solubility is one of the most important limiting factors in governing the flux across biological membranes, it is the combination of solubility and partition coefficient that influences the absorption and transport processes. It can be shown that biological activity may be dependent on concentration or dose and partition coefficient, concentration alone, solubility alone, or the product of solubility and partition coefficient.

Because of interdependence of solubility and partition coefficient, no single value for either parameters can be assigned. For example, an aqueous solubility of several micrograms/milliliter for a very potent drug requiring a few milligram dose for a therapeutic dose may suffice, but inadequate bioavailability may result for a drug with similar solubility which requires a therapeutic dose of several hundreds of milligrams. Similarly, a highly lipophilic drug may have low bioavailability because of its poor solubility and dissolution characteristics, while a drug which is too polar will probably exhibit poor transport properties. Recently, a mathematical model based on a microscopic mass balance approach, which predicts the fraction dose absorbed of suspensions of poorly soluble compounds, has been proposed.[42] It incorporates the physicochemical properties of drug and the physiological factors in the intestine into four fundamental dimensionless parameters to estimate the fraction of the dose absorbed. Several cases of fraction dose absorbed based on these parameters are presented.

Chemical and physical decomposition and degradation continually occur for most drugs and formulations. When drug formulations lose their potency by chemical degradation, the chemical potency should not fall below acceptable registered specification (usually 90% of the labeled potency). Physical appearance, including other performance characteristics, also needs to be within acceptable limits; otherwise, the products are considered subpotent and may no longer produce the desired pharmacological response. Thus, chemical and physical stability of the drug substance in solid and solution states under a variety of environmental conditions, e.g., light, humidity, temperature, pH, buffers, oxidation, solvents, and physical stress, etc. provide the limitations and opportunities for successful design and development of dosage forms. Similarly, investigations of stability of formulations under most of these conditions, including testing under accelerated conditions, is critical to successful development for early clinical evaluation as well as for ultimate marketing. Thanks to the harmonization efforts, the finalized ICH guidelines for conducting physical and chemical stability for both drug substances and products have been issued recently.[43-44] These guidelines allow uniform testing of drug substances and drug products for registration in Europe, Japan, the U.S., and Canada. Stability testing under more stringent conditions is required for marketing in tropical countries because of extreme climate conditions. Process development, optimization of formulations, and validation are other important activities that must be carried out in the later stages for large-scale manufacturing required for continued clinical evaluation or for marketing after regulatory approval. A workshop report related to scale up of oral solid dosage forms delineating key parameters for formulations and process changes affecting scale up and *in vitro* drug release requirements based on solubility and permeability considerations has recently issued.[45]

7 SUMMARY

The drug discovery and development process involves complex interplay of physicochemical, biological, dosage form, and route of administration considerations. These factors have significant impact on the biological performance of drugs by modulating transport across biological barriers as well as affecting other biochemical events. A combination of these factors may be regarded as critical for successful formulation design and pharmaceutical development. A thorough understanding and consideration of these by pharmaceutical scientists, medicinal chemists, pharmacologists, biologists, clinicians, toxicologists, and others involved in the drug discovery, design, and development process can significantly improve the rational selection or design of drug molecules for early evaluation in animals and humans.

REFERENCES

1. International Conference on Harmonization: Draft guideline on impurities in new drug substances; availability. *Fed. Reg.*, 59 (183), 48740-44, September 22, 1994.
2. Impurities in new drug substances, draft guideline at the step 2 process by the ICH steering committee, November 1, 1993.
3. FDA's policy statement for the development of new stereoisomeric drugs, *Fed. Reg.*, 57, May 27, 1992.
4. The European Community Guidelines, Good clinical practice for trials on medicinal products in the European community, 1990.
5. The European Community Guidelines, Development of pharmaceutics and process validation, April 1988.
6. Davis, S.S., Hardy, G., Fara, J.W., Transit of pharmaceutical dosage forms through the small intestine, *Gut*, 27, 886-92, 1986.
7. Christensen, F.N., Davis, S.S., Hardy, J.G., Taylor, M.J., Whalley, D.R., Wilson, C.G., The use of gamma scintigraphy to follow the gastrointestinal transit of pharmaceutical formulations, *J. Pharm. Pharmacol.*, 37, 91-95, 1985.
8. Coupe, A.J., Davis, S.S., Wilding, I.R., Variation in gastrointestinal transit of pharmaceutical dosage forms in healthy subjects, *Pharm. Res.*, 8, 360-364, 1991.
9. Dressman, J.B., Bass, P., Ritschel, W.A., Friend, D.R., Rubinstein, A., Ziv, E., Gastrointestinal parameters that influence oral medications, *J. Pharm. Sci.*, 82, 857-872, 1993.
10. Reed, K.W., Yalkowsky, S.H., Lysis of human red blood cells in the presence of various cosolvents, *J. Parenter. Sci. Technol.*, 39, 64-69, 1985.
11. Reed, K.W., Yalkowsky, S.H., Lysis of human red blood cells in the presence of various cosolvents. II. The effect of differing NaCl concentrations, *J. Parenter. Sci. Technol.*, 40, 88-94, 1986.
12. Reed, K.W., Yalkowsky. S.H., Lysis of human red blood cells in the presence of various cosolvents. III. The relationship between hemolytic potential and structure, *J. Parenter. Sci. Technol.*, 41, 37-39, 1987.

13. Obeng, E.K., Cadwallader, D.E., *In vitro* dynamic method for evaluating the hemolytic potential of intravenous solution, *J. Parenter. Sci. Technol.*, 43, 167-173, 1989.
14. Cox J.W., Sage, G.P., Wynalda, M.A., Ulrich, R.G., Larson, P.G., Su, C.C., Plasma compatibility of injectables: comparison of intravenous U74006F, a 21-aminosteroid antioxidant, with Dilantin brand of phenytoin, *J. Pharm. Sci.*, 80, 371-375, 1991.
15. Davio, S.R., McShane, M.M., Kakuk, T.J., Zaya, R.M., Cole, S.L., Precipitation of renin inhibitor ditekerin upon i.v. infusion; *in vitro* studies and their relationship to *in vivo* precipitation in the cynomolgus monkey, *Pharm. Res.*, 8, 80-83, 1991.
16. Greenfield, J.C., Loux, S.J., Sood, V.K., Jenkins, K.M., and Davio, S.R., *In vitro* evaluation of the plasma and blood compatibility of a parenteral formulation for ditekerin, a novel renin inhibitor pseudopeptide, *Pharm. Res.*, 8, 475-479, 1991.
17. Dressman, J.B., Fleisher, D., Mixing-tank model for predicting dissolution rate control or oral absorption, *J. Pharm. Sci.*, 75, 109-16, 1986.
18. Krishna, A.K., Flanagan, D.R., Micellar solubilization of a new antimalarial drug, beta-arteether, *J. Pharm. Sci.*, 78, 574-576, 1989.
19. O'Driscoll, C.M., O'Reilly, J.R., Corrigan, O.I., A comparison of the effect of synthetic and naturally occurring surfactants on the solubility and absorption of clofazimine, *Eur. J. Drug. Metab. Pharmacokinet.*, 3, 116-119, 1991.
20. Fahelelbom, K.M., Timoney, R.F., Corrigan, O.I., Micellar solubilization of clofazimine analogues in aqueous solutions of ionic and nonionic surfactants, *Pharm. Res.*, 10, 631-634, 1993.
21. Yalkowsky, S.H., Rubino, J.T., Solubilization by cosolvents. I. Organic solutes in propylene glycol-water mixtures, *J. Pharm. Sci.*, 74, 416-421, 1985.
22. Rubino, J.T., Blanchard, J., Yalkowsky, S.H., Solubilization by cosolvents. II. Phenytoin in binary and ternary solvents, *J. Parenter. Sci. Technol.*, 38, 215-221, 1984.
23. Rubino. J.T., Yalkowsky, S.H., Solubilization by cosolvents. III. Diazepam and benzocaine in binary solvents, *J. Parenter. Sci. Technol.*, 39, 106-111, 1985.
24. Rubino, J.T., Blanchard, J., Yalkowsky, S.H., Solubilization by cosolvents. IV. Benzocaine, diazepam and phenytoin in aprotic cosolvent-water mixtures, *J. Parenter. Sci. Technol.*, 41, 172-176, 1987.
25. Wang, Y.J., Korwal, R.R., Review of excipients and pHs for parenteral products used in the U.S., *J. Parenter. Drug Assoc.*, 34, 452-462, 1988.
26. Zia, H., Ma, K., O'Donnell, J.P., Luzzi, L.A., Cosolvency of dimethyl isosorbide for steroid solubility, *Pharm. Res.*, 8, 502-504, 1991.
27. Yalkowsky, S.H. and Valvani S.C., Precipitation of solubilized drugs due to injection or dilution, *Drug Intell. Clin. Pharm.*, 11, 417-419, 1977.
28. Morris, M.E., Compatibility and stability of diazepam injection following dilution with intravenous fluids, *Am. J. Hosp. Pharm.*, 35, 669-672, 1978.
29. Yalkowsky, S.H., Valvani, S.C., Johnson B.W., *In vitro* method for detecting precipitation of parenteral formulations after injection, *J. Pharm. Sci.*, 72, 1014-1017, 1983.
30. Brazeau, G.A., Fung, H.L., Physicochemical properties of binary organic cosolvent-water mixtures and their relationships to muscle damage following intramuscular injection, *J. Parenter. Sci. Technol.*, 43, 144-149, 1989.
31. Olson, W.P., Faith, M.R., Human serum albumin as a cosolvent for parenteral drugs, *J. Parenter. Sci. Technol.*, 42, 82-85, 1988.
32. Darwish, I.A., Florence, A.T., Saleh, A.M., Effects of hydrotropic agents on the solubility, precipitation, and protein binding of etoposide, *J. Pharm. Sci.*, 78, 577-581, 1989.
33. Brewster, M.E., Estes, K.S., Bodor, N., Development of a non-surfactant formulation for alfaxalone through the use of chemically-modified cyclodextrins, *J. Parenter. Sci. Technol.*, 43, 262-265, 1989.
34. Sjostrom, B., Kronberg, B., Carlfors, J., A method for the preparation of submicron particles of sparingly water-soluble drugs by precipitation in oil-in-water emulsions. I. Influence of emulsification and surfactant concentration, *J. Pharm. Sci.*, 82, 579-583, 1993.
35. Sjostrom, B., Bergenstahl, B., Kronberg, B., A method for the preparation of submicron particles of sparingly water-soluble drugs by precipitation in oil-in-water emulsions. II. Influence of the emulsifier, the solvent, and the drug substance, *J. Pharm. Sci.*, 82, 584-589, 1993.
36. Shah, K.P., Chafetz, L., Use of sparingly soluble salts to prepare oral sustained release suspensions, *Int. J. Pharm.*, 109, 271-281, 1994.
37. Anderson, B.D., Conradi, R.A., Knuth K.E., Strategies in the design of solution-stable, water-soluble prodrugs. I. A physical-organic approach to pro-moiety selection for 21-esters of corticosteroids, *J. Pharm. Sci.*, 74, 365-374, 1985.
38. Anderson, B.D., Conradi, R.A., Knuth, K.E., Nail S.L., Strategies in the design of solution-stable, water-soluble prodrugs. II. Properties of micellar prodrugs of methylprednisolone, *J. Pharm. Sci.*, 74, 375-381, 1985.
39. Anderson, B.D., Conradi, R.A., Spillman, C.H., Forbes, A.D., Strategies in the design of solution-stable, water-soluble prodrugs. III. Influence of the pro-moiety on the bioconversion of 21-esters of corticosteroids, *J. Pharm. Sci.*, 74, 382-387, 1985.
40. Sinkula, A.A., Morozowich, W., Rowe E.L., Chemical modification of clindamycin: synthesis and evaluation of selected esters, *J. Pharm. Sci.*, 62, 1106, 1973.

41. Amidon, G.L., Sinko, P.J., Fleisher, D., Estimating human oral fraction dose absorbed: A correlation using rat intestinal membrane permeability for passive and carrier-mediated compounds, *Pharm. Res.*, 5, 651-654, 1988.
42. Oh, D.M., Curl, R.L., Amidon, G.L., Estimating the fraction dose absorbed from suspensions of poorly soluble compounds in humans: A mathematical model, *Pharm. Res.*, 10, 264-270, 1993.
43. International Conference on Harmonization: Stability testing of new drug substances and products; guideline; availability, *Fed. Reg.*, 59 (183), 48754-48759, September 22, 1994.
44. Stability testing of new drug substances and products, ICH harmonized tripartite guideline endorsed by the ICH steering committee at step 4 of the ICH process, October 27, 1993.
45. Skelly, J.P., Van Buskirk, G.A., Savello, D.R., Amidon, G.L., Arbit, H.M., Dighe, S., Fawzi, M.B., Gonzalez, M.A., Malick, A.W., Malinowski, H., Nedich, R., Peck, G.E., Pearce, D.M., Shah, V., Shangraw, R.F., Schwartz, J.B., Truelove, J., Scale-up of immediate release oral solid dosage forms. AAPS/FDA Workshop Committee Report, *J. Pharm. Sci.*, 10, 313-316, 1993.

Chapter 2

The Pharmacological Background

B. J. R. Whittle, J. A. Salmon, and R. M. Ferris

CONTENTS

1 Introduction 15
2 Regulatory Requirements 16
3 Action Relevant to the Proposed Therapeutic Use: Primary Pharmacology 16
4 Other Actions Demonstrated or Sought: Secondary Pharmacology 17
4.1 Central Nervous System 17
4.2 Autonomic System 18
4.3 Cardiovascular System 18
4.4 Respiratory System 18
4.5 Gastrointestinal System 18
5 Additional Secondary Pharmacology 18
5.1 Central Nervous System 19
5.2 Autonomic System 19
5.3 Cardiovascular System 19
5.4 Respiratory System 19
5.5 Gastrointestinal System 19
5.6 Other Relevant Systems 19
5.6.1 Renal 19
5.6.2 Inflammation 19
5.6.3 Platelet Function 19
5.7 Drug Interactions 20
6 Additional Comments 20
References 20

1 INTRODUCTION

The pharmacological studies that must be conducted on a new chemical entity (NCE) to support the application for a CTX/IND or a MAA/NDA are not defined precisely by the regulatory authorities. Although most readers are probably familiar with the above abbreviations, they are defined here for clarification. Thus, the CTX is the exemption from the need to hold a full clinical trial certificate in U.K. and Europe; a similar stage of the development in the U.S. is an application to the Food and Drug Administration (FDA) for the Investigation of a New Drug (IND). At a later stage, a Marketing Authorization Application (MAA; previously known as a Product License Application) and a New Drug Application (NDA) are submitted to the U.K., European, and U.S. agencies, respectively.

The toxicological data, as well as the absorption, metabolism, distribution, and excretion (ADME) studies that are needed for submission are identified, at least in general terms, by the Department of Health in the U.K., the European Drug Regulatory Authorities and by the FDA. The regulatory agencies also require the review of suitable pharmacological-pharmacodynamic information about the NCE, although the nature and extent of the studies employed are largely the decision of the individual professional pharmacologist. The one exception is the regulatory authority in Japan. The Japanese Ministry of Health and Welfare, which is the Japanese regulatory and licensing authority, lists an extensive series of pharmacological tests which, by implication, are expected to be conducted and reported before permission for clinical study with the NCE will be granted.

In this chapter, the primary consideration will be for the development of pharmacological agents as therapeutic drugs, but a similar approach should be adopted for potential chemotherapeutic agents such as anti-viral, anti-cancer, or anti-parasitic drugs. In addition, products derived from biotechnological

0-8493-9230-6/97/$0.00+$.50
© 1997 by CRC Press, Inc.

techniques should be evaluated in a comparable fashion, but since these agents may pose specific problems, investigators will have to apply their best scientific judgment.

2 REGULATORY REQUIREMENTS

Although the U.S. and European authorities differ in their specific requirements for toxicology and ADME studies, particularly at the CTX/IND stage, there are no significant variations in their general requirements for the pharmacological-pharmacodynamic information. Furthermore, the required format of the pharmacology reports for submission to the different regulatory authorities is similar. Although the regulatory agencies do not specify in detail the pharmacological tests which should be performed, they do provide guidance for the style and format for reporting the appropriate data.

Each of the regulatory authorities require presentation of the pharmacological properties of the NCE in two separate sections: (1) The primary pharmacology, which should be concerned with the pharmacological actions relevant to the proposed therapeutic use and (2) the secondary pharmacology, which should describe other relevant activities of the NCE. These secondary tests are sometimes referred to as the "safety pharmacology evaluation," but there is some concern about the use of the word safety in this context. Thus, primary safety tests are conducted as part of the toxicological submission package and such studies must be conducted according to Good Laboratory Practice (GLP) procedures. As will be discussed later, there are different opinions as to whether the pharmacological studies need to be performed according to GLP procedures. A third section on "drug interactions," when appropriate to the NCE, is also required by the regulatory agencies.

3 ACTION RELEVANT TO THE PROPOSED THERAPEUTIC USE: PRIMARY PHARMACOLOGY

Although, the term "primary pharmacology" is employed in this section, if the NCE is, for example, an anti-viral or an anti-tumor agent, then the appropriate studies which support the primary activity for the proposed therapeutic utility of the compound should be reported. The authorities expect that the primary pharmacological properties of the NCE will be demonstrated using scientifically acceptable experimental techniques, and that these actions can be determined *in vivo* after administration by the route which will be used in the clinic.

The authorities expect to be able to review data which establish the mechanism of the principal pharmacological action. However, it may not be possible to explain fully the mechanism of action of some novel compounds. Indeed, this is particularly true for compounds that have been identified and selected using *in vivo* pharmacological models that assess the overall effects in a system rather than a precise pharmacological or biochemical effector mechanism. Although it is unlikely that a submission will fail if the pharmacological or biochemical mechanism of action is not fully elucidated, it is clearly desirable to establish the mode of action, if only for scientific and clinical reasons. Obviously the type and extent of these studies will depend on the particular NCE and this is one reason why the regulatory authorities cannot, and do not, define the precise studies which should be performed.

The authorities require appropriate validation of the experimental models and technical procedures employed. It would, therefore, be expedient to utilize procedures which are generally accepted by the scientific community as appropriate and reliable, or to present information which illustrates the validity of the techniques and data. The guidelines published by the authorities also suggest that, where possible, the evaluation of the NCE should be performed in parallel with a standard drug of the same therapeutic class. As with most of the advice given by the authorities, this approach can be regarded as good scientific policy. However, if the NCE has a novel mode of action, it may not be possible or valid to undertake such comparisons, and once again, it is anticipated that sound scientific judgment will be applied to the nature of the studies undertaken.

It is appropriate that the data should be expressed and presented in quantitative terms. The authorities not only expect to have the opportunity to review dose-related effects, but also the time-course of the activity. Thus, the relationship of the pharmacodynamics to the pharmacokinetic profile of the NCE should be considered. Indeed, there is a growing expectancy of the regulatory authorities that the pharmacological and pharmacodynamic studies should be linked closely to the pharmacokinetic evaluation, and if possible, to be conducted within the same series of experiments in the same animals. When submitting data to the European authorities at the MAA stage, one has the opportunity to draw attention to the relationship of the pharmacodynamic findings with the pharmacokinetic profile in the "Expert Report."

4 OTHER ACTIONS DEMONSTRATED OR SOUGHT: SECONDARY PHARMACOLOGY

The primary safety evaluation of the NCE will be reported in the toxicology section of the application. However, a general pharmacological profile of the NCE is also required, with special attention to any effects additional to the primary pharmacological action. The aim of the secondary pharmacological studies should be to establish the effects on the major physiological systems using a variety of experimental models. Indeed, the Japanese authorities have suggested that another scientific reason for conducting the secondary pharmacological tests could be to explore whether the NCE has other potential clinical utilities. Data on the effects of the NCE on the cardiovascular and respiratory systems and on the overall behavior of laboratory animals are expected. More extensive investigation is also required if the dose of the NCE that produces secondary effects approaches that producing the primary therapeutic effect.

The particular series of experiments for the secondary pharmacological evaluation will, to some extent, depend on the research philosophy of the pharmaceutical house. An organization which relies on random screening for discovery of drugs often includes in its submission of the NCE a large number of routine screens and tests which probably have no particular relevance to the proposed therapeutic utility. Such an example would be the determination of the anti-inflammatory properties of a new antihypertensive agent. In contrast, a company which has a focused drug discovery program will probably only conduct selected experiments considered appropriate to these needs. Good scientific judgment is therefore required to decide on the nature and profile of these pharmacological studies. Thus, if the NCE which is to be used as an anti-inflammatory agent produces notable cardiovascular effects in experimental studies *in vivo*, it would be useful and probably required, to establish the cause of such effects. In such cases, therefore additional studies may be required, such as evaluation of the NCE in specific vascular beds *in vivo* or on isolated vascular tissues *in vitro*.

The guidelines published by the U.S., the U.K., and the European authorities suggest that the secondary pharmacological activities of the NCE should be reported under the headings listed in Table 1. This list, therefore, gives an indication of the type of studies that the authorities expect to review. Although there are minor differences in the lists, principally in the terminology used to define the studies, it is probable that either list could be used as a general guide for writing reports on the NCE to be submitted to any of the drug regulatory agencies. Separate reporting on each facet of the various experimental studies on the NCE is encouraged for clarity and for ease of assimilation of the data. The studies performed as part of the secondary pharmacology evaluation of the NCE can be classified according to those which are the essential or core studies, and those which are necessary to define undesirable side effects, observed in these core experiments. It is apparent that there is a reasonable agreement within the pharmaceutical industry about what constitutes the core pharmacological test package.

4.1 Central Nervous System

Almost without exception, the pharmaceutical industry assesses the overall behavioral effects of the NCE in mice (see Irwin, 1962, 1968). Behavioral changes induced by the NCE, such as hypoactivity and ataxia are subjectively evaluated over a range of doses. Such studies in mice also serve to give an indication of the effect of the NCE on the autonomic nervous system; for example, any influence of the NCE on salivation, pupil size, penile erection, ear coloration or respiratory rate should be noted and reported. A few pharmacological laboratories do perform a similar series of tests in rats rather than in mice, yet in most instances there is no clear advantage.

Most companies monitor the interaction of the NCE with convulsant agents, as well as their effects on writhing induced by acetic acid phenylbenzoquinone or acetylcholine in mice (Siegmund et al., 1957; Koster et al., 1959; Collier et al., 1968; Follenfant et al., 1988). The effects on barbiturate-induced sleeping time (Aston, 1966) is often included as part of the CNS evaluation. This latter study can also provide a valuable early indication of the effect of the NCE on liver metabolism, since liver enzyme induction or inhibition may be indicated by a decrease or increase in sleeping time, respectively.

Table 1 Secondary Pharmacological Evaluation of New Chemical Entities

U.K. and Europe	U.S.
Central nervous system	Neuropharmacology
Autonomic system	Cardiovascular/respiratory
Cardiovascular system	Gastrointestinal
Respiratory system	Genitourinary
Gastrointestinal system	Endocrine
Other systems where relevant	Anti-inflammatory
	Immunoactive
	Chemotherapeutic
	Enzyme effects
	Other

Note: These lists and terminologies are derived from the recommendations of the respective regulatory authorities, as laid out in the *EEC Notice to Applicants*, ISBN 92-825-9503 X, and the *Guideline for the Format and Content of the Nonclinical Pharmacology/Toxicology Section of an Application.*

Center for Drugs and Biologies, Food and Drug Administration, Department of Health and Human Services, Washington, D.C., U.S. February 1987.

4.2 Autonomic System

In addition to recording any effects resulting from autonomic interactions in the behavioral studies, it is usual to evaluate the *in vivo* effects of the NCE on the autonomic nervous system in more detail using appropriate pharmacological techniques (see Davey and Reinert, 1965; Hughes and Chapple, 1965, 1981; Cavero et al. 1978).

4.3 Cardiovascular System

The majority of pharmaceutical companies evaluate the cardiovascular profile of the NCE in some detail, including changes in heart rate and systemic arterial blood pressure, in both anesthetized and conscious laboratory animals. Thus, a routine choice is to study the cardiovascular actions of these agents in both anesthetized and conscious rats and dogs using established experimental techniques (for example, see Cambridge et al., 1988). However, other species may also be used, such as cats or monkeys (see Allan et al., 1985), if it is considered appropriate or necessary to define the actions of that particular NCE in these species.

4.4 Respiratory System

The effects of the NCE on bronchopulmonary parameters including respiratory rate and tidal flow minute volume are usually determined in the conscious or anesthetized cat or dog using standard experimental approaches (see Widdicombe, 1966). Occasionally these respiratory parameters are determined in the anesthetized or conscious guinea pig (Payne et al., 1988). It can be useful to evaluate the respiratory effects in the same animals that are used to monitor the cardiovascular actions of the NCE.

4.5 Gastrointestinal System

As an overall index of gastrointestinal motility, most pharmaceutical companies investigate the effect of the NCE on the transit of a polyvinyl chloride or charcoal meal, or of phenol red along the gastrointestinal tract following oral administration in mice or rats (Green, 1959; Scarpignato et al., 1980).

5 ADDITIONAL SECONDARY PHARMACOLOGY

In addition to the core studies, a number of other studies are performed in some pharmacological laboratories, although these experiments often reflect the research interests and expertise available in the individual companies. Alternatively, they may be performed in response to particular observations made in the core studies. For example, an unexpected vascular response elicited during a cardiovascular study *in vivo* may be followed up with an assessment of the effects of the NCE on isolated preparations of heart or other organs *in vitro*, in order to establish the mechanism underlying such a response. Some of the additional studies that may be conducted are outlined below.

5.1 Central Nervous System

A few pharmaceutical companies consider that the effect of new compounds on the behavior of cats or dogs is necessary for the secondary pharmacological evaluation, although it is a general experience that the regulatory authorities are satisfied if such behavioral studies on the NCE are only conducted in rodents. Other secondary tests that are conducted under rare circumstances include more detailed evaluation of the effects of the NCE on the EEG or on tetrabenazine-induced sedation and ptosis in rats (Vernier et al., 1962).

5.2 Autonomic System

In addition to the core studies, the effect of the NCE on the autonomic nervous system may be evaluated further using suitable isolated tissue preparations and occasionally, relevant ligand binding experiments. Such tests would not, however, be considered essential.

5.3 Cardiovascular System

The most pertinent cardiovascular studies will have been conducted as part of the core package. In addition, the arrhythmogenic or anti-arrhythmic activity of the CE may be determined in mouse, rat, cat, or dog preparations (see Pool and Sonnenblick, 1967; Lawson, 1968; Wit et al., 1970; Lubbe et al., 1978). The evaluation of the NCE on isolated vascular smooth muscle is also sometimes included in the dossier submitted to the regulatory authorities.

5.4 Respiratory System

Occasionally, blood gas analysis following administration of the NCE to the rat or other species is reported in the submission.

5.5 Gastrointestinal System

The effects of new compounds on gastric acid secretion in anesthetized rats or specific measurements of gastrointestinal motility in rats or rabbits are usually only reported if the NCE is expected to have a direct effect on these parameters by virtue of its pharmacological profile. Studies of the spasmogenic actions of the NCE on isolated gastrointestinal smooth muscle may also be reported.

5.6 Other Relevant Systems

5.6.1 Renal

Many companies monitor the effect of the NCE on diuresis in salt-loaded rats as part of the routine pharmacological profile. Other companies only include these studies if an effect is predicted or has been suggested from other studies, such as following cardiovascular evaluation in conscious dogs or rats. A more detailed evaluation of the effects of the NCE on renal function, for example, in conscious dogs, should be conducted if indicated in these preliminary tests.

5.6.2 Inflammation

The general anti-inflammatory activity of the NCE is sometimes included as part of the submissions of some pharmaceutical companies. These studies may include inhibition of adjuvant-induced arthritis (Currey and Ziff, 1968) and inhibition of carrageenin-induced hyperalgesia, pain or edema in rats (Winter et al., 1962; Vinegar et al., 1973; Higgs et al., 1988). However, this information probably does not serve any major purpose unless appropriate for the anticipated clinical utility. These data on the NCE are often generated in general screening schemes, and once it is available it is felt that it should be reported. If the compound exhibits pro-inflammatory reactions, clearly this property should be reported and, if possible, examined in more detail as an indication of a potential side effect of the NCE.

5.6.3 Platelet Function

If appropriate, the activity of the NCE on human platelet aggregation can readily be assessed *in vitro* (Born, 1962; Whittle, 1987) and such an evaluation may provide useful preclinical information. Studies on platelet function *ex vivo* following administration of the NCE can also be determined (Allan et al., 1985). The effects on other hematological parameters are usually conducted as part of the toxicological investigation.

5.7 Drug Interactions

The regulatory agencies request that relevant pharmacological studies on the interaction of the NCE with other drugs that the patient is likely to receive, are reported in a separate section of the submission. Furthermore, interaction studies may also be required with respect to anticipated excipients of the drug delivery system for the NCE.

6 ADDITIONAL COMMENTS

The regulatory requirements are, by necessity, constantly evolving and being refined, but there are some trends that are emerging which deserve comment. One important question is whether the pharmacological studies should be conducted according to GLP procedures. Clearly, all work submitted to the regulatory agencies is expected to be of a high scientific standard and fully validated. The regulatory agencies have not, and do not yet, insist that pharmacological studies meet GLP requirements, although the guidelines on this aspect are vague and somewhat ambiguous. The decision to use GLP for these studies is left, at the present time, to the laboratory or company conducting the experiments, but whether this will eventually become a requirement is uncertain. There are obviously greater logistical problems in performing the primary pharmacological studies according to strict GLP procedures, and therefore, it is less likely that these studies will attract such requirements.

Another question that is receiving considerable attention at the present time is how, or if, a compound which is known to be a mixture of isomers should be developed and assessed. Obviously this is a debate of general interest which is not just confined to the pharmacological assessment of the NCE. However, it is clear that it will be important to determine whether the pharmacological activities, both primary and secondary, reside in one specific isomer. A similar question being actively discussed within the scientific and legislative community is how compounds with known impurities should be evaluated and developed.

The introduction of the Expert Report at the MAA stage will have a significant impact on the presentation of the submission to the European authorities, although there is no corresponding requirement of an "expertise" for the U.S. authorities. The European Expert Report should present a critical evaluation of the experimental studies and interpretation of the pharmacological data, with the relationship to the ADME and toxicological results adequately discussed. The Expert Report is thus a medium for justifying and explaining the preclinical development of the product. Much of the key experimental data will be expected to be included as appendices in appropriately designed tables. This may initially increase the editorial time needed to complete the dossier but the benefit of a standard presentation for the regulatory authorities should become apparent and will eventually expedite the preparation of subsequent dossiers.

The FDA has started to consider the submission of data by electronic means, for example, the computer-assisted NDA (CANDA). It is anticipated that as these systems evolve, such approaches will become the accepted method of transmitting data to regulatory agencies in the future. Therefore, it is apparent that industrial pharmacologists, as well as scientists from the other disciplines concerned with generating and submitting data for consideration by regulatory authorities, will need to keep abreast of developments in information technology.

REFERENCES

Allan, G., Follenfant, M.J., Lidbury, P., Oliver, P.L. and Whittle, B.J.R. (1985). The cardiovascular and platelet actions of 9ß-methyl carbacyclin (ciprostene), a chemically stable analogue of prostacyclin, in the dog and monkey. *Br. J. Pharm.* 85, 547-555.

Aston, R. (1966). Acute tolerance indices for pentobarbital in male and female rats. *J. Pharmacol. Exp. Ther.* 152, 350-353.

Born, G.V.R. (1962). Aggregation of blood platelets by adenosine diphosphate and its reversal. *Nature, (London)* 194, 927-929.

Cambridge, D., Whiting, M.V. and Allan, G. (1988). Cardiac and renovascular effects in the anaesthetised dog of BW A575C: a novel angiotensin converting enzyme inhibitor with adrenoceptor blocking properties. *Br. J. Pharmacol.* 93, 165-175.

Cavero, L., Fenard, S., Gomeni, R., Lefevre, F. and Roach, A.G. (1978). Studies on the mechanism of the vasodilator effects of prazosin in dogs and rabbits. *Eur. J. Pharmacol.* 49, 259-270.

Collier, H.O.J., Dinneen, L.C., Johnson, C.A. and Schneider, C. (1968). The abdominal constriction response and its suppression by analgesic drugs in the mouse. *Br. J. Pharmacol.* 32, 295-310.

Currey, H.L.F. and Ziff, M. (1968). Suppression of adjuvant disease in the rat by heterologous antilymphocyte globulin. *J. Exp. Med.* 127, 185-203.

Davey, M.J. and Reinert, H. (1965). Pharmacology of the antihypertensive, guanoxan. *Br. J. Pharmacol.* 241, 29-48.

Follenfant, R.L., Hardy, G.W., Lowe, L.A., Schneider, C. and Smith, T.W. (1988). Antinociceptive effects of the novel opioid peptide BW 443C compared with classical opiates; peripheral versus central actions. *Br. J. Pharmacol.* 93, 85-92.

Green, A.F. (1959). Comparative effects of analgesics respiratory frequency and gastrointestinal propulsion. *Chemotherapy* 14, 26-34

Higgs, G.A., Follenfant, R.L. and Garland, L.G. (1988). Selective inhibition of arachidonate 5-lipoxygenase by novel acetohydroxamic acids: effects on acute inflammatory responses. *Br. J. Pharmacol.* 94, 547-551.

Hughes, R. and Chapple, D.J. (1965). Effects of non-depolarising neuromuscular blocking agents on peripheral autonomic mechanisms in cats. *Br. J. Anaesth.* 48, 59-68.

Hughes, R. and Chapple, D.J. (1981). The pharmacology of atracurium: a new competitive neuromuscular blocking agent. *Br. J. Anaesth.* 53, 31-44.

Irwin, S. (1962). Drug screening and evaluative procedures. *Science,* 136, 123-128.

Irwin, S. (1968). Comprehensive Observational Assessment: la. A systemic, quantitative procedure for assessing the behavioural and physiologic state of the mouse. *Psychopharmacology (Berlin)* 13, 222-257.

Koster, R., Anderson, M. and de Beer, E.J. (1959). Acetic acid for analgesic screening. *Fed. Proc.* 18, 412.

Lawson, J.W. (1968). Antiarrhythmic activity of some isoquinoline derivatives determined by a rapid screening procedure in the mouse. *J. Pharmacol. Exp. Ther.* 160, 22-31.

Lubbe, W.F., Daries, P.S. and Opie, L.H. (1978). Ventricular arrhythmias associated with coronary artery occlusion and reperfusion in the isolated perfused rat heart: a model for assessment of antifibrillatory action of antiarrhythmic agents. *Cardiovasc. Res.* 12, 212-220.

Payne, A.N., Garland, L.G., Lees, I.W. and Salmon J.A. (1988). Selective inhibition of arachidonate 5-lipoxygenase by novel acetohydroxamic acids: effects on bronchial anaphylaxis in anaesthetised guinea-pigs. *Br. J. Pharmacol.* 94, 540-546.

Pool, P.E. and Sonnenblick, E.H. (1967). The mechanochemistry of cardiac muscle. I. The isometric contraction. *J. Gen. Physiol.* 50, 951-965; Scarpignato, C., Capovelle, T. and Bertaccini, G. (1980). Action of caerulein on gastric emptying of the conscious rat. *Arch. Int. Pharmacodyn.* 246, 286-294.

Siegmund, E., Cadmus, R. and Lu, G. (1957). A method for evaluating both non-narcotic and narcotic analgesics. *Proc. Soc. Exp. Biol. Med.* 95, 729-731.

Vernier, V.G., Hanson, H.M. and Stone, C.A. (1962). The pharmacodynamics of amitriptyline. In Nadine, J.H. and Moyer, J.H. (Eds). *1st Hahnemann Symposium on Psychosomatic Medicine.* Lea & Febiger, Philadelphia, pp. 683-690.

Vinegar, R., Truax, J.F. and Selph, J.L. (1973). Some quantitative temporal characteristics of carrageenan-induced pleurisy in the rat. *Proc. Soc. Exp. Biol. Med.* 143, 711-714.

Whittle, B.J.R. (1987) Aggregometry techniques for prostanoid study and evaluation. In Benedetto, C., McDonald-Gibson, R.G., Nigan S. and Slater, T.F. (Eds) *Prostaglandins and Related Substances — A Practical Approach.* IRL Press, Oxford, pp. 151-166.

Widdicombe, J.G. (1966). Action potentials in parasympathetic and sympathetic efferent fibres to the trachea and lungs of dogs and cats. *J. Physiol.* 186, 56-88.

Winter, C.A., Risley, E.A. and Nuss, G.W. (1962). Carrageanin-induced oedema in hind paw of the rat as an assay for anti-inflammatory drugs. *Proc. Soc. Exp. Biol. Med.* 111, 544-547.

Wit, A.L., Steiner, C. and Damato, A.N. (1970). Electrophysiologic effects of bretylium tosylate on single fibres of the canine specialised conducting system and ventricle. *J. Pharmacol. Exp. Ther.* 173, 344-356.

Chapter 3

The Metabolic Background

Wade J. Adams

CONTENTS

1 Introduction 23
2 Preclinical Drug Disposition Studies 25
3 General Guidelines 25
4 Prelude 26
  4.1 Analytical Methodology 26
  4.2 Physicochemical Properties 27
5 Absorption and Pharmacokinetics 27
6 Distribution 29
7 Metabolism 30
8 Excretion 31
9 Conclusions 32
References 32

1 INTRODUCTION

Preclinical bioavailability and pharmacokinetic studies in animal models are recognized to be of fundamental importance (Clark and Smith, 1984; Zbinden, 1988; Adams, 1994; Peck et al., 1992), as are metabolism and disposition studies (Zbinden, 1984, 1988; Glockin, 1982; Smith, 1988), to the interpretation and rationalization of animal pharmacology and toxicology data and the extrapolation of these data to humans. Increasingly, *in vivo* bioavailability and pharmacokinetics studies are being conducted in animal models during lead selection, usually in rodents to conserve compound, to select from among multiple leads that have potent *in vitro* or *in vivo* activity in pharmacologic screens (Adams, 1994). A major reason for conducting these *in vivo* studies is that the extent of absorption and presystemic metabolism (first-pass effect) of orally administered drugs cannot be predicted with certainty from the physicochemical and *in vitro* dissolution characteristics of drugs and drug formulations and from *in vitro* metabolism studies. Although a number of *in vitro* and *in situ* preparations have found utility in screening for absorption of closely related structural analogs and for understanding the intimate details of absorption processes (Stavchansky and McGinity, 1990), these preparations obviously do not take into account all of the absorption, distribution, metabolism, and excretion (ADME) processes of the physiologically intact animal.

As drug development progresses for a compound that is intended to be administered by an extravascular route, *in vivo* biopharmaceutics and pharmacokinetics studies are frequently conducted in animal models to obtain basic information about the physicochemical and physiological factors affecting the rate and extent of absorption. These studies are done in a species that can accommodate a human-scale dosage formulation to evaluate the solid form of the drug that is most appropriate for development (e.g., a free base or a salt), whether micronization is necessary for drug candidates that have low aqueous solubilities under the physiological conditions encountered in the gastrointestinal tract, the effect of formulation excipients on oral bioavailability, and the effect of concomitant administration of food and fluids.

Early position papers (Drug Research Board, 1969) and regulatory statements (World Health Organization, 1966; Goldenthal, 1968) stressed the importance of using, in toxicology studies, animal species that have a metabolic pattern qualitatively similar to that of humans so that test animals are broadly exposed to the same array of metabolites as humans. Because of the lack of adequate basic animal pharmacology data for many species, only a few animal species can realistically be considered for safety testing, with the rat, dog or monkey, rabbit, and mouse almost invariably used. Thus, the pronouncement

0-8493-9230-6/97/$0.00+$.50
© 1997 by CRC Press, Inc.

to use animal species that have a metabolic pattern similar to that of humans must be regarded as a reminder to consider interspecies differences in metabolism in the interpretation and rationalization of safety data, and to select from available animal species those that have metabolism most like that of humans. It has been suggested that it may be possible to take advantage of the marked strain differences in drug metabolism that exist within some species to find a strain that is more representative of the human situation (Smith, 1988). Comparative *in vitro* metabolism studies using human and animal liver tissue may provide insight into species differences in metabolism at a very early stage of drug development (Wrighton et al., 1993).

The occurrence of a rare, life-threatening ventricular arrhythmia (torsades de pointes) in an otherwise healthy young woman in 1989 led clinicians to consider the possibility that the patient's near fatal arrhythmia was caused by a drug-drug interaction involving her antihistamine (terfenadine) and her antifungal (ketoconazole) medications (Monahan et al., 1990). Subsequent investigations revealed that the arrhythmia was induced by high blood concentrations of terfenadine, which is ordinarily not detectable in blood because of its rapid metabolism, that were a result of the inhibition of the oxidative metabolism of terfenadine by the cytochrome P-450 3A4 inhibitor, ketoconazole (Honig et al., 1993; Woosley et al., 1993). As a consequence of this incident and the investigations that followed, it is now widely recognized that the identification of the human cytochrome P-450 isoforms responsible for the metabolism of a new drug using human tissues, human microsomes, or specific cytochrome P-450 enzymes (Wrighton et al., 1992, 1993) is important for the prediction of the types of compounds that might inhibit or be inhibited by the drug, and provides guidance in the selection of *in vivo* drug interaction studies (Tucker, 1992; Peck et al. 1993).

The importance of obtaining comparative metabolic and pharmacokinetic data over the dosage range of the drug in animal species has been emphasized (EEC Commission, 1980; Glockin, 1982). An assessment of the exposure of animals to the intact compound, and metabolites when appropriate, should be made in conjunction with subchronic and chronic toxicity studies. Dose alone is clearly not a satisfactory index of exposure in toxicity studies, especially when comparing across species, since the same drug dose may result in very different levels of exposure to intact drug and metabolites because of species-dependent drug absorption, distribution, metabolism, and elimination. Not only is the disposition of a drug species-dependent, but also a number of physiological, pathological, gender, genetic, and environmental factors are now known to influence the disposition of drugs in the same individual or population (Bousquet, 1970; Smith, 1988). Across-species assessments of exposure to drugs and their metabolites is best made on the basis of quantitative pharmacokinetic parameters such as maximum plasma concentration, area under plasma concentration-time curve (AUC), systemic clearance and terminal disposition half-life.

These data allow an assessment of the extent and duration of exposure to the drug and indicate whether metabolic patterns change with dosage. High dose exposure may saturate major metabolic pathways and result in alternative pathway metabolism or metabolic switching. Metabolic switching can result in a different array of metabolites or, at the very least, in a change in the relative proportions of metabolites as compared with the low dose situation. High dose exposure may also lead to nonlinear pharmacokinetics (i.e., AUC does not increase in proportion to drug dose), which may result in prolonged exposure and accumulation in test species. The use of high doses in chronic safety studies where metabolic switching and/or nonlinear pharmacokinetics can occur may confound the interpretation of data and cause major problems in safety assessment. Although high dose administration may reveal the toxic potential of drugs, particularly affected target organs, it is very difficult to use the results of such studies for safety assessment when therapeutic doses result in exposure that may be many orders of magnitude lower than where metabolic switching and/or nonlinear pharmacokinetics occur. An additional concern in chronic dosing studies is the possibility of a drug inhibiting or inducing its own metabolism. Induction of drug metabolism with chronic exposure to a drug may result in the accelerated metabolism of the drug, thereby causing a lower than expected exposure.

Ideally, drug disposition studies should be conducted at an early enough stage of drug development to allow an assessment of the validity of the animal model in terms of qualitative and quantitative dispositional behavior. The dosage and dosage regimen of the drug can then be appropriately adjusted to take into account interspecies differences in drug exposure. Comparative disposition studies may also provide insight into mechanisms of toxicity due to overexposure within particular species or to the formation of toxic or reactive metabolites. This information may provide a basis for a species-dependent toxic effect, and the relevance of this effect to the human situation can then be more readily assessed.

2 PRECLINICAL DRUG DISPOSITION STUDIES

Although *in vitro* studies are necessary to understand the intimate details of biological and biochemical processes and provide a great deal of insight into the metabolism and disposition of drugs and their mechanism of action, they cannot replace *in vivo* studies. As is schematically depicted in Figure 1, the *in vivo* situation is infinitely more complex in that (1) the administered drug must traverse tissue barriers to reach its site of action; (2) a substantial fraction of the drug may be bound to blood components in the vascular system from which it may be slowly released; (3) the drug may be metabolized to active, inactive or reactive metabolites in a variety of tissues; (4) the drug must be distributed to tissues where it exerts its pharmacological effect, but will also be distributed along with its metabolites to other body tissues from which it may be slowly released or where it may react with macromolecules; and (5) the drug and/or its metabolites are eliminated from the body by excretion. Thus, the intensity and duration of action of drugs whose pharmacological and toxicological effects are dose-dependent and reversible are governed by the rates of drug input or absorption, distribution to tissues and elimination by metabolism or excretion (Ariens, 1966). For drugs that produce their effects indirectly by depletion of pharmacologically active endogenous substances, the intensity and duration of drug response are dependent on the rate of biosynthesis of the endogenous substance.

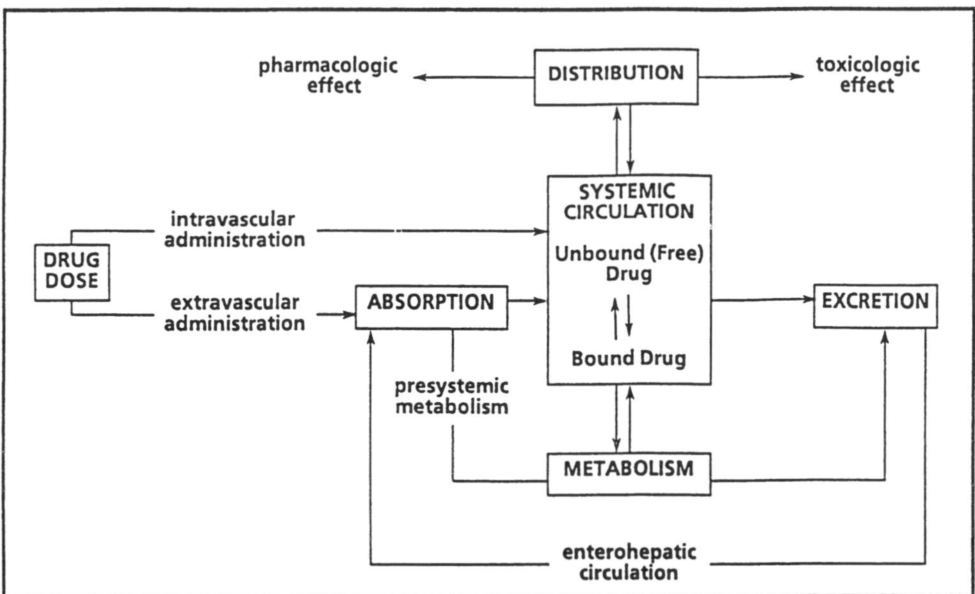

Figure 1 Schematic representation of *in vivo* absorption, distribution, metabolism, and excretion.

On the basis of the complexity of the *in vivo* situation, it is hardly surprising that the disposition of drugs is species-dependent and is affected by a broad range of physiological, pathological, genetic, and environmental factors. As a consequence, it is critical to control these factors in disposition studies and, where appropriate, study their effects. A brief description of the preclinical drug disposition studies that may be relevant to the rational pharmacological and toxicological evaluation of drugs is presented below, along with a discussion of some of the factors that affect drug disposition.

3 GENERAL GUIDELINES

The conduct of *in vivo* drug disposition studies should be viewed as an essential adjunct to pharmacology and safety studies, and not as a regulatory exercise. The establishment of a "checklist" or rigid protocol approach to the conduct of these studies is not appropriate because of the diversity in the types of drugs under investigation and their novelty. Instead, a guidelines approach to drug development is preferred, in which studies are tailored to the specific drug and its intended clinical use (Glockin, 1982; Smith, 1988). The following general guidelines should be considered when conducting drug disposition studies.

1. Disposition studies should be synchronized with acute and subchronic safety studies, prior to the initiation of chronic toxicology and carcinogenicity studies.
2. The species, strain, sex and age of animals used in metabolism and disposition studies should be consistent with those used in safety studies; but information from animals of other species, strains, ages, or altered physiological states may indicate important qualitative or quantitative differences in disposition which are important for the interpretation of pharmacological and toxicological data.
3. Drug doses administered in disposition studies are dependent on the purpose of the study but should be representative of the range of doses used in pharmacology and safety studies.
4. The routes of administration and dosage formulations used in disposition and safety studies should be comparable, except for disposition studies that are specifically conducted to evaluate the biopharmaceutical characteristics of the drug and its dosage formulations.
5. Absolute (systemic) and/or relative bioavailability studies should be conducted to determine the absorption and pharmacokinetic characteristics of different forms and formulations of the drug used in definitive safety studies.
6. Administration of drugs in safety studies as a bolus or as drug-diet mixtures should be based on the disposition characteristics of the drug, to ensure appropriate exposure to the drug.
7. When safety tests have been conducted by one route of administration and studies by a new route are proposed, the disposition characteristics of the drug by both routes should be compared to assess the extent of further safety testing required for the new route.
8. Additional disposition studies may be required if absorption problems, unusual toxic dose-response relationships or notable species differences in toxicity are observed in safety studies.

It is important to remember that guidelines are intended to identify minimal criteria for producing consistent and comparable data. Guidelines should not suppress innovative research or the conduct of special studies beyond their specifications.

4 PRELUDE

4.1 Analytical Methodology

The development of suitable analytical methodology for the identification and quantification of parent drugs and their metabolites is an essential and highly challenging component of drug disposition studies. Furthermore, it frequently represents a challenge that may extend over the entire course of drug development, since new and more sensitive analytical methodology is usually required as more is learned about the metabolism of drugs, and as ever-lower drug concentrations are encountered on progressing from acute animal toxicology studies to human efficacy studies.

Chromatographic methods that use sensitive non-radiotracer detection techniques, particularly high-performance liquid chromatography and gas chromatography, are widely used for the quantification of parent drugs and metabolites in biological specimens. The use of detection techniques that are highly sensitive and specific to the parent drug and its metabolites, and do not require derivatization, are preferred for quantitative studies. Without question, quantitative methods based on liquid chromatography with ultraviolet or fluorescence detection are most widely used, but liquid chromatography with mass spectrometric detection is rapidly gaining favor because of its high specificity and sensitivity for a broad range of compounds, including those that have no chromaphore and are nonvolatile (Siuzdak, 1994). Characterization and identification of metabolites are usually accomplished by use of mass spectrometry, particularly liquid chromatography/mass spectrometry because of its high sensitivity, and nuclear magnetic resonance spectroscopy.

The use of radioactive isotopes has been of inestimable value in the conduct of disposition studies, because of the high sensitivity, specificity to parent drug and metabolites, and absolute unit of measurement they provide (Mertel, 1979). Radioisotopes most commonly used in metabolism and disposition studies are fairly long-lived weak ß-emitters, namely ^{14}C and ^{3}H, with ^{14}C being the isotope of choice. An *in vivo* mass balance study should be conducted, usually in the rat, after the chemical stability of the radiolabeled drug has been established, to ensure that the drug has been labeled in a metabolically stable site. Loss of the radiolabel during the course of *in vivo* metabolism and disposition studies may confound the interpretation of these studies and result in excessive exposure of species to ionizing radiation. On occasion, a test drug may have to be labeled in multiple sites with different label atoms to obtain a comprehensive assessment of its metabolism and disposition.

4.2 Physicochemical Properties

Physicochemical properties such as molecular size and shape, lipid-to-water partition coefficient or lipophilicity, pK_a, and solubility have a major effect on the disposition of drugs inasmuch as drugs must gain entry to the body and/or body tissues by penetration of a succession of lipoidal membranes. Ideally, the physicochemical properties of drugs should be evaluated prior to the selection of a drug candidate for development.

Drugs and their metabolites cross membranes in one of three ways: by filtration through pores, by specialized transport systems, or by passive diffusion (Pang, 1983). Small molecular species are filtered through small pores (70 Å) in the membrane. Larger molecular species that are chemically similar to endogenous cellular substrates may be transported across membranes by specialized transport systems such as facilitated diffusion or active transport. In both facilitated diffusion and active transport, the drug is transported across the membrane as a drug-carrier complex. Both of these processes can become saturated and both are competitively inhibited by substrates that utilize the same mechanism. Most drugs penetrate membranes by passive diffusion which is dependent on the lipid-to-water partition coefficient or lipophilicity of the drug, the pK_a of the drug, and the concentration gradient of the drug between the two phases that exist on opposite sides of the membrane. In the case of drugs that are protein-bound, only the free or unbound drug can passively diffuse across the membrane. The partition coefficient has been shown to have a parabolic effect on absorption rate, analogous to its effect on the biological activity of the compound (Hansch and Clayton, 1973). As the partition coefficient approaches zero, the compound will be so insoluble in lipid that it will not cross the membrane and will remain localized in the first aqueous phase that it contacts. Conversely, as the partition coefficient becomes very large, the compound will be so insoluble in the aqueous phase that it will tend to localize or accumulate in the lipoidal membrane.

Most drugs are weak organic electrolytes that may exist in the body in ionized or nonionized form, depending on their pK_a and the pH of the medium. Since the nonionized form of the drug is more soluble in lipoidal membranes, the nonionized form of the drug is most readily transported across body membranes. Hence, the penetration of body membranes by these drugs may be predictable based on their partition coefficient, their pK_a, and the pH at the membrane surface.

Although it may not be feasible to ascertain the quantitative effect of aqueous solubility on the absorption of compounds following extravascular administration, it can provide insight into probable absorption difficulties, since a compound must be in solution before it can be transported through body membranes. As a general rule, aqueous solubilities greater than 1% (1 g/100 ml) would not be indicative of oral absorption problems due to solubility. It is important to recognize that the 1% solubility figure is arbitrary and does not represent a universal limitation on solubility. Other factors have to be considered in determining the influence of low aqueous solubility on drug absorption. These factors include the size of the therapeutic dose, the solubility and intrinsic dissolution rate as a function of pH within the physiological range, and the dissolution rate as a function of particle size or surface area of the compound (Kaplan, 1973), and the ability of the compound to exist as a supersaturated solution. Even in the case of intravascular drug administration, adequate aqueous solubility is necessary so that the drug does not precipitate *in vivo* and can be formulated in a vehicle that is well tolerated and does not cause the aggregation of vascular components.

5 ABSORPTION AND PHARMACOKINETICS

Absorption and pharmacokinetic studies should be conducted very early in the drug evaluation process in conjunction with pharmacology and toxicology studies to determine the temporal relationship between systemic drug levels and pharmacological and toxicological effects. These studies should be designed to gain insight into the rate and extent of absorption and to obtain a quantitative assessment of the extent and duration of systemic exposure to the drug. Pulmonary, intramuscular, and subcutaneous routes of administration resemble the intravenous route, although the rate of delivery into the systemic circulation will be dependent on blood flow within the specific tissues. Administration by inhalation results in the delivery of drug via both the oral and pulmonary routes, with most of the dose (approximately 90%) being delivered orally. The intraperitoneal route is frequently used in animal studies on the basis of the assumption, which is not always valid (Pang, 1983), that the entire dose will be absorbed into the portal circulation and delivered to the liver, analogous to oral absorption from the gastrointestinal tract. The oral route is most commonly used in clinical situations; consequently, it will be the focus of discussion below.

Biopharmaceutical as well as pharmacological and toxicological properties of drugs should be considered when evaluating the potential of a lead compound as a drug. In the case of orally administered drugs, the form of the drug having the greatest potential for absorption should be selected for development. After the biopharmaceutical properties of the drug have been defined, the effect of formulation variables can be determined. The formulation of the drug as a solution that can be administered intravenously is very desirable for the conduct of these studies, since a solution represents the most bioavailable formulation of the drug and is a suitable reference formulation with which all other formulations can be compared. A number of physiological factors influence oral absorption, including transit time, gastrointestinal pH, presence of food, microbial flora, and metabolic enzymes in the gut wall and liver (Kaplan, 1973; Adams, 1994). Control of these variables is important, when conducting absorption studies, to obtain consistent data. The effect of food on the rate and extent of absorption of drugs should be evaluated, since food may have an effect on both the rate and extent of absorption and/or the clearance of the compound. The conduct of bioavailability studies in animal models unquestionably provides valuable information about the biopharmaceutic and pharmacokinetic characteristics of new drugs during their development (Adams, 1994). Although little may be known during the early phases of drug development about the suitability of an animal model for bioavailability and bioequivalence assessment of human dosage formulations, a body of knowledge which is accumulated as data from multiple species becomes available from pharmacokinetics: bioavailability and dose proportionality studies; toxicokinetics studies; and absorption, distribution, metabolism, and excretion studies. Dogs, pigs, and rhesus monkeys all have simple stomachs that can readily accommodate a human-scale dosage formulation, however, from an anatomical and physiological perspective, there is no one animal species that can be predicted, *a priori*, to be the most suitable animal model for evaluation of human dosage formulations. Review of data available in the open literature from a number of comparative animal and human bioavailability studies in which common dosage formulations were administered confirmed that the *a priori* substitution of animal models for humans in definitive bioavailability studies is not warranted because no animal species was generally able to predict the bioavailability/bioequivalence of formulations in humans (Adams, 1994). Without question, the dog represents the most convenient animal species for the conduct of biopharmaceutic studies, since unit dosage formulations can be administered and serial blood specimens can be collected without difficulty. However, other animal models should be considered for these studies if the disposition of the drug class in dogs is known to differ from that in humans (Kaplan, 1973; Adams, 1994).

The most direct way of assessing drug absorption *in vivo* is to compare blood and, if possible, urinary levels of parent drug following administration of the drug by the intended route and by the intravenous route. If absorption is less than quantitative and/or presystemic metabolism of the drug occurs (e.g., in the gut wall or liver for an orally administered drug), then blood levels of intact drug will differ after extravascular and intravenous administration. The ratio between the areas under the concentration-time curves by the intended route and the intravenous route, normalized for drug dose, is defined as the systemic bioavailability and provides a quantitative measure of the extent to which the drug reaches the systemic circulation. The systemic bioavailability of drugs with nonlinear kinetics should be determined at equivalent drug doses by the intended route of administration and by the intravenous route of administration as the amount of drug in systemic circulation, and hence AUC, does not increase in proportion to drug dose.

Assessment of drug absorption is greatly facilitated by the use of radiolabeled drug, since both the intact drug and metabolites can be readily measured in blood, urine, faeces, or other excreta. These radiotracer studies are frequently referred to as mass balance or absorption and excretion studies, since they provide quantitative information about the rate and extent of drug absorption and the routes and extent to which the parent drug and its metabolites are excreted. Absorption and excretion studies are usually done sequentially in the rat and non-rodent (dog and/or monkey) prior to the administration of the drug to humans and at dosage levels that are representative of the doses used in pharmacology and subchronic toxicity studies. These studies are also conducted in other species used in the toxicological evaluation of the drug. Human radiotracer studies are only conducted after mass balance and tissue distribution studies have been conducted in animals and the tolerance of humans to single doses of the drug has been established. This ensures that safe and appropriate doses of radiotracer are administered to humans after the need to do such studies has been established. The conduct of radiotracer studies in humans should not be considered if non-radiotracer analytical methodology is available that can quantitatively account for the excretion of parent drug and metabolites. Radiotracer studies in humans are not conducted in Japan because of regulatory restrictions on the use of radioisotopes in human subjects.

Although concentration-time profiles of total radioactivity are useful for assessing the duration of exposure to drug-related material and for radiation dosimetry calculations, they are not useful for pharmacokinetic purposes. An understanding of the pharmacokinetics of a drug and its metabolites requires the specific measurement of each component, including any stereoisomers (Smith, 1988). Determination of maximum blood concentration, time at which the maximum blood concentration is achieved, AUC, systemic clearance, and terminal disposition half-life are important for a quantitative assessment of drug exposure. Information about the volume of distribution and rate and extent of elimination of the parent drug and metabolites is also of interest. Pharmacokinetic parameters should be determined over the range of doses used in pharmacology and safety studies and following administration of single and multiple doses of the drug. The key pharmacokinetic information that is necessary for the interpretation of safety data and the design of subsequent studies is whether the extent of absorption and clearance of the drug are linear over the dosage range of pharmacology and toxicology studies, since changes in absorption and/or clearance affect the extent and duration of exposure; and whether the extent and duration of exposure change when multiple doses of the drug are administered.

6 DISTRIBUTION

The distribution of parent drug and metabolites and the factors that affect this distribution are of fundamental importance, since the intensity of a pharmacological response or the onset of toxic side effects are, for most drugs, related to the concentration of the active component at the locus of action. As previously noted, the physiochemical properties of drugs have a major impact on their distribution and should be evaluated during the drug selection process. The apparent volume of distribution of drugs is highly dependent on their lipophilicity and the extent to which they are ionized at physiological pH (7.4). Thus, lipophilic drugs are extensively distributed, because they are readily transported by passive diffusion across cell membranes and have a high affinity for adipose tissue and lipid components of cells. Weak acids tend to be less extensively distributed than weak bases, because weak acids are ionized to a greater extent at physiological pH than are weak bases, which inhibits their transport across cell membranes. Polar compounds do not enter the brain readily, because of the endothelial lining that separates the brain from the circulation, unless they can take advantage of specialized transport systems. Highly polar and ionized drugs are to a great extent restricted to the vascular system and tend to have low volumes of distribution.

The extent to which drugs bind to vascular components (e.g., plasma proteins and red blood cells), cellular components, and tissues depends on the macromolecule involved in the binding and the drug and has a major impact on the extent to which a drug is distributed, since the driving force for the distribution of passively transported drugs is the concentration of unbound drug. Albumin is the major plasma protein (59%) and is the predominant macromolecule involved in the reversible binding of most drugs, especially acidic or anionic molecular species. ß-Lipoproteins are thought to play a major role in the binding of basic or cationic species. Binding to α- and γ-globulins is less important for most drugs (Pang, 1983).

The plasma-protein binding characteristics of drugs should be evaluated by standardized experimental procedures (e.g., ultrafiltration and equilibrium dialysis; Chignell, 1977), to determine the binding capacity of plasma proteins and the affinity of drugs for binding sites on these proteins. The concentration dependence of protein binding should be evaluated over the range of drug concentrations observed in pharmacology and safety studies. Because highly significant species differences in protein binding have been observed (Davidson, 1971), these studies should be done on proteins from animals used in safety studies as well as from humans. In later stages of drug development it may be useful to conduct competitive protein-binding studies to assess the effects of other drugs on the protein binding of the investigational drug, particularly if protein-binding studies have indicated that the drug is highly protein-bound. Drug interactions frequently have as their basis the competition of drugs for binding sites on proteins, some of which may be low-capacity binding sites.

The most comprehensive technique currently available for the semiquantitative determination of tissue distribution is that of whole-body autoradiography (Waddell and Marlowe, 1977). In this technique, animals are rapidly frozen in a suitable organic solvent at predetermined times after administration of radiolabeled drug and embedded in a block of carboxymethylcellulose ice prior to being sectioned in a cryostated microtome. Sagittal sections of the whole experimental animal are then placed against an X-ray film to determine the distribution of radioactivity (parent drug and metabolites) in the entire animal. Although a variety of species have been used for this technique, the most widely used animals are the mouse and the rat. Use of pregnant and post partum animals in these experiments allows an assessment of whether transplacental transfer of drug occurs and whether the drug is secreted into milk. Pigmented animal strains can also be used to evaluate binding to pigmented tissue. ^{14}C-labeled drug is ideal for nearly all autoradiography applications except those requiring high resolution, in which case ^{3}H is the isotope of choice.

Whole-body autoradiography has two unique advantages over classical tissue distribution studies, in which tissues are excised and homogenized before analysis for total radioactivity. First, tissues and fluids that ordinarily would not be sampled can be readily evaluated, and second, concentration gradients within a tissue can be detected. The latter advantage is particularly relevant to the toxicological evaluation of drugs, since highly localized concentrations of drugs in tissues may lead to tissue necrosis and toxicity. Classical tissue distribution studies and/or autoradiography studies in animals are conducted prior to the administration of radiolabeled drugs to humans to assess the extent and duration of exposure of organs and tissues to the radiolabeled material.

7 METABOLISM

The duration and intensity of action of lipophilic drugs is highly dependent on their rate of metabolism or biotransformation, since the majority of these compounds are readily reabsorbed in the kidney tubule following glomerular filtration. The liver, replete with a variety of metabolizing enzymes, cofactors, and endogenous scavengers of reactive metabolites (e.g., reduced glutathione), is the principal organ mediating the biotransformation of drugs. However, other sites in the body may play a critical role in metabolism in certain situations. Thus, the skin, lung, small intestine, and gastrointestinal flora may have a significant impact on biotransformation, depending on the drug, the drug dose, and the route of exposure (Lake and Gangolli, 1981; Selen, 1991).

Many factors are now known that affect the metabolism and, consequently, the activity of drugs. A wide variety of xenobiotics, including drugs, have the ability to induce or inhibit metabolizing enzymes, thereby altering not only their own metabolism but also that of other xenobiotics, drugs, and endogenous substances. Other factors such as dose, route, and frequency of administration, age, sex, genetic differences, and diet may profoundly affect metabolism (Lake and Gangolli, 1981). Consequently, it is extremely important to carefully control experimental conditions in metabolism studies, and, where appropriate, study the effects of these factors on the disposition of the drug.

Although the general pattern of metabolism is common to all species, the initial phase usually consisting of functionalization reactions (oxidations, reductions, and hydrolyses) and the second phase consisting of synthesis reactions (conjugations), major species differences in drug metabolism exist. It is this diversity in metabolism among species that is the major difficulty in extrapolating animal pharmacology and toxicology data to humans (Williams, 1971). The prediction of species differences in qualitative patterns of metabolism is at best an inexact science or forecast. Particularly helpful in this regard is information that has been acquired concerning species defects with respect to particular metabolic pathways and substrates (Smith, 1988).

The physicochemical characteristics of drugs should be considered in evaluating preclinical metabolism study requirements. In general, drugs that have low lipid solubility at physiological pH are not metabolized but are eliminated by excretion. A number of antibiotics and quaternary ammonium drugs, among others, fall into this category (Renwick, 1983). The pharmacological and toxicological effects of these compounds in humans can often be predicted reasonably well on the basis of animal data. Furthermore, these drugs are not likely to be affected by a broad range of factors that may affect drugs that depend on biotransformation for elimination (e.g., enzyme induction or inhibition). On the other hand, lipophilic drugs are often extensively metabolized, with the rate and extent of metabolism and pathways of metabolism species-dependent. In this situation, extensive effort will be required to characterize the metabolism and to investigate factors that may affect the metabolism of these drugs. Radioisotopically labeled drug is invariably used in these investigations to elucidate pathways of metabolism and detect low levels of potentially toxic metabolites or the reaction products of reactive metabolites.

In vitro metabolism studies, using tissue slices, isolated cell suspensions, and homogenates of tissues and subcellular fractions (e.g., microsomes), or isolated liver perfusion studies can provide a wealth of information concerning the metabolism of the drug and potential reactive, toxic metabolites and are a useful adjunct to *in vitro* and *in vivo* toxicity studies. These techniques also represent a rapid means of isolating small quantities of metabolites for further testing. Metabolites that may be pharmacologically active should be isolated and characterized early in the drug evaluation process if comparative pharmacology and pharmacokinetic data suggest the presence of active metabolites. Human liver, human microsomes, and specific cytochromes P-450 isoforms are becoming increasingly available for drug metabolism studies *in vitro* and are valuable screening tools for determination of which clinical drug-drug interaction studies are most worthwhile (Peck et al., 1993; Wrighton et al., 1992, 1993). It is now possible to determine which isoforms are involved in metabolizing drugs and which xenobiotics are most likely to interfere with the metabolism of a specific drug. These *in vitro* techniques can be applied very early in the drug development program. P-450 inhibitors (specific antibodies or chemical inhibitors) can also be used to identify the role of specific isoforms in the metabolism of a drug.

In vivo metabolism studies should be conducted in animal species and strains used in the toxicological evaluation of the drug to elucidate metabolic patterns and to ensure that metabolic switching does not occur at high doses (Glockin, 1981). Pooled or individual specimens from mass balance studies can be used for this purpose. Elucidation of metabolic patterns during preclinical testing is essential for the expeditious interpretation and rationalization of interspecies differences in toxicity that may affect the administration of the drug in humans. *In vivo* investigation of a drug's potential to induce or inhibit metabolism should also be considered, since these attributes can have a major impact on drug interactions (Conney, 1971; Peck et al., 1993).

8 EXCRETION

An assessment of the rate and routes of excretion of intact drug and metabolites is an essential component of preclinical drug evaluation. The importance of determining the proportion of intact drug and metabolites excreted (i.e., metabolic pattern) in each animal species has already been emphasized. The rate and routes of excretion are best determined by mass balance studies using radioisotopically labeled drug, as previously described. In this manner, a rapid assessment can be made of the routes of excretion and the duration of exposure to intact drug or metabolites. These excretion studies also provide valuable insight concerning the potential for drug accumulation in patients with impaired renal or hepatic function.

Quantitatively, the kidney is the most important excretory organ for compounds of low molecular weight, and the vast majority of drugs and/or their metabolites appear in the urine to some extent (Levine, 1983). Unbound drugs or metabolites having molecular weights of approximately 30,000 or less are filtered through the glomerulus, and some bound and unbound drugs and metabolites are secreted by active transport. Reabsorption of some drugs and metabolites occurs following glomerular filtration, mostly by passive diffusion and in some cases by active transport. The degree of reabsorption is dependent on lipophilicity, degree of plasma-protein binding and pK_a of the drug or its metabolites. Thus, the biotransformation of lipophilic drugs to polar metabolites enhances renal excretion. For drugs having a pK_a near the pH of urine, the rate of excretion can be increased or decreased by manipulation of urinary pH. The active transport systems for organic anions and cations are subject to competitive inhibition. For example, the half-life of a number of antibiotics can be extended by concomitant administration of probenecid, an organic anion that inhibits tubular secretion of other organic anions. Although there are notable differences in renal excretion between mammalian and non-mammalian species, tubular reabsorption appears to be a general phenomenon among common laboratory species (Trevor et al., 1971).

Although fewer drugs are excreted by humans in the bile than in urine, the hepatobiliary system ranks next in importance to the kidney as an excretory organ. The function of the hepatobiliary system in the enterohepatic circulation is responsible for the persistence of some drugs and may result in prolonged pharmacological activity or toxicity. Conjugation, particularly conjugation with glucuronic acid, appears to facilitate biliary excretion (Plaa, 1971). A molecular weight threshold appears to exist for biliary secretion of organic anions, which varies among species, with approximate thresholds of 325, 475 and 500–700 for rats, rabbits and humans, respectively. The molecular weight threshold for organic cations is approximately 200, with little or no interspecies variation apparent. Renal ligation does not increase biliary excretion of compounds below the molecular weight threshold, and bile duct ligation does not increase urinary excretion of compounds well above the molecular weight threshold. Compounds of intermediate molecular weight are excreted in both urine and bile (Hirom et al., 1976).

Drugs excreted in urine and bile are usually unbound; consequently, free drug concentrations in the urinary and biliary tract may be several orders of magnitude higher than in blood, accounting for the renal and hepatic toxicity of some highly protein-bound drugs (Clark and Smith, 1984). Furthermore, high drug and/or metabolite concentrations may be achieved in the renal cortex, even though little drug or metabolite ultimately appears in the urine. Consequently, it should not be assumed that the kidney is not exposed to high drug or metabolite concentrations simply because these compounds are not eliminated in the urine. Autoradiography or tissue distribution studies are required to reveal this phenomenon. The rate of drug administration also has an impact on renal and hepatic toxicity. Normally, bolus intravenous doses result in higher toxicity because of high drug concentrations in target organs (Clark and Smith, 1984).

Although quantitatively less important than urinary or biliary excretion, the excretion of drugs in expired air, sweat, saliva, feces, and milk may be of consequence for specific drugs and circumstances. The secretion of drugs into milk is of concern and should be examined in conjunction with reproductive toxicity studies and in humans before administration of drugs to nursing mothers.

9 CONCLUSIONS

Drug disposition studies should be conducted at an early enough stage of drug development to allow a biologically coherent evaluation of drug pharmacology and safety and to be of predictive value. The dosage and dosage regimen of the drug can then be appropriately adjusted to take into account interspecies differences in the extent and duration of drug exposure. These studies may also provide insight into mechanisms of toxicity due to overexposure within particular species or because of the formation of a toxic metabolite. This information may provide a basis for a species-dependent toxic effect, and the relevance of this effect to the human situation can be more readily assessed. Only too frequently disposition studies are done too late to be used in a beneficial manner. This may result in the development of a candidate with less than optimal properties that has a lower probability of ultimately receiving marketing approval, or in the rejection of drug candidates that might prove to be useful therapeutic agents. In the last analysis, what is required in terms of preclinical evaluation is a research program that is scientifically appropriate to the drug under investigation and its intended clinical use. This evaluation should allow an assessment of the benefit; risk ratio of a new therapeutic agent which can be compared with similar ratios for already established drugs.

REFERENCES

Adams, W. J. (1994). In Jackson, A. J. (Ed.). *Generics and Bioequivalence.* CRC Press, Boca Raton, pp. 139-177.

Ariens, E. J. (1966). Receptor theory and structure-action relationships. *Adv. Drug Res.*, 3, 235-85.

Bousquet, W. F. (1970). In Swarbrick. J. (Ed.). *Current Concepts in the Pharmaceutical Sciences: Biopharmaceutics.* Lea & Febiger, Philadelphia, pp. 151-95.

Clark, B. and Smith, D. A. (1984). Pharmacokinetics and toxicity testing. *CRC Crit. Rev. Toxicol.*, 12, 343-85.

Chignell, C. F. (1977). In Garrett, E. R. and Hirtz, J. L. (Eds.), *Drug Fate and Metabolism*, Volume 1, Marcel Dekker, New York, pp. 187-228.

Conney, A. H. (1971). In LaDu, B. N., Mandel, H. G. and Way, E. L. (Eds.), *Fundamentals of Drug Metabolism and Drug Disposition.* Williams & Wilkins, Baltimore, pp. 253-78.

Davidson, C. (1971). In LaDu, B. N., Mandel, H. G. and Way, E. L. (Eds.), *Fundamentals of Drug Metabolism and Drug Disposition.* Williams & Wilkins, Baltimore. pp. 63-75.

Drug Research Board. National Academy of Sciences/National Research Council (1969). Application of metabolic data to the evaluation of drugs. *Clin. Pharmacol. Ther.*, 10, 607-34.

EEC Commission (1980). Proposal for a council recommendation concerning tests relating to the placing on the market of proprietary medicinal products, *Off. J. Eur. Commun.*, No. C355/6-29.

Glockin, V. C. (1982). General considerations for studies of the metabolism of drugs and other chemicals. *Drug Metab. Rev.*, 13, 929-39.

Goldenthal, E. I. (1968). FDA papers, May 3, 1968, U.S. Food and Drug Administration, Washington, D.C.

Hansch, C. and Clayton, J. M. (1973). Lipophilic character and biological activity of drugs. II. The parabolic case. *J. Pharm. Sci.*, 62, 1-21.

Hirom, P. C., Millburn, P. and Smith, R. L. (1976). Bile and urine as complementary pathways for the excretion of foreign organic compounds. *Xenobiotica*, 6, 55-64.

Kaplan, S. A. (1973). In Swarbrick, J. (Ed.), *Current Concepts in the Pharmaceutical Sciences: Dosage Form Design and Bioavailability.* Lea & Febiger, Philadelphia, pp. 1-30.

Lake, B. G. and Gangolli, S. D. (1981). In Jenner, P. and Testa, B. (Eds.), *Concepts in Drug Metabolism,* Part B, Marcel Dekker, New York, pp. 167-218.

Levine, W. G. (1983). In Caldwell, J. and Jakoby, W. B. (Eds.), *Biological Basis of Detoxication.* Academic Press, New York, pp. 251-85.

Mertel, H. E. (1979). In Garrett, E. R. and Hirtz, J. L. (Eds.), *Drug Fate and Metabolism,* Volume 3, Marcel Dekker, New York, pp. 133-91.

Monahan, B. P., Ferguson, C.L., Killeavy, E.S., Lloyd, B. K. Troy, J. and Cantilena, L. R. (1990). *JAMA*, 264, 2788-2790.

Pang, K. S. (1983). In Caldwell, J. and Jakoby, W. B. (Eds.), *Biological Basis of Detoxication*. Academic Press, New York, pp. 213-50.

Peck, C. C., Barr, W. H., Benet, L. Z., Collins, J., Desjardins, R. E., Furst, D. E., Harter, J. G., Levy, G., Ludden, T., Rodman, J. H., Sanathanan, L., Schentag, J. J., Shah, V. P., Sheiner, L. B., Skelly, J. P., Stanski, D. R., Temple, R. J., Viswanathan, C. T., Weissinger, J. and Yacobi, A. (1992). Opportunities for integration of pharmacokinetics, pharmacodynamics, toxicokinetics in rational drug development. *Pharm. Res.*, 9, 826-833.

Peck, C. C., Temple, R. and Collins, J. M. (1993). Understanding consequences of concurrent therapies. *JAMA*, 269, 1550-1552.

Plang, G. L. (1971). In LaDu, B. N., Mandel, H. G. and Way, E. L. (Eds.), *Fundamentals of Drug Metabolism and Drug Disposition*. Williams & Wilkins, Baltimore, pp. 131-45.

Renwick, A. G. (1983). In Caldwell, J. and Jakoby, W. B. (Eds.), *Biological Basis of Detoxication*. Academic Press, New York, pp. 151-79.

Selen, A. (1991). In Welling, P. G., Tse, F. L. S. and Dighe, S. V. (Eds.), *Pharmaceutical Bioequivalence*. Marcel Dekker, New York, pp. 117-148.

Siuzdak, G. (1994). The emergence of mass spectrometry in biochemical research. *Proc. Natl. Acad. Sci. U.S.A.*, 91, 11290-11297.

Smith, R. L. (1988). The role of metabolism and disposition studies in the safety assessment of pharmaceuticals. *Xenobiotica*, 18, 89-96.

Stavchansky, S. A. and McGinity, J. W. (1990). In Lieberman, H. A., Lachman, L. and Schwartz, J. B. (Eds.), *Pharmaceutical Dosage Forms*, Volume 2, 2nd edition, Marcel Dekker, New York, pp. 349-569.

Trevor, A., Rowland, M. and Way, E. L. (1971). In LaDu, B. N., Mandel, H. G. and Way, E. L. (Eds.), *Fundamentals of Drug Metabolism and Drug Disposition*, Williams & Wilkins, Baltimore, pp. 369-99.

Tucker, G. T. (1992). The rational selection of drug interaction studies: implications of recent advances in drug metabolism. *Int. J. Clin. Pharmacol. Ther. Toxicol.*, 30, 550-553.

Waddell, W. J. and Marlowe, C. (1977). In Garrett, E. R. and Hirtz, J. L. (Eds.), *Drug Fate and Metabolism*, Volume 1, Marcel Dekker, New York, pp. 1-25.

Williams, R. T. (1971). In LaDu, B. N., Mandel, H. G. and Way, E. L. (Eds.), *Fundamentals of Drug Metabolism and Drug Disposition*, Williams & Wilkins, Baltimore, pp. 187-205.

Woosley, R. L., Chen, Y., Frieman, J.P. and Gillis, R. A. (1993). Mechanism of the cardiotoxic actions of terfenadine. *JAMA*, 269, 1532-1536.

World Health Organization (1966). Principles for pre-clinical testing of drug safety. *W.H.O. Tech. Rep. Ser.*, 341.

Wrighton, S. A. and Stevens, J. C. (1992). The human hepatic cytochromes P450 involved in drug metabolism. *CRC Crit. Rev. Toxicol.*, 22, 1-21.

Wrighton, S. A., Vandenbranden, M., Stevens, J., Shipley, L. A. and Ring, B. J. (1993). *In vitro* methods for assessing human hepatic drug metabolism: their use in drug development. *Drug Metab. Rev.*, 25, 453-484.

Zbinden, G. (1984). In Caldwell, J. and Paulson, G. D. (Eds.), *Foreign Compound Metabolism*, Taylor & Francis, Philadelphia, pp. 203-211.

Zbinden, G. (1988). Biopharmaceutical studies, a key to better toxicology. *Xenobiotica*, 18, 9-14.

Chapter 4

Animal Tests as Predictors of Human Response

Darryl Wood and Peter I. Folb

CONTENTS

1 Introduction 36
2 Limits to Extrapolating Animal Data in Predicting the Human Response 36
3 Classic Acute Toxicity Testing 36
3.1 Direct Toxic Effects on Tissues 36
3.1.1 Skin 36
3.1.2 Eyes 36
3.1.3 Mucosal Surfaces 36
3.2 The Lethal Dose 50 (LD_{50}) Test 37
3.2.1 The Value of the LD_{50} Test 37
3.2.2 Limits to Extrapolation 37
3.3 Testing for Systemic Toxicity 37
4 Classic Chronic (Long-Term) Toxicity Testing 37
4.1 Mechanisms of Long-Term Drug Injury 38
4.2 Dose Considerations 38
4.3 Frequency of Administration 38
4.4 Route of Administration 38
4.5 Duration of the Study 38
4.6 U.K. Guidelines 39
5 Carcinogenicity Testing 39
5.1 Database Required for Carcinogenicity Risk Assessment 39
5.2 *In Vivo* Systems for Carcinogenicity Testing 40
5.3 Special Issues in Extrapolating Carcinogenicity Data 40
6 Hypersensitivity Testing and Immunological Studies 40
7 Reproductive and Developmental Toxicity Testing 41
8 Neurotoxicity Testing 41
9 Categorizing the Toxicological Response 42
10 Recommendations for Improving the Relevance of Toxicology Testing 42
11 Ethical and Moral Issues 42
12 Refining Animal Experiments 43
13 The Four Rs 45
13.1 Reduction 45
13.2 Refinement 45
13.3 Replacement 45
13.4 Responsibility 45
14 New Strategies for Toxicity Testing 46
14.1 Limit Test 46
14.2 Fixed-Dose Oral Toxicity Testing 46
14.3 Sequential Studies and a Decision Tree 46
14.4 *In Vitro* Toxicity Testing 46
14.5 Computer-Based Systems 47
15 Aging Studies 47
16 Physiological Measurements 47
References 47

0-8493-9230-6/97/$0.00+$.50
© 1997 by CRC Press, Inc.

1 INTRODUCTION

Many serious toxic reactions caused by new chemical entities may be detected reliably by routine toxicological testing. Experience has shown that predictable, "dose- and time-dependent" reactions are likely to be revealed in animal experiments. It is the detail of these that forms the basis of the experimental toxicology that is applied to new drug development. Unpredictable idiosyncratic adverse effects, not related to time or dose, are considerably more difficult to identify in preclinical drug evaluation.

2 LIMITS TO EXTRAPOLATING ANIMAL DATA IN PREDICTING THE HUMAN RESPONSE

The limitations inherent in extrapolating animal toxicology data to prediction of the human response (Balazs, 1974; Zbinden, 1980) include the following:

1. Pharmacokinetic differences between test animals and humans.
2. Idiosyncratic adverse events in humans, the mechanisms of which are poorly understood, and are not normally demonstrable in animals by standard toxicological investigation.
3. Underlying pathological condition – drugs may exacerbate underlying diseases in humans which do not exist in healthy animals. Relationships that might exist between the drug and its metabolites on the one hand, and an underlying disease on the other, cannot adequately be investigated or predicted from studies which has been conducted in healthy animals.
4. Species differences in anatomy and physiological functions (see Zbinden, 1980).
5. Species differences in tolerance and enzyme induction (see Balazs, 1974).
6. Adverse drug events that can only be communicated verbally by the patient are not normally recognized in animals.

3 CLASSIC ACUTE TOXICITY TESTING

Acute exposure of experimental animals to a toxic agent may express itself either directly in one or more tissues and/or systemically following absorption from a local site (Brown, 1987).

3.1 Direct Toxic Effects on Tissues

The skin, eyes, gastrointestinal mucosa, vagina, and respiratory tract are at greatest risk of topical toxic effects of drugs. When a substance is known to be locally irritant or corrosive, it is not normally necessary for animal tests to be conducted in order to confirm what is already established. On the other hand, local irritation may be materially influenced by the conditions of exposure, such as local pH. Topical toxicity testing is required to determine this.

3.1.1 Skin

In order to evaluate the degree of skin irritation that may be exerted by a potentially toxic substance, it is necessary to examine the effect in human subjects. Due to enormous variability in the response of the skin of different animal species to toxic chemicals, there is little value in skin irritancy testing that requires extrapolation of findings from one species to another.

3.1.2 Eyes

As a general rule, any chemical with irritant or corrosive properties when applied to the skin is also likely to be irritant to the cornea and conjunctiva, and ocular irritancy tests need not be carried out. The most widely used predicting test for ophthalmological irritancy is still the Draize test in rabbits (Draize et al., 1944).

3.1.3 Mucosal Surfaces

Irritancy testing of mucosal surfaces is necessary when substances are designed for application to particular surfaces, such as the vagina, where local factors such as pH have to be considered. There is comparatively little difference between species, and indeed between individuals, in mucosal responses to toxic injury.

3.2 The Lethal Dose 50 (LD_{50}) Test

The LD_{50} test (Zbinden and Flury-Roversi, 1981; Paget, 1983; Rowan, 1983) is aimed at determining the dose of a toxic substance that kills 50% of the animals that receive it. It forms a traditional part of the early assessment of a new medicine, and it also makes it possible to study precisely the nature of the acute toxicity of a compound. Nevertheless, the concept of killing animals in this way has proved repugnant to many, and this has necessitated a critical review of the justification for the LD_{50}.

3.2.1 *The Value of the LD_{50} Test*

The value of the LD_{50} test in acute toxicity testing is as follows (Paget, 1983):

1. Therapeutic margin — the margin between the effective dose and the toxic dose can be determined in this manner. Compounds may be compared, allowing for those with the widest margin of safety to be selected for further development. When significant species variation is found this is regarded as having implications for human use.
2. Toxokinetic evaluation — the LD_{50} test makes it possible for lethal effects to be compared with blood levels of the active principle and with the findings obtained in repeated dosing studies.

3.2.2 *Limits to Extrapolation*

It is important that the objections that have been raised to the LD_{50} test, and the caveats to extrapolation of data derived from it, should be carefully considered (Zbinden and Flury-Roversi, 1981). Even when conducted with great care, the results of the LD_{50} test should be regarded as an isolated finding. The results need to be considered in conjunction with other findings from acute toxicity testing. Zbinden has proposed the following guidelines for the use of the LD_{50} test, and these have been widely accepted.

1. LD_{50} data should always be considered in conjunction with other relevant information, not in isolation.
2. Conduct of the LD_{50} test on large animals should be discontinued; a test on a limited number of small animals, including detailed recording of symptomatology and pathology, should be done instead.
3. No LD_{50} test should be conducted with pharmacologically inert substances (a maximum dose of 5 g/kg for oral administration and 2 g/kg for parenteral administration should be sufficient if death or acute symptoms are not produced).
4. The test should not be conducted in newborn animals.

In summary, it is important in acute toxicity testing of a new drug that full understanding be obtained of the nature of the acute toxic injury. In the foreseeable future it is unlikely that the whole animal will be replaced by simpler models. The LD_{50} test represents a comparatively small part of the information that can be gained from acute toxicity studies. If the test is carefully performed, with appropriate concern for the humane issues that are associated with it, it can provide valuable information about the biological and toxicological properties of a new chemical entity.

3.3 Testing for Systemic Toxicity

Systemic effects resulting from short-term exposure to chemicals may develop either rapidly or after delayed onset and the result may be transient, prolonged, or irreversible. The systemic toxicity of any substance is likely to be determined by the combined effects of the exposure, the route of administration, and the physical presentation of the product to the target organ. For an animal model to provide meaningful results, it is necessary that it be comparable physiologically with humans, and that there should be toxokinetic similarities in the new chemical entity in the test animal and in humans.

4 CLASSIC CHRONIC (LONG-TERM) TOXICITY TESTING

The value of chronic toxicity testing in animals (Aldridge, 1976; Dayan, 1986; Frederick 1986; Glockin, 1986; Jackson, 1986; McLean, 1986; Rawlins, 1986; Worden, 1986; Worden and Walker, 1987) has been seriously questioned for many years, and it has been hoped that a more complete understanding of the relevant pharmacology, and of the physiological changes caused by acute exposure to a new drug, might provide sufficient information to anticipate adverse long-term effects. This has not been achieved, and there remains for the time being no better alternative.

Dayan (1986) has pointed out that with repeated-dose testing most structural lesions that are likely to be produced should be identifiable, and that knowledge can also be gained of functional disturbances, although the latter are unlikely to be quantifiable. Long-term animal studies only partly reveal functional

Table 1 Weights of Organs in the Mouse, Rat, Rabbit, Rhesus Monkey, Dog, and Human

Animal	Adrenal	Brain	Lung	Liver	Kidney	Heart	Spleen
Mouse (0.02 kg)	0.36	1.75	0.32	0.08	0.1	0.004	0.12
Rat (0.25 kg)	1.8	10.0	2.0	1.0	0.75	0.05	1.5
Rabbit (2.5 kg)	14	77	13	5	1	0.5	18
Rhesus Monkey (5 kg)	90	150	25	18.5	8	1.2	33
Dog (10 kg)	80	320	50	80	25	1	100
Human (70 kg)	1400	1800	310	330	180	14	1000

Note: Organ weights (g)

From Davies, B. and Morris, T. (1993). *Pharm. Res.*, 10, 1093. With permission.

disorders, and the influence on toxicity of drugs of factors such as aging, disease, and diet remains uncertain.

4.1 Mechanisms of Long-Term Drug Injury

In planning and evaluating long-term toxicity studies in animals, various mechanisms of drug injury are considered (McLean, 1986).

1. Accumulation of the parent drug, and/or its metabolite(s), in the tissues, with consequent toxic injury.
2. Repeated or low-grade continuous injury may occur to DNA, or to the hereditable DNA expression which is found during cell differentiation.
3. The adaptive synthesis of cell receptors may be disturbed.
4. Damage to repair responses may occur, and such an animal may be extremely sensitive to an additional toxic insult.

4.2 Dose Considerations

The normal practice is to employ a minimum of three treatment groups, divided according to dose, and one control group. An additional group may be added if it is necessary to examine a toxic effect in relation to a particular dose. The lowest dose is conventionally set at the equivalent of five times the projected therapeutic dose, to establish a nontoxic dose level. The mid-dose usually represents the geometric mean between the low and high doses, but pharmacokinetic considerations have to be considered when selecting this. The high-dose level is calculated so as to identify toxic effects but not to a degree that might jeopardize successful completion of the study.

4.3 Frequency of Administration

In general, adequate exposure of the experimental animal to a drug is achieved by once-daily dosing, seven days a week, but more frequent administration may be necessary in the case of drugs with a very short half-life or brief duration of action.

4.4 Route of Administration

The route of administration in animal studies of an investigational new drug should be the same as that which is proposed for clinical use (Jackson, 1986). This can be problematic if a high dose is required, which cannot be tolerated when given by a particular route. If use of an alternative route is inevitable, comparative pharmacokinetic data will be required.

4.5 Duration of the Study

In rodents, the number of incidental (spontaneous) lesions begins to rise from 15 to 18 months of age onward (Dyan, 1986). This reduces the discriminative power of any study, because of the lesions themselves, and the impairment that they might cause to the normal response of the animals. In the dog and primate, and other non-rodent species, on the other hand, an 18-month-old animal might not yet have reached the pubertal stage of development.

Glockin (1986) has explained the U.S. Food and Drug Administration (FDA) requirement for 12-month, long-term animal toxicity studies. This refers to rodent as well as non-rodent studies. The study

Table 2 Volumes of Various Body Fluids and Organs in the Mouse, Rat, Rabbit, Monkey, Dog, and Human[a]

Organ	Mouse	Rat	Rabbit	Monkey	Dog	Human
Brain	—	1.2	—	—	72	1450
Liver	1.3	19.6	100	135	480	1690
Kidneys	0.34	3.7	15	30	60	280
Heart	0.10	1.2	6	17	120	310
Spleen	0.1	1.3	1	—	36	192
Lungs	0.1	2.1	17	—	120	1170
Gut	1.5	11.3	120	230	480	1650
Muscle	10.0	245	1350	2500	5530	35000
Adipose tissue	—	10.0	120	—	—	10000
Skin	2.9	40.0	110	500	—	7800
Blood	1.7	13.5	165	367	900	5200
TBW	14.5	167	1790	3465	6036	42000
ICF	—	92.8	1165	2425	3276	23800
ECF	—	74.2	625	1040	2760	18200
Plasma volume	1.0	7.8	110	224	515	3000

[a] The same weights for the various species are assumed as for Table 1. Organ volume is given in milliliters.

Note: Key: TBW = total body water, ICF = intracellular fluid, and ECF = extracellular fluid.

From Davies, B. and Morris, T. (1993). *Pharm. Res.*, 10, 1093. With permission.

should be extended beyond 12 months when warranted by a specific concern or by an unusual condition of use.

Lumley and Walker (1985b) and Worden (1986) have suggested that a six-month study should be sufficient to establish the toxicity profile of new drugs, and that no-effect levels can also be predicted within that period. This is only true if reliance is not placed solely on histopathological changes.

4.6 U.K. Guidelines

Grahame-Smith (1986) has provided in broad outline the requirements of the U.K. authorities for the conduct of repeated-dose studies in animals, except for carcinogenicity and reproductive studies, for which the duration of testing is determined by the likely duration of treatment with the agent in humans.

5 CARCINOGENICITY TESTING

The majority of human carcinogens have also been shown to be carcinogenic in animals, and virtually all, when tested appropriately, induce cancer in several animal species (Gait et al., 1979; Kodell et al., 1982; Hoel et al., 1983; IARC, 1984; Purchase, 1987; Weisburger, 1987). It is not unusual for 80-100% of the test animals to be affected with a relatively short latent period of 12-18 months. Human carcinogens that are genotoxic (most are) also reliably display activity in the standard short-term *in vitro* mutagenicity tests.

Conversely, a chemical which (1) is consistently genotoxic in a number (not just one) of short-term *in vitro* tests, (2) is active in several *in vivo* bioassay systems (high yield of tumors, latent period less than 18 months), and (3) exhibits such activity over a range of dose levels, is a probable human cancer risk.

When an unknown test chemical is active only in a single bioassay system or in a small number of *in vitro* systems, its classification as a genotoxin requires careful analysis of the positive and negative data. It may be that in the intact mammalian system (i.e., the whole animal), biochemical defense systems adequately protect against reactive radicals, giving a negative test result, despite the evidence of genotoxicity that may be found with *in vitro* testing (Weisburger, 1987).

5.1 Database Required for Carcinogenicity Risk Assessment

The database required for carcinogenicity risk assessment of new chemical entities involves assessment of the following factors.

1. The structure-activity relationships of the chemical and its similarity to known carcinogens.
2. The results of short-term genotoxicity tests.
3. The outcome of *in vivo* studies in which evidence is sought in mice, rats, and/or hamsters of a statistically significant incidence of cancer. (Whole animal studies are selected on the basis of comprehensive assessment of the probable mechanism(s) of action, whether genotoxic or promoting, of the chemical under consideration. Carcinogenesis is often organ-specific, as a result of the formation of locally produced reactive metabolites.)

It is most improbable that any human carcinogen will yield negative results for all three components of this screening procedure.

5.2 *In Vivo* Systems for Carcinogenicity Testing

The investigations that have proved most practical for predicting chemical carcinogenesis in humans are those in which mitotic lesions are induced in the livers of rats and skin tumors in mice, mammary tumors in Sprague-Dawley female rats, and pulmonary tumors in certain sensitive strains of mice. The majority of such tumors are induced in less than one year. The test compound is compared with a known positive control, if possible, at several dose levels, so as to provide an estimate of the dose-response relationship.

Agents which are thought to act as promoters are administered together with a genotoxic carcinogen appropriate for the relevant target organ. The test substance is administered in four or five dose levels. Comparison with the appropriate positive control will provide an indication of the relative potency of the test substance.

Some workers (Gart et al., 1979; Kodell et al., 1982) have indicated how important it is in the evaluation of the data that there should be comprehensive pathological and toxicological assessment of individual animals in carcinogenicity testing, including comparison with controls, and evaluation of the "case history."

Squire (1981) has pointed out that the response in intact experimental animals reflects at best a potential for human risk, but not an order of risk.

5.3 Special Issues in Extrapolating Carcinogenicity Data

Purchase (1987) found in a study of the carcinogenicity potential of 250 compounds that both the specificity (the prediction of carcinogenicity) and the sensitivity (the prediction of noncarcinogenicity) in rat and mouse studies were approximately 85%. Of the chemicals, 64% consistently produced cancer at the same site.

The chemical and the host are each involved in the expression of a carcinogen. The potency may vary between hosts, depending on tumor type, nutritional status, environmental conditions, and other variables. This explains differences that are found between laboratories and in different test systems.

It is generally accepted that chemicals should be tested under constraints that minimize the number of false-negative results. The maximum dose chosen is usually larger than the dose that is likely to be given to humans. The group sizes are usually in the range of 50-100 animals. Results are extrapolated to humans on the (erroneous) assumption that the most sensitive outcome, from the most sensitive species, is appropriate to man, and that a simple quantitative correlation can be made. Animal data are neither quantitatively not qualitatively reliable for such extrapolation, and the dose-response relationship cannot be assumed to be linear at low levels of exposure.

6 HYPERSENSITIVITY TESTING AND IMMUNOLOGICAL STUDIES

The assessment of the effect on immune function of a new chemical entity for human use seems to be a logical and long overdue part of new drug testing. A number of immunological assays are now available which make it possible to assess the degree of cellular injury and immune functional impairment resulting from drug toxicity (Dean et al., 1982).

Miller and Nicklin (1987) have proposed a minimum screening panel for defining immune alteration after chemical exposure in rodents.

Pathotoxicology: Hematology profile, complete blood count, and differential; total body weight and organ weights — spleen, thymus, liver, kidney, brain.

Host resistance: Susceptibility to transplantable syngeneic tumor.

Delayed cutaneous hypersensitivity: T-cell-dependent antigen response.

Lymphocyte function: Lymphocyte blastogenesis to phytohemagglutinin or concanavalin A, lipopolysaccharide, and allogeneic lymphocytes (mixed lymphocyte culture).

Humoral immunity: Immunoglobulin levels (IgG, IgM, IgA); antibody response to sheep erythrocytes.

There is, at present, no suitable animal model for assessing the risk from inhaled, ingested, or injected drugs of acute hypersensitivity reactions.

7 REPRODUCTIVE AND DEVELOPMENTAL TOXICITY TESTING

The consequences of human and animal exposure to teratogens depend on the extent, duration, and time of exposure and the chemical entity concerned. The results may be various: impaired ability of the female to conceive, abortion, dysmorphogenesis, premature birth, low birth weight, perinatal mortality and morbidity, cancer, and dysfunctional growth and development after birth (Wilson, 1959; Koeter, 1983; Lasagna, 1984; Miller et al., 1985; Lansdown, 1987; Messite and Bond, 1988).

Hundreds of chemical agents are teratogenic to the experimental animal. These include poisons, therapeutic agents, and industrial and agricultural chemicals. However, proof of dysmorphogenic and other teratogenic effects on the human fetus has been shown for only a very small number of chemicals — thalidomide, androgens, virilizing progestagens, cytotoxic drugs, antithyroid drugs, and certain anticonvulsants.

For a number of reasons, reproductive toxicity data derived from animal experiments are not necessarily applicable to humans. These are as follows:

1. Species differences in drug distribution and action, and in tissue and organ responses.
2. Differences with regard to the method of dosing and the route and duration of administration. Doses which are excessive may invalidate the test by killing the animals, while doses which are too low may give a misleading impression of safety. Humans may be 2-50 times more sensitive than animals on a dose-per-weight basis.
3. The epidemiological method is imprecise when applied to evaluation of human teratogenicity, compared with more exact animal experimental data. The effects of "low-grade" human teratogens are frequently not discernible from the normal background incidence of major congenital malformations (2-3%). The problems of extrapolation are compounded by the lack of accurate information commonly encountered when the time of exposure of the pregnant mother to the suspected teratogen is reported. The matter is further complicated by some agents that may act to enable expression of the primary offender (for example, cigarette smoking, alcohol, and food additives).
4. A variety of teratogens may produce the same malformation and, conversely, a variety of malformations may be produced by the same teratogen. Moreover, an established teratogen is not necessarily deleterious with every exposure. In such circumstances attribution of causation can be very complex.
5. No clear relationship exists between a particular chemical or pharmacological class and specific effects on the embryo. For example, one sulfonylurea may cause a high percentage of malformations in animals, while another has little or no such effect.

8 NEUROTOXICITY TESTING

Neurotoxicity evaluation (Silbergeld, 1982; Dewar, 1987) has become an important part of toxicology, with the recognition that the nervous system is a critical target for hazardous substances. This has been made possible by advances in the neurosciences, but limitations remain in techniques and methods of evaluation.

Behavioral change is likely to be the earliest detectable expression of toxic injury to the nervous system, as adverse biochemical or pathological effects exceed the homeostatic capacity of the central nervous system (Dewar, 1987). It may be very difficult, or impossible, to detect intellectual impairment (a common expression of neurotoxicity in man) by animal tests, particularly as distinctions are relative rather than absolute.

Age is another complicating issue in assessing toxic insult to the central nervous system. The immature and developing brain is especially susceptible to toxic injury at the time of active cellular proliferation, myelination, and synaptogenesis. The aging central nervous system is also very vulnerable.

9 CATEGORIZING THE TOXICOLOGICAL RESPONSE

The outcome of a toxicological study in animals may fall into one of four categories (based on the International Agency for Research on Cancer, IARC, 1984).

1. Sufficient evidence exists of an association between the toxic agent and the purported outcome. This is based on findings in multiple species or strains, or in multiple experiments, preferably with different routes of administration, or different doses, or both; or the incidence of the finding is unusual in degrees, site, type, or age of onset. There may be additional data on dose-response effects, short-term studies, and chemical structure.
2. Limited evidence. The data suggest a causative effect, but are insufficient because (a) only a single species or strain was examined, or the results were derived from a single experiment; (b) the experiments were conducted with inadequate dosage levels, too brief duration of exposure, inadequate period of follow-up, poor animal survival and too few animals, or the reporting was inadequate; or (c) the lesions produced often occur spontaneously.
3. Inadequate evidence. Because of major qualitative or quantitative limitations the studies cannot be interpreted as showing either the presence or absence of an effect; or, within the limits of the test, the chemical has not been shown conclusively to produce the lesions concerned.
4. No data are available.

The first two categories provide an indication only of the strength of the experimental evidence, and not of the extent of the activity of the chemical entity under review or the mechanism of its toxic effect. The classification may change as other information becomes available.

10 RECOMMENDATIONS FOR IMPROVING THE RELEVANCE OF TOXICOLOGY TESTING

A number of recommendations have been made for improving the relevance of toxicology testing in animals (Litchfield, 1962; Fletcher, 1978; Zbinden, 1980; Lumley and Walker, 1985; Zbinden, 1987a,b). These include:

1. The establishment of databanks for collection of results, which could provide a valuable resource for analysis and for the design of future experiments (Lumley and Walker, 1985a).
2. The methodology in experimental toxicology should develop to the extent that subjective effects in humans, such as hallucinations, dizziness, difficulty in concentrating, and disturbance in memory, might be assessed in animals by behavioral testing (Zbinden, 1980).
3. Improved systems of comparative evaluation of anatomical structure, physiological function, and pathology, in test animals and in humans, including patients with the diseases for which the medicine is intended, should improve extrapolation and reduce the difficulties produced by species differences in metabolism, distribution, and elimination.

11 ETHICAL AND MORAL ISSUES

In the U.S. five different regulatory institutions protect against mistreatment of animals. These are the federal government, certain state legislatures, independent non-governmental organizations, professional societies, and other institutions concerned for animal safety and welfare.

Stanford University utilizes a model of checks and balances that protect animals against unnecessary suffering. Any prospective researcher is required to submit a rationale and detailed protocol for using animals. The proposal is required to include a complete list of drugs to be used and an inventory of surgical procedures. The university's administrative panel on laboratory animal care reviews each proposal. No animal studies may proceed without the approval of the panel. Strict adherence to the protocol of investigation throughout the study is required. Although such measures do not provide certain protection against abuse of animals for research, they do decrease the risk, and they provide for sanctions if there are transgressions (Thomas et al., 1988).

Animals are only one of the various systems available for biomedical research, which range from inanimate devices such as computers and mechanical models to *in vitro* culture systems (microbes, organ tissue) and plants. The choice of an appropriate test depends on the nature and stage of the research. The decision should be guided by three criteria:

Table 3 Flow of Blood Through the Major Organs and Other Fluids in the Mouse, Rat, Rabbit, Monkey, Dog, and Human[a]

Blood Flow	Mouse	Rat	Rabbit	Monkey	Dog	Human
Brain	—	1.3	—	72	45	700
Liver	1.8	13.8	177	218	309	1450
Kidneys	1.3	9.2	80	138	216	1240
Heart	0.28	3.9	16	60	54	240
Spleen	0.09	0.6	9	21	25	77
Gut	1.5	7.5	111	125	216	1100
Muscle	0.91	7.5	155	90	250	750
Adipose tissue	—	0.4	32	20	35	260
Skin	0.41	5.8	—	54	100	300
Hepatic artery	0.35	2.0	37	51	79	300
Portal vein	1.45	9.8	140	167	230	1150
Cardiac output	8.0	74.0	530	1086	1200	5600
Urine flow	1.0	50.0	150	375	300	1400
Bile flow	2.0	22.5	300	125	120	350
GFR	0.28	1.3	7.8	10.4	61.3	125

[a] The same weights for the various species are assumed as for Table 1. Blood flow is expressed in ml/min, except where indicated otherwise.

Note: Key: GFR = glomerular filtration rate. Measurements of urine flow and bile flow are given in ml/day. The GFR is given in ml/min.

From Davies, B. and Morris, T. (1993). *Pharm. Res.*, 10, 1093. With permission.

1. The likelihood that the study will answer the scientific question being asked.
2. The social attitudes, legal codes, and ethical standards that are affected by the study.
3. Economic considerations.

The use of research animals is expensive while non-animal models tend to be less so, and the latter are simpler to control and they provide fewer ethical hurdles. Almost no economic consideration favors the use of animals, compared with non-animal methods. Before commencing animal studies, the investigator needs to pose a specific question and describe the expected answer, to be familiar with the relevant scientific literature, and to be able to show that the available model(s) can answer the scientific question being posed.

If the proposed study offers little chance of providing meaningful information, the investigator is required to find a more appropriate system. If several models provide a reasonable prospect of useful information, the researcher needs to decide which is likely to be the best. Protocols of study should include animal care and management guidelines, even though these are time-consuming and expensive.

It has been argued that research animals deserve greater moral consideration than has been afforded them in the past, and that animals should have certain rights even if they do not qualify for the right not to be used in experimental work. Others have suggested that animals have comparable rights to human beings, which proscribe their use in research. Finally, there are those who feel that animals do not qualify for rights, and that it is permissible for them to be used in experiments under defined circumstances. A common position is the principle of humane treatment. This places the researcher under an obligation to prevent undue pain and suffering, but does not confront the issue of animal rights. It denies the view of animals' rights being equal to those of humans, and it admits that certain things done to animals may not be done to humans. "Humane treatment" establishes a double standard for animals and humans (Cohen, 1986).

12 REFINING ANIMAL EXPERIMENTS

Pakes (1990) has pointed out that good science and good conscience go hand in hand with sound care of experimental animals. Animals' feelings such as pain and distress affect the subjects' physiological responses. The researcher needs to be on the lookout for disturbances of these including: sleeping, drinking, feeding, locomotion, grooming, exploration, learning, mating, and reproduction. Physiological signs include pupil dilation, increased blood pressure and heart rate, increased respiration, and an arousal response on the EEG. When an animal experiences acute pain, signs such as guarding, moving away, biting, self-mutilation, restlessness, salivation, impaired ambulation, changes in respiration, and assuming abnormal positions may give the researcher some idea of the feelings of an animal. Animals experiencing chronic pain may become quiet and withdrawn, lose appetite and weight, change their urinary and bowel activity, and develop abnormal grooming behavior. Chronic pain is more difficult to recognize than acute pain.

Laboratory veterinarians play an important role in detecting and minimizing the pain and distress that animals may experience, and they are required for the planning and supervision of studies, and for maintaining a watching brief for the humane and sensitive treatment of the animals. There are numerous ways in which pain may be avoided or minimized including: reducing the level of surrounding noxious stimuli, avoiding stressful and other situations that lower the threshold of animals' pain tolerance, and improving methods and procedures so that pain tolerance is raised. Veterinarians should review protocols routinely to ensure that procedures are as untraumatic as possible, to anticipate problems, and to develop informed responses. The level of anxiety is important in this regard. Gentle handling and special attention such as petting and talking to the test animal go a long way in reducing stress levels. If an animal has to be restrained, it is necessary that the restraining devices are the correct size for the animal and that they are as comfortable as possible. The animal needs to be conditioned to the environment prior to the start of the experiment. Records should be kept of the entire procedure.

Table 4 Transit Time, pH and Enzyme Activity of the Gastrointestinal Tract of the Mouse, Rat, Rabbit, Monkey, Dog, and Human[a]

Transit Time	Mouse	Rat	Rabbit	Monkey	Dog	Human
Stomach		—	—	—	96	78
Small intestine	—	88	—	—	110	238
Whole gut	—	—	—	—	770	2350
pH (fed)						
Stomach:						
Anterior	4.5	5.0	1.9	4.8	5.5	—
Posterior	3.1	3.8	1.9	2.8	3.4	5.0
Small intestine:						
Beginning	—	6.5	6.0	5.6	6.2	5.4
End	—	7.1	8.0	6.0	7.5	7.5
Cecum	—	6.8	6.6	5.0	6.4	6.0
Colon	—	6.6	7.2	5.1	6.5	7.5
Feces	—	6.9	7.2	5.5	6.2	—
Beta-glucuronidation activity (nmol substrate/h/g of contents):						
Prox. small intestine	1200	304	2.4	—	—	0.02
Distal small intestine	5015	1341	45.4	—	—	0.9

[a] The same weights for the various species are assumed as for Table 1. Transit time is given in minutes.

From Davies, B. and Morris, T. (1993). *Pharm. Res.*, 10, 1093. With permission.

Recent studies have shown that handling or maternal contact stimulates growth and decreases blood levels of beta-endorphins in rat pups. This reduces variance of data and increases the level of significance of observed changes. However, certain species do not react positively to handling; for example, young hamsters may react adversely. Thus, handling can significantly influence physiological responses such as release of prolactin, corticosterone, thyroxine, and other hormones. Heart function and hematological values may also be affected. Stress causes an elevation in circulating catecholamines, which in turn mobilize fats from adipose tissues, with a resultant rise in free fatty acids in the blood (Rowan, 1990).

Environmental factors that can affect the outcome of an animal experiment include physical (temperature, light, noise), chemical (food, water, detergents, pesticides, gases), biological (disease), and social (isolation, grouping, handling, and maternal influences).

Another consideration is the choice of the most appropriate animal. Species, strain, and gender are important. Other necessary considerations are specific disease profiles such as tumor type, which may vary between animal species, strain, gender, and age.

Traditional methods of assessment and measurement need to be re-examined. For example, death need not be the end-point of a study. Specific signs of disease or illness, such as impaired ambulation, muscle atrophy, rapid weight loss, paralysis, and central nervous system disturbances may suffice in many cases.

The route of administration of a test substance is important, and it can affect the pain and stress of the animal. As far as possible, this should closely mimic the anticipated human exposure, balancing this against the discomfort and pain that it might cause to the animal.

Table 5 Miscellaneous Physiological Parameters of the Mouse, Rat, Rabbit, Monkey, Dog, and Human[a]

	Mouse	Rat	Rabbit	Monkey	Dog	Human
Surface area (m^2)	0.008	0.023	0.17	0.32	0.51	1.85
Mean lifespan potential (y)	2.7	4.7	8.0	22	20	93
Total plasma protein (g/100 ml)	6.2	6.7	5.7	8.8	9.0	7.4
Plasma albumin (g/100 ml)	3.27	3.16	3.87	4.93	2.63	4.18
Plasma a-1-AGP (g/100 ml)	1.25	1.81	0.13	0.24	0.37	0.18
Hematocrit (%)	45	46	36	41	42	44
Total ventilation (l/min)	0.025	0.12	0.80	1.67	1.50	7.98
Respiratory rate (per/min)	163	85	51	38	23	12
Heart rate (beats/min)	624	362	213	192	96	65
Oxygen consumption (ml/h/g bw)	1.59	0.84	0.48	0.43	0.34	0.20

[a] The same weights for the various species are assumed as for Table 1.

From Davies, B. and Morris, T. (1993). *Pharm. Res.*, 10, 1093. With permission.

13 THE FOUR RS

It has been suggested that the modern approach to toxicological testing should be based on the four Rs — reduction, refinement, replacement, and responsibility (Gad, 1990; Pakes, 1990; Rowan, 1990). This is aimed at optimizing the balance between the needs of society and the welfare of animals.

13.1 Reduction

The number of animals should be reduced to the absolute minimum that will achieve the necessary result, by placing greater focus on the objectives of the study, achieving better experimental design, and minimizing the need for repeat studies. Reassessing lethal tests (the LD_{50} test), using prescreening, using *in vitro* tests where possible, and promoting greater sharing and dissemination of test data worldwide, will contribute to reduction of animal testing. Re-using animals, or using them for multiple tests (for example, ocular and dermal), might be considered.

13.2 Refinement

Adjustments to study designs and techniques have led to a reduction in the number of animals used, and in many cases they have made testing more humane, without compromising scientific validity, and in some cases improving it. Examples include the "fixed dose" scheme adopted by the British Toxicological Society, limit tests, and modifications to eye irritation tests (the low volume test, a tiered approach, and the use of prescreens and sequential tests).

13.3 Replacement

A number of alternative tests have been studied, and significant progress has been made in developing *in vitro* replacement models. These currently include eye, muscle and skin irritation, phototoxicity, photosensitization, and target organ toxicity testing.

13.4 Responsibility

This refers to the need for toxicologists and other researchers to reduce animal suffering and to treat the animals as well as possible.

14 NEW STRATEGIES FOR TOXICITY TESTING

14.1 Limit Test

A simple method has been proposed for the screening assessment of acute oral and dermal toxicity, using only three rats and mice of each sex at each dose level. Animals are first treated with chemicals at a dose of 2000 mg/kg and carefully observed for compound-related morbidity and mortality. If none of the animals die, subsequent toxicity tests are suspended. If some die, toxicity tests are performed at doses of 200 and 20 mg/kg, respectively. The approximate LD_{50} values are calculated by this method; they show little difference between laboratories, and are in close agreement with LD_{50} values reported for the same chemicals in the literature. The LD_{50} values that were estimated by extrapolation using this method were approximately 2 to 2.5 times the maximum non-lethal dose (MNLD) determined in acute oral and dermal toxicity testing. This means that a chemical may be regarded as having an LD_{50} of 4000 mg/kg or higher when there is no mortality at 2000 mg/kg. A chemical with such low toxicity does not require further testing for lethal effects. This method serves as a limit test, and it obviates the need for a full LD_{50} test (Yamanaka et al., 1990).

In the guidelines of the U.S. Environmental Protection Agency (USEPA, 1984), 2000 mg/kg is an acceptable limit test for the dermal route, and 5000 mg/kg is the accepted dose for testing via the oral route. This simple test permits important information such as signs of intoxication, identification of target organs, and reversibility of toxicity to be obtained from careful observation in a small number of animals.

14.2 Fixed-Dose Oral Toxicity Testing

In an international study involving 33 laboratories in 11 countries, the acute oral toxicity of rats to 20 substances was evaluated using a fixed-dose procedure (Van den Heuvel et al., 1990). The results were compared with those obtained for the test materials using the standard LD_{50} test. The study showed that fixed-dose testing:

1. Produces consistent results that are not seriously affected by interlaboratory variation.
2. Provides adequate information for risk assessment of acute toxicity, including its nature, time to onset, duration and outcome, for the substances concerned.
3. Makes use of fewer animals than the current internationally agreed procedures.
4. Subjects animals to less pain and distress than the LD_{50} test, and causes less compound-related mortality.
5. Enables substances and preparations to be ranked according to standard classification systems, and to their acute oral toxicity; such ranking being consistent with that allocated by the results of standard LD_{50} studies.

14.3 Sequential Studies and a Decision Tree

Gad et al. (1984) have reported their experience over 4 years, in which they have conducted 124 acute systemic toxicity studies (64 oral, 39 dermal, and 21 inhalational), throughout which they have altered study and program designs with the purpose of maximizing information and minimizing animal usage. By employing dose selection strategies, probes and lethality limits instead of the LD_{50}, with staggered sequential dosing, and by conducting studies in batteries, animal usage was reduced by 48% below the average number regarded as necessary for an LD_{50} study. They suggested that the combined use of a neurobehavioral screen, adjunct studies, and flexible study design has resulted in significant improvement in the information obtained from these studies.

The use of a decision tree approach for selecting tissues for histopathology was developed by the same workers (Gad et al., 1984). Specific indicators (such as organ weights) for selecting organs for microscopic examination were evaluated. The overall result has been to increase the flexibility of the standard appoach to the design and conduct of acute systemic toxicity studies, and to subject standard procedures to more critical consideration. The authors' experience has been widely accepted by regulatory authorities, being regarded as providing all the necessary information.

14.4 *In Vitro* Toxicity Testing

It has been predicted that *in vitro* toxicity tests will play an increasingly important role in chemical safety evaluation. They will be used as screens to provide data for product development priorities, and they will be incorporated into drug regulatory testing. They will maximize the opportunities for identifying highly toxic materials at an early stage in the process of evaluation and reduce the excessive need for *in vivo* testing (Frazier, 1993).

An evaluation process that is provided entirely by *in vitro* testing requires a far deeper knowledge base than is presently available. *In vitro* toxicity and toxicokinetic studies, combined with physiologically based toxicokinetic modeling and quantitative structure-activity testing, will form the basis for such an approach. It has been suggested that every effort needs to be made to develop scientifically sound testing systems aimed at minimizing the need for *in vivo* animal testing (Frazier, 1993).

14.5 Computer-Based Systems

Computer-based structure-activity relationships combined with cell culture testing systems provide valuable toxicological data for hazard and risk assessments, and in *in vitro* systems allow for more rapid identification of toxic compounds (DelRaso, 1993). They can also be utilized to study mechanisms of toxicity at cellular and subcellular levels. The data derived from these studies can be used to improve the predictability of standard animal models for chemical and drug toxicity.

It is not realistic to expect that *in vitro* methods will entirely replace testing in the whole animal. There are numerous interrelationships between structure, function, and behavior in toxicology that require the intact animal. Examples include the measurement of the neurobehavioral effects of toxic substances, strain and species differences with regard to the metabolic fate of test compounds, the role of the intestinal flora and enterohepatic circulation in influencing metabolic pathways of test compounds, and differential distribution within an organ of xenobiotic biotransformation due to variations in organ architecture and cell polarity.

15 AGING STUDIES

Recently, there has been increasing attention paid to models and systems for research into aging, to conduct studies that cannot be done in humans for ethical, legal, or technical reasons, and which are indispensable for progress in biomedical research into aging (Hazzard et al., 1991). It seems clear that there are diverse processes of senescence that have the common outcome of accelerating mortality rates in different animal species. The use of a broad range of animal models is important to allow for generalization of findings, and to make possible the discovery of primary aging processes. Equally important may be the discovery of a process unique to the aging of a particular class of animals.

A variety of animal models exist that have advantages or special features which may contribute to research on aging. The appropriate choice of a model will require a number of conditions, the most important of which should allow for manipulation of the genetic system, characterization of physiological data, and easy and affordable husbandry.

16 PHYSIOLOGICAL MEASUREMENTS

Physiological parameters for different laboratory animal species are diverse and difficult to quantify. The work of Davies and Morris (1993), which is reproduced here with permission, is helpful in assisting researchers to make practical physiological and biochemical decisions when testing animals.

REFERENCES

Aldridge, W. N. (1976). Chronic toxicity as an acute phenomenon: introduction to symposium, *Proc. Eur. Soc. Toxicol.*, 17, 5-6.

Balazs, T. (1974). Development of tissue resistance to toxic effects of chemicals. *Toxicology,* 2, 247-55.

Brown, V. K. (1987). Animal models of responses resulting from short-term exposures. In Worden, A., Parke, D. and Marks, J. (Eds.), *The Future of Predictive Safety Evaluation,* Volume 2, MTP Press, Lancaster, pp. 47-55.

Cohen, C. (1986). The case for the use of animals in biochemical research, *N. Engl. J. Med.*, 315, 865.

Davies, B. and Morris, T. (1993). Physiological parameters in laboratory animals and humans. *Pharm. Res.,* 10, 1093.

Dayan, A. D. (1986). The scientific basis for long-term animal studies — what can and cannot be detected. In Walker, S. R. and Dayan, A. D. (Eds.), *Long-Term Animal Studies: Their Predictive Value for Man,* MTP Press, Lancaster, pp. 3-7.

Dean, J. H., Luster, M. I., Boorman, G. A. and Lauer, L. D. (1982). Procedures available to examine the immunotoxicity of chemicals and drugs. *Pharmacol. Rev.*, 34, 137-48.

DelRaso, N. J. (1993). *In vitro* methodologies for enhanced toxicity testing. *Toxicol. Lett.*, 68, 91.

Dewar, A. J. (1987). Neurotoxicity. In Worden, A., Parke, D. and Marks, J. (Eds.), *The Future of Predictive Safety Evaluation,* Volume 2. MTP Press, Lancaster, pp. 107-28.

Draize, J. H., Woodard, G. and Calvery, H. O. (1944). Methods for the study of irritation and toxicity of substances applied topically to the skin and mucous membrane. *J. Pharmacol.*, 82, 377-90.

Fletcher, A. P. (1978). Drug safety tests and subsequent clinical experience. *J. R. Soc. Med.*, 71, 693-6.

Frazier, J. M. (1993). *In vitro* models for toxicological research and testing. *Toxicol. Lett.*, 68, 73.

Frederick, G. L. (1986). The evidence supporting 18 month animal studies. In Walker, S. R. and Dayan, A. D. (Eds.), *Long-Term Animal Studies: Their Predictive Value for Man.* MTP Press, Lancaster, pp. 65-76.

Gad, S. C. (1990). Recent developments in replacing, reducing, and refining animal use in toxicologic research and testing. *Fund. Appl. Toxicol.*, 15, 8.

Gad, S. C., Smith, A. C., Cramp, A. L. et al. (1984). Innovative designs and practices for acute systemic toxicity studies. *Drug Chem. Toxicol.*, 7, 423.

Gart, J. J., Chu, K. C. and Tarone, R. E. (1979). Statistical issues in interpretation of chronic bioassay tests for carcinogenicity. *J. Natl. Cancer Inst.*, 62, 957-74.

Glockin, V. C. (1986). Justification for 12 month animal studies. In Walker, S. R. and Dayan, A. D. (Eds.), *Long-Term Animal Studies: Their Predictive Value for Man.* MTP Press, Lancaster, pp. 77-82.

Grahame-Smith, D. (1986). What is expected from repeated-dose studies by the regulatory authorities. In Walker, S. R. and Dayan, A. D. (Eds.), *Long-Term Animal Studies: Their Predictive Value for Man.* MTP Press, Lancaster, pp. 23-7.

Hazzard, D. G., Warner, H. R. and Finch, C. E. (1991). National Institute on Aging, NIH: workshop on alternative animal models for research on aging. *Exp. Gerontol.*, 26, 411.

Hoel, D. G., Kaplan, N. L. and Anderson, M. W. (1983). Implication of nonlinear kinetics on risk estimation in carcinogenesis. *Science*, 219, 1032-7.

IARC Monographs on the Evaluation of the Carcinogenic Risk of Chemicals to Humans. (1984). Supplement 4, Chemicals, Industrial Processes and Industries Associated with Cancer in Humans. IARC Monographs, International Agency for Research on Cancer, Lyon, Volumes 1-29.

Jackson, M. R. (1986). Conventional design of long-term toxicity studies in the pharmaceutical industry. In Walker, S. P. and Dayan, A. D. (Eds.), *Long-Term Animal Studies: Their Predictive Value for Man.* MTP Press, Lancaster, pp. 35-44.

Kodell, R. L., Farmer, J. H., Gaylot, D. W. and Cameron, A. M. (1982). Influence of cause of death assignment on time-to-tumor analyses in animal carcinogenesis studies. *J. Natl. Cancer Inst.*, 69, 659-64.

Koeter, H. B. W. M. (1983). Relevance of parameters related to fertility and reproduction in toxicity testing. *Am. J. Ind. Med.*, 4, 81-6.

Lansdown, A. B. G. (1987). Testing for reproductive toxicity. In Worden, A. N., Parke, D. V. and Marks, J. (Eds.), *The Future of Predictive Safety Evaluation,* Volume 2. MTP Press, Lancaster, pp. 77-106.

Lasagna, L. (1984). Regulatory agencies, drugs and the pregnant patient. In Stern, L. (Ed.), *Drug Use in Pregnancy.* Adis Health Science Press, Sydney, pp. 12-16.

Litchfield, J. T. (1962). Evaluation of the safety of new drugs by means of tests in animals. *Clin. Pharmacol. Ther.*, 3, 665-81.

Lumley, C. E. and Walker, S. R. (1985a). A toxicology databank based on animal safety evaluation studies of pharmaceutical compounds. *Hum. Toxicol.*, 4, 447-60.

Lumley, C. E. and Walker, S. R. (1985b). What is the value of animal toxicology studies beyond 6 months? *Br. J. Pharmacol.*, 84, Suppl., 117P.

McLean, A. E. M. (1986). The relationship between animal and human responses. In Walker, S. R. and Dayan, A. D. (Eds.), *Long-Term Animal Studies: Their Predictive Value for Man.* MTP Press, Lancaster, pp. 99-104.

Messite, J. and Bond, M. B. (1988). Reproductive toxicology and occupational exposure. In Zenz, C. (Ed.), *Occupational Medicine: Principles and Practical Applications.* Year Book Medical Publishers, Chicago, pp. 847-903.

Miller, K. and Nicklin, S. (1987). Immunological aspects. In Worden, A., Parke, D. and Marks, J. (Eds.), *The Future of Predictive Safety Evaluation,* Volume 1. MTP Press, Lancaster, pp. 181-94.

Miller, R. K., Mattison, D. R., Filler, R. S. and Rice, J. M. (1985). Reproductive and developmental toxicology. In Eskes, T. K. A. B. and Finster, M. (Eds.), *Drug Therapy During Pregnancy,* Butterworths, London, pp. 215-24.

Paget, E. (1983). The LD_{50} test. *Acta Pharmacol. Toxicol.*, 52, Suppl. 2, 6-19.

Pakes, S. P. (1990). Contributions of the laboratory animal veterinarian to refining animal experiments in toxicology. *Fund. Appl. Toxicol.*, 15, 17.

Purchase, I. F. H. (1987). Carcinogenic risk assessment: Are animals good surrogates for man? In Bannasch, P. (Ed.), *Cancer Risks: Strategies for Elimination.* Springer-Verlag, Berlin, pp. 65-79.

Rawlins, M. D. (1986). What is expected from repeated-dose studies by clinical pharmacologists. In Walker, S. R. and Dayan, A. D. (Eds.), *Long-Term Animal Studies: Their Predictive Value for Man.* MTP Press, Lancaster, pp. 17-22.

Rowan, A. (1983). Shortcomings of LD_{50} values and acute toxicity testing in animals. *Acta Pharmacol. Toxicol.*, 52, 52-64.

Rowan, A. N. (1990). Refinement of animal research technique and validity of research data. *Fund. Appl. Toxicol.*, 15, 25.

Silbergeld, E. K. (1982). Current status of neurotoxicology, basic and applied. *Trends Neurosci.*, 5, 291-4.

Squire, R. A. (1981). Ranking animal carcinogens: A proposed regulatory approach. *Science*, 214, 877-80.

Thomas, J. A., Ham, T. E., Perkins, P. L. and Raffin, T. A. (1988). Animal research at Stanford University, *N. Engl. J. Med.*, 318, 1630.

Van den Heuvel, M. J., Clark, D. G., Fielder, R. J. et al. (1990). The international validation of a fixed dose procedure as an alternative to the classical LD_{50} test. *Fd. Chem. Toxicol.*, 28, 469.

Weil, C. S. and Scala, R. A. (1971). Study of intra- and interlaboratory variability in the results of rabbit eye and skin irritation tests. *Toxicol. Appl. Pharmacol.*, 19, 276-360.

Weisburger, J. H. (1987). Safety evaluation — carcinogenic risks. In Worden, A., Parke, D. and Marks, J. (Eds.), *The Future of Predictive Safety Evaluation,* Volume 2. MTP Press, Lancaster, pp. 129-52.

Wilson, J. G. (1959). Experimental studies on congenital malformations. *J. Chron. Dis.,* 10, 111-30.

Worden, A. N. (1986). The evidence supporting 6-month animal studies. In Walker, S. R. and Dayan, A. D. (Eds.), *Long-Term Animal Studies: Their Predictive Value for Man.* MTP Press, Lancaster, pp. 83-6.

Worden, A. N. and Walker, S. R. (1987). Animal models for long term toxic effects. In Worden, A., Parke, D. and Marks, J. (Eds.), *The Future of Predictive Safety Evaluation,* Volume 2, MTP Press, Lancaster, pp. 57-64.

Yamanaka, S., Hashimoto, M., Tobe, M. et al. (1990). A simple method for screening assessment of acute toxicity of chemicals, *Arch. Toxicol.,* 64, 262.

Zbinden, G. (1980). Predictive value of pre-clinical drug safety evaluation. In Turner, P. (Ed.), *Proceedings of Plenary Lectures Symposia and Therapeutic Sessions of the First World Conference on Clinical Pharmacology and Therapeutics.* Macmillan Press, London.

Zbinden, G. (1987a). Risks predicted from animal studies. In Walker, S. R. and Asscher, A. W. (Eds.), *Medicines and Risk/Benefit Decision.* MTP Press, Lancaster, pp. 49-56.

Zbinden, G. (1987b). Predictive value of animal studies in toxicology. Centre for Medicines Research, Carshalton.

Zbinden, G. and Flury-Roversi, M. (1981). Significance of the LD_{50}-test for the toxicological evaluation of chemical substances. *Arch. Toxicol.,* 47, 77-99.

Chapter 5

The *In Vitro* Assessment of Human Hepatic Drug Metabolism

G. T. Tucker

CONTENTS

1 Introduction 51
2 The Enzymes 52
  2.1 Cytochromes P-450 52
    2.1.1 Probe Substrates, Inhibitors, and Inducers 52
  2.2 Flavin-Containing Monooxygenases (FMO) 53
  2.3 Conjugation (Phase II) Enzymes 53
3 Experimental Systems 54
  3.1 Human Liver Tissue 54
    3.1.1 Microsomes 54
    3.1.2 Hepatocytes 55
    3.1.3 Slices 55
  3.2 Heterologous Expression Systems 55
  3.3 Molecular Models 55
4 Applications of Relevance to the Early Clinical Assessment of New Drugs 55
  4.1 Prediction of *In Vivo* Drug Clearance 55
  4.2 Identification of Enzyme Isoforms 56
  4.3 Understanding of Drug Side Effects 57
  4.4 Prediction of Drug Interactions 58
    4.4.1 Substrate and/or Inhibitor or Inducer? 58
    4.4.2 Screening for Interaction Potential 59
    4.4.3 *In Vitro-In Vivo* Extrapolation 59
    4.4.4 Case Studies 60
      4.4.4.1 SSRIs and Tricyclic Antidepressants 60
      4.4.4.2 Terfenadine-Ketoconazole 60
5 Conclusions 60
References 61

1 INTRODUCTION

Several factors have led to a recent surge of interest in using *in vitro* methods to study human drug metabolism. These include the rapid increase in knowledge of the enzymes involved based on application of the techniques of molecular biology, a wider appreciation of the limitations of animal data and the pressure to find alternatives to animal experimentation, and an increased availability of human tissue for this kind of research. Understandably, investigation has concentrated on hepatic drug metabolism, as the liver is the main site of metabolism for most drugs, and encompasses the use of subcellular fractions (especially microsomes), hepatocytes (primary suspension culture and monolayer culture), and precision-cut tissue slices. These techniques are also being supplemented and extended by the development of heterologous expression systems for single and multiple enzymes, and by the elaboration of molecular models of active sites.

In the context of drug development, information derived from the *in vitro* study of human drug metabolism is of potential benefit to the pharmacologist, the toxicologist, and the clinician. Thus, it should help in the following ways:

1. To identify and isolate drug metabolites for subsequent evaluation of pharmacological activity
2. To identify potentially toxic metabolites and to evaluate their activity using cellular markers

0-8493-9230-6/97/$0.00+$.50
© 1997 by CRC Press, Inc.

3. To compare products and patterns of drug metabolism with those in other species, thereby facilitating the choice of animal species for pharmacological and toxicity testing or, at least, the *post hoc* rationalization of such studies with respect to exposure to drug and metabolites
4. To predict *in vivo* drug clearance in man (*in vitro-in vivo* scaling), as an aid to the selection of dosage in phase I studies
5. To predict the influence of genetic, environmental, and clinical factors on the clearance of a new drug *in vivo* by identification of specific enzyme isoforms mediating its metabolism
6. To identify drug-drug interactions, caused by induction or inhibition of specific enzyme activities, which should be studied in phase I volunteer studies (more importantly, perhaps, to eliminate unnecessary drug interaction studies)

Ultimately, as understanding of the relationships between chemical structure and metabolism improves, knowledge of the routes and rates of drug metabolism should become a fully integrated part of drug design.

2 THE ENZYMES

2.1 Cytochromes P-450

The cytochrome P-450 monooxygenases comprise the most important class of enzymes with respect to drug metabolism. This is a superfamily of enzymes, grouped across species according to their amino acid sequence into families and subfamilies. A greater than 40% homology defines a family and a greater than 55% homology defines a subfamily. The symbol CYP is used to denote both the human cytochrome P-450 gene and enzyme. This is followed by an arabic numeral denoting the family, a capital letter designating the subfamily and then another arabic numeral representing the individual gene/enzyme.[1] For example, CYP2D6 refers to debrisoquine hydroxylase, a human form of cytochrome P-450 which shows a marked genetic polymorphism. In humans five CYP subfamilies appear to be principally involved in hepatic drug metabolism, namely CYP's 1A, 2C, 2D, 2E, and 3A. Specific isoforms of importance within these groups are CYP's 1A2, 2C8-10, 2C19, 2D6, 2E1, and 3A3, 4, 5. CYP's 2A6 and 2B6 appear to play a minor role. Collectively, these enzymes represent about 70% of total immunodetectable cytochrome P-450; estimates of their average relative abundance in adult liver are shown in Figure 1. CYP3A7 is specific to fetal liver where it is the major form.[3]

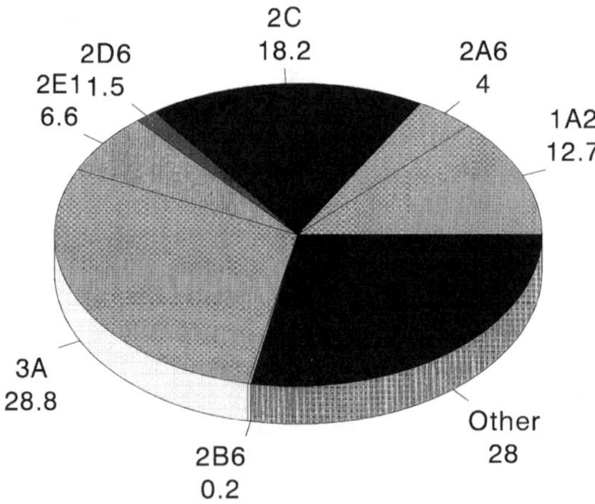

Figure 1 Average relative abundance of individual cytochrome P-450 isoforms determined immunochemically in microsomes from 60 human livers. (From Shimada, T., Yamazaki, H., Mimura, M., Inui, K. and Guengerich, F. P., *J. Pharmacol. Exp. Ther.*, 270, 414, 1974. With permission.)

2.1.1 Probe Substrates, Inhibitors, and Inducers

A list of selective substrates and inhibitors of the main human CYP isoforms is shown in Table 1, along with an indication of enzyme inducers and whether the isoform shows marked genetic polymorphism. It should be noted that the list includes many of the low therapeutic index drugs of concern with regard to drug interactions, thus, in principle, it is increasingly possible to predict which kinds of compounds a new drug might or might not interact with at the level of metabolism. The selectivity of enzyme inducers is rather less than that of inhibitors. CYP2D6 is only weakly inducible, polycyclic hydrocarbons induce 1A, phenobarbitone and rifampicin induce 2C, ethanol induces 2E1 and dexamethasone, rifampicin and phenytoin induce 3A. CYP's 2D6 and 2C19 exhibit marked genetic polymorphism.

Table 1 Xenobiotic Substrate Probes, Selective Inhibitors and Regulation of Human Cytochrome P-450 Isoforms

Isoform	Model Substrate/Activity	Selective Inhibitors	Inducers/Genetic Polymorphism
1A1	Benzo(a)pyrene-hydroxylation		Induced by cigarette smoke, omeprazole Not constitutively expressed in human liver
1A2	Caffeine-3-demethylase Phenacetin-*O*-deethylase	Furafylline	Induced by cigarette smoke, omeprazole
2A6	Coumarin-7-hydroxylase	8-methoxypsoralen	
2C9/10	Tolbutamide-hydroxylase Phenytoin-hydroxylase S-warfarin-7-hydroxylase	Sulfaphenazole	Induced by rifampicin, phenobarbitone
2C19	S-mephenytoin-4′-hydroxylase Omeprazole-hydroxylase Proguanil-cyclase		Genetic polymorphism (3%PM in C; 20% in O)
2D6	Debrisoquine-4-hydroxylase Sparteine-oxidase Metoprolol α-hydroxylase-*O*-demethylase Dextromethorphan-*O*-demethylase	Quinidine	Genetic polymorphism (8% PM in C; <1% in O)
2E1	Chlorzoxazone-6-hydroxylase *N*-nitroso-dimethylamine-*N*-demethylase 4-nitrophenol-hydroxylation	Diethyldithiocarbamate	Induced by ethanol, isoniazid
3A3/4/5	Testosterone-6-hydroxylase Erythromycin-*N*-demethylase Nifedipine-oxidase	Ketoconazole (low conc.) Gestodene Quercetin Troleandomycin	Induced by dexamethasone, rifampicin Barbiturates, phenytoin
	Cyclosporine-oxidase		3A5-polymorphic (present in 30% livers)
	Lignocaine-*N*-deethylase Midazolam-hydroxylase Ethynylestradiol-hydroxylation		

Note: PM = poor metabolizer phenotype; C = Caucasian; O = Oriental.

From Birkett, D. J., McKenzie, P. I., Verones, M. E. and Miners, J. O., *Trends Pharmacol. Sci.*, 14, 292, 1993. With permission. Also from Wrighton, S. A., Vandenbranden, M., Stevens, J. C., Shipley, L. A. and Ring, B. J., *Drug Metab. Rev.*, 25, 453, 1993. With permission.

The broad structural characteristics of substrates for each of the main CYP isoforms involved in human drug metabolism are indicated in Table 2.

2.2 Flavin-Containing Monooxygenases (FMO)

In contrast to cytochromes P-450, which primarily carry out C-oxidations, the FMOs catalyze oxidation at nucleophilic N, S, and P atoms. Multiple forms of FMO have been identified in human liver,[7] but systematic studies of substrate structure-activity relationships are lacking. Nicotine-*N′*-oxidation has been used as a general probe reaction for FMO activity in human liver microsomes.[5]

2.3 Conjugation (Phase II) Enzymes

Phase II enzymes include UDP-glucuronosyltransferases (microsomal), sulfotransferases (cytosolic), glutathione S-transferases (microsomal and cytosolic), methyl transferases (cytosolic), and N-acetyl transferases (cytosolic).

Table 2 Substrate Structure-Activity Relationships of Cytochrome P-450 Isoforms

CYP1A	Neutral, flat aromatic compounds, tricyclic and above
CYP2A	Neutral, bicyclic planar compounds with a minimum of one aromatic ring
CYP2C9	Neutral or acidic molecules with a site of oxidation 5-8 Å from H-bond donor heteroatom
CYP2D6	Arylalkylamines with site of oxidation 5-7 Å from protonated hydrogen
CYP2E1	Small, polar molecules. Lower rotational and tumbling energy for binding at nonspecific site
CYP3A	Neutral or basic molecules with site of oxidation determined by ease of electron or hydrogen atom abstraction

From Smith, D. A. and Jones, B. C., *Biochem. Pharmacol.*, 44, 2089, 1992. With permission. Also from Smith, D. A., personal communication.

The UDP-glucuronosyltransferases (UDPGT) represent the family of phase II enzymes with probably the most members, although it appears that the diversity is not as extensive as in the case of cytochromes P-450. Also, substrate structure-activity relationships are not as well delineated as with the P-450s.[8,9] Based upon inhibition studies, morphine and paracetamol, which might be regarded as typical probe drug substrates, are glucuronidated by two distinct sets of at least two human liver UDPGTs.[9] Like cytochromes P-450, different forms of UDPGT may be differentiated by their response to inducing agents.[10]

Microsomal epoxide hydrolases may be loosely regarded as phase II enzymes in that they add (conjugate) water to epoxides. These important postoxidative detoxification enzymes may be probed using styrene or carbamazepine epoxide as model substrates.[11]

3 EXPERIMENTAL SYSTEMS

3.1 Human Liver Tissue

Despite considerable amino acid sequence similarity in enzymes across species, even small differences can alter the catalytic activity dramatically. For example, the 6- and 8-hydroxylation of warfarin is catalyzed by CYP1A1 in the rat but not in the mouse, despite 93% homology in the enzyme sequence.[12] S-mephenytoin is 4-hydroxylated by CYP2C19 in man, but this reaction is mediated by CYP3A in the rat.[13,14] Thus, prediction of the role of specific enzyme isoforms mediating drug metabolism in man from animal data and, consequently, genetic, environmental, and clinical influences on enzyme activity, are generally inadequate. Hence, the necessity for studies with human tissue and enzymes. However, in turn, this raises issues of availability and ethics.[15,16] While these issues are under debate, ready access to human liver tissue is possible currently through nonprofit making sources in the U.S.

When assessing drug metabolism it is clearly important to study a sufficiently wide range of samples from different livers to ensure that results are representative. A typical "liver bank" should contain at least 15–20 specimens characterized as fully as possible with respect to donor age, sex, and drug and medical histories and a range of different drug metabolizing activities. It is also vital to establish that the samples were obtained as soon as possible after surgery then stored rapidly at –80°C. Under these conditions loss of metabolic activity is not a problem.[5] Shimada et al.[2] have characterized individual variations in the level and activity of the major human CYPs in liver microsomes from 60 patients. In general, activities varied by about 10-fold and were relatively independent of age, sex, and race (Japanese/Caucasian). For those enzymes, such as CYP2D6, which show marked genetic polymorphism the availability of genotyped liver samples facilitates diagnosis of the role of the enzyme in the metabolism of a compound.[17]

3.1.1 Microsomes

Microsomes are easy to prepare and characterize. With addition of the appropriate co-factors they can be used to study both phase I and II metabolism, although assessment of the full extent of glucuronidation also requires addition of detergent to optimize exposure of substrate to the enzyme. Apart from the obvious lack of cellular integrity, the limitations of using microsomes include a short incubation time, necessitating the development of sensitive assays for metabolites of slowly metabolized compounds, inability to study induction, and the difficulty of assessing the contribution of metabolism to net drug clearance without independent data on other pathways of drug elimination.

3.1.2 Hepatocytes

A major advantage of using hepatocytes is the ability to study enzyme induction. However, a considerable disadvantage at the present time is that when used fresh in suspension the cells do not survive for more than a few hours, and standard primary culture techniques preserve differentiated CYP function poorly. However, progress in cryopreservation and methods of culture which retain intercellular contacts and tissue architecture is anticipated.[18]

3.1.3 Slices

Recent developments in methods of preparing thin, precision-cut liver slices have helped to minimize the limitation of poor diffusion of substrate to the enzyme site.[19] However, concerns about viability with time require careful validation of the conditions of use.

3.2 Heterologous Expression Systems

A variety of cellular systems (mammalian cell lines, insect cells — baculovirus, yeast, and bacteria) expressing single or multiple human CYPs and other drug metabolizing enzymes are now available, each with distinctive advantages and limitations.[20] Once validated, their use can confirm rapidly the participation of a single enzyme in the metabolism of a compound. However, although expression systems can show that a compound is metabolized by a particular enzyme, it is important to remember that the reaction may be carried out by more than one isoenzyme in the liver. Therefore, any assessment of the quantitative contribution of a single enzyme to net metabolite production requires comparison of the activity of each isoenzyme involved with respect to its specific content in the liver (Figure 1). This may be difficult if the relative efficiency of the heterologous expression of each isoenzyme is not known. Perhaps in the future an array of expressed human enzymes, present together in relation to their appropriate abundance, may be used as an "artificial liver" for studying drug metabolism. Transgenic animals expressing human drug metabolizing enzymes are also on the horizon.

3.3 Molecular Models

Models of the active sites of several of the cytochromes P-450 are in the process of being refined. For example, in the case of CYP2D6 these range from templates based upon structure-metabolism relationships to representations based upon protein structure.[21] Ultimately, a combination of approaches including systematic structure-activity studies, single-enzyme expression systems, site-directed mutagenesis, and molecular modeling will improve our ability to visualize the topography of active sites and, thereby, to predict drug metabolism *in computro*.

4 APPLICATIONS OF RELEVANCE TO THE EARLY CLINICAL ASSESSMENT OF NEW DRUGS

4.1 Prediction of *In Vivo* Drug Clearance

Extending earlier investigations of Rane et al.[22] and others, Houston[23] has proposed a general strategy for the prediction of *in vivo* drug clearance from data obtained using liver microsomes and hepatocytes.

The method proceeds in four steps, as summarized in Figure 2. The first stage is to obtain estimates of Vmax and Km of the substrate either from initial rates of metabolite formation or drug loss or by fitting the Michaelis-Menten equation to the time-course of drug loss. Correction of Km for nonspecific partition binding to microsomal protein may be required. Division of Vmax by Km gives the *in vitro* intrinsic clearance. This value is then scaled to an *in vivo* estimate using liver weight and protein content (for microsomes) or cell number (for hepatocytes). In stage 3 a model of hepatic drug clearance must be assumed (e.g., a "well-stirred liver") such that net metabolic clearance can be calculated from intrinsic metabolic clearance, the free fraction of drug in plasma and hepatic blood flow. This scales the kinetic data in terms of circulating plasma drug concentration rather than the concentration of drug within the liver. Finally, total body clearance is estimated by combining metabolic clearance with clearance values estimated independently for other elimination mechanisms (extrahepatic metabolism, biliary and renal excretion). Using this approach, predictions were made using data taken from the literature on 25 drugs studied using both rat liver microsomes and hepatocytes.[23] Considering that the data were from a variety of sources and covered a range of chemical structures metabolized by different P-450 isoforms, the predictions were remarkably good (Figure 3). The precision of the method needs to be evaluated further but, in principle, it should be equally applicable to human *in vitro* data, even that derived from heterologous expression systems. Along with the use of allometric scaling, *in vitro* estimates of metabolic

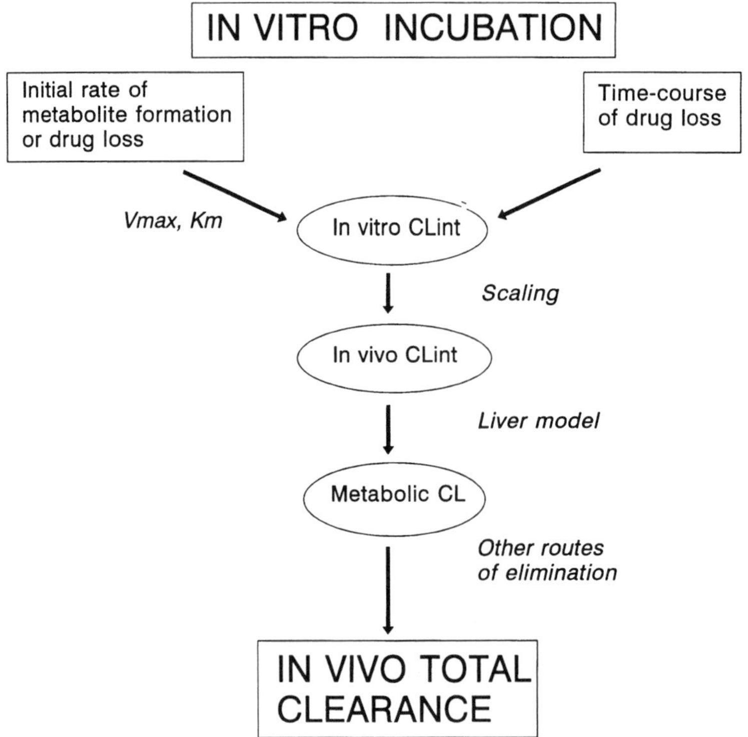

Figure 2 A strategy for the extrapolation of *in vitro* drug metabolism data to estimate *in vivo* drug clearance. (Adapted from Houston, J. B., *Biochem. Pharmacol.*, 47, 1469, 1994. With permission).

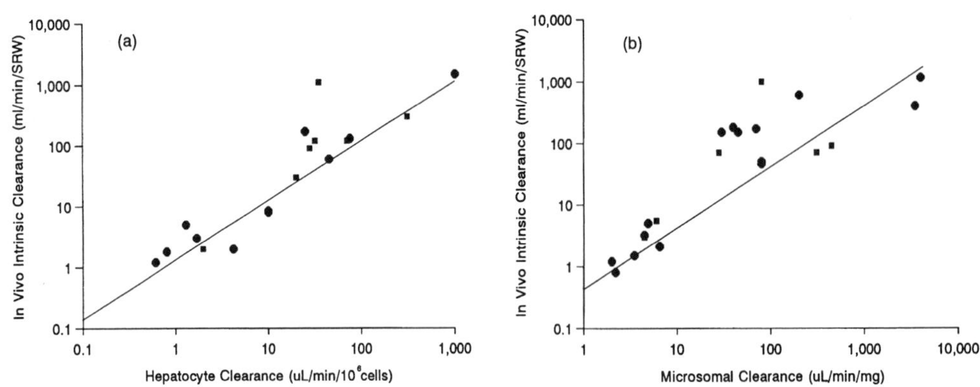

Figure 3 Relationships between *in vivo* intrinsic hepatic clearance of drugs metabolized by cytochromes P-450 and (a) hepatocyte clearance and (b) hepatic microsomal clearance in the rat. Circles refer to *in vitro* data obtained from metabolite formation; squares refer to *in vitro* data obtained from loss of substrate. The lines represent scaling factors (1.5×10^9 cells/standard rat weight; SRW and 500 mg microsomal protein/SRW, respectively). (Adapted from Houston, J. B., *Biochem. Pharmacol.*, 47, 1469, 1994. With permission).

clearance in man relative to that in animal species should provide guidance for the selection of safe and effective doses in phase I studies.

4.2 Identification of Enzyme Isoforms

A systematic approach to the identification of the isoforms of cytochrome P-450 involved in the metabolism of a compound is possible because this superfamily is well-characterized compared to other drug metabolizing enzymes. A typical procedure based on the use of human liver microsomes is as follows:

1. Identification of metabolites.
2. Development of metabolite assays.
3. Characterization of enzyme kinetics using microsomes from a small number of livers, metabolite formation should be studied under linear conditions with respect to protein and time, and over a sufficient range of substrate concentration to determine the possibility that more than one isoenzyme is involved in the same pathway. This enables the most appropriate substrate concentrations to be selected for subsequent studies.
4. Correlation experiments. Using microsomes from each sample in the liver bank, metabolite formation is correlated with previously determined activities for the range of CYP isoforms, established using model substrates and specific antibodies. A high correlation coefficient provides evidence for a significant contribution to metabolism from a particular CYP.
5. Inhibition experiments. The effects of various selective inhibitors/substrates (Table 1) on the formation of metabolite is assessed. Potent inhibition by a probe compound is evidence for a significant contribution to metabolism from a particular CYP. In addition, inhibitory antibodies raised against particular CYPs can be used, provided that their specificity is validated.
6. Confirmation with expression systems. Presence or absence of metabolite formation is assessed using either whole cells or microsomes from an array of validated single enzyme expression systems.

A model example of the use of stages 1 through 5 of the above approach is described by Andersson et al.,[24] who identified the CYP isoforms involved in the metabolism of omeprazole. Data for the major hydroxy-product are shown in Figure 4. At clinically relevant drug concentrations, it was concluded that most of this reaction is mediated by CYP2C19 (S-mephenytoin hydroxylase) as a high affinity site, with some contribution from CYP3A4 as a low affinity site. However, in some individuals the role of CYP3A4 might be dominant to the extent that it is an inducible enzyme. Furthermore, the gut has considerable CYP3A4 activity.[25] Neverthless, the *in vitro* findings predict earlier *in vivo* observations that omeprazole exhibits polymorphic metabolism co-segregating with the oxidation of S-mephenytoin, and that it inhibits the metabolism of diazepam, another 2C19 substrate.[26,27] In an extension to their investigation of the enzymes involved in the metabolism of omeprazole itself, Andersson et al.[28] have also elucidated the P-450 isoforms which mediate the formation of secondary from primary omeprazole metabolites. Secondary metabolites are often observed *in vivo*, but cannot be studied adequately from *in vitro* incubations of parent drug because secondary pathways mediated by the same enzyme tend to be inhibited in the presence of saturating concentrations of parent drug. Therefore, the primary metabolites must be added to incubations as initial substrates.

The role of CYP2D6 in metabolism is particularly easy to establish using microsomes from both "poor" and "extensive" metabolizers, quinidine as a highly selective chemical inhibitor, the specific anti-LKM_1 inhibitory antibody,[29] and a validated yeast expression system.[30] In addition, a simple two-dimensional template model, in which the site of oxidation is located 5-7A from a basic nitrogen (Table 2), is generally diagnostic, with further improvements in molecular modeling imminent. Based on the two-dimensional model, Koymans et al.[31] predicted that 4 out of 14 potential metabolic routes for 4 drugs developed by the Janssen Company should be CYP2D6 mediated. The CYP2D6 pathways were confirmed by *in vitro* and *in vivo* studies for all but one route for one compound.

4.3 Understanding Drug Side Effects

Side effects not predicted from animal toxicology may occur during the early clinical use of a new compound. In some cases it may be possible to rationalize or preempt these observations based upon *in vitro* metabolism studies with human tissue. For example, in preclinical safety studies using rats and dogs there was no evidence of hepatoxicity from tacrine, yet 20-50% of patients during clinical trials developed dose-dependent, asymptomatic elevations in serum enzymes associated with impaired liver function.[32] Subsequent investigations showed that tacrine undergoes metabolic activation to protein-reactive and cytotoxic metabolites to a much greater extent when incubated with human liver microsomes compared to those from noninduced rats.[33,34] Although a cause-and-effect relationship is not established, these findings emphasize the importance of using human tissue for examining potential mechanisms relating drug metabolism and toxicity.

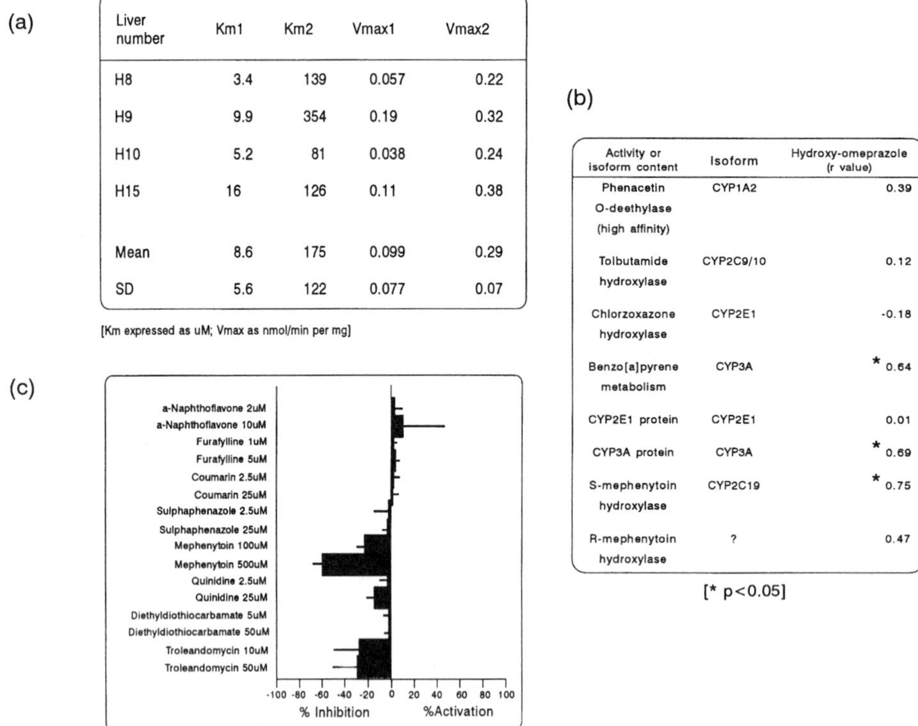
(a)

Liver number	Km1	Km2	Vmax1	Vmax2
H8	3.4	139	0.057	0.22
H9	9.9	354	0.19	0.32
H10	5.2	81	0.038	0.24
H15	16	126	0.11	0.38
Mean	8.6	175	0.099	0.29
SD	5.6	122	0.077	0.07

[Km expressed as uM; Vmax as nmol/min per mg]

(b)

Activity or isoform content	Isoform	Hydroxy-omeprazole (r value)
Phenacetin O-deethylase (high affinity)	CYP1A2	0.39
Tolbutamide hydroxylase	CYP2C9/10	0.12
Chlorzoxazone hydroxylase	CYP2E1	-0.18
Benzo[a]pyrene metabolism	CYP3A	* 0.64
CYP2E1 protein	CYP2E1	0.01
CYP3A protein	CYP3A	* 0.69
S-mephenytoin hydroxylase	CYP2C19	* 0.75
R-mephenytoin hydroxylase	?	0.47

[* p<0.05]

(c)

Figure 4 Identification of human liver cytochrome P-450 isoforms mediating the hydroxylation of omeprazole. (a) Michaelis-Menten parameters for a two-site model of metabolite formation in liver microsomes; (b) Spearman rank correlations (r) between the formation velocity of hydroxyomeprazole in liver microsomes and specific CYP activities and isoform contents; and (c) effects of various selective CYP inhibitors and/or substrates on the formation of hydroxyomeprazole in liver microsomes. [α-naphthoflavone (CYP1A2 inhibitor — low concentration; CYP3A activator — high concentration); furafylline (CYP1A2); coumarin (CYP2A6); sulfaphenazole (CYP2C9/10); quinidine (CYP2D6); and diethyldithiocarbamate (CYP2E1); troleandomycin (CYP3A)]. (Adapted from Andersson, T. et al., *Br. J. Clin. Pharmacol.*, 36, 521, 1993. With permission).

4.4 Prediction of Drug Interactions

In drug development the selection of *in vivo* drug interaction studies is usually based upon two main criteria — the likelihood of co-prescription and therapeutic index. Traditionally, studies are done using antipyrine as a model inhibitee and cimetidine as a ubiquitous cimetidine, while the list of low therapeutic index compounds that are of concern includes warfarin, oral contraceptives, phenytoin, theophylline, and cyclosporin. The problem with this approach is "how long is a ball of string?", where does the list end? Alternatively, rather than carrying out extensive "box-ticking" volunteer studies with "classical" compounds such as antipyrine (where understanding of isoenzyme selectivity is incomplete), prior *in vitro* studies should direct phase I studies to the interactions that might be relevant, and give confidence to assess the less likely ones by population kinetic screens in patients.[35]

It should also be pointed out that *in vitro* studies may also identify desirable drug interactions. For example, the demonstration of selective inhibition by cimetidine of the N-hydroxylation of dapsone in human liver microsomes suggested that its co-administration *in vivo* might increase the therapeutic ratio of dapsone by suppressing methemoglobin formation.[36,37]

4.4.1 Substrate and/or Inhibitor or Inducer?

Clearly, once the major human enzyme isoforms involved in the metabolism of drug X have been identified, this will flag likely effects of other drugs on drug X and vice versa. However, in addition to establishing any inhibitory/inductive effect of probe compounds on drug X as described already, it is also necessary to assess the opposite effect experimentally. This is particularly important in view of the fact that inhibitors/inducers of specific enzymes are not necessarily substrates for those enzymes. For example, quinidine inhibits CYP2D6 but is apparently not metabolized by it, while being a substrate and a less potent inhibitor of CYP3A4. Many beta-blockers inhibit CYP2D6 in relation to their lipid-solubility, but not all are substrates of the enzyme.[38,39] Mexiletine is a substrate for CYP2D6, yet inhibits the metabolism of theophylline, a substrate of CYP1A2.[40] As discussed previously, omeprazole is metabolized primarily by CYP's 2C19 and 3A4, yet it is a weak inducer of CYP's 1A1 and 1A2.[41,42]

A unique characteristic of the CYP3A subfamily of enzymes is their ability to be activated or autoactivated by certain compounds (e.g., 7,8-benzoflavone, α-naphthoflavone), independent of a classical induction mechanism. This suggests that the catalytic site can accommodate activator and substrate molecules simultaneously, a possibility that should also be considered as a mechanism for drug interactions.[43]

4.4.2 Screening for Interaction Potential

A particularly comprehensive *in vitro* study screening drugs for interaction with a single substrate was reported by Pichard et al.,[44] who used human liver microsomes and hepatocytes to allocate 59 drugs representative of 17 different therapeutic classes as inhibitors or inducers of or non-interactors with the CYP3A4-mediated metabolism of cyclosporin.

Fuhr et al.[45] provide an excellent illustration of how *in vitro* drug interaction data can be assimilated into drug design. Thus, they defined relationships between the structures of quinolone antibacterials, their effects on bacterial growth, and their ability to inhibit CYP1A2-mediated caffeine 3-demethylation. An optimal structure which maximized antibacterial effect while minimizing the potential for drug interactions involving inhibition of CYP1A2 was suggested.

Studies of the potential effects of drugs on the glucuronidation of zidovudine by human liver microsomes exemplify the extension of *in vitro* screening to phase II pathways.[46,47]

4.4.3 In Vitro-In Vivo Extrapolation

A number of factors must be considered when extrapolating the results of *in vitro* studies of drug interactions to expectations *in vivo*.

Equation 1 indicates that, assuming competitive inhibition, the decrease in clearance of an inhibitee, and hence its steady-state plasma concentration (C_{ss}), will depend critically on the fraction of the dose normally metabolized by the pathway that is inhibited (fm), and the ratio of the concentration of the inhibitor at the enzyme site (I) to the inhibition constant (K_i).[48]

$$\frac{C_{ss}(\text{inhibited})}{C_{ss}(\text{normal})} = \frac{1}{\left[\text{fm}/\left(1+(\text{I})/\text{K}_i\right)+(1-\text{fm})\right]} \tag{1}$$

This equation emphasizes the insensitivity of net drug clearance to inhibition when fm is less than 0.5. Therefore, any interpretation of *in vitro* data must take into account the contribution of the metabolic pathway to net drug clearance, although even a low value of fm will clearly be of significance if the metabolite itself has potent pharmacological activity or toxicity.

It could be argued that, ideally, the (I)/K_i ratio should be expressed in terms of free inhibitor and inhibitee concentrations at the enzyme site. Although free plasma concentration of inhibitor at steady-state (Cu_{ss}) is likely to approximate to that at the enzyme site *in vivo*, there are difficulties in equating total concentrations of substrate and inhibitor added to an *in vitro* incubate with those at the enzyme site because of partitioning into the lipid environment of the enzyme and nonspecific binding.[49] Thus, the K_i value obtained *in vitro* will reflect the partition characteristics of both inhibitor and inhibitee. Further complications arise if it is considered that concentrations "seen" by the enzyme are not those in the aqueous phase. The enzyme binding site may be aqueous- or lipid-facing or, more likely, a mixture of both.[49]

The mechanism of inhibition by many compounds is not competitive, but is mediated by a metabolite, an intermediate complex, or involves covalent binding. For this reason, when using some probe inhibitors *in vitro*, such as furafylline[50-52] and cimetidine,[53] it is necessary to pre-incubate them to allow adequate formation of the inhibiting species.

Thus, scaling of *in vitro* to *in vivo* (I)/K_i ratios is not straightforward. Nevertheless, a knowledge of *in vitro* inhibitor concentrations relative to Cu_{ss} values can be of prognostic value provided that the difficulties are appreciated. A final point to consider is that enzymes will be subjected to much higher drug concentrations during "first-pass" through the liver after oral drug administration than steady-state

Cu_{ss} values. These high concentrations should also be taken into account when extrapolating from *in vitro* data. A reasonable estimate of drug concentration going to the liver via the portal vein may be obtained from the product of the fraction of the dose crossing the gut wall as intact drug and the absorption rate constant divided by assumed hepatic portal blood flow.

4.4.4 Case Studies

Two examples will now be discussed where information from *in vitro* screens might have prevented some dangerous drug interactions following the introduction of new drugs into clinical practice.

4.4.4.1 SSRIs and Tricyclic Antidepressants

The standard "package" of metabolism and pharmacokinetic studies carried out during the development of paroxetine (a selective serotonin reuptake inhibitor, SSRI), indicated that its kinetics were complex, that it is not a general inducer or inhibitor of hepatic drug oxidation, and that it has little or no effect on the pharmacokinetics of other drugs examined.[54] Unfortunately, the latter compounds were classical nonspecific *in vivo* probes such as antipyrine and warfarin. Subsequently, just prior to registration, it was shown both *in vitro* and *in vivo* that paroxetine is oxidized by CYP2D6 and that it is also a potent inhibitor of this enzyme.[55-58] Thus, an appropriate proactive warning about interactions with other substrates of CYP2D6 was formulated for the U.K. Data Sheet. In contrast, fluoxetine which, along with its major active nor-metabolite, also inhibits CYP2D6,[55,59] was introduced into clinical practice without the benefit of this knowledge. If this information had been available earlier perhaps a number of cases of severe cardiotoxicity resulting from co-administration of fluoxetine with tricyclic antidepressants might have been avoided.[60] Many tricyclic antidepressants are metabolized to a significant extent by CYP2D6, explaining why the addition of fluoxetine to therapy increased their plasma concentrations by up to 300%, with subsequent toxicity.

4.4.4.2 Terfenadine-Ketoconazole

In 1989 astute clinical observation linked the occurrence of a rare, life-threatening ventricular arrhythmia (torsades de pointe) in an otherwise healthy woman with an interaction between her antihistamine (terfenadine) and antifungal (ketoconazole) medication.[61] Additional cases were identified through the FDA's spontaneous reporting system, leading to the circulation of "Dear Doctor" letters in August 1990 in the U.S. and in July 1992 in the U.K.

There would be little reason to suspect an interaction between terfenadine and ketoconazole on the basis of their respective pharmacological actions. However, in retrospect, it is clear that an important interaction should have been predictable from a knowledge of drug metabolism and an appropriate appreciation of the cardiovascular effects of terfenadine. Terfenadine is a pro-drug which undergoes extensive biotransformation on first-pass through the liver. Thus, plasma concentrations of parent drug are virtually undetectable under normal conditions, and the combination of antihistaminic activity and minimal sedation is due to a zwitterionic C-oxidation product which does not pass the blood-brain barrier. Using human liver microsomes it has been shown that both C-oxidation and N-dealkylation of terfenadine are mediated by CYP3A4.[62] *In vitro* studies have also shown that, at concentrations below about 10 μM, ketoconazole is a potent and selective inhibitor of this enzyme.[63] Therefore, when ketoconazole is co-administered with terfenadine its systemic availability becomes appreciable, resulting in arrhythmia mediated by the parent compound.[64]

Unlike ketoconazole, fluconazole is a much less potent inhibitor of CYP3A4. Inhibition constants with respect to the oxidation of cyclosporine by human liver microsomes are 0.3 and 63 μM, respectively.[63] Therefore, it comes as no surprise to learn that during co-administration of terfenadine with the recommended daily 200 mg dose of fluconazole, plasma concentrations of unchanged terfenadine remain undetectable and there are no significant changes in cardiac repolarization.[65]

5 CONCLUSIONS

A case can be made for early *in vitro* studies of drug metabolism using human liver tissue and enzymes during the course of drug development. Although interpretation of such data is not without its problems, this information does promise to minimize the box-ticking approach to selection of some studies in healthy volunteers. While identifying the enzymes involved in the metabolism of drug X may itself become a "box" to tick, it is a relatively cheap box compared to those involving volunteer or patient studies. By helping to focus on relevant *in vivo* investigations, *in vitro* screens could have significant economic and ethical advantages for drug development.

REFERENCES

1. Nelson, D. R., Kamataki, T., Waxman, D. J., Guengerich, F. P., Estabrook, R. W., Feyereisen, R., Gonzalez, F. J., Coon, M. J., Gunsalus, I. C., Gotoh, O., Okuda, K. and Nebert, D. W., The P-450 superfamily: Update on new sequences, gene mapping, accession numbers, early trivial names of enzymes, and nomenclature, *DNA Cell Biol.*, 12, 1, 1993.
2. Shimada, T., Yamazaki, H., Mimura, M., Inui, K. and Guengerich, F. P., Interindividual variations in human liver cytochrome P-450 enzymes involved in the oxidation of drugs, carcinogens and toxic chemicals: Studies with liver microsomes of 30 Japanese and 30 Caucasians, *J. Pharmacol. Exp. Ther.*, 270, 414, 1994.
3. Kitada, M., Kamataki, K., Itahashi, K., Rikihisa, T., Kato, R. and Kanakubo, Y., Purification and properties of cytochrome P-450 from homogenates of human fetal livers, *Arch. Biochem. Biophys.*, 241, 275, 1985.
4. Birkett, D. J., Mackenzie, P. I., Verones, M. E. and Miners, J. O., *In vitro* approaches can predict human drug metabolism, *Trends Pharmacol. Sci.*, 14, 292, 1993.
5. Wrighton, S. A., Vandenbranden, M., Stevens, J. C., Shipley, L. A. and Ring, B. J., *In vitro* methods for assessing human hepatic drug metabolism: Their use in drug development, *Drug Metab. Rev.*, 25, 453, 1993.
6. Smith, D. A. and Jones, B. C., Speculations on the substrate structure-activity relationship (SSAR) of cytochrome P-450 enzymes, *Biochem. Pharmacol.*, 44, 2089, 1992.
7. Lawton, M. P. and Philpot, R. M., Molecular genetics of the flavin-dependent monooxygenases, *Pharmacogenetics*, 3, 40, 1993.
8. Tephly, T. R. and Burchell, B., UDP-glucuronosyltransferases: a family of detoxifying enzymes, *Trends Pharmacol. Sci.*, 11, 276, 1990.
9. Miners, J. O. and Mackenzie, P. I., Drug glucuronidation in humans, *Pharmacol. Ther.*, 51, 347, 1991.
10. Boutin, J. A., Antoine, B. and Siest, G., Heterogeneity of hepatic microsomal UDP-glucuronosyltransferase(s) activities: A new kinetic approach for the study of induction and specificity, *J. Pharm. Sci.*, 83, 591, 1994.
11. Kroetz, D. L., Loiseau, P., Guyot, M. and Levy, R. H., *In vivo* and *in vitro* correlation of microsomal epoxide hydrolase inhibition of progabide, *Clin. Pharmacol. Ther.*, 54, 485, 1993.
12. Kaminsky, L. S., Dannan, G. A. and Guengerich, F. P., Composition of cytochrome P-450 isozymes from hepatic microsomes of C57BL/6 and DBA/2 mice assessed by warfarin metabolism, immunoinhibition, and immunoelectrophoresis (with anti-rat cytochrome P-450), *Eur. J. Biochem.*, 141, 141, 1984.
13. Shimada, T. and Guengerich, F. P., Participation of a rat liver cytochrome P-450 induced by pregnenolone 16 alpha-carbonitrile and other compounds in the 4-hydroxylation of mephenytoin, *Mol. Pharmacol.*, 28, 215, 1985.
14. Shimada, T., Misono, K. S. and Guengerich, F. P., Human liver microsomal cytochrome P-450 mephenytoin 4-hydroxylase, a prototype of genetic polymorphism in oxidative drug metabolism: purification and characterization of two similar forms involved in the reaction, *J. Biol. Chem.*, 261, 909, 1986.
15. Bardsley, J. S., Establishment of human tissue banks, *Hum. Exp. Toxicol.*, 13, 435, 1994.
16. Fenton, J. H., The use of human tissues in *in vitro* toxicology, Stirling, 28/29 April 1993. Summary of general discussions, *Hum. Exp. Toxicol.*, 13, 446, 1994.
17. Otton, S. V., Crewe, H. K., Lennard, M. S., Tucker, G. T. and Woods, H. F., Use of quinidine inhibition to define the role of sparteine/debrisoquine cytcochrome P-450 in metoprolol oxidation by human liver microsomes, *J. Pharmacol. Exp. Ther.*, 247, 242, 1988.
18. Koebe, H.-G., Pahernik, S., Eyer, P. and Schildberg, F.-W., Collagen gel immobilization: a useful cell culture technique for long-term metabolic studies on human hepatocytes, *Xenobiotica*, 24, 95, 1994.
19. Barr, J., Weir, A. J., Brendel, K. and Sipes, I. G., Liver slices in dynamic organ culture. II. An *in vitro* cellular technique for the study of integrated drug metabolism using human tissue, *Xenobiotica*, 21, 341, 1991.
20. Numerous authors, Special Issue: Application of cellular systems in drug metabolism and toxicity studies, *Toxicology*, 82, Nos. 1-3, 1-262, 1993.
21. Koymans, L., den Kelder, G. M. D. O., te Koppele, J. M. and Vermeulen, N. P. E., Cytochromes P-450: Their active-site structure and mechanism of oxidation, *Drug Metab. Rev.*, 25, 325, 1993.
22. Rane, A., Wilkinson, G.R. and Shand, D. G., Prediction of hepatic extraction ratio from *in vitro* measurement of intrinsic clearance, *J. Pharmacol. Exp. Ther.*, 200, 420, 1977.
23. Houston, J. B., Utility of *in vitro* drug metabolism data in predicting *in vivo* metabolic clearance, *Biochem. Pharmacol.*, 47, 1469, 1994.
24. Andersson, T., Miners, J. O., Veronese, M. E., Tassaneeyakul, T. W., Meyer, U. A. and Birkett, D. J., Identification of human liver cytochrome P-450 isoforms mediating omeprazole metabolism, *Br. J. Clin. Pharmacol.*, 36, 521, 1993.
25. Kolars, J. C., Awni, W. M., Merion, R. M. and Watkins, P. B., First-pass metabolism of cyclosporin by the gut, *Lancet*, 338, 1488, 1991.
26. Andersson, T., Regardh, C.-G., Dahl-Puustinen, M. L. and Bertilsson, L., Slow omeprazole metabolizers are also poor S-mephenytoin hydroxylators, *Ther. Drug Monit.*, 12, 415, 1990.
27. Andersson, T., Cederberg, C., Edvarsson, G., Heggelund, A. and Lundborg, P., Effect of omeprazole treatment on diazepam plasma levels in slow versus normal rapid metabolizers of omeprazole, *Clin. Pharmacol. Ther.*, 47, 79, 1990.
28. Andersson, T., Miners, J. O., Veronese, M. E. and Birkett, D. J., Identification of human liver cytochrome P-450 isoforms mediating secondary omeprazole metabolism, *Br. J. Clin. Pharmacol.*, 37, 597, 1994.

29. Zanger, W. M., Hauri, H. P., Loeper, J., Homberg, J. C. and Meyer, U. A., Antibodies against human cytochrome P-450db1 in autoimmune hepatitis type II, *Proc. Natl. Acad. Sci. U.S.A.*, 27, 8256, 1988.
30. Ellis, S. W., Ching, M. S., Watson, P., Lennard, M. S., Tucker, G. T. and Woods, H. F., Catalytic activity of human debrisoquine 4-hydroxylase (CYP2D6) heterologously expressed in *Saccharomyces cerevisiae*, *Biochem. Pharmacol.*, 44, 617, 1992.
31. Koymans, L., Vermeulen, N. P. E., van Acker, S. A. B. E., te Koppele, J. M., Heykants, J. J. P., Lavrijsen, K., Meuldermans, W. and den Kelder, G. M. D. O., A predictive model of substrates of cytochrome P-450-debrisoquine (2D6), *Chem. Res. Toxicol.*, 5, 211, 1992.
32. Farlow, M., Gracon, S. I., Hershey, L. A., Lewis, K. W., Sadowsky, C. H. and Dolan-Ureno, J., A controlled trial of tacrine in Alzheimer's disease, *J. Am. Med. Assoc.*, 268, 2523, 1992.
33. Woolf, T. F., Pool, W. F., Bjorge, S. M., Chang, T., Goel, O. P., Purchase, C. F., Schroeder, M. C., Kunze, K. L. and Trager, W. F., Bioactivation and irreversible binding of the cognition activator tacrine using human and rat liver microsomal preparations, *Drug Metab. Dispos.*, 21, 874, 1993.
34. Spaldin, V., Madden, S., Pool, W. F., Woolf, T. F. and Park, B. K., The effect of enzyme inhibition on the metabolism and activation of tacrine by human liver microsomes, *Br. J. Clin. Pharmacol.*, 38, 15, 1994.
35. Tucker, G. T., The rational selection of drug interaction studies: Implications of recent advances in drug metabolism, *Internat. J. Clin. Pharmacol. Ther., Toxicol.*, 30, 550, 1992.
36. Tingle, M. D., Coleman, M. D. and Park, B. K., The effect of pre-incubation with cimetidine on the N-hydroxylation of dapsone by human liver microsomes, *Br. J. Clin. Pharmacol.*, 32, 120, 1991.
37. Coleman, M. D., Scott, A. K., Breckenridge, A. M. and Park, B. K., The use of cimetidine as a selective inhibitor of dapsone N-hydroxylation in man, *Br. J. Clin. Pharmacol.*, 30, 761, 1990.
38. Al-Asady, S. A. H., Black, G. L., Lennard, M. S., Tucker, G. T. and Woods, H. F., Inhibition of lignocaine metabolism by beta-adrenoceptor antagonists in rat and human liver microsomes, *Xenobiotica*, 19, 929, 1989.
39. Ferrari, S., Lemman, T. and Dayer, P., The role of lipophilicity in the inhibition of polymorphic cytochrome P-450IID6 oxidation by beta-blocking agents *in vitro*, *Life Sci.*, 48, 2259, 1991.
40. Hurwitz, A., Vacek, J. L., Botteron, G. W., Sztern, M. I., Hughes, E. M. and Jayaraj, A., Mexiletine effects on theophylline disposition, *Clin. Pharmacol. Ther.*, 50, 299, 1991.
41. Diaz, D., Fabre, I., Daujat, M., Saint Aubert, B., Bories, P., Michel, H. and Maurel, P., Omeprazole is an aryl hydrocarbon-like inducer of human hepatic cytochrome P-450, *Gastroenterology*, 99, 737, 1990.
42. McDonnell, W. M., Scheiman, J. M. and Traber, P. G., Induction of cytochrome P-4501A genes (CYP1A) by omeprazole in the human alimentary tract, *Gastroenterology*, 103, 1509, 1992.
43. Shou, M., Grogan, J., Mancewicz, J. A., Krausz, K. W., Gonzalez, F. J., Gelboin, H. V. and Korzekwa, K. R., Activation of CYP3A4: Evidence for the simultaneous binding of two substrates in a cytochrome P-450 active site, *Biochemistry*, 33, 6450, 1994.
44. Pichard, L., Fabre, I., Fabre, G., Domerque, J., Aubers, B. S., Morad, G. and Maurel, P., Cyclosporin A drug interactions. Screening for inducers and inhibitors of cytochrome P-450 (cyclosporin A oxidase) in primary cultures of human hepatocytes and in liver microsomes, *Drug Metab. Dispos.*, 18, 595, 1990.
45. Fuhr, U., Strobl, G., Manaut, F., Anders, E.-M., Sorgel, F., Lopez-de-Brinas, E., Chu, D. T. W., Pernet, A. G., Mahr, G., Sanz, F. and Staib, A. H., Quinolone antibacterial agents: Relationship between structure and *in vitro* inhibition of the human cytochrome P-450 isoform CYP1A2, *Mol. Pharmacol.*, 43, 191, 1993.
46. Sim, S. M., Back, D. J. and Breckenridge, A. M., The effect of various drugs on the glucuronidation of zidovudine (azidothymidine; AZT) by human liver microsomes, *Br. J. Clin. Pharmacol.*, 32, 17, 1991.
47. Rajaonarison, J. F., Lacarelle, B., Catalin, J., Durand, A. and Cano, J.-P., Effect of anticancer drugs on the glucuronidation of 3′-azido-3′-deoxythymidine in human liver microsomes, *Drug Metab. Dispos.*, 21, 823, 1993.
48. Rowland, M. and Matin, S. B., Kinetics of drug-drug interactions, *J. Pharmacokin. Biopharm.*, 1, 553, 1973.
49. Parry, G., Palmer, D. N. and Williams, D. J., Ligand partitioning into membranes: Its significance in determining Km and Ks values for cytochrome P-450 and other membrane bound receptors and enzymes, *FEBS Lett.*, 67, 123, 1976.
50. Sesardic, S., Boobis, A. R., Murray, B. P., Murray, S., Segura, J., De La Torre, R. and Davies, D. S., Furafylline is a potent and selective inhibitor of cytochrome P-450 1A2 in man, *Br. J. Clin. Pharmacol.*, 29, 651, 1990.
51. Kunze, K. L. and Trager, W. F., Isoform-selective mechanism-based inhibition of human cytochrome P-450 1A2 by furafylline, *Chem. Res. Toxicol.*, 6, 649, 1993.
52. Clarke, S. E., Ayrton, A. D. and Chenery, R. J., Characterization of the inhibition of P-450 1A2 by furafylline, *Xenobiotica*, 24, 517, 1994.
53. Jensen, J. C. and Gugler, R., Cimetidine interaction with liver microsomes *in vitro* and *in vivo*. Involvement of an activated complex with cytochrome P-450, *Biochem. Pharmacol.*, 34, 2141, 1985.
54. Kaye, C. M., Haddock, R. E., Langley, P. F., Mellows, G., Tasker, T. C. G., Zussman, B. D. and Greb, W. H., A review of the metabolism and pharmacokinetics of paroxetine in man, *Acta Psychiatr. Scand.*, 80 (Suppl. 350), 60, 1989.
55. Crewe, H. K., Lennard, M. S., Tucker, G. T., Woods, F. R. and Haddock, R. E., The effect of selective serotonin reuptake inhibitors on cytochrome P-4502D6 (CYP2D6) activity in human liver microsomes, *Br. J. Clin. Pharmacol.*, 34, 262, 1992.

56. Skjelbo, E. and Brosen, K., Inhibitors of imipramine metabolism by human liver microsomes, *Br. J. Clin. Pharmacol.*, 34, 256, 1992.
57. Bloomer, J. C., Woods, F. R., Haddock, R. E., Lennard, M. S. and Tucker, G. T., The role of cytochrome P-450 2D6 in the metabolism of paroxetine by human liver microsomes, *Br. J. Clin. Pharmacol.*, 33, 521, 1992.
58. Sindrup, S. H., Brosen, K. and Gram, L. F., Pharmacokinetics of the selective serotonin reuptake inhibitor paroxetine: Nonlinearity and relation to the sparteine oxidation polymorphism, *Clin. Pharmacol. Ther.*, 51, 288, 1992.
59. Otton, S. V., Wu, D., Joffe, R. T., Cheung, S. W. and Sellers, E. M., Inhibition by fluoxetine of cytochrome P-450 2D6 activity, *Clin. Pharmacol. Ther.*, 53, 401, 1993.
60. Westermeyer, J., Fluoxetine-induced tricyclic toxicity: Extent and duration, *J. Clin. Pharmacol.*, 31, 388, 1991.
61. Peck, C. C., Temple, R. and Collins, J. M., Understanding consequences of concurrent therapies, *J. Am. Med. Assoc.*, 269, 1550, 1993.
62. Yun, C.-H., Okerholm, R. A. and Guengerich, F. P., Oxidation of the antihistaminic drug terfenadine in human liver microsomes. Role of cytochrome P-450 3A(4) in N-dealkylation and C-hydroxylation, *Drug Metab. Dispos.*, 21, 403, 1993.
63. Maurice, M., Pichard, L., Duajat, M., Babre, I., Joyeux, H., Domergue, J. and Maurel, P., Effects of imidazole derivatives on cytochromes P-450 from human hepatocytes in primary culture, *FASEB J.*, 6, 752, 1992.
64. Honig, P. K., Wirtham, D. C., Zamani, K., Conner, D. P., Mullin, J. C. and Cantilena, L. R., Terfenadine-ketoconazole interaction. Pharmacokinetic and electrocardiographic consequences, *J. Am. Med. Assoc.*, 269, 1513, 1993.
65. Honig, P. K., Wortham, D. C., Zamani, K., Mullin, J. C., Conner, D. P. and Cantilena, L. R., The effect of fluconazole on the steady-state pharmacokinetics and electrocardiographic pharmacodynamics of terfenadine in humans, *Clin. Pharmacol. Ther.*, 53, 630, 1993.

Part II. Organization and Decision Making

Chapter 6

Decision Points in Human Drug Development

Stots B. Reele

CONTENTS

1 Introduction 67
2 Entry-Into-Man 68
3 Tolerability Studies 69
3.1 Should the First Study Be Performed in Healthy Volunteers or Patients and in the Young or Elderly? 69
3.2 What Is the Initial Dose that Should Be Administered in the Entry-Into-Man Protocol? 70
3.3 How Should the Subsequent Doses Be Escalated? 70
3.4 What Safety Parameters Should Be Followed? 71
3.5 Which Parameters Can Be Measured to Ascertain if the Drug Is Likely to Have the Expected Effect in Humans? 72
3.6 What Is the Dose/Response and Time-Course of the Pharmacodynamic Effects of the New Drug? 72
3.7 What Should Be the Top Dose that Will Be Administered to Subjects? 74
3.8 From the Single-Dose Tolerability Studies, What Information Will Be Required to Start the Multiple-Dose Tolerability Study? 74
3.9 In a Multiple-Dose Tolerability Study, What Should Be the Duration of Drug Administration? 74
3.10 What Duration of Followup Will Be Required to Ensure the Safety of the Subjects after the Last Dose Has Been Administered? 75
3.11 Should the Drug Be Administered in the Fed or Fasted State? 75
4 First Efficacy Studies 75
4.1 How Does One Determine Clinical Efficacy in a Manageable Period of Time? 75
4.2 Do the Pharmacologic Properties of the Drug Translate into Clinical Benefit? 76
4.3 What Is the Dose/Plasma Concentration/Effect Relationship? 76
5 Clinical Pharmacology Studies beyond the First Single- and Multiple-Dose Studies 77
5.1 Drug Interactions 77
5.2 The Need to Modify the Dose in Special Patient Populations 78
5.3 Effect of Food, Antacids, Sucralfate, etc. 78
6 What Information Is Required to Discontinue Drug Development? 78
References 79

1 INTRODUCTION

The drug development process could be characterized as the creation of an ever-changing *informational database*. Ideally, this database would answer all questions posed by the patient and the medical practitioner, allowing the rational use of a new medication. Questions like, "Is the drug effective and safe?" "What is the best route to administer the drug (i.e., orally, transdermally)?" and "What is the dose and frequency of administration?" invite other questions. "Is the drug effective for all patients or only a special subset of patients?" "How does the efficacy of this drug compare to other drugs or treatment modalities?" "What are the most common adverse events associated with the use of this drug?" or "What are the most serious adverse events?" "Is there a subpopulation of patients (for instance, elderly subjects or patients with renal failure) at increased risk for adverse events?" "What is the lowest or initial dose that should be prescribed?" "What is the highest tolerated dose?" "Which patients need a modified dose?" "Can the drug be given with food or other drugs?" Phases I and II in drug development generate the essential framework for answering many of these questions.

0-8493-9230-6/97/$0.00+$.50
© 1997 by CRC Press, Inc.

Though this informational database is theoretically built during the complete drug development process, the decision points during phases I and II are critical — not only to the process of drug development itself but also to the effective use of the drug in human trials and post-market evaluation. We know that, beginning with the initial preclinical pharmacologic data, the process of drug development is not complete until regulatory approval has been granted by governmental authorities (who have acted as surrogates on behalf of both the patient and practitioner) and actual marketplace performance has been demonstrated. Even then, there is a need for continued vigilance in answering the essential questions of safety and appropriate usage after the drug has been introduced into the general medical *armamentarium.* This fact is illustrated by the revisions of dosing recommendations for approximately 15% of all new chemical entities marketed and in general use in the 1980s.[1]

The above list of questions is not exhaustive; there is no list that can be all-inclusive for all drugs. Based on an individualized, acceptable risk/benefit ratio for the patient population being treated, the natural course of the disease, and the availability of alternative therapies, the list of important questions requires constant modification. This chapter will introduce the questions typically encountered during phase I and II drug development and will explore the information required to develop the answers.

2 ENTRY-INTO-MAN

One of the most exciting times in the drug development process is the initial introduction of a new chemical entity into man. Here, the clinician must turn to his colleagues in preclinical pharmacology and toxicology to obtain the necessary information to formulate the entry-into-man studies. The clinician would like to know the answer to questions like (see Figure 1):

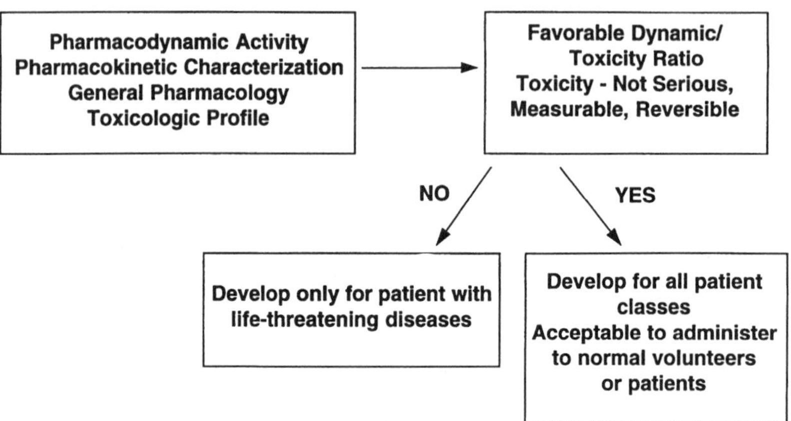

Figure 1 Entry-into-man.

1. What are the pharmacodynamic properties of the compound?
2. What methodologies are available to measure the pharmacodynamic effects in man? Can these effects be measured in healthy volunteers or can they only be measured in patients?
3. What is the target organ for toxicologic effects? How can patients or volunteers be monitored to detect these effects as early as possible?
4. What was the non-effect and first toxic dose (or alternatively the exposure) in the toxicologic studies?
5. Based on this information, what would be the predicted concentration/dose producing toxicologic effects in man?

Today, the major goal of rational drug development is to demonstrate the beneficial effects of a chemical entity in humans predicted by the pharmacologic properties identified in preclinical research. (This approach differs from the older development paradigm in which drugs were chosen for development by massive screening of potentially active compounds using animal disease models.) Now, the preclinical scientist seeks to formulate and test compounds with specific pharmacologic activity; ideally, the compounds are chosen to have a predictable and specific pharmacologic mechanism. As part of the preclinical development process, multiple organ systems are monitored to determine the compound's effects on the normal animal physiology. The same physiologic effects are anticipated to occur in man and a primary objective of the initial clinical studies is to demonstrate the pharmacologic properties of a new compound on the targeted organ systems of volunteers (either healthy subjects or patients).

It is also important to study and understand the toxicologic profile of a new compound to establish the risk/benefit relationship — serious adverse effects that might be unacceptable in the context of trivial disease might be totally acceptable in patients with serious (e.g., fatal, nontreatable) diseases. Thus, the toxicologic findings must be considered in light of an acceptable therapeutic index in the proposed patient population.

The first dose in humans is usually a fraction of the dose that caused no effects in toxicologic studies. (This precaution allows for a margin of safety if man is found to be more sensitive than the species used for preclinical evaluation.) A further discussion of how the first dose is selected to be administered to man appears below.

3 TOLERABILITY STUDIES

The objectives of the first studies are to characterize the pharmacodynamic and pharmacokinetic profiles and (potentially) dose-limiting adverse events of a new compound. Unfortunately, the number of subjects in the initial studies is too small to allow for the full adverse event profile to be ascertained. There are many important questions to be asked and they are discussed in the following subsections.

3.1 Should the First Study Be Performed in Healthy Volunteers or Patients and in the Young or Elderly?

Before this question can be answered (Figure 2), the benefits and risks of administering a drug to a healthy volunteer compared to a patient must be considered. The decision should be based on the preclinical toxicology rather than on the envisioned targeted patient population. All drugs should be considered as potentially toxic provided the dose is high enough. Toxic effects on major organ systems do not necessarily preclude the introduction of studies in healthy volunteers.

The potential reversibility of the preclinical toxicologic observations should contribute to the decision on whether to use healthy or patient volunteers, as should the possibility to detect effects before they become severe. As healthy volunteers would not receive a clinical benefit they should not be exposed to adverse events that could cause permanent damage. On the other hand, many oncologic or anti-AIDS compounds were routinely introduced only into patients even though the toxic effects were reversible and predictable, and this need not be the case. If the above conditions of safety are met, there is no reason not to use healthy volunteers in the first study.

With recent advances in biotechnology, new chemical entities based on naturally occurring proteins are being introduced into clinical trials. These compounds create unprecedented and unique issues in determining whether the first study should be administered to healthy volunteers. The most salient problem with administering proteins is that most proteins, when administered to man, may potentially induce antibody formation. There is then a possibility that the antibody will crossreact with the naturally occurring protein, conceivably neutralizing the physiologic effects of that naturally occurring protein. Among other factors, the potential consequences of antibody formation must be considered in determining whether initial studies should be performed in healthy volunteers or patients.

Performing the tolerability studies in healthy volunteers offers several advantages. First, studying healthy subjects usually allows rapid enrollment and completion of the studies. Furthermore, they may have a greater physiologic reserve then the intended patients. If an adverse event were to occur, the healthy volunteer would be more likely to recover without suffering long-term negative consequences. Also, frequent measurements and a greater volume of blood (to measure the drug's pharmacokinetic and pharmacodynamic parameters) may be more acceptable in a healthy volunteer than from a patient. A complete and unencumbered picture of the compound could be obtained because the observations are not confounded by the effects of any underlying diseases or concomitant treatment.

On the other hand, pharmacodynamic effects of the drug may be measurable only in patients. This is exemplified by antihypertensive medications such as nifedipine having little or no effect on blood pressure in normotensive subjects.[2] In addition, the tolerability of a drug may differ between healthy volunteers and patients, favoring the enrollment of patients in the initial studies. For example, many antipsychotic medications are tolerated by patients at significantly higher doses than by healthy volunteers (see Part VII, Assessment of Drug Effects on the CNS).

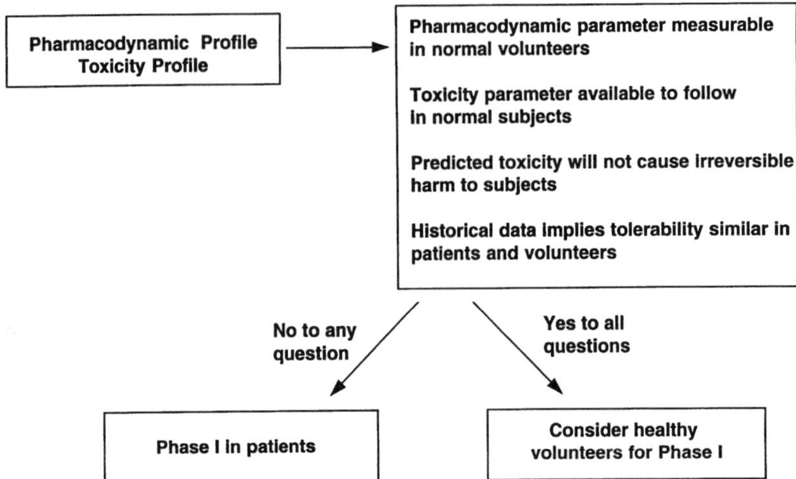

Figure 2 Phase I design issues.

Traditionally, the first studies have been performed in young, rather than elderly subjects. The rationale underlying this paradigm is that elderly subjects have a higher incidence of occult diseases that would put them at an increased risk if adverse events were to transpire. There may also be the physiological decrement of many organ systems (such as a decline in renal and pulmonary functions) that could influence their ability to eliminate the drug.

In general, the tolerability of a compound should be similar in young and elderly provided that the exposure is comparable in both groups. Consequently, dosing may need to be modified in the elderly so that equivalent exposures are observed. For some compounds, however, the tolerability is different in elderly subjects compared to younger subjects. A notable example of this is the increased central nervous system sensitivity of the elderly compared to young subjects.[3] For such compounds, elderly subjects should be enrolled in the initial studies.

3.2 What Is the Initial Dose that Should Be Administered in the Entry-Into-Man Protocol?

Traditionally, the first dose has been chosen as a fraction of the "clean" or "no-effect" dose observed in the toxicology studies. The typical unwritten rule was that the dose should be 1/25 to 1/100 of the no-effect dose in mg/kg. Today, though, it is recognized that drug exposure is a better indicator of cross-species toxicity than the administered dose. From the animal data, most clinical pharmacologists will try to extrapolate the human exposure using allometric scaling. A discussion of these techniques is beyond the scope of this chapter.

For oncologic drugs, the first studies are often performed in patients who have failed to respond to conventional therapy with the hope that the patients may obtain a clinical benefit from the trial. Hence, the oncologists are frequently more aggressive in choosing the first dose to administer to patients. Typically the first dose is based on the experience of administering the compound to mice. A dose 1/3 to 1/5 that which is lethal to 10% of the animals (LD_{10}) expressed as mg/m^2 has been chosen as the first dose to administer to patients.[7] The compounds are frequently also studied in a second species, and if the second species is more sensitive to the toxicologic effects of the drug, then the dose is further reduced.

3.3 How Should the Subsequent Doses Be Escalated?

Three different schemes have been generally employed in developing a dose-escalation paradigm for the first study: increasing the dose in a logarithmic manner; doubling the dose; or using the Fibonacci scheme. The first two schemes recognize that pharmacologic effects are usually related to the logarithm of the dose or concentration, so a progressively larger increase in the dose will not cause a sudden increase in the pharmacologic activity. The Fibonacci scheme or the modified scheme has been utilized by oncologists[5] (see Figure 3).

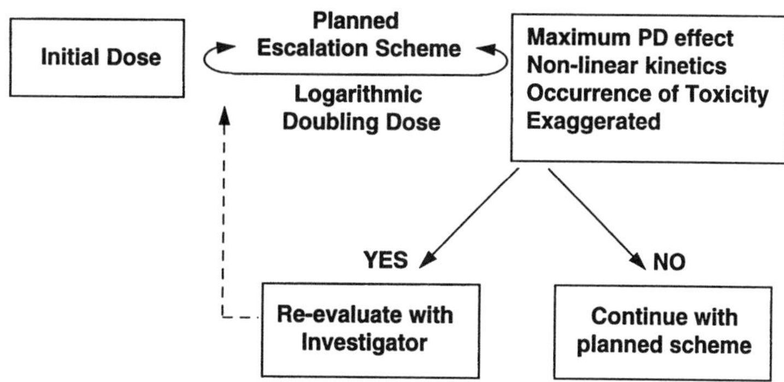

Figure 3 Dose Escalation.

The Fibonacci scheme was developed for cytotoxic drugs initially administered to cancer patients. To offer a clinical benefit to their patients, oncologists wanted to achieve a therapeutic dose as rapidly as possible. As described above, the initial dose was chosen based on the LD_{10} in mice.[6] The dose was rapidly increased in the initial dose levels, then progressively smaller steps in the escalation scheme were utilized (expressed, based on the original dose, as 2x, 3.3x, 5x, 7x, 9x, 12x, and 16x or the increases were 100, 67, 50, 40, and each subsequent step 33.3%) until dose limiting toxicity is observed. The basis of the scheme was that the pharmacologist could predict both the clinically beneficial and toxic doses. However, recent experience with oncological drugs has demonstrated that using this scheme, from 1 to over 10 dose levels has been required to reach the maximum tolerated dose (MTD).[7]

The sponsor and the investigator require frequent communication to insure that the entry-into-man dose-escalation protocol is modified if necessary as observations are made during the progression of the study. *Any evidence of pharmacologic effect requires the reevaluation of the dose-escalation scheme.* If serious toxicity has been observed to occur with little warning in the preclinical studies, then the increases should be made in small increments. Conversely, if the preclinical data indicates that the toxicity will be non-serious and reversible with a large safety margin, the dose-escalation scheme can be more aggressive.

During the initial entry-into-man dose-escalation study, the sponsor should strive for rapid turnaround of pharmacokinetic samples. Ideally, the samples from a group of subjects should be assayed before the next group is enrolled into the study. If there appears to be nonlinearity of the pharmacokinetics, then the dose escalation should be cautious.

Equally important in performing the entry-into-man studies, if it appears that with an increase in the dose there is no increase in drug exposure, the sponsor should consider termination of the study. Such an event could occur if there is lack of solubility of the compound or saturation of a drug-absorption process.

3.4 What Safety Parameters Should Be Followed?

In designing the tolerability trials, two categories of safety issues may be anticipated. The first is the result of an extension of the therapeutic effects of the drug, such as the hypotensive effects of vasodilators, or prolonged bleeding time with an antiplatelet drug. These effects are predictable and should be carefully monitored. Such effects should be related to the exposure or plasma concentration of the drug so that rational dosage schemes for clinical trials and eventual clinical use can be established.

It is possible that a drug could have an effect on a physiologic system that may not be observed in a healthy volunteer but which may become apparent in a patient with a compromised physiologic reserve. Here, the counterregulatory system of the healthy volunteer may have compensated for the pharmacologic effects of the drug; a patient with limited physiologic reserve may not be able to marshal the counter-regulatory activity. Beta adrenergic blockers, for example, are well tolerated in terms of respiratory effects by healthy subjects, but not by asthmatic patients.

The second category of safety issues concerns the toxicologic profile of the drug. Toxicity may be of two types, those in parallel with the preclinical observations and those which are unexpected. In the design of the trial, the sponsor must always consider that man may be the most sensitive species when compared to the species utilized in toxicologic studies. An important objective of entry-into-man studies is to monitor for an early signal of more severe toxicity. It is essential to monitor function of the critical organs identified in the toxicology studies. One should, however, consider the occurrence of unexpected and unpredictable effects not related to the type of toxicity observed during the preclinical evaluation of the compound.

Early studies should monitor important organ systems and should include the drug's effects on the cardiovascular system (vital signs, electrocardiograms), pulmonary function, hepatic, renal, and hematologic systems. In addition, as noted, safety monitoring should encompass any other organ system indicated as a "target" organ based on the preclinical pharmacologic and toxicologic studies.

Safety monitoring should be initially broad but if changes in these parameters are not observed in the first studies, it would be extremely unlikely for the parameters to change later without a concomitant change in a primary organ system. Hence, the range of parameters may be pruned during later development stages. For example, if a drug does not change lipid metabolism (cholesterol and triglyceride concentrations) in the first studies, then it would be highly unlikely for such changes to occur in subsequent studies (assuming there is the same plasma concentration as in the initial studies) without effects on other organs. The sudden appearance of hypercholesterolemia would be an unexpected observation during phase III development if it were not observed in phase I or early phase II studies unless the changes were secondary to toxicity in a major organ system, such as renal toxicity with the development of the nephrotic syndrome. As urinalysis and serum creatinine concentrations are more specific and sensitive parameters of renal abnormalities, measurement of serum cholesterol as part of the later-stage safety parameters usually would be unwarranted.

3.5 Which Parameters Can Be Measured to Ascertain if the Drug Is Likely to Have the Expected Effect in Humans?

The value of the old paradigm of developing drugs by massive screenings using animal disease models has been drastically reduced in today's pharmaceutical industry. The drug development models of the major pharmaceutical companies are based predominantly on rational drug development which focuses on developing drugs that are designed to interfere with a specific physiologic process as either agonists or antagonists of naturally occurring pathways. The sponsor needs to determine how the pharmacologic properties can be measured during the first human studies and whether these effects occur at dose levels that are tolerated in man. Often, with antagonists, pharmacologic activity can only be demonstrated with a provocative challenge to the volunteer or patient if the targeted pathway is operative only in a disease state. For example, leukotriene has no effect on bronchopulmonary function of normal volunteers, but inhibits bronchoconstriction after challenges with leukotriene D_4.[8,9]

3.6 What Is the Dose/Response and Time-Course of the Pharmacodynamic Effects of the New Drug?

Before this question can be answered, one must consider if the desired pharmacologic effect of the drug is a direct consequence of the drug or a secondary event. An antagonist with immediate effects on receptors — as seen in the effects of calcium channel blockers on cardiac conduction — exemplifies a direct pharmacologic effect. An example of an immediate agonistic effect is the bronchodilation induced by the inhalation of a beta agonist. If the immediate pharmacologic effect is related to a disease process, then a simple correlation between pharmacologic antagonism or agonism activity and clinical benefit is assumed. When possible, observation of the maximum pharmacologic activity is desired in modeling a dose/plasma concentration effect relationship. However, in some situations, the maximum effect cannot safely be determined, such as in the excessive hypotension observed with potent vasodilators like nitroprusside, minoxidil, and diazoxide.

The observation that every drug has a maximum effect is rational when one considers that at some dose/concentration an antagonist will achieve maximum inhibition of the naturally occurring intrinsic activity. If the drug works as an agonist, at some dose one may presume that it will have saturated the receptor(s) and maximally stimulated the natural response (which can be either stimulatory or inhibitory). This implies that, if a large enough dose/plasma concentration range is studied, the dose-response relationship should fit a classic E_{max} relationship. Thus, if there are no safety concerns, it is desirable during the initial studies to measure the maximum drug effect and relate that to the plasma concentrations. Knowing the concentration associated with the maximum effect (C_{max}), baseline effect before drug is present (Co), and the concentration associated with half maximum effect (EC_{50}) one can characterize the concentration effect relationship of the drug using the sigmoid E_{max} equation.

$$C = C_0 + \frac{C_{max} D^{\gamma}}{EC_{50}^{\gamma} + C^{\gamma}} \tag{1}$$

Another consequence of the sigmoid E_{max} equation is demonstrated on a typical plot of concentration vs. effect (see Figure 4). When this data is plotted on a semi-logarithmic plot of log concentration vs. effect, around the EC_{50} there is a straight line. Hence, in this area of effect (between about the EC_{20} and EC_{80}), doubling the dose will increase the pharmacodynamic effect only by the natural logarithm of 2 (ln 2 = 0.693) and increasing a dose by threefold will have only about double the pharmacologic effects (ln 3 = 1.10).

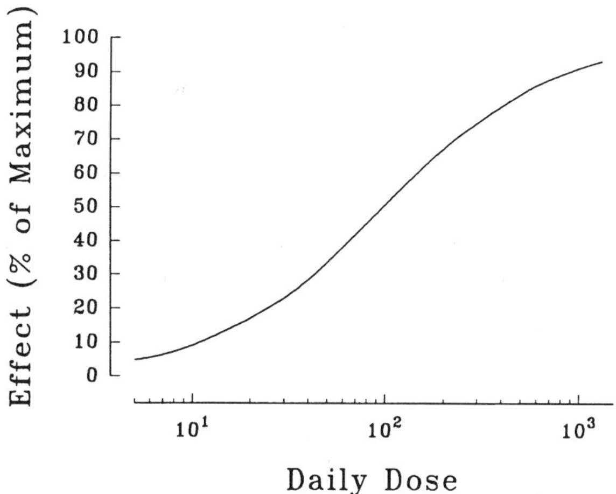

Figure 4 Plot of concentration vs. effect.

Many of the newer drugs, however, derive their therapeutic benefit indirectly by, for instance, activating a cellular cascade which results in beneficial effects. In this case, there may be many intrinsic factors affecting the target cell, such as other mediators and "feedback loops." A clear dose-response relationship may be more difficult to ascertain, but if a drug has a clinical benefit, and even though there might be a time dissociation between concentration and effect, a dose-response relationship must exist. There is some dose at which a clinical benefit is observed and a lower dose without clinical effect. Between these doses must be a dose with partial effects, thus a dose-response relationship. For some drugs, the determination may be extremely difficult. Drugs with marginal clinical benefit would require the study of many patients to demonstrate a dose-response relationship.

As mentioned above, due to the time-course of transport of a drug from the central plasma compartment to the site of its activity, or the time needed to change a physiological cascade, concentration-effect relationships may show a delay between the plasma concentrations and the measured pharmacologic effects, a hysteresis. If present, drugs of very similar activities may have different hysteresis properties based on minor chemical differences. This has been demonstrated with administration of the benzodiazepines midazolam and diazepam.[10]

A thorough understanding of the preclinical pharmacology often will give the clinician insight into these complex relationships. Taking this information into consideration, dose-response and time-course relationships of the drug can often be determined as part of the single or multiple dose tolerability trials. If not, specially designed studies may be required to obtain this information.

Developing a drug with a novel pharmacologic mechanism can be challenging. The intensity and duration of the pharmacologic effect required to achieve a clinical benefit is unknown at the start of development. The broad dose-response relationship can be determined and it is a major objective of phase II therapeutic dose-finding studies to define the clinically meaningful dose or concentratiom range.

Time-course considerations are important in providing regulatory authorities with a rationale for the dosing intervals selected in therapeutic studies. One aspect of this requirement is to determine the pharmacodynamic dose-response relationship at the trough of the desired dosing interval.

3.7 What Should Be the Top Dose that Will Be Administered to Subjects?

As described earlier, it is easier to phrase the question as a "clinical" dose, but today the answer revolves around exposures. There is no universal rule, but the sponsor and the investigator must consider the risk/benefit ratio and the patient population to be studied. By custom, with healthy volunteers, the highest exposure usually is a fraction (1/5 to 1/25) of the exposure in animals that had no pharmacologic or toxicologic effects (the "no-effect" dose). The safer the drug appears (interpreted as if the preclinical effects were to occur in man, only minor, nonlife-threatening, fully reversible effects would be observed), then a higher dose can be administered. In some situations, the highest exposure in man may even be higher then in some of the preclinical animals, if the effects are mild, reversible, and easily monitored.

In patients where there is a strong likelihood that the drug will offer a benefit compared to the risk, the highest dose administered may be related to the acceptable toxicity in the patient population. This is common with chemotherapeutic agents administered to cancer patients, in which toxicity is the norm and doses or exposures that cause WHO grade III or IV toxicities are not infrequently observed.

A concept frequently described is the maximum tolerated dose (MTD). In the treatment of nonlife-threatening disease, with other therapeutic options, this is a dose that is well tolerated in most if not all of the patients. In order to determine this dose, a dose needs to be administered which will cause some ill effects. The lower dose or exposure level is then the MTD. If the highest anticipated therapeutic dose can be determined and is well-tolerated, it is acceptable to establish an acceptable "safety margin" beyond that dose without defining an MTD.

An accompanying concept is the "therapeutic index." Ideally, the dose or exposure that has a clinical benefit will be below the MTD. The ratio of dose or exposure that has a therapeutic benefit to the MTD or exposure is the therapeutic index. In the chronic treatment of nonlife threatening disease, a large therapeutic index is desired. With a large index, the same dose can be administered to a diverse patient population without the need for individualized dosage modification. The drug-related adverse events should be minimal. With a narrow therapeutic index, individualized dosage recommendations are required. The dose may be individualized based on the demographic and clinical characteristics of the patient (i.e., age, sex, renal function) or through therapeutic drug monitoring.

3.8 From the Single-Dose Tolerability Studies, What Information Will Be Required to Start the Multiple-Dose Tolerability Study?

The major objectives of the single-dose study are to lay the foundation for the multiple-dose tolerability study, provided the drug is intended for multiple-dose administration. Information required to adequately design the multiple-dose study should allow a recommendation of the dosing frequency and the duration of dosing. Recommendations on dosing frequency often translate to determining the presence of pharmacodynamic effects at the trough plasma concentrations (about the time of the administration of the next dose). From the single-dose tolerability study, the duration of pharmacodynamic effects can often be predicted. Just as there is some drug accumulation with multiple dosing compared to single-dose data, there can be accumulation of pharmacodynamic effects with multiple doses. If the pharmacokinetic parameters predict significant drug accumulation after multiple dosing with the chosen dosing interval, then pharmacokinetic/pharmacodynamic modeling to predict multiple-dose trough dynamic effects would be helpful in supporting the dosing interval chosen.

3.9 In a Multiple Dose Tolerability Study, What Should Be the Duration of Drug Administration?

The major objective of the multiple-dose study is to determine the tolerability of the drug during repeated dosing and to observe the time-course of the pharmacokinetic and pharmacodynamic parameters. By convention, for drugs with short elimination times ($t_{1/2}$ of less than a day), drugs are frequently administered until steady-state plasma concentrations are observed (about 4 to 5 times the $t_{1/2}$), plus another one to two days after steady state is reached. For drugs with long elimination times, most sponsors will dose the drug for 10 to 14 days. For these drugs with a very long half-life, the rate of accumulation after these time periods will be slow (assuming linear pharmacokinetic properties). With the close supervision of these studies (the subjects are often housed for the duration of the dosing) and the frequent observations made, any sudden onset of adverse events related to accumulation of the drug will be observed, allowing for corrective measures to be rapidly implemented. With these characteristics, it is unlikely that sudden unexpected toxicities will be exhibited when the drug is administered to outpatients over a longer period of time with more infrequent observation periods. The time lost by waiting for the achievement of steady state may be overcome by utilizing a loading dose, followed by maintenance doses to replace eliminated drug.

3.10 What Duration of Followup Will Be Required to Ensure the Safety of the Subjects After the Last Dose Has Been Administered?

The duration of follow-up for subjects that have been enrolled in a study should be based on two characteristics, the time period in which an adverse event may become manifested, and the time in which the subjects still have significant drug exposure. The latter is usually taken as 4 to 5 times the elimination half-life of the drug. The former requires information on the target organ. For most drugs, adverse events will be evident within a short period after they occur; but infrequently late toxicity has been observed as occurred with FIAU administered to patients with hepatitis.[11] A further example of a possible delay in the appearance of the toxicologic effects is in the hemopoietic system. For example, anemia may not be manifested until weeks after drug exposure when there has been enough of a turnover of the red cell population for the anemia to be detected. With the above considerations, most sponsors will follow participants in the early clinical trials for the time of exposure with a follow-up visit scheduled at the equivalent of 4 to 5 times the half-life of the drug. It is usually suggested to the investigator that any serious adverse event that they become aware of within the 4 weeks after dosing be also reported.

3.11 Should the Drug Be Administered in the Fed or Fasted State?

This is a simple question but one that needs to be answered early. Traditionally, the early studies are performed with the subjects in the fasted state. The most common food drug interactions observed are a retardation and increased variability of absorption. A fasting subject will allow for an easier quantification of the pharmacokinetic and pharmacodynamic effects of the drug. For a few drugs in which animal data indicates that the absorption is greater in the fed state, all of the initial studies should be performed with the subjects fed. With very fat soluble drugs, meals have significantly increased the absorption of the compounds. Accutane bioavailability increases up to twofold in the presence of food compared to the fasted state.[12]

A formal food interaction study is not required in the early drug development scheme. Instead, the presence of major effects should be determined early. This is often accomplished by having a separate group of subjects take the medication in the alternative food state after the completion of planned ascending dose tolerability studies.

4 FIRST EFFICACY STUDIES

Results of the initial entry-into-man studies set the platform for the initial efficacy studies (see Table 1). These studies are designed to answer the following questions.

Table 1 Data Needed to Start Efficacy Study

Determination of primary efficacy parameter
Surrogate
Clinical endpoint
Dose or plasma concentration associated with range
Lowest pharmacodynamic effects
Maximum dose or concentration
Maximum tolerated dose
Maximum dynamic effect over dosing interval
Dosing interval
Based on pharmacokinetics
Based on pharmacodynamics
Patient criteria
Likely limitations based on drug or disease interactions
Method of administration — fasted or fed

4.1 How Does One Determine Clinical Efficacy in a Manageable Period of Time?

Surrogate endpoints are parameters which are believed to track the clinical course of a disease. A beneficial drug effect on the surrogate endpoint should translate into a clinical benefit. Ideally, the chosen surrogate endpoint should have been validated for the disease being studied. Validation requires that the surrogate endpoint should predict the outcome of the disease in a patient. A change in the clinical status of the patient should be reflected in a change in the surrogate endpoint and vice versa. For many diseases, clinical benefit requires months or years of treatment, while changes of surrogate endpoints may be evident in a short period of time.

To validate a surrogate endpoint, a correlation of a measurement with outcome needs to be demonstrated. Next, a successful intervention should occur and both a positive clinical outcome and a correlated effect on the surrogate should also be observed. The problem then becomes apparent, because if there is no effective therapy then it would be almost impossible to validate a surrogate endpoint. Likewise, a surrogate endpoint validated with a drug with a given mechanism of action may not be an appropriate surrogate for a drug utilizing another mechanism of action. An example of this contradiction is the antiarrhythmic therapy of premature ventricular contractions. For many years, it was commonly believed that suppression of these was a surrogate endpoint for the prevention of fatal arrhythmias, but the Cardiac Arrhythmia Suppression Trial (CAST) study disproved this notion.[13,14] However, other data has indicated that newer classes of antiarrhythmic medications as exemplified by amiodarone, may benefit patients with life-threatening arrhythmias.[15,16]

4.2 Do the Pharmacologic Properties of the Drug Translate into Clinical Benefit?

There are several ways of demonstrating clinical benefit. For certain diseases, regression of the disease does not occur or is considered so rare that any regression of the disease is taken as demonstration of benefit. This has most notability been utilized in oncologic therapy in which regression of tumor size during therapy confirms clinical benefit.

For most other types of therapy, the most convincing method is to demonstrate a clinical benefit of the drug when compared to patients receiving placebo. A clinical benefit of the new drug over standard therapy would be extremely convincing evidence of a drug's clinical benefit, but this usually requires the enrollment of a large number of patients and is rarely possible especially during Phase II studies. When the administration of placebo is not acceptable, the demonstration of statistical benefit of a drug compared to a very low dose offers convincing demonstration of benefit.

Many physicians have argued that if a drug can be demonstrated to be equivalent to a standard treatment regimen, then benefit has been demonstrated, but there are a number of problems with this paradigm. First, statistically, there are no methods that allow two treatments to be demonstrated as equivalent. Instead, statistics can only demonstrate differences. But it is statistically possible to demonstrate that two treatments do not differ by some predetermined magnitude. Clinically, the first step would be to determine what magnitude of difference would be clinically important. Also, it has been suggested that with poorly designed studies, it is easier to demonstrate that two drugs are equivalent then different.[17]

With poorly designed studies, an increase in variability will make it impossible to demonstrate differences. The other problem with trying to demonstrate that two therapies are equivalent is that, even for effective treatments, in some studies benefit will be demonstrated while in other studies there will be a lack of benefit. In the study designed to show how two drugs are equivalent, it would be impossible to know whether the comparator drug actually had a benefit. In this situation, it is conceivable that the comparator drug did not show benefit in the trial and the new therapy is actually just *equivalent to an ineffective therapy.*

A further method to demonstrate efficacy is the demonstration of a statistically significant dose-response relationship. This has been accepted by regulatory authorities as significant demonstration that a drug has clinical benefit and is discussed below.[18]

4.3 What Is the Dose/Plasma Concentration/Effect Relationship?

If the therapeutic benefits are shown to increase in a dose/plasma concentration response relationship, there is very strong evidence that the drug is effective. Most drugs will have a maximum effect, and there will be a dose that has no pharmacologic effects. If the data is fitted to a mathematical E_{max} model, this results in a sigmoid-shaped curve. Frequently, though, a full curve cannot be studied because adverse events prevent the administration of high doses. In this case, the data often can be plotted to a logarithm-linear relationship. A correlation of a clinical benefit fitted to either of these types of curves is considered by regulatory authorities and scientists as strong evidence of clinical benefit of the treatment.

In fitting the data to the E_{max} model, the maximum effect needs to be determined. To demonstrate this benefit, two doses/plasma concentrations that are significantly different (e.g., fourfold different) should have the same clinical benefit. Also, the no-effect dose needs to be determined. For many diseases, placebo treatment will result in some clinical benefit so the administration of placebo helps to determine the no-effect baseline relationship. If not, two low (but different) doses/plasma concentrations (at least fourfold different) that have the same effects are strong evidence of the no-effect relationship.

Clinically, it is not important to determine the no-effect dose, but to find the initial dose to be administered to patients. If the disease requires immediate efficacy, then the dose must be effective in all patients, as, for example, with antibiotics. On the other hand, with chronic diseases, it is often possible for the physician to titrate the patient to the effective dose. In this situation, it is desirable to give a dose that has a clinical benefit in a significant number of patients but not all patients. Those patients demonstrating a clinical benefit with the lower dose would not require a higher dose and be spared an increased risk of adverse events that may be associated with a higher dose. Hence, it is not desirable to start all of the patients on the high dose. There will be some patients who require a higher dose, but these patients can be titrated to that dose over a period of time.

It is important to try to determine the dose/plasma concentration relationship of the individual patients compared to the whole population. The relationship of the whole population gives a general guide to the range of doses that should be explored by the physicians, but the individual patient may have a dose/plasma concentration relationship that is different and steeper. This would occur if there is a large variation in the patient's ED_{50}s (see Figure 5). If the patient's dose/plasma concentration curves are steep and when a clinical effect is first observed, the dose/plasma concentrations need to be increased in small steps.

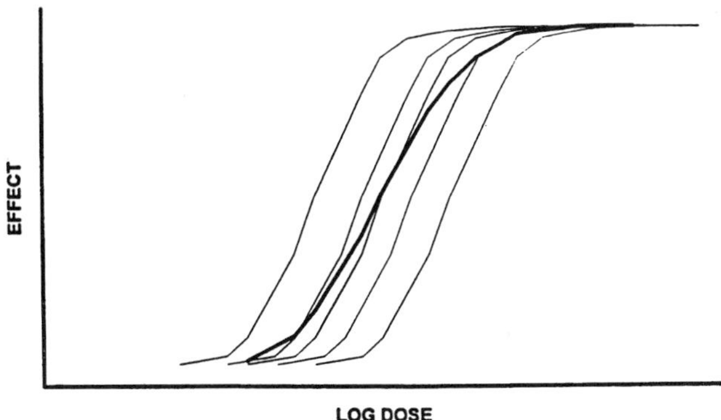

Figure 5 Thin lines represent individual dose-response relationships while thick line represents a less steep mean dose-response relationship.

To adequately answer this question, individual patients must be studied at different doses/targeted plasma concentrations. This is possible only if there is a relatively short time frame to demonstrate the clinical benefit of the drug and there are little or no carryover effects to other doses/plasma concentrations. This allows for patients to be treated at different doses/plasma concentrations and individualized dose-response relationships to be determined.

The individual patient responses can not be dissected from the classic parallel dose-response studies, as individual patients are not treated at different dose levels. Therefore, whenever possible, both the group parallel study and titration of individual patients should be part of the drug development plans. Using multiregression analysis, it may be possible to determine the individual and patient dose-response relationships from the same study as long as some of the patients are treated at different doses.

5 CLINICAL PHARMACOLOGY STUDIES BEYOND THE FIRST SINGLE- AND MULTIPLE-DOSE STUDIES

During phase II, in addition to the efficacy studies, the clinical pharmacology program needs to be continued to determine the information base required to facilitate treatment of the general population once clinical benefit is demonstrated. Typical studies that may be required are discussed below.

5.1 Drug Interactions

It is important to determine whether drug dosage needs to be adapted in the presence of concomitant medication. There are two interactions that must be considered. Does the experimental drug affect the pharmacokinetics of a standard drug? Does a concomitant drug affect the pharmacokinetics of the experimental drug? As a general rule, drug interactions need to be considered only with drugs that have a narrow therapeutic index, such as the antiepileptics, antiarrhythmics, digoxin, warfarin, and theophylline.

A frequent error in drug development is an excessive concentration on commonly prescribed drugs that may be administered concomitantly to treat the indication being studied, rather than considering a scientific rationale and the therapeutic index.

By understanding the pharmacokinetics of the experimental drug, it may be possible to predict drug interactions and metabolism using, for instance, in *vitro* metabolic studies such as with hepatic microsomes or liver slices. If a drug is metabolized by the cytochrome P-450 3A4 pathway then drugs such as erythromycin, cimetidine, and ketoconazole need to be examined. Renal clearance of a drug with a clearance rate greater than the glomerular filtration rate implies that the drug is tubularly secreted. The possibility of drug interactions with other renally tubularly secreted drugs such as cimetidine or probenecid needs to be examined. The protein binding for drugs can also be assessed *in vitro* and the potential for displacement interactions predicted.

5.2 The Need to Modify the Dose in Special Patient Populations

Problems can often be anticipated by knowing the metabolic pathway of the experimental medication. Renal failure generally impairs a drug's elimination if a major excretion route is through renal mechanisms. The decrease in renal clearance is proportional to the decrease in renal function.

$$Cl_{tot} = Cl_{Ren} + Cl_{Non}$$

$$Cl_{Ren} = Cl_{Ren}^{*} \ (Cl_{cr}/Cl_{cr}^{*})$$

Cl_{tot}, Cl_{Ren}, Cl_{Non}, Cl_{cr} is the patient's total renal, nonrenal, and creatinine clearance and Cl_{Ren}^{*} and Cl_{cr}^{*} are the renal and creatinine clearance in the healthy population.

Using these formulas in patients with renal disease, it is possible to predict if a significant interaction will occur.

Most of the drug interaction studies in patients with liver disease have been performed in cirrhotics. Cirrhosis rarely effects drug metabolism until the patient's disease is endstage. Congestive heart failure may affect drug metabolism by a decrease in renal perfusion and hence renal clearance of a drug. Also, with severe congestive heart failure, perfusion of the liver may be impaired and the metabolism of highly cleared drugs may be effected.

5.3 Effect of Food, Antacids, Sucralfate, etc.

Patients often take their medications with meals (the bottle on the table is a convenient reminder to take medication), and therefore the effect of food should be considered as part of the initial clinical pharmacology program. In the early stages of drug development, significant interactions need to be determined, for example, does food cause a major increase or decrease in drug absorption? Significant interactions can often be determined by studying a small number of subjects ingesting the drug with a standard meal (typically a high fat breakfast such as eggs, bacon, toast with butter, and milk) added to the initial tolerability studies.

6 WHAT INFORMATION IS REQUIRED TO DISCONTINUE DRUG DEVELOPMENT?

In the typical development paradigm, only 10 to 20% of the new chemical entities undergoing clinical investigation are eventually registered as drugs. One of the objectives of early drug development is to identify and eliminate compounds that will not be registered. The development team should create a set of minimal criteria for the development of a compound, such as the required dosing frequency and an acceptable therapeutic ratio. With these criteria, any new chemical entity that does not meet the criteria would be a candidate for discontinuation of development.

Even with drug-specific development criteria, a number of generalizations is possible. To consider a drug for continued development, pharmacodynamic activity should be present at tolerable doses in the first studies. If this does not occur, then there is no scientific rationale for continued development.

A further requirement would be a minimal duration of pharmacodynamic effects that would allow for an acceptable dosing frequency. For oral drugs, this would imply a duration of effect that is long enough to allow an acceptable duration between doses. Compliance decreases with dosing more frequently than twice daily and is very low with dosing more frequently than four times daily.[19] The typical oral drug should require administration no more than four times daily and dosing is more desirable on a twice or once daily schedule. On the other hand, for an intravenous drug it is often desirable to titrate a drug to an effect and have the effects dissipate very rapidly on termination of the infusion. For intravenous drugs, a short half-life may be desirable.

In determining dosing frequency, the pharmacodynamic effects need to be linked to the pharmacokinetics of the compound. However, this is often difficult. As a surrogate for duration of pharmacodynamic effects, an acceptable kinetic profile is often sought. Such a profile would include a relatively long and consistent half-life. For a number of drugs in which the expected therapeutic effect is the result of a downstream cascade effect from the initiating pharmacodynamic effect, the pharmacokinetic half-life may not translate directly into the duration of pharmacodynamic effects. For example, interferon has a short half-life (about 2 to 4 h), but *in vitro*, when interferon is added to a cell culture, the antiviral effects can be demonstrated up to 72 h after the removal of the drug from the cultures. Clinical efficacy in the treatment of hepatitis has been demonstrated with the administration of the drug only three times per week.[20]

For orally administered drugs, very low and erratic bioavailability makes drug development extremely difficult. Erratic absorption with large intra- and intersubject variability is common with drugs of very low bioavailability. In this situation, it is not possible to control the patients' drug exposure, so clinical efficacy and the presence of adverse events would be erratic, making effective treatment either extremely difficult or impossible. This has been accomplished almost exclusively with drugs which have a very large therapeutic index. Hence, it would be possible to overdose most of the patients most of the time, such that with the erratic absorption, efficacy would be still present even if a patient were to have extremely low bioavailability of the drug.

For most drugs, the presence of unpredictable and possibly serious adverse events would cause drug development to be terminated. In making this determination, the risk/benefit ratio needs to be considered. Obviously, for diseases that are either nonfatal or have acceptable established therapy, a new drug that causes serious adverse events, even if uncommon, is not acceptable. But if a fatal and nontreatable disease is the target indication (such as cancer and AIDS), continued drug development is possible.

Finally, if at any time the data indicate that the drug will have a less then desirable therapeutic ratio, then continued development needs to be reassessed.

REFERENCES

1. Peck, C., personal communication, 1994.
2. Pedersen, O. L., Christensen, N. J., Ramsch, K. D.; Comparison of acute effects of nifedipine in normotensive and hypertensive man; *J. Cardiovasc. Pharmacol.* 2, 357; 1980.
3. Food and Drug Administration Guideline on Studies in Support of Special Populations; Geriatrics; Availability; Notice; July 1994.
4. Ings, R. M. J.; Interspecies scaling and comparisons in drug development and toxicokinetics; *Xenobiotica.* 20(11), 1201; 1990.
5. Graham, M. A., Kaye, S. B.; New approaches in preclinical and clinical pharmacokinetics; *Pharmacokin. Cancer Chemother.* 17, 27; 1993.
6. Penta, J. S., Rozencweig, M., Guarino, A. M., Muggia, F. M.; Mouse and large-animal toxicology studies of twelve antitumor agents: relevance to starting dose for phase I clinical trials; *Cancer Chemother. Pharmacol.* 3, 97; 1979.
7. Collins, J. M., Grieshaber, C. K., Chabner, B. A.; Pharmacologically guided phase I clinical trials based upon preclinical drug development; *J. Natl. Cancer Inst.* 82, 1321; 1990.
8. Smith, L. J., Geller, S., Ebright, L., Glass, M., Thyrum, P. T.; Inhibition of leukotriene D_4-induced bronchoconstriction in normal subjects by the oral LTD_4 receptor antagonist ICI 204, 219; *Am. Rev. Respir. Dis.* 141, 988; 1990.
9. Kips, J. C., Joos, G. F., De Lepeleire, I., Margolskee, D. J., Buntinx, A., Pauwels, R. A.; Van Der Straeten, M. E.; MK-571, a potent antagonist of leukotriene D_4-induced bronchconstriction in the human; *Am. Rev. Respir. Dis.* 144, 617; 1991.
10. Buhrer, M., Maitre, P. O., Crevoisier, C., Stanski, D. R.; Electroencephalographic effects of benzodiazepines. II. Pharmacodynamic modeling of the electroencephalographic effects of midazolam and diazepam; *Clin. Pharmacol. Ther.* 48(5), 555; 1990.
11. Macilwain, C.; NIH, FDA seek lessons from hepatits B drug trial deaths; *Nature.* 364, 275; July 1993.

12. Colburn, W. A., Gibson, D. M., Wiens, R. E., Hanigan, J. J.; Food increases the bioavailability of isotretinoin; *J. Clin. Pharmacol.* 23, 534; 1983.
13. The Cardiac Arrhythmia Suppression Trial (CAST) Investigators Preliminary Report; Effect of encainide and flecanide on mortality in a randomized trial of arrhythmia suppression after myocardial infarction; *N. Engl. J. Med.* 324, 781; 1991.
14. The Cardiac Arrhythmia Suppression Trial II Investigators; Effect of the anti-arrhythmia agent moricizine on survival after myocardial infarction, *N. Eng. J. Med.* 327, 227; 1992.
15. Cairns, J. A., Connolly, S. J., Gent, M., Roberts, R.; Post-myocardial infarction mortality in patients with ventricular premature depolarizations: Canadian Amiodarone Myocardial Infarction Arrhythmia Trial Pilot Study; *Circulation.* 84, 550; 1991.
16. Ceremuzynski, L., Kleczar, E., Krzeminska-Pakula, M.; Effect of amiodarone on mortality after myocardial infarction: a double-blind, placebo-controlled, pilot study; *J. Am. Coll. Cardiol.* 20, 1056; 1992.
17. Leber, P. D.; Hazards of inference: the active control investigation; *Epilepsia.* 30 (1), S57; 1989.
18. International Conference on Harmonization/Efficacy Tripartite Guideline on "Dose Response Information to Support Drug Registration;" October 1993.
19. Wright, E. C.; Non-compliance — or how many aunts has Matilda; *Lancet.* 342, 909; 1993.
20. Stewart II, W. E.; *The Interferon System*; Springer-Verlag, Vienna; p. 199; 1981.

Chapter 7

Principles in Costing and Administration

Mark Hovde

CONTENTS

1 Introduction ... 81
2 Complexity of Clinical Research ... 82
3 PICAS/CROCAS Database ... 82
4 The Trade Off between Costs and Time in Clinical Development ... 82
5 Managing for Higher Quality and Faster Execution Time by Economizing Program Structures ... 83
6 Stratifying Institutions by Cost, Quality, and Speed ... 85
7 Setting and Budgeting Investigator Fees ... 85
8 Setting Relative Payment Levels: Company Policy, Strategic Pricing, and Compound Novelty ... 89
9 Pricing Investigator Grants when the Investigator is an Opinion Leader ... 90
10 Managing Hospital Overheads ... 90
11 Incremental Pricing ... 91
12 Country-Specific Pricing ... 91
13 Conclusions ... 91
References ... 92

1 INTRODUCTION

This chapter discusses innovations in the costing and administration of phase I and phase II trials. It is only a small overgeneralization to say that previously, costing and administration of clinical trials was an undermanaged area. Most companies had plenty of money and there were few tools to support the systematic analysis of study costs, quality, and the factors that drive them. Today that is changing as the pharmaceutical industry comes under intense margin pressures and new tools have arisen in the form of sophisticated databases for the analysis of clinical research programs. Using these databases clinical managers can now make important contributions to improving the quality, time-to-market, and cost of clinical research programs. Accordingly, this chapter is organized under the following three broad themes:

1. Economizing program structures. The number of patients, number of visits, clinical assessments and procedures, time-in-treatment, and other important aspects of a clinical program can be compared in the database to other programs in the same indication, thus revealing areas of unnecessary complexity and effort. Once the program structure is economized, higher quality, lower costs, and faster time-to-market result.
2. Optimizing institution and CRO Selection. Databases can be used to target investigational sites and CROs with relevant project experience, staff capabilities, facilities, and patient flow. Employing more sites and more capable sites reduces data errors and time-to-market.
3. Setting appropriate fees and improving the accuracy of clinical budgeting. Managers can improve the accuracy of long range cost planning (before a protocol is written) by considering the study location (i.e., country), phase, therapeutic area, investigator affiliation (e.g., CRO, GP, or hospital), and study objective (e.g., PK/Bioavailablity). Once the protocol is written, the structure of the protocol and the intended center's pricing should be incorporated into the analysis to improve the precision and accuracy of study budgets and enhance the sponsor's power in investigator negotiations.

Databases (commercially available and those created by individual sponsors) can be used to improve the quality of long and short range planning and budgeting. With these tools, sponsors can address other important costing and administrative issues such as:

0-8493-9230-6/97/$0.00+$.50
© 1997 by CRC Press, Inc.

1. Setting a relative payment policy ("strategic" pricing) consistent with the priority and novelty of the compound
2. Establishing guidelines for payments to investigators who are opinion leaders vs. others
3. Managing hospital overheads
4. Pricing incrementally to avoid paying for patient information gathered in the normal course of treatment
5. Setting investigator payments at an appropriate level relative to the prevailing rates in the country and region where the work will be conducted
6. Setting healthy volunteer reimbursement at an appropriate level

2 COMPLEXITY OF CLINICAL RESEARCH

The inherent complexity of clinical research is the main difficulty facing those responsible for the planning and administration of clinical research projects. The human body is tremendously complex, with over 105 proteins, 104 biochemical pathways, and 30,000 ICD-9 coded diseases. Depending on the selected efficacy parameters, the study assessments may be painless, noninvasive, and inexpensive (blood pressure) or invasive and costly (colonoscopy). The number of visits may vary from one (anesthetics) to dozens over the course of months or years (growth hormones). Finding, recruiting, and retaining suitable subjects may be straightforward (asthmatics) or difficult (recipients of bone marrow transplants). Compliance in placebo-controlled study designs may be problematical in studies attracting politically or socially motivated subjects (HIV positives). These and other factors make it difficult for planners and administrators to accumulate the experience necessary to accurately forecast clinical costs.

3 PICAS/CROCAS DATABASE

The findings for this chapter stem from the ongoing PICAS/CROCAS* database project. This database consists of information on study structures, costs, and timings collected from over 60 large pharmaceutical companies and 400 CROs in the U.S. and Europe. Currently the database contains over 8000 protocols and 40,000 investigator contracts, with information on over 400 disease indications and 3000 hospitals and other institutions conducting clinical research.

4 THE TRADE OFF BETWEEN COSTS AND TIME IN CLINICAL DEVELOPMENT

As has been mentioned above, time (meaning critical path time) is a commodity that should be managed carefully in the administration of clinical trials. Critical path time is very valuable because project delay can mean slower time to market, lost sales, and a reduced ability to build the product's brand franchise. In addition, the shorter the critical path, the smaller the portfolio must be to support a given number of registrations per year.

Administrators, however, function in a world where the direct cost they can incur to pay for a reduction in their consumption of critical path time is also a precious commodity, because their budgets are generally fixed as a percentage of their firm's sales. As a result, clinical managers are constantly trading off time and money.

To shed light on the time-cost trade off, it is necessary to define the strategic aims of a modern drug development organization. One important aim is achieving a product's registration quickly to yield the highest number of sales years before patent expiry. A second objective is to minimize costs per compound to accommodate the largest portfolio possible within a fixed budget, so that pre-expiry sales for all products can be maximized.

(Another important objective is to create the right information in the registration package so that sales throughout the marketing life of the product are optimized. The fastest route to registration is not always the best. For example, the addition of mortality data to the development plan may delay registration but add greatly to sales once the product is approved.)

Suppose a U.S. development organization managing 5 compounds is performing at the industry average of about 12 years in development. If each of its 5 compounds achieves registration, then each

* PICAS™ is an acronym for Pharmaceutical Investigator Cost Analysis Service. It is database of clinical costs, program structures, and timings, marketed by the commercial company DataEdge, Inc., Ft. Washington, PA, U.S., and Walton-on-Thames, Surrey, U.K. CROCAS™ is an acronym for Contract Research Organization Capability Assessment Service. CROCAS is jointly produced and marketed by DataEdge and Technomark Consulting Services Limited, London.

will have 5 years of sales before patent expiry at 17 years. The organization will have thus generated a total of 25 pre-expiry sales years from its portfolio. Suppose that by spending 25% more per compound the time to market can be expedited by half a year, from 12 years to 11.5. Is this a sound trade off? At first glance, the faster development will generate an extra half year's pre-expiry sales for each product, increasing the total years achieved to 27.5 from the original 25. But in most companies, the direct cost budget of the R & D organization is static; management is committed to spending a fixed percentage of sales, say 15%, and no more. Spending 25% more per compound thus means that one of the five compounds will have to be dropped, and the portfolio will shrink to four compounds. Four compounds achieving 5.5 years each is a total of 22 years of pre-expiry sales. In this simple example, the 25% direct cost premium paid to achieve faster development time was not worth it.[3]

(A more complex example might incorporate factors such as the benefit realized from out-licensing the dropped compound, the time value of money, the disproportionately high value of early sales years when compounds are first in their therapeutic category, and the fact that many submitted compounds fail to achieve registration.)

In contrast, consider the opportunity afforded by reducing direct costs per compound by 20%, with no change in development time. With the lower per compound costs, a sixth compound can be supported within the original budget. Six compounds achieving 5 years each is a total of 30 years of pre-expiry sales from the portfolio. The PICAS database offers evidence that investigator fees — a major component of direct costs — can in fact be reduced without compromising development times. A preliminary review of enrollment rates from over 700 U.S. centers shows no difference in the rates achieved by centers paid at the 75th percentile vs. those paid at the 35th. Since the absolute cost difference between these two percentiles is large, this implies that many companies can substantially reduce investigator fees without sacrificing study completion time.

While the foregoing examples show that direct cost management and time management can have an important impact on the strategic outputs of the development organization, it is important to note that the management skills necessary to improve time and direct cost performance are very different. Put bluntly, it is easier to be cheap than fast. Time is hard to manage for a number of reasons. First, there is no common language and convention system for the starting and endpoints of many key clinical research activities (i.e., when does "preparing the clinical development plan" start?). There are no generally accepted accounting principles for time, and there are no chartered accountants of time. Secondly, it is hard to reliably determine the true critical path when multiple projects may be winding their way through a clinical research process encompassing hundreds of potentially rate-limiting activities. The manager may spend to improve the speed of an apparently rate-limiting step, only to find later that the step was not in fact rate limiting. For example, he pays a premium to expedite the supplies, but an unforeseen delay in the packaging negates the impact of the expedited supplies. In contrast, saving money works anywhere you can do so without prolonging a critical activity, and accounting systems capture and measure costs very accurately.

5 MANAGING FOR HIGHER QUALITY AND FASTER EXECUTION TIME BY ECONOMIZING PROGRAM STRUCTURES

Perhaps the most fundamental way to speed development while reducing cost and improving quality is to remove unnecessary complexity from protocols. The complexity of phase I protocols has increased over the past several years. Clinical protocol complexity as measured by the number of procedures conducted on each patient shows an increase of over 20% in the past 3 years (see Figure 1).

Reducing procedures per patient has a number of important benefits to the quality and speed of the overall development process:

1. Simpler, shorter CRF (faster design, faster data entry)
2. Lower investigator fees (investigators are being asked to perform less work)
3. Less source document verification, SDV (faster monitoring visits, fewer data errors)

Clinical research is difficult to plan and budget for because clinical studies are so variable and complex. The underlying variability in clinical research studies can be illustrated by examining the number of patients and the number of visits found in typical drug indications. For example, in phase II studies of hypertension compounds the number of patients and the number of visits vary greatly (Figures 2 and 3).

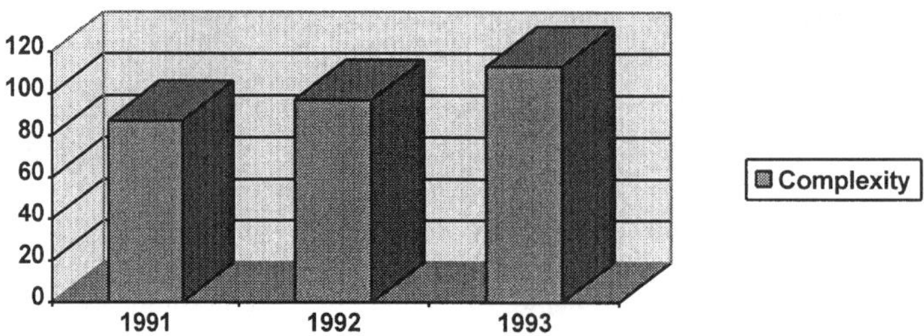

Figure 1 Phase I protocol complexity, 1991-93.

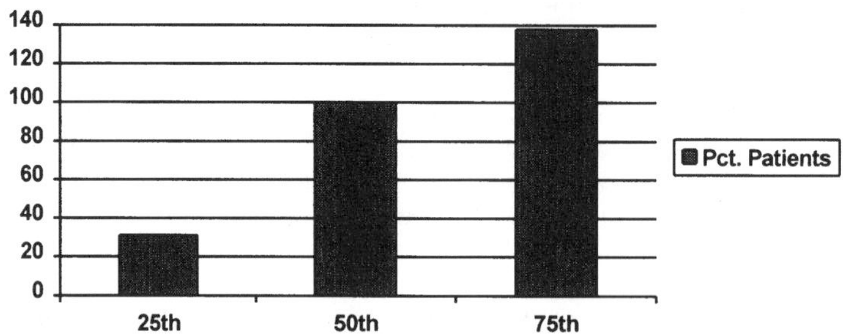

Figure 2 Indexed number of patients in phase II hypertension trials (50th percentile = 100%). Pct = percentage.

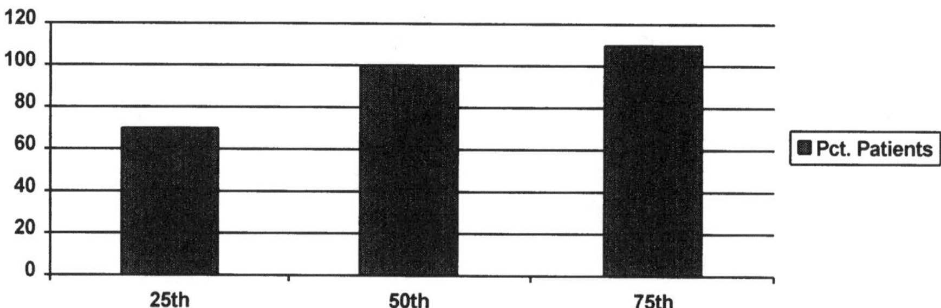

Figure 3 Indexed number of visits in phase II hypertension trials (50th percentile = 100%). Pct = percentage.

Patients, visits, and the procedures and assessments per patient drive monitoring and the data handling effort. Total monitoring and data handling effort increases as a multiplicative function of patients, visits, and procedures per visit (a study involving 50% more patients, 50% more visits, and 50% more procedures per visit will generate about 237% more CRF processing). Furthermore, the number of procedures per patient, defined here as protocol complexity, is a major driver of overall completion time.

Those responsible for study administration and costing can use databases such as the PICAS/CROCAS database to identify protocols falling outside industry ranges for their number of patients, visits, or procedures. Structural issues can then be raised with medical staff to see whether the reasons for the higher study inputs can be substantiated. Often there are excellent reasons for higher inputs, but just as frequently the reason is "because we've always done it that way." Regardless, administrators and medical staff alike can learn from asking the questions.

Beyond the number of patients, visits, and study timings, databases can be used to determine which procedures and assessments are within industry practice and which are not. For example, the database shows that the following 6 procedures are employed in more than 25% of outpatient phase I PK/bioavailability studies (shown in parentheses are the frequencies of each procedure in protocols where the procedure appears):

1. ECG (2 times)
2. Urinalysis (3 times)
3. Hemogram (3 times)
4. Urine drug screen (2 times)
5. SMAC (19 or more automated blood chemistries; 3 times)
6. Visits: initial history and physical (1 time), routine visit (2 times), brief visit (8 times)

In addition to these procedures, which might be termed the basics, the database also shows 150 procedures which appear in 25% or fewer of all such studies. Clearly, the design variability of even PK/bioavailability studies is high.

6 STRATIFYING INSTITUTIONS BY COST, QUALITY, AND SPEED

Companies are under increasing pressure in early and late phase clinical studies to find centers that can deliver the highest quality data in the shortest time. Because the impact of faster study execution and higher data quality is so high, direct cost is usually a secondary criterion in center selection. A recent paper[1] quantified the potential impact of superior center selection on study quality and speed. In a phase III CNS study, the authors ranked 16 centers on their performance in data quality (CRF errors), speed (enrollment rate), and direct costs (investigator fees). They found that removing the 5 worst performing centers and replacing these with 5 excellent centers resulted in 7000 fewer CRF errors, a 5-week reduction in project completion time, and $23,000 lower in direct costs. While the findings related to a phase III study, the implications for earlier phase work are equally compelling.

Study administrators can contribute to more intelligent center selection by screening centers for the capabilities likely to contribute to high quality performance before beginning negotiations. Centers can be screened using databases developed in-house or by using commercially available databases designed for this purpose. For example, in one such database (CROCAS), CROs and contract investigational sites can be screened based on the expertise and experience of the particular staff involved, even to the level of individual cardiovascular studies (CVs) from CROs and investigational sites. It is also possible to scan for specific project experience by drug indication, number of patients, and study start/stop date. In CRO studies, experience in the same drug indication is a good indicator of likely enrollment success because the CRO will be able to rapidly contact the best investigators from the prior work.

Direct costs can be analyzed in detail at an institutional level. Databases can provide costs of specific procedures, hospital overheads, and other charges such as equipment purchases, advertising, and study coordinator fees. The administrator can thus prescreen hospitals and academic centers for various factors that contribute to center quality and speed while understanding in detail the likely level of direct costs.

7 SETTING AND BUDGETING INVESTIGATOR FEES

Clinical managers often prepare cost estimates for development programs several years into the future. These estimates support the preparation of long range clinical budgets and contribute to the economic evaluation of drug candidates. Investigator costs are a major portion of total clinical costs (typically 30-50%). Estimates of investigator costs are difficult to prepare because the costs vary depending on the study location (i.e., country), phase, therapeutic area, investigator affiliation (GP or hospital), and study objective (e.g., PK/bioavailablity), and because managers and companies have experience that may be limited across one or more of these dimensions.

The largest percentage of investigator contracts in the U.S. and Europe are set up in phase III (Figure 4).

Because most contracts are in phase III, most investigator cost (and company experience) is in phase III. Experience in phase III trials can be misleading when applied to phases I and II. When the median investigator cost per patient of studies in phases I, II, and III, with phase III is indexed to 100%, the median phase I patient costs 48% more than the median phase III patient, while the median phase II patient costs 35% more (Figure 5).

The cost differences observed for the phases depend in turn on the purpose of the study, the health parameters measured in it, its duration in patient visits, and the location of the investigator. Most phase II and III studies in PICAS/CROCAS state an objective of efficacy and safety measurement. In phase I, studies show a variety of objectives: (1) PK/bioavailability; (2) safety and dose ranging; and (3) studies in a special patient population (Figure 6).

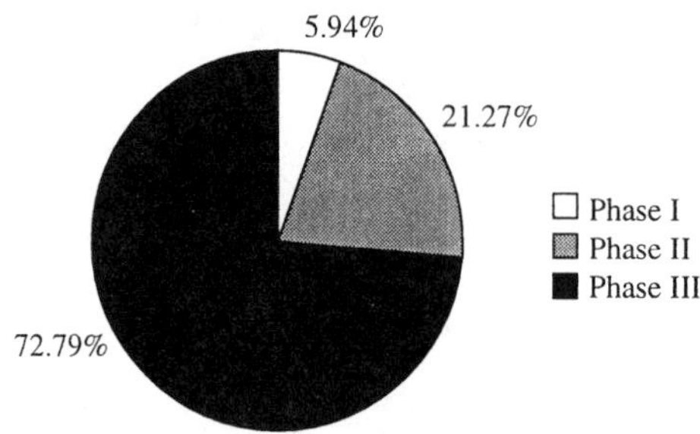

Figure 4 Percent investigator contracts by phase.

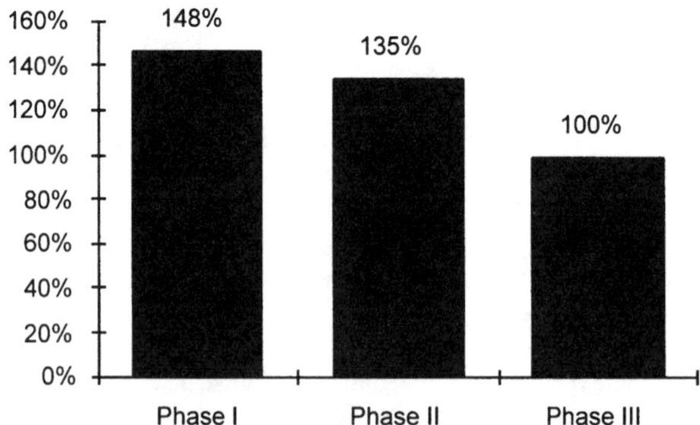

Figure 5 Indexed per patient investigator costs by phase (phase III = 100%).

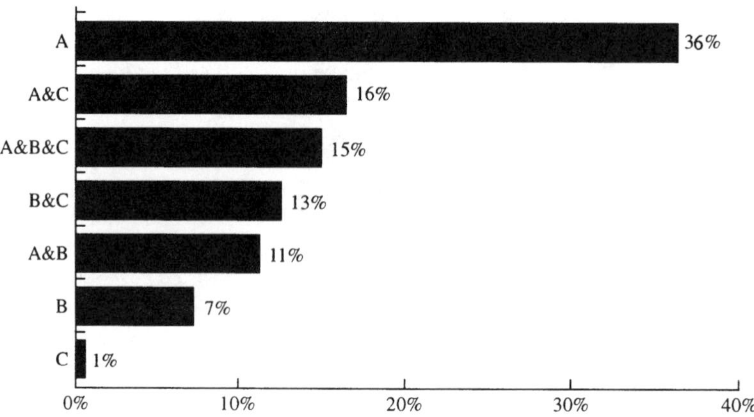

Figure 6 Percent phase I studies by study objective.

Because of differences in the difficulty of recruiting suitable patients, adding the requirement of a special patient population adds cost. Dose ranging also adds cost. Studies incorporating combination objectives such as safety/dose ranging studies in special patient populations are the most expensive (Figure 7).

In phase II studies, cost variance within countries depends on the therapeutic area and underlying study design. Phase II studies are generally distributed in seven major therapeutic areas (Figure 8).

Cardiovascular is the largest phase II therapeutic area by number of investigators, followed closely by CNS. Immunomodulation is the smallest. Over half of phase II studies are in the three areas of

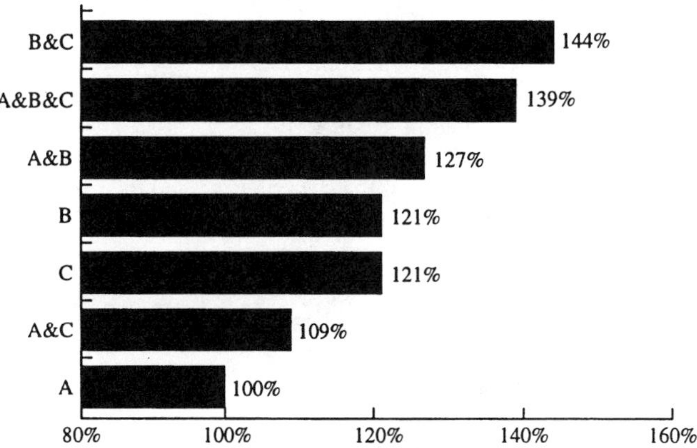

Figure 7 Indexed phase I cost per patient by study objective (PK/bioavailability = 100%).

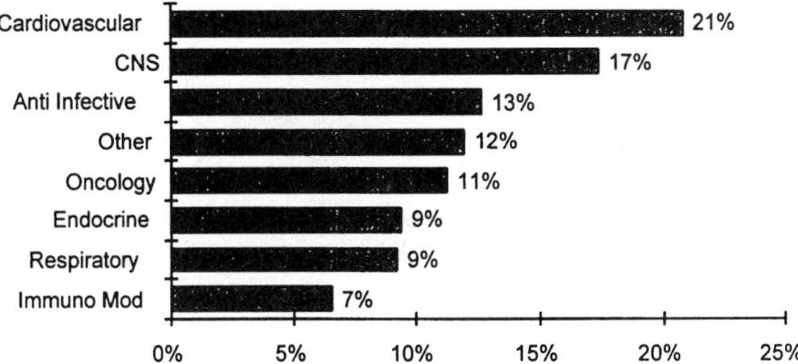

Figure 8 Percent phase II studies by therapeutic area.

cardiovascular, CNS, and anti-infective. The "other" area (12% of studies) includes dermatology, hematology, pain and anesthesia, and ophthalmology.

Phase II costs per patient vary by therapeutic area (Figure 9). Part of the variance is due to differences in the supply of and demand for investigators. For example, CNS investigators are in short supply because of the large number of companies conducting studies in this area.

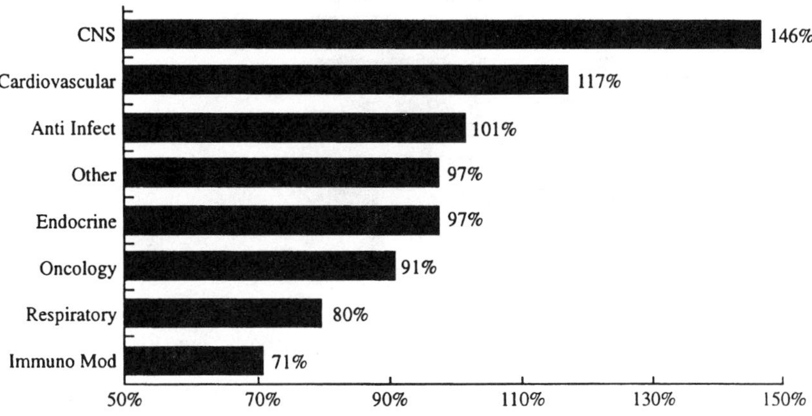

Figure 9 Indexed phase II cost per patient by therapeutic area (CV median = 100%).

Clearly, those planning long-range clinical budgets should, at a minimum, consider the phase and therapeutic area of the intended study. For example, a manager familiar with cost levels in phase II immunomodulation studies will find his experience almost completely irrelevant in a phase II CNS study, where costs per patient are likely to run 100% or more higher. Some managers take their analysis a step further and incorporate data at the indication group level. As shown above, CVs make up 21% of all phase II studies. Within CV, there are 9 large indication groups, and the percent distribution of CV studies within these groups differs widely with the hypertensive and dysrhythmia groups being by far the largest, with nearly 50% of the total CV activity within them (Figure 10).

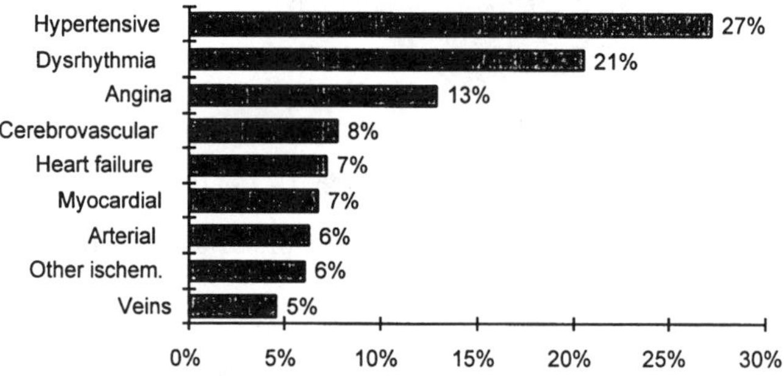

Figure 10 Percent phase II studies by CV indication group.

While costs vary between therapeutic areas by up to 100%, costs vary even more by group within a therapeutic area. Therefore those developing long-range budgets and spending plans should, where possible, take indication group into account. The highest per patient costs are seen in groups where studies require extraordinary resources for activities such as intense patient monitoring or the accommodation of unpredictable or irregular recruitment. For example, some studies of thrombolytic drugs require dosing within a few minutes or hours after a myocardial infarction, so companies may face the cost of funding around-the-clock study support staff to screen and enroll patients admitted late at night. Further adding to costs is the fact that these studies may also require expensive and repeated imaging procedures performed at frequencies far beyond that accompanying the normal course of treatment (Figure 11).

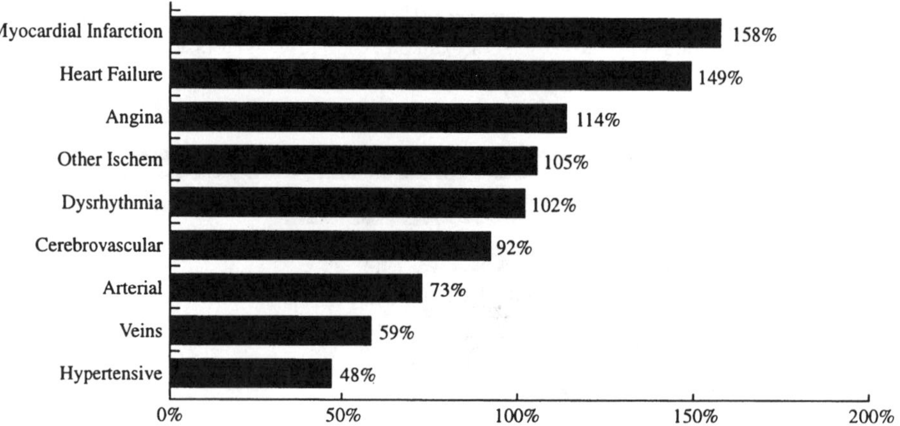

Figure 11 Indexed phase II cost per patient by CV indication group (CV median = 100%).

Within the CV area, the highest cost groups are myocardial infarction and heart failure. The cost per patient for studies in the myocardial infarction group is three times higher than studies in the hypertensive group. Because investigator costs are such a large proportion of total clinical spending, budgets and forecasts that the indication group take into account will be more accurate than those using therapeutic area data only.

The foregoing analysis estimates only the cost per patient for various phases, study designs, and disease groups. Databases such as the PICAS/CROCAS database can also be used to increase the accuracy and credibility of estimates of other important drivers of overall costs such as the number of patients, the number of patient visits, and the cost per patient visit. This is particularly important when protocol details are unavailable at the time the long-range plan is being developed.

Study quality and speed of completion continue to dominate costs as considerations in the administration and planning of clinical trials. The long-term financial consequences of delayed study completion can be immense, dwarfing the small economies that might be obtained by micormanaging investigator costs. Until recently study costs have not been an important consideration in most pharmaceutical companies. Today, however, pricing and profitability pressures on the pharmaceutical industry are forcing companies to increase their scrutiny of all costs. In this environment managing overall drug development and individual study costs has become important as R & D operations struggle with tighter budgets, fewer headcount, and increasing costs.

Illustrative of these cost increases are phase I grant costs in Europe. Part of the cost growth is due to increases in study complexity (defined as the number of procedures performed on a patient who attends all visits) over time, but using multiple classification analysis (MCA) it is possible to correct for changes in complexity. Costs have oncreased by over 30% per patient since 1991 in 6 key European countries (Figure 12).

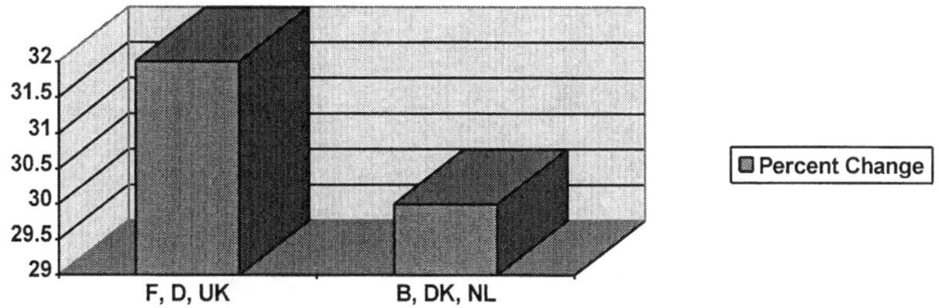

Figure 12 Percent change in phase I costs, 1991-93 in six key European countries.

All of the countries are important venues for European clinical studies. Even the smaller markets show strong increases in cost per patient over the period in question.

8 SETTING RELATIVE PAYMENT LEVELS: COMPANY POLICY, STRATEGIC PRICING, AND COMPOUND NOVELTY

Industry databases of clinical investigator costs can be used to analyze relative levels of investigator payments. Companies can examine such a database to determine whether their payments are low or high in relation to the payments of other companies for similar studies. "Similar" means alike in phase, indication, investigator location (country), study setting (GP vs. hospital), number of visits, and procedure content.

Once it knows its relative payment standing, a company can set a target level for future spending. Some managers have compared this to the salary policy, where a company determines it will pay, for example, in the top quartile in its region or industry. Of course, a salary database does not tell a company what it should pay; it only shows the range of what other companies actually do pay. Each company must set its own policy consistent with its resources and aims. In the same way, companies can now set an investigator payment policy, so that future payments will fall within a predetermined range relative to industry. Some companies plan for spending that is high in relation to industry, believing that they are buying higher quality or faster execution with the extra spending. Other companies reject this notion and plan to pay at industry median or lower. Unpublished data from the PICAS database suggests that study execution speed (as measured by enrollment rates) is not enhanced by overpaying, although enrollment does appear to be slowed by severely underpaying.

Setting a policy for overall relative investigator spending levels is important because investigator costs are such a large cost. R & D spending in large pharmaceutical companies comprises about 15-17% of sales, clinical research about 6%, with investigator costs about 2%.

Once an overall relative payment policy has been established company wide, clinical managers may set a corresponding pricing strategy for each compound in the portfolio. In the best companies, there is an attempt made to correlate relative spending with compound priority. In many cases, however, there is no correlation. For example, compound X may have a high priority in the company's development plan, but the investigator reimbursements are low in relation to peer payments for comparable studies.

At the heart of strategic pricing is compound prioritization. Compound prioritization in many companies is a major analytical exercise requiring collaboration and input from marketing and R & D. The participants have much at stake personally because an unfunded or underfunded compound can trap its professionals in a downward career spiral.

After prioritizing its development portfolio, one company examined its relative payment levels in an industry database of investigator costs (PICAS). It found little correlation between compound priority and relative payment levels. In particular, one high priority phase II compound showed unusually low payment levels. On further examination management realized that one reason for the low payments was the medical novelty of the compound, which had attracted much scientific interest from the investigator community. Therefore the company decided that both the compound priority and the novelty of the compound should be taken into account in setting a relative payment range for investigator payments in a particular project. Each compound can be arrayed in a priority/novelty matrix (Figure 13).

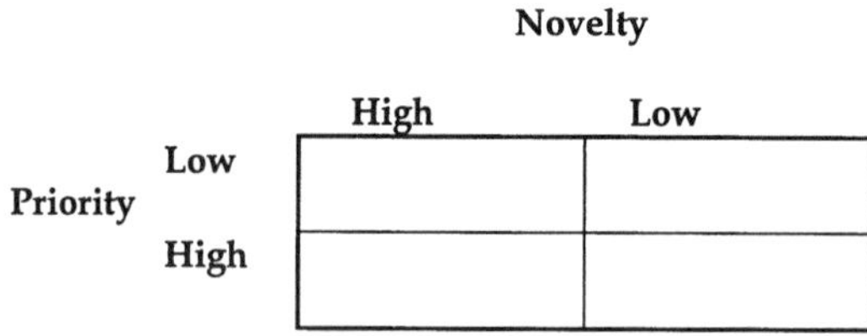

Figure 13 Compound novelty/priority matrix.

Higher relative payments were slated for compounds with low novelty and high priority, on the basis that investigators would be less scientifically, and more economically, motivated in these studies. Lower payments were planned for low priority compounds, especially those with some element of novelty.

9 PRICING INVESTIGATOR GRANTS WHEN THE INVESTIGATOR IS AN OPINION LEADER

Often an important opinion leader will be included in a study for marketing and/or regulatory reasons. This practice is common in phase IIIb and IV studies, but occurs also in phase II. Problems in grant negotiations may arise where the opinion leader commands an investigator fee above that normally prevailing with ordinary investigators. One approach is to pay a rate to all investigators reflecting the opinion leader's fee, but this will increase per patient costs across the entire study and hence overall study costs. To get around this, some companies attempt to remunerate the opinion leader off-grant, so that his basic grant reflects the same rate per patient as other investigators in that country, but there is a side contribution, say, for equipment to provide additional remuneration.

10 MANAGING HOSPITAL OVERHEADS

Broadly, clinical grant costs can be split into three parts: procedure charges (charges for ECGs, chest x-rays, etc), other activity-based charges such as physician's fees, study coordinator fees, advertising, and overheads (usually levied as a percentage of the first two types of charges). Hospital or institutional overheads can add 5-30% to the overall cost of an investigator grant. For the administrator, perhaps the most frustrating aspect of overheads is the inability of most institutions to defend the level of overhead charged. Sometimes the hospital or research institution does not understand its own cost structure, and the number is arbitrary. At a large hospital in Sweden, for example, a senior administrator admitted to the author that *the procedure prices and overhead rate used by the hospital had been recently made up by a committee, with no basis in actual costs because the hospital did not know its actual costs.* PICAS data show that some companies consistently pay lower overheads than others. A review of the most effective overhead management practices among major pharmaceutical companies shows four steps that can contribute to lower overheads.[2]

First, it is important to document existing overhead practices to find and exploit areas of inconsistency. In some cases, the company may find that one therapeutic area is paying one rate at an institution, while other therapeutic areas have negotiated a lower rate at the same institution. A second step is to look at rates paid by other companies using a database such as PICAS. It may be that the lowest rate paid in one company is still higher than the rate paid by others. A third step is to ask the institution for a breakdown of the components of its overhead calculation. The company can then see whether the full rate makes sense for every grant, or whether a partial application of the rate might be more appropriate because the rate duplicates charges already built into the grant. For example, one component of the overall rate might be a charge to cover the use of the institution's physical facilities, while the grant itself may include a charge for the use of an endoscopy exam room. Similarly, one part of the overhead might go to cover the pharmacy operation, while the grant may include explicit per visit pharmacy fees to cover the costs of warehousing and dispensing the study medication.

Some companies go a step further to determine the basis of the overhead calculation. Some institutions charge on all direct costs, while some charge on just non-lab costs or just salaries. Obviously, the basis is an important and generally negotiable part of the calculation that can have an important effect on the overall overhead paid.

Finally, experience from PICAS users shows that overhead rates can be negotiated below what industry generally pays when so-called preferred provider rates are established. A company establishes preferred provider rates by negotiating one overhead rate for all work done at that institution. Furthermore, institutions can be grouped to increase negotiating leverage. The Harvard Health System is one such group including several hospitals in the Boston area. While some companies negotiate separate overheads with these hospitals, others negotiate one rate for all work done in the hospital group.

11 INCREMENTAL PRICING

The information captured in the CRFs can be viewed in two parts. The first part is information that arises in the normal course of the patient's treatment. The second part is information required by the protocol but not required by the normal course of treatment. For example, suppose a protocol for an antiarrhythmic requires six ECGs. A doctor admitting a patient presenting with an arrhythmia will probably order some ECGs anyway, say four, regardless of whether the patient is included in the protocol. Incremental pricing distinguishes between the four ECGs ordered in the ordinary course of the patient's treatment and those extra (or incremental) two ordered especially for protocol purposes. The incremental pricer seeks to pay only for the two ECGs, on the theory that the doctor is already being reimbursed for the first four by the patient's insurance or by the national health scheme. The incremental pricer seeks to pay only for the extra work his protocol creates.

For most companies, incremental pricing represents a vast and underutilized area of savings, especially in phase II and III studies.

12 COUNTRY-SPECIFIC PRICING

Country-specific pricing recognizes real differences in the prevailing rates for medical care between countries. Some companies found they were budgeting and paying one rate regardless of country, in effect paying the highest rates possible and setting high precedents for their own single country studies. When comparing the distribution of investigator cost ratios between the U.S. and U.K. for phase III studies in 100 major disease indications, it was found that for 40% of the 100 disease groups, per patient costs in the U.K. are less than half the per patient costs in the U.S. (Figure 14). These data are probably also true for phase I and II studies.

By setting investigator fees in relation to local rates, clinical administrators can save considerable fees for their companies. In one recent example, a U.K. company saved £4 million by paying local (U.K.) rather than German rates on a single phase III protocol.

13 CONCLUSIONS

Clinical administrators are responding to the forces shaping the drug industry with new approaches to the complex trade offs between the timings and costs of clinical research programs. This chapter has

Falling into 4 Ranges vs. US Costs

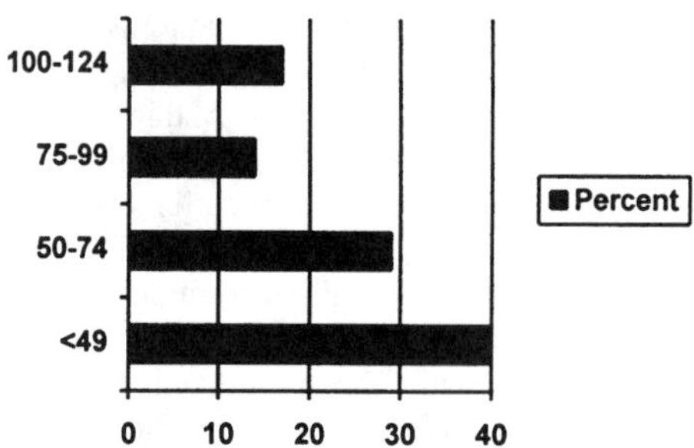

Figure 14 Percent U.K. disease groups falling into four Ranges vs. U.S. costs.

reviewed how some companies are using information from their own companies and from industry databases to economize program structures, optimize the selection of institutions and CROs, and set appropriate investigator fees to get the most for every unit of clinical spending.

REFERENCES

1. Getz, K., Brookman, S., and Fisher, S. (1994). Managing Research Centers as a Portfolio of Strategic Resources: Optimizing the Site Selection Process. DIA Poster Session Presentation, June 1994, Washington, D.C.
2. Glass, H. and Laughlin, J. (1994) Understanding and controlling institutional clinical grant overhead costs. *App. Clin. Trials,* 3(7), 42-45.

Chapter 8

Biotechnology

Peter A. Harris

CONTENTS

1 Introduction 93
2 Background 94
3 Technical Support: The Tool-Kit 95
3.1 Transgenic Animals 95
3.2 Cell Separation Techniques 96
3.2.1 Fluorescence-Activated Cell Sorting 96
3.2.2 Physical Parameter Selection 96
3.3 Immuno-Adsorption Techniques 96
3.3.1 Panning 96
3.3.2 Immune Adsorption Ferromagnetic Beads 96
3.3.3 Column Chromatography 96
3.4 Polymerase Chain Reaction (PCR) 96
3.5 DNA/RNA Probes 97
4 Perspective 97
5 Gene Therapy — Sense and Antisense 97
5.1 Sense 97
5.2 Antisense 99
6 Conclusions 99
References 100

1 INTRODUCTION

The biotechnology industry is enjoying continuing successes along with excellent long-term potential for major contribution to healthcare management. There are close to 2000 U.S.-based biotech companies and nearly 400 in Europe; over half of these are involved in healthcare of some sort, particularly therapeutics. With two blockbusters (erythropoietin, Epogen, and G-CSF, Neupogen) to its credit, Amgen became the first biotech company to join the fortune 500 list of companies.

The first products in protein therapeutics were simply identical to those long ago identified in humans, such as insulin. With advances in the production of proteins using genetically modified organism cultures, such as E. coli, and genetically modified cell cultures, such as CHO cells, it became possible to generate quantities of other naturally occurring proteins which are normally present in only very minute quantities; with such technology rt-PA, the interferons, erythropoietin, the colony-stimulating factors, and others have been explored, developed, and brought into therapeutic use.

Advances in molecular biology have also increased our knowledge about the genetic causes of disease. So even while the early experiments on the *ex vivo* manipulation of hemopoietic cells, including stem cells, were being conducted, parallel experiments with gene insertion into such cells *ex vivo* were proceeding apace. Having successfully treated two severe combined immuno-deficient disease (SCID) patients born with adenosine deaminase (ADA) deficiency by the use of *ex vivo* genetically modified autologous lymphocytes, Blease and Anderson of the National Institutes of Health (NIH), Bethesda, MD, have now shown that similarly modified autologous hemopoietic stem cells may be effective in the longer term, but it is early yet.

0-8493-9230-6/97/$0.00+$.50
© 1997 by CRC Press, Inc.

2 BACKGROUND

In 1975, Kohler and Milstein developed monoclonal antibody production technology, and in 1981 the first monoclonal antibody kit was approved. In 1977, Sanger in the U.K. reported rapid sequencing techniques for DNA, and only 5 years later the FDA was to approve Humulin®, a human insulin manufactured by recombinant DNA technology. In 1982 the gene for human tissue-type plasminogen activator (t-PA) was cloned and expressed and less than 2 years later recombinant human t-PA (rt-PA) was first administered to a patient; more extraordinary still was the marketing approval of rt-PA 3 years later, in 1987. Notwithstanding any debate over the clinical endpoints (i.e., clot lysis vs. longer term survival), this reflects a remarkably rapid and successful clinical development program in a technically complex area.

Other selected milestones during the last decade are:

1985 — Recombinant human growth hormone approved by FDA
1987 — Recombinant human t-PA approved
1989 — Erythropoietin approved by FDA
1991 — Granulocyte-colony stimulating factor approved
1992 — GM-CSF approved
1992 — IL-2 approved for treatment of renal cell carcinoma

Not every development succeeds, of course. The IL-1 antagonist, Antril (anakinra), was withdrawn from development for the treatment of severe sepsis when the phase III study failed to show adequate efficacy. As IL-1 may have other effects, Antril is currently in phase II in rheumatoid arthritis studies.

But why are biotechnology products different, or are they? Often they are. All the standard phase I/II clinical trials conducted as per the system-organ classes are relevant and important. They still represent important decision-making studies. Clear differences, however, exist with regard to the relevance of preclinical and safety studies, the toolkit required, and the effects on the immune system.

Classical pharmacology models are often irrelevant. While some proteins, such as human G-CSF, clearly express their activities across some other species, other proteins, such as the interferons, can be much more species specific. Neither poor results nor good results need be predictive of effects in humans. As such, the preclinical work overall may bear scant resemblance to a classical development program; this can be, of course, an opportunity for fast-tracking, rather than a problem.

There may well be difficulties with the toxicology, particularly if the animal develops neutralizing antibodies; long-term administration in such cases is meaningless. The effects of impurities, especially foreign proteins, may assume greater relevance in these compounds, because of antibody generation, for example. Qualitative batch-to-batch variation of impurities must be avoided. In terms of the route of administration, in most cases the product will be administered by injection. While many of the naturally occurring molecules do exist free in the blood or extracellular space, it may still be far from natural for the concentration gradient to be highest in the blood and lower intracellularly, while population densities of receptors will be expected to change dramatically and other homeostatic mechanisms may come into play.

There are important broader factors involving the unraveling of disease processes using these techniques, as well as the nature of the preclinical/paraclinical "toolkit" used for exploring and developing biotechnology products which impacts significantly on the important decision-making processes of program design.

There is an intense link between the experimental unraveling of the pathobiology with the attempts at correcting this with development candidates. Many companies have originally set up biotechnology groups with the intention of modeling the disease processes in order to design screening and selection models for their relatively classical small molecule research programs; others have done likewise but with the intention of rational structural design with the aid, for example, of receptor cloning, computer-aided molecular graphics, etc. Perhaps in the area of cytokines it is most apparent how the unraveling of a disease process such as sepsis, and the exploration of the role of tumor necrosis factor (TNF) led to the development of anti-TNF antibodies as potential therapy. Equally, in the area of single gene inherited disease, Gaucher's disease is a good example, where treatment has evolved from symptomatic management to the extraction from placentae and administration of naturally occurring glucocerebrosidase, to the production and approval for marketing of the recombinant product, and now finally, the attempts to insert the gene into autologous hematopoietic stem cells and others.

3 TECHNICAL SUPPORT: THE TOOL-KIT

Technical support systems are of critical importance for doing studies. While certain of these, such as transgenic animals, have their maximum impact on the preclinical phases, as a group they are essential for successful clinical development. By definition, if a candidate product is to enter development following in-house research, all the necessary preclinical support would have been available and successful; but there would also be a need to establish the protocol requirements for their use in the clinical development program, including timely availability and budget.

With a licensed candidate it would be essential to establish the support required, to confirm its quality and availability, and to budget and schedule its use. Although on a system-organ basis the clinical methodology may well mimic that needed for the development of a small molecule, the laboratory based backup is highly likely to differ widely. Many of the diagnoses will be made at a molecular level as well as based on clinical parameters. Equally, while the "usual" biochemistry and hematology monitoring will proceed, other candidate-specific laboratory measures such as cytokine levels, antibody levels, and receptor densities will be critical to the trials.

3.1 Transgenic Animals

In addition to their much-publicized uses in the production of humanized proteins, transgenic animals have become highly relevant to the understanding of the disease itself as well as to its treatment. Genes have been inserted into the mammalian germ cell line by direct physical techniques or retroviral transduction; the recipients have been one-cell embryos, cleavage-stage embryos, or even embryonic stem cells.

Ignoring any subtleties of the regulatory control regions, gene insertion can add or delete function. In germ cells the addition of function is frequently dominant in the expression of the phenotype whereas loss of function is usually recessive, requiring both alleles to be inactivated. This can be achieved by interbreeding the heterozygotic animals, with the production of "knockout" animals. With these knockout methods various inherited metabolic diseases can be simulated. In the mouse, deletion of function of the hypoxanthine-guanine phosphoribosyl-transferase (HPRT) gene produces a model for Lesch-Nyhan syndrome.[1] Many other metabolic models have also been generated.

In skin disease, one of the key problems for researchers is that while many skin disorders share similar symptoms they are genetically heterogeneous.[2] Transgenic models enable the determination of the contribution of a particular gene mutation to a given phenotype. With this methodology models of epidermolysis bullosa simplex, epidermolytic hyperkeratoses, the over expression of TGF-alpha and TGF-beta, and the actions of various oncogenes and tumor suppressor genes, for example, are being explored.

Given both the genetic contribution to diseases such as in leukemias and genetic neutropenias, as well as the use of hemopoietic stem cells harvested from the peripheral blood as alternatives to bone marrow transplantation in the management of malignancy, hemopoiesis is a key area for exploration. Here the roles of the cytokines such as G-CSF, GM-CSF, SCF, IL-3, IL-6 and so on, are critical. Although there exists a naturally occurring model of Kostmann's syndrome in the collie dog, other models of under- or overexpression of these cytokines need to be developed. For example, Metcalf[3] has explored the overproduction of GM-CSF in a transgenic mouse model in which excessive transcription of GM-CSF occurs in transgenic macrophages. While these mice tend to die prematurely in middle age, it has been noted that none have developed myeloid leukemia, a counter to the concern that the administration of CSFs in man may itself lead to leukemic transformation.

Another notable area of study of transgenic animals is neoplasia. While it is important to recognize that tumors in transgenic animals cannot be used as strict analogs of naturally occurring tumors,[4] oncogenes and proto-oncogenes have been used to generate tumor-bearing animals. Such models afford the possibilities, not only of drug candidate screening, but also the important area of surrogate marker detection in an attempt to predict therapeutic benefit.

It is important to note that, as the single gene manipulative techniques become more routine, strategies are developing involving the combination of candidate transgenes. For example, Barrett and Mullins[5] note that with the introduction of rat renin and angiotensinogen transgenes into the mouse, neither transgene alone affected blood pressure but in combination they caused hypertension. These authors feel that further experiments will give insight into the components of blood pressure regulation.

What is the relevance of transgenic animals for early phase clinical trials? First, an established model will reassure both in-house, as well as external ethics committees, regulators, etc. that the proposed work is justified in terms of potential efficacy and safety. More importantly and directly, however, the measurement of change in the model will contribute useful data in the difficult areas of dose-selection and therapeutic ratios in human studies.

There is always a tendency to measure "everything in sight" in early phase studies; such measurements are frequently useful when an occurrence in a later study needs explanation or corroboration; more frequently, however, they are simply a data-management burden, with the risk of outlying values which are difficult to explain, and causing concern to all parties. Using the knowledge gleaned from the transgenic animal model one can safely target the primary variables and limit the collection of data of secondary importance.

Equally important is the potential to correlate changes in the molecular biology with those of the pathology and symptomatology. Notwithstanding the reticence of regulators to accept surrogate endpoints; with the majority of diseases such endpoints form a basis for dose selection and titration in phase II studies. Only in the longer term phase III studies can the surrogates be tested against disease outcomes.

3.2 Cell Separation Techniques

In general, cells can be separated out of a mixed population by using techniques based on antigenic properties and structural and physical differences. Separation can be negative (deplete contaminants) or positive. Of major importance is the ability to select CD 34+ hemopoietic progenitor cells for techniques such as *ex vivo* expansion and autologous transfusion in oncology regimens, as well as for gene therapy.

3.2.1 Fluorescence-Activated Cell Sorting (FACS)

This technique uses cell structure and morphology. Cells flow through a sensing zone where optical and/or electrical signals are generated or measured. This is combined with the use of specific antigenic and morphological properties which allows separation of a highly purified cell population. The length of the procedure and the dilution of the target population are disadvantages, and cell viability and any possible effects of laser light have raised questions.

3.2.2 Physical Parameter Selection

Density gradient centrifugation and centrifugal counter flow elution (using size as well as density) can be costly but very effective in, for example, depleting T cells and pre-purifying bone marrow.

3.3 Immuno-Adsorption Techniques

3.3.1 Panning

After initial density gradient centrifugation, target cells are immobilized by specific antibodies fixed to the reaction site. This technique is still relatively labor intensive with multiple washing cycles and releasing the cells without damage can prove difficult.

3.3.2 Immune Adsorption Ferromagnetic Beads

This technique uses micro, middle-sized, or large beads, with a combination of labeling with antibody and superparamagnetic beads and separation via magnetic fields to trap target cells. The equipment is less expensive but it is difficult to detach all the magnetic beads from the selected cells, even with the use of an enzyme or competing polyclonal antibody.

3.3.3 Column Chromatography

Cells are labeled with biotinylated antibody and then passed under continuous flow through an avidin-treated column. A gentle agitation then releases the selected cells from the avidin-biotin-antibody complex. This technique is reliable and reproducible with high viability and functionality of the cells, and is available in "kit" form (Ceprate® from Cellpro®). The ability to select up to 10^9 cells in a few hours is making this an increasingly popular tool.

3.4 Polymerase Chain Reaction (PCR)

The availability of PCR to amplify DNA has revolutionized DNA manipulation and represents a major advance in molecular biology.[6] Using PCR it is possible to selectively synthesize regions of DNA, amplifying genes for genetic screening, diagnosing viral diseases (e.g., hepatitis C and HIV), HLA subtype, etc. Beginning with a single molecule of DNA, the PCR can generate 100 billion similar molecules in a few hours. PCR technology has changed the relevance of certain endpoints in clinical studies. For example, studies of interferons in hepatitis C relied primarily upon liver function tests to determine efficacy; while this is still so, it is equally clear that the presence or absence of the viral particles can be shown with great sensitivity using PCR and could influence treatment algorithms. Now that quantitative PCR is routinely available, antiviral studies in particular have a reliable measure of change in viral load; a technique much valued in HIV studies.

3.5 DNA/RNA Probes

To identify an individual gene directly from genetic material requires a very specific probe that reacts only with that particular sequence. The usual technique is to use a radioactive probe whose hybridization with the gene is assayed by autoradiography. Although originally mRNA itself was used as a probe, this has now been superseded by the use of a cloned cDNA copy of the mRNA. The DNA of the genome is broken down with a restriction digest and then electrophoresed on agarose gel. After "blotting" of the gel onto nitrocellulose, and hybridization with the radioactive probe for the particular sequence, autoradiography identifies the reacting sequences. When performed with DNA it is known as Southern blotting after its inventor. For RNA, with changes in the technique, it is known as Northern blotting.

4 PERSPECTIVE

A review of published literature shows wide variation in the approaches taken during phase I/II studies of biotechnology products. It could help to have seen a clear unifying strategy in therapeutic approaches, but this has not emerged to date. With the exception of the technical and preclinical elements noted above it seems that thus far, no other common factors clearly dictate the best route for clinical development.

In the early stage of biotech product development, there is, without exception, a putative biological mechanism of action and a defined site of action at a molecular level. It is critical to establish in phase I the delivery to the proposed site of action using autoradiograph studies in animals and pharmacokinetic studies in humans. Fortunately, most biotech molecules reach their target following intravenous injection. However, in certain treatments of tumors, and in some specific CVS indications such as restenosis, local administration is essential either to reduce systemic effects and/or to reach the desired site.

5 GENE THERAPY — SENSE AND ANTISENSE

To demonstrate the wide diversity of approaches of phase I/II work a selected area of biotech development will be examined. Perhaps the area of gene therapy, arguably as far away from the classical small molecule work as currently possible, will serve this purpose.

5.1 Sense

Early initiatives in gene therapy have been twofold; gene insertion to identify cells (gene-marking protocols) and gene therapy itself, targeted at diseases caused by single gene defects. The first approved clinical gene transfer took place in May 1989 when the NeoR (the neomycin resistance gene obtained from *E. coli*) was transduced into tumor infiltrating lymphocytes (TIL) using a retroviral vector. After *ex vivo* cell expansion the TIL were reinfused into the patients suffering with advanced cancer, along with similarly derived and expanded but unmarked TIL. Blood sampling, PCR, and NeoR probes indicated the safe and effective expression of the gene over a time-course of about three weeks.[7] Note that the cells were treated *ex vivo*, thus allowing sampling in order to show cell viability and active gene expression. When readministered to man the questions to answer included:

Do the cells stay viable?
Is their intravascular disposition modified in any way?
Did the inserted gene remain active, and for how long?
Was there an immune response, and to what?

The first therapeutic protocol was approved and conducted in the NIH and involved two young girls suffering from ADA deficient SCID. The defect originates on chromosome 20 and causes high levels of adenosine and deoxyadenosine which is toxic to T and B lymphocytes. Although weekly injections of pegylated bovine ADA have been shown to reduce systemic deoxyadenosine levels and reduce the frequency and severity of infections, it is felt to be important to produce ADA within the T cells themselves to better correct the disease phenotype.[8] The initial protocol used autologous T cells transduced with a retroviral vector (LASN) that expressed the human ADA and NeoR. The corrected T cells were detectable for 6 months after the cell infusions were stopped. A later protocol in ADA is, in addition, transferring autologous hemopoietic stem cells transduced with a different, hence differentiable, vector (G2NaSvAd). It is hoped that the T cells from the stem cells will continue to be produced long term and that any deficiencies in the immune repertoire from the initial limited variety of T cells will eventually be overcome.

Decisions in this area involve disease targets, gene transfer vectors, and target tissues. The disease targets will range from single gene defects such as cystic fibrosis (cystic fibrosis transmembrane conductance regulator gene), ADA, Gaucher's disease (glucocerebrosidase gene), muscular dystrophy (dystrophin gene), etc. through to approaches in the management of cancer. Sikora[9] reviews six cancer strategies under development:

1. Genetic tagging: can help decision making, e.g., detecting the source of failure in autologous bone marrow transplantation. Phase I/II studies also need to address the reliability (false-positives, false-negatives) as well as the safety of these techniques.
2. Enhancing tumor immunogenicity. *Ex vivo* modified tumor cells can be used as and anti-tumor "vaccine." Phase I/II studies must map the immune response to such vaccines, and explore its specificity to the tumor cells.
3. Vectoring cytokines to tumors. The TNF gene can, for example, be inserted into TIL targeted at melanoma cells.
4. Inserting drug-activating genes. Promoters of tumor gene can be coupled with an enzyme such as cytosine deaminase to metabolize intracellular flucytosine to fluorouracil. Specificity and leakage from tumor cells causing systemic toxicity need to be assessed.
5. Suppressing oncogenes-antisense (see below). In this area, studies need to examine whether it reaches the cell and the gene, and specifically inactivates it.
6. Replacing defective tumor suppressor genes.

To this list can be added supportive therapy such as the addition of the multidrug resistance gene (MDR1) to autologous stem cells to protect them from chemotherapy. Many questions arise. Are such cells immortal? Is the MDR1 effective enough to allow higher/longer chemotherapy and to what benefit? Is the chemotherapy still limited by, e.g., mucositis, diarrhea, etc?

Looking at the transfer vectors the majority of approved studies have used retroviral vectors for transduction. The viral genes are disabled or removed so that viral proteins are not produced in infected cells. An adenovirus vector was used to deliver the CTFR gene to the airway epithelium, the most important site in terms of health of the CF patient. Early successes in animals have included liposome-mediated transfer, hepatocyte receptor complexing and internalization, and targeting the transferrin receptor.

Miller states the advantages and disadvantages as follows:

Retroviral vector:	High efficiency of transfer into dividing cells
	Gene transferred into cellular DNA but:
	No transfer to nondividing cells
	Cannot be purified to homogeneity
	Potential for helper virus production
	Safety and production issues
Adenoviral vector:	Potential to carry larger segments of DNA
	Can infect nonreplicating cells
	Can infect *in situ* (e.g., lung) but:
	Does not integrate into chromosomal DNA
	May stimulate immune system
	Safety and production issues
Nonviral:	Can be purified to homogeneity
	Can target cell-specific receptor but:
	Not yet as efficient as the virus at entering nuclei and entering cells, and becoming integrated

The target cells thus far transduced include, for example, T cells, TIL, hemopoietic stem cells, hepatocytes, muscle cells, and tumor cells, but many others are being explored. Interestingly, genes can be transferred into muscle cells by direct injection of DNA, and experiments are now exploring the use of myoblasts and stem cells from other tissues.

Apart from the largely historic concerns noted about viral vectors, there is another safety risk involved when material is "blindly" inserted into chromosomes; namely that of insertional mutagenesis and activation of oncogenes. Although the calculations suggest the risk is extremely low, it is a factor not yet eliminated from the equation and emphasizes the need for long-term followup. Lifetime followup is required by the GTAC. Concerns have also been voiced over the overproduction of, for example, a cytokine. Although from a therapeutic point of view there might be more reasons to fear under- or nonproduction, strategies are being put in place, some with drug-activating enzymes, to eliminate the treated cells should this be desirable.

The long-term goals of gene therapy must encompass the safe and effective *in vivo* delivery of genes into specific cell types, the regulation of which is under natural physiological control.

5.2 Antisense

In the antisense approach, modified oligonucleotides (oligos, for short) are used to block mRNA actions. A key application here is the unraveling of functionality as well as the potential for therapy. It is clearly important to distinguish between gene products that are simply associated with a functional state as opposed to those that regulate function.[10] Three strategies are available:[11]

1. Binding to mRNA, cytoplasmic mRNA, or nuclear localized precursor hnRNA (antisense)
2. Binding at DNA to form a triple helix (antigene)
3. Anti-protein agents, preventing recognition of nucleic acid sequences by proteins

Stein and Cheng in their excellent review[12] have identified six criteria that therapeutic oligos binding to cytoplamic RNA must fulfil:

1. Easy bulk synthesis
2. Stable *in vivo*
3. Able to enter target cell
4. Retained by target cell
5. Interact with cellular targets
6. Do not interact in a nonsequence-specific manner with other macromolecules.

Phase I trials to evaluate the safety of these compounds have started in cancer patients. A phosphothioateoligo complimentary to the p53 mRNA has been administered to a patient with refractory myelogenous leukemia. Another trial using a methylphosphonate oligo for purging autologous marrow in myelogenous leukemia has been designed. An antisense c-myb 18-mer blocked accumulation of intimal smooth muscle cells in a rat with left carotid injury, raising the possibility of a mechanism to block restenosis after coronary artery angioplasty.[13] Finally, experiments have shown success using viral-suppressive oligos, e.g., offering potential in HIV-1 RT.

Questions remain surrounding the duration of action, effectiveness of long-term treatment, usefulness of action in solid tumors, and absorbability for topical viral therapy. Good animal models of human malignancy will be essential and, in particular, knowledge of which oncogenes are dominant, before useful cancer management will become possible.

6 CONCLUSIONS

Gabbay[14] has conducted a pilot survey with a sample of companies involved with biotech developments; interestingly it detected issues which raised as much concern as it suggested opportunity. Interviewees stressed that biotech compounds are all different and that it was often hard to predict the clinical indications. Companies agreed that the major safety issues surround antigenicity. Although they felt that more toxicology was performed than necessary, there was concern expressed over possible genotoxic effects.

In the preclinical arena, the tracking of naturally occurring molecules causes difficulties, and the need for validated animal models remains.

In the clinic, the wide diversity of potential clinical indications may lead to defocusing. Furthermore, many of the diseases studied lack good surrogates and have inadequate outcome measures. Some respondees asked for more guidelines.

In conclusion, it seems wisest to approach the development of biotech compounds with cautious optimism directed mainly by the clinical indication under study. Close cooperation with the in-house scientists will facilitate both the preclinical work (including animal models) as well as ensuring that the technical support for clinical work is available at the correct time. Finally, it is worth emphasizing that significant input in the design and running of the phase I/II trials needs to come from the bench scientists who built the molecule.

REFERENCES

1. Hooper ML, Hardy K, Handyside A et al., HPRT-deficient (Lesch-Nyhan) mouse embryos derived from germline colonization by cultured cells. *Nature,* 1987; 326:292-295.
2. Rothnagel JA, Greenhalgh DA, Wang X-J et al., Transgenic models of skin diseases. *Arch. Dermatol.,* 1993; 129:1430-1436.
3. Metcalf D. Transgenic mice as models of hemopoiesis. *Cancer,* 1991, Suppl. May 15; 67:2695-2699.
4. Liggitt HD and Reddington GM. Transgenic animals etc. *Xenobiotica,* 1992; 22 (9/10):1043-1054.
5. Barrett GL and Mullins JJ. Strategies towards a transgenic model of essential hypertension. *Biochem. Pharmacol.,* 1992; 43(5):925-930.
6. Markham AF. The polymerase chain reaction: a tool for molecular medicine. *BMJ,* 1993; 306:441-446.
7. Anderson WF. Human gene therapy. *Science,* 1992; 256:808-813.
8. Miller AD. Human gene therapy comes of age. *Nature,* 1992; 357:455-460.
9. Sikora K. Genes, dreams and cancer. *Br. Med. J.,* 1994; 308:1217-1221.
10. Ferrari S, Manfredini R, Grande A, and Torelli U. Antisense strategies to characterise the role of genes and oncogenes involved in myeloid differentiation. *Ann. N.Y. Acad. Sci.,* .
11. Carter G and Lemoine NR. Antisense technology for cancer therapy; does it make sense? *Br. J. Cancer,* 1993; 67:869-876.
12. Stein CA and Cheng Y-C. Antisense oligonucleotides as therapeutic agents — is the bullet really magical? *Science,* 19XX; 261:1004-1012.
13. Simons M, Edelman ER, DeKeyser J-L et al., Antisense c-myb ligonucleotides inhibit intimal arterial smooth muscle cell accumulation *in vivo. Nature,* 1992; 359:67-70.
14. Gabbay FJ. Drug development and Regulatory issues with Biotechnology. Paper presented at ICPM, in Rome, April 1994.

Part III. Ethical and Legal Considerations

Chapter 9

Ethical Aspects of Research in Healthy Volunteers

Steven J. Warrington

CONTENTS

1 Introduction 103
2 Justice 103
3 Beneficence 104
4 Non-Maleficence 104
5 Respect for Autonomy 105
5.1 Consent 105
6 Payment 106
7 Recruitment 107
8 Special Groups 108
8.1 Students 108
8.2 Staff 108
8.3 The Impoverished 108
8.4 Children 109
8.5 Women of Childbearing Potential 109
8.6 Elderly 109
8.7 Prisoners 109
References 109

1 INTRODUCTION

Let us begin by making a series of statements with which no reasonable person is likely to disagree:

1. Society derives great benefit from our existing stock of medicines, many of which have been generated by research programs which include experiments done in healthy volunteers.
2. Present and future research programs will yield new medicines which will be of great value to society.
3. The development of medicines would be slower, more difficult, and more expensive without the participation of healthy volunteers, but it could be done, nevertheless.
4. Delay in development of medicines is to the disadvantage of patients.
5. The extra costs of development of drugs are borne by patients, consumers, and taxpayers, not by the manufacturer.

Thus, we cannot escape the early conclusion that research in healthy volunteers can yield benefits for society. If it were not so, further discussion of the ethics of such research would be pointless, since an activity which entails even an infinitesimal risk to life or health but which produces no benefits for anyone must be unethical. The real ethical difficulties arise in the consideration of how studies in volunteers should be organized and executed. Before confronting these problems, I shall consider how some general ethical principles impinge upon research in volunteers.

Ethics are a reasoned analysis of moral duty. For the purpose of this discussion, we might take our moral duties to be as follows (Beauchamp and Childress, 1983): justice — being fair; beneficence — doing good; non-maleficence — not doing harm; and respect for autonomy — allowing the individual to determine what happens to him or her.

2 JUSTICE

The moral duty of justice requires us to be fair in our treatment of others. Thus, our treatment of volunteers should be equitable: they should be compensated adequately for inconvenience, discomfort,

0-8493-9230-6/97/$0.00+$.50
© 1997 by CRC Press, Inc.

and loss of time when participating in studies, and this is an ethical justification for the payment of research subjects. The duty to be just also clearly requires us to ensure that volunteers are properly and promptly compensated for any injury arising from their participation in a study, irrespective of the question of legal liability. Thus, justice here gives the individual rights in addition to any to which he is entitled under the law.

The principle of fairness may also require us to study volunteers instead of, or in addition to, patients. Should not we healthy members of society share with victims of disease the burden of helping in the development of medicines from which there is no certainty that those victims will benefit?

3 BENEFICENCE

Beneficence requires that our actions should, when possible, benefit others. While it is clear that conducting research in healthy volunteers complies with this requirement in so far as the wider community is concerned, it might seem at first sight that we fail in our duty to do good to the individual volunteer. In fact, the volunteer may benefit in several ways. Most obviously, she (or he, as I shall write from now onward) gains financially. Furthermore, the experience of participation in a study may well be socially rewarding in that it involves contact with doctors, nurses, technical staff, and other volunteers. And is it not pleasant sometimes to be the center of attention, and to have one's slightest complaints taken seriously and recorded for posterity? Nor is it flippant to suggest that volunteers may regard as a benefit the opportunity to contribute to the welfare of others. In the special case of medical students, participation in a research study allows them to gain insight into the experiences of their patients — so benefiting both the student and his future patients.

Beneficence imposes upon us a powerful ethical obligation to maintain the highest standards in the design and execution of research. A badly designed study is unethical because it fails to yield as much useful data as a well-designed one. A badly executed project is even worse; it offends against both beneficence and non-maleficence, for not only will the yield of the experiment be less than it might have been, but also the risk of injury to the volunteers must be greater.

A final consideration is that beneficence requires us to be nice to our volunteers, just as we should be nice to our patients (Gillon, 1986). None of us can claim to be nice to all of our patients or volunteers all of the time, and it follows that we are each more or less frequently guilty of (mildly) unethical behavior. Because we are not generally condemned because of these lapses, it follows that occasional unethical behavior is condoned. Presumably the medical duty of beneficence is realistically regarded as an ideal to which we should aspire, rather than as a norm to which we must conform.

4 NON-MALEFICENCE

At first sight, observance of the duty not to harm others might appear to preclude the use of healthy volunteers in research, since no study can be entirely without risk. Indeed, if the principle of non-maleficence is accepted as absolute *(primum non nocere* — above all, do no harm), then almost all medical activities would cease. Clearly, non-maleficence must be linked with beneficence and cannot have complete priority over it. The risk of causing harm has always to be seen relative to the benefits to be derived, and *primum non nocere* has to be rejected as a strict instruction, although it remains a useful and pithy reminder of the dangers of medical intervention. Thus, the duty of the physician conducting research in healthy volunteers must be to minimize the risks and to maximize the benefits. If risks are to be minimized, the investigator must be highly trained, experienced, and conscientious. Similarly, beneficence requires extreme competence in the investigator in order that the obligation to do good may be fulfilled.

Although non-maleficence cannot be an absolute principle, it clearly is a crucial one when the ethics of research in volunteers are considered. All agree that the risk of injury to volunteers in research should be kept to an extremely low level, and the safety record to date does appear to be good (Cardon et al., 1976; Royle and Snell, 1986; Vere, 1988; Orme et al., 1989). However, problems do arise in defining what is meant by an "extremely low" level of risk. Should participation in a research study be as safe as crossing the road (what road? at traffic lights? on a pedestrian crossing? in rain or sunshine?), smoking ten cigarettes (low, middle, or high tar? inhaled or not?), traveling in a passenger aircraft (how far? how many take offs and landings?), or working in a mine or on a construction site?

Cardon et al. (1976) deduced that the risks of participation in nontherapeutic research were no greater than those in everyday life, as follows. Annual rates for accidental injuries that were temporarily disabling, permanently disabling, and fatal were, respectively, 50, 2, and 0.6 per 1000 Americans. The corresponding figures for a population of nearly 100,000 U.S. research subjects were 0.37, 0.01, and 0 per 1000. These authors reasoned that, since the average duration of a study might be about one hundredth of a year, the risks of nontherapeutic studies were similar to those of everyday life. The only real weakness in this argument is that the incidence of adverse events in nontherapeutic research was probably underestimated: the authors used a postal questionnaire and telephone calls to investigators to quantify adverse events occurring during the previous 3 years, and this would surely lead to substantial under reporting. Furthermore, the 15% of investigators classified as "nonresponders" might well have encountered more adverse events than those who did respond.

These workers' findings, although not above criticism, are at least corroborated by surveys of volunteer studies in the U.K. (Royle and Snell, 1986; Orme et al., 1989). A finding common to both U.S. and U.K. studies was the high frequency of minor adverse symptoms occurring in relation to research studies, but Reidenberg and Lowenthal (1968) found a remarkably similar frequency of such symptoms in people who had not received either active medication or placebo.

Balancing non-maleficence against beneficence in volunteer studies is by no means the same thing as balancing risks and benefits in the treatment of patients. The crucial difference is that no volunteer research is ethically acceptable if it entails more than a tiny risk of injury, and this remains true however large the rewards to the volunteer and however great the value of the project to society in general. In contrast, extreme risks may be taken quite ethically in the therapy of a life-threatening condition — although such risks should be accepted only with the patient's knowledge and consent (in other words, with due respect for autonomy). Non-maleficence obliges us to keep risk of injury in any experiment to an extremely low level, while beneficence requires that we maximize the benefit that is derived from research.

5 RESPECT FOR AUTONOMY

Respect for autonomy signifies our obligation to preserve the right of the individual to determine what should or should not be done to him. In the context of our moral duties to healthy volunteers, this obligation clearly has priority over justice, beneficence, and non-maleficence. We cannot, for example, ethically coerce anyone to participate in a research study on the grounds either that enormous benefits would flow from such participation or that great harm would ensue if the experiment were not done. Nor can we insist that justice requires that the subject share with others the burden of developing a drug or testing a hypothesis.

5.1 Consent

Respect for autonomy is almost tangibly expressed in the universal requirement that a person must give his consent to participate as a volunteer in a research project. The obtaining of consent is one area in which ethical obligations coincide with legal requirements (Dodds-Smith, 1985). The autonomy of the volunteer is manifestly abused if he is pressed into agreement to participate, or if he gives consent on the basis of inadequate information; if it is to be valid, consent must be both informed and freely given. We must give the subject a fair description of what will be done to him and what the risks of discomfort or injury are. The information has to be given in a form that the volunteer can understand; we fail in our ethical duties if we supply comprehensive but incomprehensible explanations. One potentially satisfactory way to inform volunteers about a study is to provide them with a detailed leaflet, the contents of which have been reviewed by both medical and nonmedical assessors, and some ethical committees can provide invaluable help with such a review. Verbal explanation of a study may be ethically satisfactory but has two severe drawbacks: it is inaccessible to critical review, and it is unlikely to be as fresh after multiple repetition as it was when first propounded. Written information is, of course, valuable, but the volunteer must also have the opportunity to ask questions of the investigator.

The subject must also be of sufficient maturity and intelligence to understand the implications of the study; I shall return later to the ethical problems of nontherapeutic research in children, who by their very nature lack maturity (if not intelligence). Whereas the investigator may have little difficulty in assessing approximately the level of a volunteer's intelligence, the detection of psychopathology is a knottier problem altogether. How many physicians responsible for phase I units would claim to be able at the prestudy examination to spot, say, a patient with treated schizophrenia? Such patients are sometimes said to appear more normal than normal people. Not only is the validity of such a patient's consent in serious doubt, but also the long-term medication of psychiatric illness may interact — perhaps fatally

(Darragh et al., 1985) — with the drug being studied. Invalid consent offends against the principle of respect for autonomy, and placing the volunteer at appreciable risk offends against non-maleficence to a degree which surely none would find acceptable. The investigator is therefore ethically bound to notify the volunteer's personal physician of the subject's intended participation in a study. In the U.K., at least, individuals must very rarely receive treatment for chronic illness without their general practitioner's knowledge.

The validity of consent is perhaps most often questioned on the grounds that the potential subject is not adequately informed. However, we should also question whether consent is truly "freely given." Does the promise of a large financial reward compromise the volunteer's autonomy by inducing him to consent to procedures which he would otherwise be too afraid to want to undergo? If a teacher suggests to his student that participation in a study might be interesting and worthwhile, can the student's consent subsequently be regarded as valid? Similar reservations must be held about the use of junior staff in research projects, in both academic and industrial environments. I shall return to these questions when considering the problems of recruitment and payment of special groups of volunteers.

6 PAYMENT

There is no fundamental objection to the payment of volunteers; for example, in the armed forces volunteers have never been rewarded any less than conscripts. Failure to reward volunteers for their efforts would offend against justice and beneficence, whereas excessive reward must compromise the subject's autonomy. Relating the reward to the perceived risk would not in itself be ethically wrong; many U.K. readers will recall that, in the debate on the remuneration of coal-miners, the risks to which these workers are exposed were generally accepted as a justification for paying them well. It is rather the exposure of volunteers to anything other than negligible risk which would be unacceptable, offending as it does against justice and non-maleficence.

The issue, then, is not whether volunteers should be rewarded, but how much they should be given. I find it helpful to regard participation in a study as analogous to doing part-time unskilled work — although lawyers would object to such an analogy on the grounds that volunteers lack all the legal rights (and obligations) which have been granted to employees. If we pay our volunteers at rates similar to those which apply locally to part-time unskilled workers, then the individual has, except in time or areas of high unemployment, the freedom to choose between a research study and (say) lugging carpets around a warehouse. Participation in a research study carries a risk of mild and moderate adverse symptoms, and a very small risk of severe injury, but so, too, do most unskilled jobs. For example, work on a construction site is notoriously dangerous, and even in a warehouse one might be crushed by a falling roll of carpet or transfixed by a forklift truck. Payment of volunteers at locally available rates for part-time work should help us to fulfill the moral duties of justice and respect for autonomy. Beneficence, on the other hand, might encourage us to reward the volunteers at higher rates, and such generosity may surely be ethically acceptable on occasion; the difficulty is in deciding at what point the size of the reward compromises the subject's autonomy and becomes ethically dubious. Furthermore, the analogy with part-time work is not helpful in assessing the correct level of reward for undergoing a safe but uncomfortable procedure such as swallowing an orogastric or nasogastric tube. The opinion of lay people, including lay members of ethical committees, may be a valuable guide.

One unexpected problem associated with large payments is that the very size of the payment may make the volunteer believe that the study involves a substantial risk, even when it is quite safe. Medical students at least "expected to be rewarded for taking risks as well as for inconvenience" (Chaput de Saintonge et al., 1988). As investigators, we concern ourselves mainly with what we believe to be the actual risks of the study; for the volunteers, in contrast, it is the perceived rather than the actual risk which may do the damage.

What are the moral duties of the investigator whose valuable (and ethical) research is stymied because the supply of volunteers is inadequate? If he follows the analogy with part-time work, he should simply increase the size of the reward until sufficient volunteers come forward. Is this ethical? The answer is not straightforward. I have already concluded (and you will have agreed) that the research must involve no more than a tiny risk of severe injury, and that volunteers may be rewarded for both time spent and discomfort suffered. If insufficient volunteers come forward, should the project be delayed or abandoned, or should it be more widely advertised, or should the payment be increased? What should be the attitude of the ethics committee to this problem? Abandoning a valuable project offends against beneficence; wider advertising has its own problems (see below), and increasing the payment may compromise the subject's autonomy, particularly in the case of the impoverished. The reader of this book may find it hard to believe that such a modest sum as t:600 (about $1000) could persuade anyone to submit himself to a research procedure against his inclination and better judgment, but a straw poll of students in London suggested that this might indeed be the case. The argument that the "reluctant volunteer" is happy with his money, and that his health has not been placed at risk, is not tenable; we know, albeit from anecdotal reports, that some volunteers do regret their participation and feel guilty that they risked (as they see it) their health in return for a reward.

The resolution of these difficulties must lie in a compromise between the investigator's conflicting ethical duties. This may mean some delay in finishing the project, which may, in turn, delay or reduce the good which is achieved, somewhat wider advertising and higher payments, which may compromise the autonomy of susceptible individuals. Ethics committees can be genuinely valuable in helping the investigator to balance these conflicting issues, although researchers often feel that the committees underestimate the value of their projects and that they function mainly as guardians of the volunteer's welfare.

Some investigators attempt to circumvent or diminish the ethical difficulties of payments to volunteers by making payment "in kind" — that is, with goods rather than cash. This maneuver is clearly ludicrous (although not necessarily unethical), because goods which are desirable in the volunteers' eyes are as much of an inducement as cash; and if the goods provided are not desirable to the volunteer, he will feel cheated, and valuable research funds will have been wasted. Thus, the investigator fails miserably in his duties of justice, beneficence, and non-maleficence.

Another ploy which aims to reduce the ethical difficulties of paying volunteers is not to announce the payment until the study is completed. This is not so disastrous a scheme as payment in kind, but nevertheless creates more ethical problems than it solves. Potential volunteers learn mainly from their peers of the existence of research units, and thus are well aware of the "going rate" for participation in studies. If the volunteer is genuinely in ignorance of the likely payment until the very end of the study, what are we to do if he is profoundly dissatisfied with what he receives? Will the volunteer correctly accuse us of failing in our obligations to be just, beneficent, and non-maleficent (though he will probably use more blunt terminology)? "Ah yes", you may say, "but we will avoid such a scene by paying our subjects so well that no one will be disgruntled"; but this, too, is ethically unsound, since payments which *everyone* would regard as generous must surely be an excessive inducement to a sizable minority.

Subjects who have to withdraw from a study for medical reasons relating to the medication or procedures are normally given payment in full, which seems fair. Should subjects be told in advance that they will be treated thus? If they are told, might they not be inclined to magnify (or even invent) adverse symptoms in order to receive their fee earlier and in return for less effort ("work")? This would lead to misleading conclusions about the drug, which might be to the detriment of the manufacturer, other volunteers, and future patients. On the other hand, if the volunteer believes that he has to complete the study in order to receive full payment, he might stoically minimize and endure unpleasant symptoms — to the detriment of both himself and (possibly) future recipients of the drug. Thus, neither policy is free from offense against justice, non-maleficence, and respect for autonomy. One compromise might be not to inform the subject that he will receive full payment if he has to be withdrawn, unless and until he experiences anything more than trivial adverse symptoms; this places a heavy responsibility upon the investigator to enquire energetically into any hint that the volunteer might be suffering unduly. This is evidently not entirely satisfactory, but then neither are the alternatives.

7 RECRUITMENT

Volunteers should be recruited by means of a general notice rather than by direct approach, which might compromise the subject's autonomy — particularly in the case of students or staff within the researcher's institution. However, I see no ethical objection to supplying, by letter or telephone call, information about forthcoming studies to individuals who have previously participated in research projects — the so-called "volunteer panel." General advertising for volunteers is often regarded as suspect and is, remarkably, condemned without explanation in the current Association of the British Pharmaceutical Industry *Guidelines for Medical Experiments in Non-Patient Volunteers* (ABPI, 1988); perhaps this is a reflection of the restrictions upon doctors' freedom to advertise. In fact, there is strong ethical justification for advertising for volunteers. The duty of justice surely obliges us to distribute the opportunity to volunteer equally among those who might wish to do so, and it is hard to see how this offends against beneficence, non-maleficence, or respect for autonomy. The "targeting" of advertising at the impoverished is unethical, not because it is wrong to offer to the poor the opportunity to volunteer, but because it is wrong to deprive others of the same opportunity.

Advertisements for volunteers may reasonably mention payment, but should not give any indication of the amount. Failure to mention the fact of payment is ethically unsatisfactory, because it deprives the individual of information which is important in forming a decision about whether to volunteer. On the other hand, the size of the payment cannot be correctly interpreted by the subject unless it is accompanied by the full details of the study, and such details are unlikely to be contained in any advertisement.

8 SPECIAL GROUPS

8.1 Students

Students have long been used as research subjects in the study of both pharmacology and physiology. I have already alluded to the question of whether consent can be deemed to be freely given when the volunteer is a student and the investigator his teacher, but this is not the only ethical objection. The student might also feel undue pressure not to disappoint the teacher/investigator by withdrawing from the study, or might be diffident about "giving up" in front of his classmates or friends. In class experiments, the subject might well be reluctant to divulge full medical information. The widespread use of students in studies at their own teaching hospital seems to be an example of a practice which continues mainly because it has gone on for so long that the ethical issues are not given the consideration which they deserve (Vere, 1986). An acceptable solution in the case of volunteer studies is for researchers to use students from other institutions only, although the arrangement is much less convenient for everyone.

8.2 Staff

The use by academic departments or pharmaceutical companies of their own staff as volunteers raises ethical difficulties similar to those encountered with students. The relationship between the junior and senior staff in an academic unit is not unlike that between student and teacher, but the head of department has even greater control over the destiny of his juniors than does the teacher over his students. Thus, questions must arise in relation to respect for autonomy; the validity of consent and freedom to withdraw from the study are particularly threatened.

The ethical considerations are no less troublesome if junior staff volunteer to participate in their colleagues' studies. Beneficence requires that we help our peers whenever we can do so, and justice seems to demand that the action of volunteering be reciprocated. These duties may lead to disturbing or intolerable conflict with autonomy both at the stage of consent ("He agreed to participate in my paracetamol single-dose pharmacokinetic study; am I not therefore obliged to help him similarly with his air embolism tolerance project?") and when the volunteer wishes to withdraw ("If I pull out now, this final study for his Ph.D. thesis will not be finished before he returns to Matabeleland").

Pharmaceutical manufacturers are no doubt scrupulously careful not to exert any pressures upon employees to act as volunteers, and to recruit subjects by general notice only. Furthermore, justice might seem to demand that the employees should share the burden of testing a drug from which they might ultimately derive benefit in the form of greater success for their company. On the other hand, there must at least occasionally be a risk that the staff-volunteer's autonomy will be threatened at the stage of consent (when full medical information might not be divulged) or of withdrawal from the study. A further (perhaps purely theoretical) problem is that the status of an employee by its nature requires some surrendering of autonomy, whereas in research respect for the autonomy of the volunteer should be paramount.

8.3 The Impoverished

Justice surely requires not only that the poor should be given opportunity equally with others to act as volunteer subjects, but also that they should receive the same rewards. Furthermore, is not our duty of beneficence better satisfied by the distribution of rewards to the poor than by giving similar rewards to the rich? Unfortunately, there is at least one real ethical problem in the use of impoverished subjects in research: a level of payment which is judged appropriate by normal criteria (see Section 6) might be an excessive inducement to the impecunious. Thus, autonomy might be compromised at the stage of obtaining consent, and non-maleficence when the subject later experiences regret or guilt. The worst possible solution to this ethical conflict would be to lower the level of payment so that only the poor would consider it worthwhile to volunteer, since they would then bear a disproportionate burden and in return would receive a reward which was less than the job demanded. The best that we can do is: to set payments at a level which an ordinary person would consider to be reasonable; to inform the subjects fully, even when they are overeager to complete the formalities and start earning the money; to remain sensitive to any indication that the volunteer is having second thoughts about the wisdom of continuing; and to treat subjects generously if they do decide that participation in research is not for them.

The directing of advertising at the poor or unemployed has been condemned (ABPI, 1988), but is only objectionable on ethical grounds in so far as it implies that the well-to-do and employed are deprived of adequate information. It would be intolerably patronizing to keep the poor in ignorance in order that the ethical issues might simply be "ducked".

8.4 Children

It is impossible to see how children could be considered as true volunteers, because of their inability to give valid consent. The parents' consent to their children's participation could not be accepted, because even a child surely has some expectation of autonomy. Could the "volunteering" of progeny even be a form of "child abuse by proxy"? Justice also demands that the child be rewarded for his efforts, and there are several methods of ensuring that money paid can be kept for the benefit of the child when full age is reached.

8.5 Women of Childbearing Potential

There are no ethical problems which are peculiar to women volunteers; the issues are concerned with safety. Participation in a research study should involve no more than minimal risk, and women of childbearing potential must be excluded from any study which entails risk to the individual or her future offspring. Because these risks are often unquantified until late in the development of the drug, most early studies are done in men. This is regrettable because it offends against the principle of justice and may appear insulting to women who are certain that they intend never to bear any children. Unfortunately, women (and men, of course) are notorious for changing their minds as time goes by.

8.6 Elderly

Because the risk of any given study must inevitably be higher in the elderly than in the young, we should only ask the elderly to volunteer if the risk remains acceptably minute and if the project could not be done equally well in the young. Studies in the elderly may be required by the regulatory authorities, but there must be some doubt as to whether they are always needed. Much is already known about changes in drug disposition with age, and most problems of drug toxicity in the elderly in recent times could have been predicted from studies in the young. The investigator's ethical duties, then, are to ensure that the experiment is really necessary and that the risks are truly negligible. Poverty and mental incapacity may, perhaps, be more common in old age, but the ethical problems arising therefrom are not confined to the elderly.

8.7 Prisoners

Use of prisoners as "volunteers" is now impossible in the U.K., and there is little point in agonizing here over the ethics of the matter. However, the issues involved are most interesting and challenging, and the reader is invited to debate them alone or with others, forearmed with the prejudices formed while reading the preceding pages.

REFERENCES

Association of the British pharmaceutical Industry (1988). *Guidelines for Medical Experiments in Non-Patient Human Volunteers*. ABPI, London.

Beauchamp, T. L. and Childress, J. F. (1983). *Principles of Biomedical Ethics*, 2nd ed. Oxford University Press, Oxford, pp. 148-58.

Cardon, P.-V., Dommel, F. W. Jr. and Trumble, R. R. (1976). Injuries to research subjects — a survey of investigators. *New Engl. J. Med.*, 295, 650-4.

Chaput de Saintonge, D. M., Crane, G. J., Rust, N. D., Karadia, S. and Whittam, L. R. (1988). Modelling determinants of expected rewards in healthy volunteers. *Pharm. Med.*, 3, 45-54.

Darragh, A., Kenny, M., Lambe, R. and Brick, I. (1985). Sudden death of a volunteer. *Lancet*, 1, 93-4.

Dodds-Smith, I. C. (1985). The legal implications of studies in healthy volunteers. *BIRA Jl.*, 4, 88-91.

Gillon, R. (1986). Philosophical medical ethics: Doctors and patients. *Br. Med. J.*, 292, 466-9.

Orme, M., Harry, J. Routledge, P. and Hobson, S. (1989). Healthy volunteer studies in Great Britain: the results of a survey into 12 months' activity in this field. *Br. J. Clin. Pharmacol.*, 27, 125-33.

Reidenberg, M. M. and Lowenthal, D. T. (1968). Adverse nondrug reactions. *New Engl. J. Med.*, 279, 678-9.

Royle, J. M. and Snell, E. S. (1986). Medical research on normal volunteers. *Br. J. Clin. Pharmacol.*, 21, 548-9.

Vere, D. W. (1986). Ethics. In Glenny, H. and Nelmes, P. (Eds.), *Handbook of Clinical Drug Research.* Blackwell Scientific, Oxford, pp. 1-32.

Vere, D. W. (1988). The ethics of adverse drug reactions. *Adverse Drug Reaction Bulletin* No. 128, 480-3.

Chapter 10

Bioethics and Industry: Ethical Aspects of Research in Patients

Frank Wells

CONTENTS

1 Introduction 111
2 Research Ethics Committees 112
3 Informed Consent 113
4 U.K. Department of Health Guidelines 114
5 Good Clinical (Research) Practice 115
6 Fraud and Misconduct in the Context of Clinical Research 115
7 The Reasons for Fraud 115
8 The Detection of Fraud 116
9 The Prosecution of Fraud 117
10 The Ethics of Promotion 117
References 118
Appendix 1 Guidelines for Ethical Approval of Human Pharmacology Studies Carried Out by Pharmaceutical Companies 118
Appendix 2 Guidelines for Research Ethics Committees Considering Studies Conducted in Healthy Volunteers by Pharmaceutical Companies 120

1 INTRODUCTION

Medicines owe their existence to research carried out by pharmaceutical companies, or on their behalf, or to the development of the results of academic research. Before a medicine can be marketed, the pharmaceutical company will have accumulated a great deal of toxicological, pharmacological, and clinical evidence, and will have met all the statutory requirements for the testing, manufacture, and marketing of that product. Quite apart from their voluntary commitment to undertake research and promotion to high ethical standards, companies are required to conform with the comprehensive legislation which exists to safeguard the public by ensuring that all medicines meet standards of quality, efficacy, and safety which are acceptable in the light of present knowledge and experience.

The involvement of patients in clinical trials, which are, to all intents and purposes, experiments, is, understandably, an emotive issue. However, although most members of the public are vaguely aware that clinical trials take place so that medicines can come onto the market, few of them are aware of the full licensing procedure for medicines; equally few of them are aware of the extent to which the pharmaceutical industry collectively is committed to a clinical research program; and only a very small proportion of the population of the countries where research is conducted are aware of their own potential personal involvement. The issue of ethical review of projects and of informed consent is thus of great importance.

Historically, our forebears had a very robust attitude toward medical experimentation; for example, the condemned prisoners in Newgate Gaol in 1721 who volunteered for experimental variolation in return for their freedom (if they survived) probably had few second thoughts. Auto-experiments, which were also popular with physicians in the 19th century, remained in vogue in some departments of physiology until very recently. The major drug disasters of the first half of the 20th century arose because inadequate experimentation was carried out before the medicines came onto the market (A). Two classic examples are the U.S. elixir scandal, in which an untested ethylene glycol solution of sulfanilamide was marketed, and killed over 100 patients, and the similar large-scale disaster which occurred in France when Stanilon, an untested organic compound of tin, was marketed for the treatment of furunculosis. The ethylene glycol tragedy, incidentally, led directly to the establishment in the U.S. of the Food and

0-8493-9230-6/97/$0.00+$.50
© 1997 by CRC Press, Inc.

Drug Administration (FDA). The universal view held now, therefore, is that safeguards — not previously thought necessary — must be in place to protect the interests of the experimental subject.

There is absolute agreement within the pharmaceutical industry that research investigations on human subjects must be conducted in accordance with scientific and ethical codes which are recognized internationally — in particular the Declaration of Helsinki of the World Medical Association, as subsequently modified, most recently at the 41st World Medical Assembly which took place in Hong Kong in 1989.

There are certain statements in this declaration which are highly relevant in this context in which it is appropriate to quote in full:

> The purpose of biomedical research involving human subjects must be to improve diagnostic, therapeutic or prophylactic procedures and the understanding of the aetiology and pathogenesis of disease.
> The design and performance of each experimental procedure involving human subjects should be clearly formulated in an experimental protocol which should be transmitted for consideration, comment and guidance to a specially appointed committee independent of the investigator and the sponsor.
> The research protocol should always contain a statement of the ethical considerations involved and should indicate that the principles enunciated in the present Declaration are complied with.

Because there are so many mixed emotional reactions to the idea of being involved as a guinea pig when ill, ethical guidance and approval is essential before any clinical research involving patients is begun. This is recognized as being most appropriately given by a research ethics committee, or, in the U.S., an institutional review board.

2 RESEARCH ETHICS COMMITTEES

The independent committees referred to in the Declaration of Helsinki perform a pivotal role; neither investigators nor sponsors should be the sole judges of whether their research projects conform to generally accepted guidelines, and therefore all protocols must be submitted for independent review to a research ethics committee. The objectives of such committees are essentially to protect the subjects who are used experimentally in research projects, to preserve or safeguard their rights, and to provide public reassurance. Approval by a research ethics committee not only of protocols for clinical trials but also of investigators conducting such trials also protects these investigators and the institutions where such trials are carried out.

The definitive report on research ethics committees in the U.K. was published in 1990 by the Royal College of Physicians,[9] and is supported by the Association of the British Pharmaceutical Industry (ABPI), which represents virtually all the research-based pharmaceutical companies in the country. Although local research ethics committees have been established within the U.K. for at least the past two decades, their constitution and performance have been very variable. This criticism was recently spelled out in an important report written by Rabbi Julia Neuberger, and published by the Kings Fund Institute, where she has been a visiting fellow for two years.[10]

Research ethics committees, with the unqualified support of the industry, should always consider the following points:

1. Whether the scientific quality of the protocol has been properly assessed; by definition, any study which is unscientific is also unethical, and on both counts should be rejected.
2. Whether the investigator and any other persons who will be involved in carrying out the trial are competent, and whether their facilities are adequate.
3. The possible hazards to the trial subjects involved and the precautions taken to deal with them.
4. That appropriate informed consent will be obtained.
5. That adequate compensation arrangements are in place in the event of medicine-induced injury, or any other damage to the subject arising from the conduct of the trial.
6. The methods of recruitment, details of the information to be given to the subjects, and of any payments which may be made to them (usually out-of-pocket expenses for patient subjects, plus payment for pain, suffering, and inconvenience for non-patient volunteers).
7. The payments which may be made to the investigators.

With regard to the conduct of non-patient volunteer studies, the pharmaceutical industry held the view until about five years ago that only new experimental designs such as the administration of a new chemical entity required the program of work envisaged to be approved by an independent and properly constituted research ethics committee. By 1988 that had changed, and it is now agreed that all studies involving the administration of substances to non-patient volunteers must have a written protocol, submitted to, and approved by, a research ethics committee before the study begins. The ABPI report on the ethical approval of such studies is of fundamental importance in this regard; published in 1989, it has withstood the test of time and appears as an appendix to this chapter.

The report of the Royal College of Physicians referred to earlier rightly emphasizes the importance of the independence of research ethics committees, and states that any such committees set up by pharmaceutical or other industrial companies to review the testing of their own products pose particular problems in obtaining high quality members who are truly independent and of general credibility.

There are special circumstances which exist in the context of projects using non-patient volunteers which require their protocols to be considered by research ethics committees set up by the company. The circumstances which particularly apply are:

1. The need to have a committee with members of adequate expertise to deal with the special circumstances of "first-time" drug studies in human subjects.
2. The need for a guaranteed "turn round time" of protocols as most studies in this category are on the critical path for drug development, and as many as 60 protocols may be submitted by any one company during a single year.
3. The need for research ethics committees to be convened at short notice to review protocol amendments.
4. The need for confidentiality concerning the commercial details of the studies.

Pharmaceutical companies contracting outside establishments to conduct volunteer studies on their behalf must ensure that protocols have been submitted to, and approved by, an independent research ethics committee. Once ethical approval has been given for the study, its supervision becomes the sole responsibility of the named registered medical practitioners sponsoring and supervising the study. However, major protocol amendments should be referred to the research ethics committee, or its chairman, and no further test substances should be administered before approval is received.

3 INFORMED CONSENT

The concept of informed consent was first discussed early in this century, in the context of surgery. Current standards are those set out in the revised Declaration of Helsinki. It can be defined as the process whereby explicit information is provided to enable a patient or experimental subject to decide whether or not to have a particular treatment or to take part in a particular clinical trial. It has to be genuinely "informed," voluntary, and competent.

It can also be described as the willing obligation of the investigator, to the best of his or her knowledge, to inform the experimental subject about the personal benefit and risk which that subject faces in the proposed experiment, the significance of the experiment for the advancement of human knowledge and welfare, and the stakes involved for the investigator him- or herself.[2] This means that the most honest effort possible must be made by the investigator to guarantee the freedom of the subject to decide whether to agree or to refuse to take part in a clinical trial. This effort must be made with unreserved sincerity and is the antithesis of negligence. It is also a counsel of perfection, though it can and should be achieved.

Having stated that, however, it is a fact that a great deal of criticism has been written or spoken in the media — and indeed by doctors themselves — on the ineffective way in which informed consent has been sought in the past.

A recent leading article in the *Lancet*[3] refers to the "central dogma" which now seems to prevail that whatever is done for the sake of medical science is alien to the treatment of the individual and should therefore be labeled an experiment, necessitating informed consent by the patient and adjudication by an ethics committee. This dogma is in contrast to the ancient and natural process whereby doctors learn from the experience they gain when treating patients; the beneficiary is the next patient.

The *Lancet* editorial was concerned that the need to protect the interests of the patient, which must nevertheless always be upheld, was being taken to impractical extremes, whereby, for example, it may not in some countries (including the U.S.) be permissible merely to look at medical records for the purpose of selecting cases for an observational study without obtaining informed consent. Thus, it was argued, that at least for observational research, where the patient is essentially a nonparticipant, ethical approval and informed consent were not necessary, given the time-honored guarantee of medical confidentiality.

Walshe followed up this editorial with a supportive letter particularly referring to orphan drugs.[4] This distinguished physician refers to his considerable experience in introducing three new therapies over a period of 35 years for the treatment of the fatal condition Wilson's disease. He is an advocate of auto-experimentation, having taken all three substances himself, and is concerned that the therapies would never have passed a research ethics committee, and therefore would not have been allowed to be given, even under experimental conditions, to patients. Such a rejection would, he states, have resulted in the loss of several lives (subsequently saved by the use of the three substances to which he refers; penicillamine, trientine, or ammonium tetrathiomolybdate) with no blame attributable to the ethics committee.

These views were subsequently challenged in another letter, sent by the chairman of a research ethics committee,[5] who pointed out that in those 35 years important changes had taken place, not least the shift in public perception, which objects to medical paternalism, arising from some notoriously ill-advised trials on a number of ill-informed patients. Research ethics committees are, it must be recognized, here to stay, and their activities have undoubtedly stimulated better communication between investigator and the subjects of research, though at the same time the continued requirement for every research project to be vetted by such a committee has tended to increase and to perpetuate an attitude of mistrust toward scientists and doctors.

With regard to patient studies, all protocols for clinical trials should be reviewed and approved by a properly constituted independent research ethics committee. This approval should be obtained by the investigator, but a copy should be held by the sponsor. The objectives of the ethics committee are to protect subjects of research, to preserve their rights, and to provide public reassurance. Ethics committee approval also protects investigators and institutions.

All clinical trials in general practice must equally have the protocol approved. Where the study is to be carried out within a local area only, approval should be sought from the relevant local research ethical committee. Where the study is to be carried out in a wider area, it may be appropriate to seek approval from a central research ethics committee, such as that established by the Royal College of General Practitioners; however, if approval is granted by such a committee, then that information should be made known to the local research ethics committees in whose areas the research is to be carried out. These local committees may, if there are particular local issues bearing upon the research, also require to give approval to the local investigator. Similarly, a local investigator invited to participate in a research project to which ethical approval has been given by a distant ethics committee should, if he or she feels there are local issues to be considered, submit the protocol to the relevant local committee before agreeing to take part in the study. For the industry, the involvement of the local committee is an important point, as approval of the investigator by the local research ethics committee is sometimes even more important than approval of the protocol, and where this has not happened some problems have arisen.

4 U.K. DEPARTMENT OF HEALTH GUIDELINES

Following the publication of the so-called "Red Book" on guidelines for local research ethics committees (LRECs),[11] the activities of such committees increased considerably. However, these activities were uncoordinated and haphazard, and the arrival of further guidelines from the NHS Training Division[12] in September 1994 was particularly timely. These guidelines were published in three parts: a set of standards; a set of standard operating procedures (SOPs); and a bridging document describing how the standards should be used.

The documents from the NHS Training Division were produced on behalf of the Department of Health to support LRECs in performing the tasks outlined in the "Red Book" and arrived none too soon. They are particularly intended to supplement, not to replace, the *Manual for Research Ethics Committees*[13] produced by the Department of Medical Law and Ethics at Kings College, London — a particularly useful manual, but with no status with regard to standardizing operational procedures.

The first section of the new guidelines introduces the use of a Framework in describing what the LREC should be able to do, and the second is a set of SOPs which demonstrate — and will hopefully stimulate — a common approach to the problems of ethical review of research procedures. Thus the Framework refers to the outcome of the procedures of the LREC, and the SOPs refer to the processes themselves which are necessary to ensure that a satisfactory outcome is attained. Only time will tell whether these documents, and the training on their usage, bring about the collective improvement in LREC performance which is so necessary at the time of writing this chapter.

5 GOOD CLINICAL (RESEARCH) PRACTICE

Following publication of the industry guidelines on Good Clinical Research Practice (GC(R)P) by the ABPI in 1988,[1] much time and effort has been spent in explaining the principles of good clinical research practice to the leaders of the medical profession, and to individual investigators. The guidelines underline the importance of monitoring and of audit procedures. More recently, the European Commission has approved the guidelines on GC(R)P produced by the Committee on Proprietary Medicinal Products (CPMP). These have been operative from July 1, 1991, and covered by a directive since January 1, 1992. The need for this information to be promulgated and for investigators to be trained in the principles of GC(R)P continues.

Soon after the acceptance of these guidelines, the commission issued a discussion document on the need for a directive, with a number of points for consideration. These began by referring to the detection in the U.S., by the FDA, of a number of cases of fraudulent results relating to bioavailability studies for generic products. In other words, this concern arose because of the wickedness of a company rather than the wickedness of an investigator. Both parties obviously have to be equally honest in the generation and submission of data.

6 FRAUD AND MISCONDUCT IN THE CONTEXT OF CLINICAL RESEARCH

The conduct of most clinical research is honest and honorable. Just occasionally, however, the sponsor of a clinical study may be faced with data which are suspect. Such data might or might not be fraudulent. It is vitally important for society in general, and for the pharmaceutical industry in particular, that fraudulent research is eliminated. The ABPI recently published a report to alert member companies and others to fraud and to provide guidelines for its detection, investigation, prosecution, and prevention.[7] Many companies already have SOPs in place which outline the steps to be adopted by any employees suspecting fraud and emphasize the philosophy and management commitment of the company. This report was therefore also intended to stimulate and assist companies in establishing SOPs.

Ideally, fraud should not occur; agreed high ethical standards must be set for clinical research, to which all interested parties should adhere. However, procedures must also be in place if fraud is suspected despite the existence of these standards. Within the pharmaceutical industry, such standards for clinical research already exist[6] and have been accepted by virtually all U.K. pharmaceutical companies and members of the Association of Independent Clinical Research Contractors (AICRC). European Commission GC(R)P guidelines are now covered by a directive, and have therefore assumed the status of "rules," as from July 1991.[8]

The ABPI working party began its deliberations against a background of increasing confidence on the part of pharmaceutical companies to take action against doctors found to have submitted fraudulent data, but uncertain how best to investigate or to handle suspicions that such data might be fraudulent. The working party recognized that what was needed was a mechanism which could make it easier for member companies to pursue such suspicions without prejudice.

One method could have been the appointment of a "screener" who would decide whether or not an allegation should be investigated. To enable that decision to be made, the screener would first receive and consider a detailed confidential statement in support of the allegation. If it were clear that the suspicion was justified, then an investigation should be conducted to enable a case, if proved, to be presented to a court of law, or, in the U.K., to the General Medical Council. If, however, it were not found that the allegation was substantiated, then an informal enquiry would be conducted, subject to the utmost degree of confidentiality, by a panel of three "appropriate" persons. The enquiry would either lead to the allegation being withdrawn or to it proceeding to an investigation, as above. Fraud is most likely to be prevented if investigators and their colleagues are fully aware of GC(R)P standards, of the requirement for the industry to operate to them, and of the ethical commitment of companies to act vigorously against any irregularities.

7 THE REASONS FOR FRAUD

Despite GC(R)P, there is always a possibility that investigators will deliver unsatisfactory clinical data. This can be for a number of reasons including, for example, pressure of work or fatigue. Occasionally, it can be because of carelessness. Careful, meticulous, clinical investigators who are trustworthy are essential. It is the responsibility of the pharmaceutical physician, in cooperation with the clinical trial monitor, to ensure that only reliable investigators are recruited. Potential investigators who are over busy, or who, for whatever reason, are not motivated to take part in a clinical research project, should be avoided. Companies should reject any potential investigators about whom there are doubts arising from their past involvement in a research project.

There are many reasons why for the wrong reasons doctors may volunteer to become investigators. For some it may be pressure to publish, though recent industry experience does not indicate this. However, it is well known that doctors in training, ultimately hoping to obtain consultant appointments, seek to enhance their list of published papers, which will be closely scrutinized when they come to apply for a career post. Also, doctors in academic departments undoubtedly believe that an impressive list of publications will help when, for example, they apply for extra staff or for scarce additional research grants.

Some doctors might wish to take part in a clinical trial because of, to them, the excessively routine nature of day-to-day clinical practice. Involvement in a research project injects a break into that routine, and such doctors may produce very good data because they have been stimulated by their involvement in research. But it is also recognized that a doctor who has become bored may well have difficulty in maintaining standards, and the involvement of such a doctor in a research project must be monitored with care.

Some doctors will admit that they offer to take part in clinical trials primarily because of the money they will earn for doing so. Such doctors are particularly likely to take short cuts or to produce fraudulent data. In the light of recent experience, it is they who undertake too many clinical trials with the patient population or the time at their disposal and are tempted to invent patients or to invent data attributed to genuine patients. Some doctors may be emotionally disturbed (on more than one occasion recently used as an excuse for fraudulent data) or frankly mentally ill; bizarre aberrations of data may be supplied by a doctor who is suffering from a psychotic illness. Some doctors are motivated by the incentive of vanity; they need their partners or their colleagues or the world at large to see how busy or how clever they are, without having any real commitment to undertaking clinical research in accordance with the principles of GC(R)P.

8 THE DETECTION OF FRAUD

Most investigators conduct research projects entirely satisfactorily. However, despite careful selection of investigators, occasionally standards slip, and if these are insidious they can be exceedingly difficult to detect. Sometimes, for example, data which appear to be meticulous are found to be too good to be true. An extreme case of fraudulent research in the U.S. was first investigated after the research team at a pharmaceutical company became suspicious when the data submitted by a specialist physician were found to be "too perfect."

The general principles for the detection of fraud are all common sense, but it is often the complexity of clinical trials that makes the application of common sense difficult and fraud hard to detect. It is essential that the exact methods used by companies for the detection of fraud be kept secret; detection may often depend on a particular way of selecting numbers or patterns within written text which are easy for potential forgers to avoid if they are forewarned.

Fraud is often detected by the field monitor or clinical research associate, who may well be junior staff entering their first professional post after obtaining a degree. They must be trained that if they have the slightest concern that something is not right with the center or investigator it is ethically appropriate that this should be communicated to the responsible person within the company. Many new graduates find this very difficult to put into practice, particularly if dealing with well-known investigators or centers, and strong reassurance must be given on the importance of this issue. If basic and refresher training programs for clinical trial monitors and clinical research associates discuss fraud case studies, all staff will learn to pick up signs which lead them to accept that they should be suspicious of an investigator or center. There have also been cases of fraud where there has been collusion between a company employee or department and the clinical investigator. This is obviously totally unacceptable and it is therefore critical that methods for communicating doubts about the integrity of any data should take this into account.

A whole range of methods of looking at data derived from clinical trials, including medication consumption, can be developed, aimed at detecting patterns which arouse suspicion. Once numerical data has been loaded into a database its comprehensive analysis becomes possible. The fundamental question being asked is whether there are any groups of patients whose data are atypical compared with other patients within the same center or from the other centers within the study. Routine statistical and graphic systems can readily be established to allow such comparisons to be run on a regular basis as part of a quality control audit check.

A far greater difficulty is the detection of a single fraudulent entry or series of entries relating to a particular visit. This situation can occur if a patient misses a follow-up appointment for any reason and the data for that visit is invented. The detection of this type of fraud is very difficult, provided the investigator has inserted clinically sensible values, taking into account previous and subsequent results. However, the audit procedures and requirements for source documentation verification inherent in GC(R)P may reveal discrepancies which require further investigation. Although these techniques may help the pharmaceutical industry in the detection and management of fraud, it requires vigilance from trial monitors and the consistent application of quality control checks to minimize the risk.

9 THE PROSECUTION OF FRAUD

Once an investigator has been shown beyond all reasonable shadow of doubt to have submitted fraudulent data to a pharmaceutical company or contract house, it is essential in the interests of the public, the profession, and the industry that that doctor should be referred to the General Medical Council (GMC) for possible consideration by the professional conduct committee. Alternatively, the doctor could be prosecuted for the criminal offense of fraud. In the U.K. the former alternative is preferable as it is a more rapid procedure than the courts of law.

If a company decides for whatever reason that it does not wish to use the GMC procedure, or if, for example, in another European country, a company wishes to prosecute a doctor who is not registered with the GMC, it is always open to that company to use a legal process. The GMC has made it clear that it would not seek to usurp the proper authority of the police or of the Crown Prosecution Service where a criminal offense may have been committed. Alternatively, a company which considered itself fraudulently exploited by a doctor could take out a civil prosecution. A prosecution, however, would take considerably longer to process through to conviction than the GMC procedure, and, if successful, would automatically (in the U.K.) lead to the GMC disciplinary procedure being invoked. The ABPI therefore strongly recommends that companies should consider it most appropriate that offending doctors in the U.K. should be submitted to the professional disciplinary proceedings laid down by law for the GMC.

The question was also raised as to whether there should be free exchange of information about detected, or even suspected, fraud between member states. My own view is that there should, though I rather doubt whether it will be of much value outside the member state concerned, because there is in practice very little movement of doctors between member states.

The situation facing the industry in this regard, therefore, is the probability of much more frequent site inspections than previously — a situation which must be explained to, and understood by, the doctors likely to be visited. However, the medical profession in general should have been made aware of the need to uphold standards by virtue of the publicity now being given to the prosecution of fraud, and will hopefully accept the various procedures needed to ensure that standards are of the highest.

Labeling is important in the interests of patient-subject safety. Certain items of information must appear on the label of a clinical trial product, including the location of manufacture, batch and serial numbers, storage and handling particulars, expiry date, and disposal instructions are specified in the discussion document. That list leaves out one of the most important items which I personally feel must be included, on which there is an ABPI policy; that is the contact telephone number, if telephoning the manufacturer at the location given on the label does not give access to someone who is able to provide additional information which may be needed in an emergency. A facility must exist whereby a doctor (such as a casualty officer) treating a patient (in an emergency), who happens to be taking part in a clinical trial, can obtain information about trial medication within an hour, even if it is double blind, and there is no information about who the investigator might be. There are several ways in which this can be done, but it would be unethical if an appropriate facility were not in place.

10 THE ETHICS OF PROMOTION

Just as the pharmaceutical industry is committed to high ethical stands of research, so it is committed to high ethical standards of promotion. The situation in the U.K. exemplifies this, where there is a Code of Practice which owes its origin to the determination of the ABPI to secure the acceptance and adoption of high standards of conduct in the marketing of medicines designed for use under medical supervision.

The International Federation of Pharmaceutical Manufacturers' Associations (IFPMA) also operates a Code of Practice which applies to the promotion of medicines particularly in the developing world.

As has already been stated in the first part of this article, marketed medicines owe their existence to successful research. Once a medicine has been licensed, however, it is necessary for a pharmaceutical company to promote it, given that the company operates in a keenly competitive industrial environment and that the professionals who use its products have freedom of choice. It could be argued that it would be quite unethical not to make available — and promote — medicines which offer greater opportunities for treatment. These Codes of Practice emphasize the importance in the public interest of providing accurate, fair, and objective information to doctors about medicines which they are entitled to prescribe. Contravention of the codes is unacceptable, and breaches are publicized; however, most companies bend over backwards to try not to breach the codes accepting that it is poor marketing practice, as well as unethical, to promote any medicine inappropriately.

REFERENCES

1. Bankowski Z. and Howard-Jones N. Eds. Human experimentation and medical ethics; 1982. Council for International Organisation of Medical Sciences, Geneva.
2. Guttentag O. Ethical problems in human experimentation. In: Torrey E. F. Ed. *Ethical Issues in Medicine*; 1968; Little, Brown; Oxford.
3. **Anon.** Medical ethics: should medicine turn the other cheek? *Lancet* 1990; ii: 846-847.
4. Walshe J. M. Ethical committees? (L) *Lancet* 1990; ii: 1194.
5. Powell D. E. B. Ethics committees (L) *Lancet* 1990; ii; 1448.
6. Wells F. O. Ed. *Medicines: Good Practice Guidelines.* 1990; Queens University Press; Belfast.
7. ABPI Medical Committee Working Party. Fraud and malpractice in the context of clinical research; 1992. Association of the British Pharmaceutical Industry, London.
8. European Commission. Good Clinical Practice Guideline. Brussels: EC, 1991, in press.
9. Royal College of Physicians of London Working Party. The role and functions of research ethics committees; 1990. Royal College of Physicians, London.
10. Neuberger J. Ethics and health care: the role of research ethics committees in the U.K.; 1992. King's Fund Institute, London.
11. Department of Health. Guidance for Local Research Ethics Committees; 1991. HMSO, London.
12. NHS Training Division. Standards for Local Research Ethics Committees; 1994. HMSO, London.
13. Foster, C. G. Ed. *Manual for Local Research Ethics Committees,* 1993. Kings College, Department of Medical Law and Ethics, London.

APPENDIX 1

GUIDELINES FOR ETHICAL APPROVAL OF HUMAN PHARMACOLOGY STUDIES CARRIED OUT BY PHARMACEUTICAL COMPANIES

INTRODUCTION

There is general agreement that research investigations on human subjects should conform with codes which are internationally recognized, such as the Declaration of Helsinki of the World Medical Association (as subsequently modified) and the guidance issued by the World Health Organization and its associated bodies. Such research includes experiments conducted on non-patient volunteers.

There is also general agreement that neither investigators nor sponsors should be the sole judges of whether their research conforms to such guidelines, but that all protocols should be submitted for independent review by a research ethics committee.

For nearly 30 years, since the publication of the Stuart-Harris report, the pharmaceutical industry, through the ABPI, has operated guidelines for the conduct of non-patient volunteer studies. More recently, the ABPI has published definitive policy guidelines for the conduct of medical experiments in non-patient volunteers (1988) and on the facilities which should exist where such studies are carried out (1989). The 1988 guidelines include a brief section on ethics committees.

The Royal College of Physicians has also issued reports on the conduct of research on humans and on the practice of research ethics committees, most recently in January 1990. The European Commission and the World Health Organization have also issued definitive guidelines on Good Clinical (Research) Practice, intended to cover all four phases of clinical research.

In its ethics committee report, the Royal College of Physicians states that research ethics committees set up by pharmaceutical or other industrial companies to review the testing of their own products pose particular problems of obtaining high quality independent members and of general credibility. However, the ABPI believes that, for studies carried out by pharmaceutical companies on non-patient volunteers in the course of their own research, special circumstances exist that normally require the protocols for such studies to be considered by research ethics committees set up by the company; and the evidence presented by individual companies does not support the view that they have difficulty in recruiting independent members of very high caliber.

The circumstances which particularly apply are:

- The need to have a committee with members of adequate expertise to deal with the special circumstances of "first-time" drug studies in human objects.
- The need for guaranteed "turn round time" of protocols as most studies in this category are on the critical path for drug development, and as many as 60 protocols may be submitted by any one company during a single year.
- The need for research ethics committees to be convened at short notice to review protocol amendments.
- The need for confidentiality concerning the commercial details of the studies.

The 1988 ABPI guidelines for the conduct of non-patient volunteer studies include the following section on ethics committees.

- All studies involving the administration of substances to non-patient volunteers must have a written protocol submitted to and approved in writing by an appropriate independent ethics committee before the study begins.
- Pharmaceutical companies contracting outside establishments to conduct volunteer studies on their behalf must ensure that protocols have been submitted to and approved by an independent ethics committee.
- Once ethical approval has been given for the study, the supervision of the study becomes the sole responsibility of the named registered medical practitioners sponsoring and supervising the study. However, major protocol amendments should be referred to the committee or its chairman, and no further test substances should be administered before approval is received.

The above three clauses from the 1988 guidelines were intended to apply to research ethics committees set up by companies, for the reasons stated in clause 1.5.

The Royal College of Physicians guidelines on the practice of research ethics committees emphasizes that every member of such a committee should serve as an individual and not as a delegate taking instruction from other bodies or reporting to them. Thus the affiliation of individual members to a particular institution should be considered irrelevant to their independent judgement.

It is nevertheless recognized that the establishment of research ethics committees by pharmaceutical companies, even if solely to assess human pharmacology studies, might provoke the criticism that they are not truly independent. It is therefore recommended that each company should conform to agreed standard operating procedures for its research ethics committee which should only by authorized to consider studies in non-patient volunteers. This document sets out guidelines which may be used as the basis for the drafting of such standard operating procedures by each company. They therefore augment the conclusions of the Royal College of Physicians report on ethics committees, and the ABPI guidelines on the conduct of non-patient volunteer studies, and specifically refer to those studies conducted in a company facility by company staff on healthy volunteers.

The ABPI supports the view of the Royal College of Physicians that the legitimate concern of the public and the profession that led to the setting up of research ethics committees cannot be satisfied by anything less than mandatory review.

APPENDIX 2

GUIDELINES FOR RESEARCH ETHICS COMMITTEES CONSIDERING STUDIES CONDUCTED IN HEALTHY VOLUNTEERS BY PHARMACEUTICAL COMPANIES

1 BACKGROUND

1.1 In accordance with the guidelines issued by the ABPI and the European Commission on Good Clinical (Research) Practice, all medical research involving human subjects should undergo ethical review and be approved by an independent body, (called a research ethics committee) before it commences, in accordance with the principle that sponsors and investigators should not be the sole judges of whether their research raises ethical issues.

2 CONSTITUTION OF THE RESEARCH ETHICS COMMITTEE

2.1 Chairman

2.1.1 The chairman of the ethics committee must be independent of the company, and must not be a company employee nor have any financial interest in the company other than as a shareholder. The holding of shares must be declared. He/she must have sufficiently broad medical and scientific experience to guide committee members through the complex issues involved in initial clinical studies.

2.2 Membership

2.2.1 As the Royal College of Physicians report points out, the World Health Organization advises that there are two principles on the membership of research ethics committees:

> "committees must command the technical competence and judgement to attempt to reconcile the physical and psychological consequences of participation with both the welfare of the subjects and the objectives of the investigation."
> "they may also with advantage, accommodate respected lay opinion in a manner that provides effective representation of community as well as of medical interest."

2.2.2 It is believed that these principles also apply to research ethics committees associated with pharmaceutical companies.

2.2.3 The voting membership, which includes the chairman, should consist of at least 6 and not more than 12 people independent of, not employed by, and with no financial interest, in the company other than as a shareholder. The holding of shares must be declared. The membership should include:

a) medical members, of which at least one should be a general practitioner, with at least one other medically qualified person occupied with both clinical care and clinical research.
b) at least one nurse, preferably in active practice with patients.
c) at least two lay members each of whom should be independent of the company.
d) both sexes should be represented on the committee.
e) as it is not practicable for the committee to include specialists in all fields of medicine and science about which they will be called upon to judge, the committee should have the power to co-opt personnel from the medical and scientific areas of the company and elsewhere. This includes the co-option of suitably qualified persons to comment on the science of the pre-human research for each specific study. Co-opted members will not become voting members as a result of their co-option, and their co-option will cease when the protocol for which they have been co-opted has been considered.

3 FUNCTIONS AND TERMS OF REFERENCE

3.1 The research ethics committee should review the ethics of all protocols for in-house studies undertaken by the company involving healthy volunteers. Its geographical area should be specified.

3.2 The committee should consider the following points:
a) whether the scientific quality of the proposal has been properly assessed.
b) the competence of the staff who will carry out the procedures and the adequacy of their facilities.
c) the possible hazards to the subjects involved and the precautions taken to deal with them.
d) the degree of discomfort or distress which may be entailed by the procedures.
e) the appropriate informed consent will be obtained.
f) that the subject's general practitioner will be informed.
g) the methods of recruitment, details of the proposed information to be given to the volunteers and the payments to be made to them, in accordance with the ABPI guidelines on the conduct of non-patient volunteer studies.

4 MEETINGS

4.1 It is considered essential that the committee actually meets to consider the majority of protocols. To work principally by mail, by telephone, or by chairman's decision is unacceptable.

4.2 The location of the meetings may be on the company's premises, so long as the voting members of the committees are enabled to meet in private. The meetings should be held outside the company's premises if the voting members of the committee so wish.

4.3 Secretarial support (arranging meetings, preparing agendas, writing minutes, and preparing reports) may be provided by the company but strict confidentiality must be maintained.

4.4 The debate as well as the outcome of consideration of protocols for ethical consideration and approval should be minuted.

4.5 The agreements between the membership of the committee and the company should be such that the company is guaranteed regular and timely meetings by a committee that is quorate. A quorum will be specified and must be defined in the standard operating procedures. Any proposed change to protocols must be submitted to the chairman who will decide whether it can be approved by the chairman him or herself, or whether, as the major changes, it requires a full additional meeting of the committee. The definition of "major change" will be specified.

5 DECISIONS

5.1 All members of the committee, other than co-opted members, shall be voting members and unanimous agreement amongst those present must be obtained.

6 REMUNERATION

6.1 It is important to recognize the status of members of the committee on whom a considerable amount of work is imposed. A free structure is therefore appropriate, whereby members are paid in annual honorarium, with or without an attendance allowance per meeting. Traveling expenses actually incurred may also be paid, but no other expenses shall be paid. The principle of remuneration should be such that if the details become public neither the committee nor the company are embarrassed.

7 CONFIDENTIALITY

7.1 All members of the committee should sign a confidentiality agreement in which they agree not to disclose any of the contents of the meetings. Agendas and minutes should only be available to the chairman and members of the committee; additionally, agendas should only be available to the relevant company personnel.

8 INDEMNITY

8.1 Members of the committee will be indemnified by the company should they be individually or severally be subject to legal action arising from their committee membership.

9 REPORTS

9.1 To the Committee

9.1.1 The Committee should receive confidential reports on the outcome of the studies they have approved. Any deviation from the original protocol must be reported to the chairman for consideration. Major adverse events or study termination must be reported immediately to the chairman.

9.2 By the Committee

9.2.1 The committee should keep a register of all studies considered and the outcome of their discussion on a simple approval/non-approval/requires modification basis. In accordance with the Royal College of Physicians guidelines on the practice of ethics committees, a report should be prepared annually, which may be made generally available.

FOW
July 1994

Chapter 11

Legal Liabilities in Clinical Trials

Ian C. Dodds-Smith

CONTENTS

1 Introduction ... 123
2 Definition ... 124
3 Law and Ethics ... 124
4 Legal Regulation Under General Principles of Law ... 127
5 The Legal Obligations of the Manufacturer ... 127
  5.1 In Relation to the Investigator ... 127
  5.2 In Relation to the Research Subject ... 128
    5.2.1 Negligence ... 128
    5.2.2 Strict Liability ... 129
    5.2.3 Criminal Liability ... 130
6 The Legal Obligations of the Investigator ... 130
  6.1 Consent ... 132
    6.1.1 Consent and Trespass to Person ... 132
    6.1.2 Consent in Children and the Mentally Handicapped ... 133
      6.1.2.1 Children ... 133
      6.1.2.2 The Mentally Handicapped ... 133
    6.1.3 Consent and Negligence ... 134
    6.1.4 The Doctrine of Informed Consent ... 135
    6.1.5 Disclosure of Risks and Research ... 135
  6.2 Randomization and Placebo Controls ... 138
  6.3 Consent Forms ... 138
7 The Liability of Other Parties to Research ... 139
  7.1 Ethics Committees ... 139
  7.2 Regulatory Authorities ... 140
8 Compensation for Injury ... 140
  8.1 Healthy Volunteers ... 143
  8.2 Patient Volunteers ... 143
9 Proof of Causation ... 144
10 Indemnities for Investigators and Others Connected with Research ... 145
References ... 146
Appendix 1 ABPI Clinical Trial Compensation Guidelines ... 149
Appendix 2 ABPI/Department of Health Form of Indemnity for Clinical Studies ... 151

1 INTRODUCTION

There is voluminous literature on legal issues in clinical research and, more particularly, the relationship between law and ethics. Medicine is international but the law often varies from country to country. This chapter must, therefore, inevitably be less than comprehensive and the approach will essentially be to indicate how the main issues are addressed by English law, making comparisons with other jurisdictions only where these are particularly striking or relevant to the likely development of English and European Community law.

2 DEFINITION

There is no universally accepted definition of clinical trials. In this chapter the term will be used in the widest sense as meaning the scientific study of drugs in man. It therefore encompasses several different types of study falling within clinical pharmacology, ranging from those involving therapy in circumstances where there is no accepted mode of treatment but where the aim is to help the particular patient and at the same time advance medical science, to those involving non-patient volunteers where no prospect of personal benefit arises. It will be seen that the very different nature of the volunteers carries with it important legal consequences. Non-patient volunteers are often referred to as healthy volunteers but this is a misleading expression, as any group of people will include the normal percentage in any population who suffer from allergies and other minor illnesses and abnormalities. However, the expression is widely used and will be used in this chapter to describe a person who has no significant illness relevant to a proposed study and agrees to participate other than with a view to personal medical benefit. Volunteers enrolling with a view to treatment will be termed "patient volunteers" and the term "clinical research" will be used to denote both fields of research.

3 LAW AND ETHICS

The medical profession has traditionally had to conduct clinical research against the background of a society that desires and applauds new drug treatments for disease but at the same time has a deeply suspicious view of the use of human beings in medical experimentation. The appalling examples of prisoners used for experimentation during World War II did little to allay that suspicion, but at least provoked the first serious set of international ethical guidelines on a subject where both the law and medical ethics was notoriously vague.[1] For once, the law has an excuse for being vague. Legal rules tend to reflect the decisions within society as to what is ethically right and proper; therefore, until the medical profession and society at large has established the ethical framework within which medical research should be conducted, the law is bound to be hamstrung.

The ethics of many aspects of medical research remain controversial and the law on the subject is unsatisfactory. Indeed, the main feature of the law is its very limited intervention in the form of specific legal rules. Even where the courts have explored the legal requirements of a particular aspect of research — such as consent — the decisions of the judges have often been conflicting. Even as late as the 1950s there was some doubt as to the legality of certain research, with Regan noting that although it was the duty of a physician to ensure that his practices reflected changing knowledge, it was also his duty "to refrain from experiments."[2]

If this statement were to be taken at face value, clinical trials could not take place, for the randomized controlled clinical trial is the very essence of an "experiment." However, there is now no doubt that most controlled clinical trials are both ethical and legal. Legislatures the world over have formally accepted that only experimentation in patients produces reliable information and helps to protect the public at large from ineffective and unsafe medicines. Results from increasingly sophisticated trials of this nature are now a legal requirement for the registration of new medicinal products throughout the Western world.

In contrast, the same legislatures have been slow to establish detailed rules relating to the manner in which clinical research is to be performed. Thus, the European Directives[3] relating to marketing authorizations and the Medicines Act legislation in the U.K. applicable to dealings in medicinal products[4] require applicants for licenses to produce clinical trial data, and most Member States require some type of approval before commencing trials and the reporting of adverse events encountered. However, such legislation does not normally provide detailed guidance on matters such as trial design and patient consent. Directive 75/318/EEC sets out the form of the particulars relating to a product that must be submitted under Directive 65/65/EEC when a marketing authorization is sought and must be examined by the competent authorities. The Annex to Directive 75/318 provides details of *inter alia*, the clinical trial data to be provided. The current Annex (adopted by Directive 91/507/EEC) provides in Part 4 that trials must comply with GCP but no particular form of GCP is referenced. Compliance with the Declaration of Helsinki and "in principle" the freely given informed consent of each trial subject must be obtained and documented. Ethics committee approval must be given in writing before the trial begins. It is noted that "in general" the clinical trials should be controlled and, if possible, randomized. Compensation and indemnity issues are not specifically addressed.

In 1991 a discussion paper was issued by the European Commission[5] on the need for a directive on clinical trials. Issues of fraud in research, inspection of sites, monitoring by regulatory authority, adequacy of preclinical testing, manufacturing and labeling standards, and archiving were raised. However, liabilities were not addressed and as yet no directive has been adopted. More recently the fashion for adopting a principle of "subsidiarity" allowing Member States to control lower levels of regulation may discourage progress in harmonizing research practice which frequently raises difficult ethical issues.

In the meantime, Member States have different regulatory regimes for clinical research. Some require approval for clinical trials and others mere notification. In the U.K. the supply of drugs for healthy volunteer studies remains wholly unregulated by statute. A committee set up in the U.K. after the thalidomide catastrophe in the 1960s to recommend what legislation was required relating to the safety and efficacy of drugs declared that "responsibility for the experimental laboratory testing of new drugs before they are used in clinical trials should remain with the individual pharmaceutical manufacturer."[6] Records of debates in Parliament at that time reflect the fact that the primary concern was to ensure that new drugs were not put on the market before possible harmful side effects had been evaluated rather than to protect the rights of either patients or healthy volunteers. The unwritten assumption was that the medical profession could be relied upon to look after the former and the latter were well able to look after themselves.

Since that time such an assumption has increasingly been questioned in the U.K. The requirement since 1967 that all clinical research conducted in institutions within the National Health Service should be referred by the investigator for vetting by an independent ethics committee,[7] and the fact that such a practice is now also standard in respect of research conducted in private institutions and companies, has only partly alleviated public concern. In October 1989, the Department of Health in the U.K. began consultation[8] on revised guidance to research ethics committees in the face of "widespread uncertainty about requirements and a great variance in operational procedures." This in part responded to reports in the media of patients enrolled in clinical trials without being fully aware of this fact, and widespread criticism within and outside the medical profession of the increasing commercialization of healthy volunteer studies. Emotive headlines such as "Students are cancer drug guinea pigs" and "Tests go on at drug death clinic"[9] not only typify the approach of a media keen to sensationalize any issue concerning drugs, but also underline more general misgivings about the notion that self-regulation by the pharmaceutical industry and the professions offers adequate safeguards to volunteers in the absence of clear ethical or legal rules in conformity with which clinical research will be conducted. In 1991, the Department of Health issued guidelines[10] relating to the constitution and ethical principles applicable to the work of local research ethics committees. As much clinical research in the U.K. involves patients treated in the National Health Service, very many research proposals will be considered against the provisions of this document. However, these matters are still not regulated by legislation.

To date, the pressure for change in the U.K. has been limited by the fact that, despite the ethical and legal confusion, very few people are injured in clinical research.[11] Care in selection of subjects and the high level of monitoring of subjects have led to a dearth of cases to test the legal waters. However, faced with a more litigious society, even the medical profession is increasingly troubled by the legal uncertainties that periodically envelop them and recognize that a more formal framework would provide benefits in terms of their own legal protection. However, all legislatures face a dilemma. They recognize the need for some statutory intervention to protect both the volunteer and the investigator, but the difficulty of developing rules that on the one hand are practical to apply in a field as disparate as clinical research, and on the other not so restrictive as to encourage overdefensive medicine, has thus far been difficult to resolve. For the present, in the U.K. at least, fears about defensive medicine appear dominant and a bill entitled "Unethical Experiments" failed to get a second reading in Parliament when introduced in 1977.

For some years the U.K. position was not exceptional, but in the last few years the majority of Member States have taken initiatives to control the performance of clinical research by statute. Early steps were taken in Germany as the German Drug Law of 1976[12] contains some provisions specific to clinical research and the Republic of Ireland embraced more detailed statutory control through the Control of Clinical Trials Act 1987,[13] but only after several requirements of the draft bill were watered down in the face of major opposition from the medical profession concerning several impractical features. In France a new law for the Protection of Persons Undergoing Biomedical Research was passed in 1988, but did not come fully into effect until 1991. This provided for mandatory ethics committee review and notification of research to the Ministry of Health. In addition, special compensation arrangements for volunteers injured in research are required. The definition of biomedical research and the different requirements applicable to healthy volunteer, as opposed to patient volunteer trials, have caused some confusion. In France, a clause in the French Constitution which declared illegal the use of one's body for profit for a long time hindered the use of healthy volunteers in research. Despite the new law directed at the protection of volunteers, there has been strong opposition in France to such studies in some parts of the medical profession.[14] In 1994 the social affairs inspectorate suggested an amendment to exclude phase IV from the law as the procedural complexities were hindering performance of trials without clear benefit to subjects. A full review of the clinical trials law has been commissioned by the French government.

Undeterred by the problems encountered when countries sought to legislate others have followed suit in the 1990s. Spain promulgated new laws in 1990 requiring a negative clearance system for healthy volunteer and patient volunteer studies, adherence to the Declaration of Helsinki and compliance with GCP as well as extensive insurance requirements.[15] Portugal passed a new law in 1992 governing trials conducted to support subsequent applications for marketing authorizations which requires compliance with the Declaration of Helsinki and GCP; it was followed by a decree on clinical trials in April 1994.[16] Italy passed a decree in 1992 requiring approval of clinical research and compliance with GCP guidelines including arrangements for appropriate compensation for injured subjects.[17] Finland issued a circular under its Medicines Act in 1987 requiring notification of clinical trials to the National Agency for Welfare and Health and adherence to the Nordic GCP guidelines; in practice, ethics committee approval is required and will not be granted without evidence of insurance for trial subject.[18]

Outside the European Union (EU), Switzerland passed regulations on clinical trials effective in January 1995 which have the effect of requiring compliance with GCP and ethics committee approval that will not normally be obtained without compensation provisions and insurance for injury for subjects.[19] Japanese guidelines for GCP were notified by the Director of the Pharmaceutical Affairs Bureau of the Ministry of Health and Welfare in 1989. They are not backed by legislation but de facto require compliance with GCP and have been followed up with further general guidelines on clinical evaluation of new drugs issued in 1992.[20]

Although the focus for many legal initiatives relating to the marketing of pharmaceuticals has switched to harmonization within Europe, attempts to fill the vacuum from that quarter have suffered from the inevitable problem of getting agreement on what is, or is not, ethically acceptable within countries where medical and social traditions are markedly different. The first attempt at some form of European harmonization related to GCP guidelines and was the Report of July 1987 from the EEC/CPMP Working Party on Efficacy of Drugs, which drafted a "Recommended Basis" for the "Conduct of Clinical Trials of Medicinal Products" within the community.[21] The CPMP guidelines — described by one member of the Working Party[22] as "a modest start toward common regulation in this field" — were based upon international codes of practice and sought to provide a common basis for clinical evaluation of new chemical entities, in order to promote the development of safe products at lowest possible risks. The guidelines covered all phases of clinical trials and made recommendations for everything, from the qualifications of investigators, design of protocols and ethics committee approval, to issues of consent and liability for injury to subjects. In 1990 the commission published detailed CPMP guidelines entitled "Good Clinical Practice for Trials on Medicinal Products in the European Community."[23] These are now the controlling guidelines in the EU and are hereafter referred to as the CPMP Guidelines. They set out principles of GCP applicable to all four phases of clinical research. The document notes that:

> "Pre-established, systematic written procedures for the organisation, conduct, data collection, documentation and verification of clinical trials are necessary to ensure that the rights and integrity of the trial subjects are thoroughly protected and to establish, scientific and technical quality of trials."

The CPMP Guidelines are worded often rather vaguely but address the protection of trial subjects and include an analysis of the responsibilities of each party to research. Ethics committee approvals must be sought that include vetting of the documentation used to obtain informed consent from subjects. The Ethics committee is to receive information on serious or unexpected adverse events so as to be able to reassess its approval, as appropriate. It is also stated that the committee should specifically consider the rights to compensation and treatment of a volunteer in the case of injury due to the trial and the terms of any insurance or indemnity covering the liability of the investigator and sponsor. Some countries like Italy have adopted these guidelines in national law but in most Member States the CPMP Guidelines remain one of several sets of guidelines in circulation on GCP matters.

In April 1996 a pre-consultation draft of an EC Directive on Clinical Trials was prepared by the EC Commission which incorporates a requirement for approval (not simply notification) of all clinical research (including Phase I) and a database of trials accessible only by competent authorities. Ethics

Committee approval would be mandatory and the Directive sets out the Committee's function and a proposal for a single approval for multi-center trials in each Member State. Manufacturing, labeling and adverse event reporting standards for investigational products are defined and the Directive provides for site inspections by Community inspectors. There is no requirement for special compensation or insurance arrangements for injured subjects but this is a matter to be considered by the Ethics Committee. Finalization, adoption, and implementation of the Directive will probably not happen quickly.

4 LEGAL REGULATION UNDER GENERAL PRINCIPLES OF LAW

Codes of Practice ranging from international initiatives such as the Nuremberg Code and Declaration of Helsinki[24] to the many guidelines from national institutions, industrial associations, and professional bodies provide rules which reflect (albeit inconsistently) the three fundamental ethical principles; namely the requirement of respect for persons, the requirement to minimize the risk of harm, and the requirement to treat persons fairly. For persons seeking to establish that certain behavior was, or was not, contrary to general principles of law, guidelines based on these principles may have evidential value through indicating prevailing standards of medical practice. In the U.K., guidelines on GCP were issued by the Association of the British Pharmaceutical Industry (ABPI) in 1992[25] that reflect the CPMP Guidelines. Separate guidelines were issued in 1993 for phase IV studies.[26] In Germany, France, and the Republic of Ireland the statutory provisions clearly draw heavily on GCP guidelines.

In the U.K., as in many other countries, none of these principles are yet mirrored in comprehensive and clearly defined legal requirements relating to research. Nevertheless, civil law codes or principles of judge made general law — "common law" — establishing a duty to avoid causing injury through lack of care, have general application and in a wider sense regulate all the activities of those initiating or conducting clinical research, from the selection of volunteers and the organization and execution of the study to the counseling of volunteers and their rights (if any) to compensation in the event of injury. In the U.K., despite the lack of specific laws, research has not been noticeably impeded except perhaps in a few areas where the lack of clear judicial authority (e.g., in relation to the capacity of children or the mentally incapacitated to give consent) has had an inhibiting effect. Equally, little guidance can be found from the decisions of the courts of other countries, as few cases relating specifically to planned medical research have come to trial anywhere in the world. This absence of authority means that any description of the legal obligations of the parties to research must normally be extrapolated from general principles of law such as negligence and trespass to person. These principles are, broadly speaking, common to all parts of Europe, although their basis (common law or code), as well as their detailed application, vary.

5 THE LEGAL OBLIGATIONS OF THE MANUFACTURER

5.1 In Relation to the Investigator

The legal relationship between the sponsoring company (invariably the manufacturer of the drug under study) and the investigator will be governed primarily by the terms of the contract they enter into. In most cases of research in healthy volunteers or patient volunteers it is desirable that there be a written contract between the sponsor and the investigator; this is the case whether the latter be an individual physician contracting to perform the research or a contract research establishment. The express terms of the contract may be supplemented by conditions implied by operation of law. Thus, under English law, in any contract for services there are implied terms relating to the exercise of reasonable care and skill and the need to complete the work in a reasonable time.[27] Furthermore, statutory provisions may limit the extent to which liability on the happening of certain events may be excluded by either party.[28] A Directive on Unfair Contract Terms which seeks to harmonize law within the EU was adopted in 1994.[29]

Deciding what legal obligations are to be accepted by each party and thereafter translated into specific terms of the agreement are essentially commercial matters, and while some guidance[30] on issues to consider has been issued by the ABPI, a standard form of agreement has not been developed. However, these usually define, at the very least, the protocol to be followed, the information to be made available in relation to the compound to be studied, the time limit for the study, the fee for carrying out the work, the reporting procedure for adverse events, confidentiality and publication of results, intellectual property rights, and liability for injury to subjects. None of these matters give rise to particular difficulties, except perhaps the question of liability for injury to volunteers and indemnities, which are considered later in this chapter.

5.2 In Relation to the Research Subject

Under English law, the sponsor will typically not be in a contractual relationship with the research subject, although ethical guidelines relating to compensation for injury may require a contractually binding undertaking on this question to be given by the sponsor to a healthy volunteer. However, independent of contract, the sponsor has long been exposed to liability for negligence and more recently in strict liability. A similar legal remedy in negligence exists in each of the Member States of the EU, although the burden of proof in relation to establishing it varies and the strict liability provisions are not uniform.

5.2.1 Negligence

The sponsoring manufacturer under English law owes the research subject an obligation to exercise reasonable skill and care, and any careless act or omission that leads to injury may expose the sponsor to liability to pay compensation.[31] Such an act or omission could in theory arise in a number of ways touching upon the supply of the test compound.

He will be exposed if a defect (such as contamination) arises in the course of the process of manufacturing the drug. Such cases are very rare, as quality control standards are very high in the industry. More likely is the possibility of some harmful propensity of the drug, implicit in its design, going undetected prior to administration to humans. This will always be a major concern for a manufacturer, but the manufacturer's exposure to liability is, in fact, limited. His duty in this regard is to carry out reasonable preclinical research with a view to establishing that it is safe to proceed from administration to animals to administration to humans. When assessing later whether the manufacturer exercised the standard of care required, the courts will judge the likelihood of harm — and therefore his decision to proceed — by reference to the state of scientific knowledge at the time or the "state of the art" as it is commonly known. The state of the art would essentially comprise prevailing knowledge of both animal and human toxicology as gleaned from both the international literature on the compound in question (or the class of compounds of which it is a member) and the preclinical research conducted by the manufacturer. Any preliminary clinical data already obtained by the company or an associated company may also be relevant.

A research subject who is injured and brings a claim for compensation will need to establish that the manufacturer had insufficient evidence to justify introducing the drug into humans or that he should have established the harmful propensity of the drug by virtue of the observations which were made, or should have been made, in the course of the preclinical work or from the published literature. Failure to follow authoritative guidelines relating to the type and extent of testing results to be available before administration to humans may be used as evidence of negligence, although each case will turn on its particular facts. Such an inquiry is rarely simple, and the outcome in terms of liability may ultimately depend upon who carries the burden of proof. Under English law the burden is upon the injured research subject. The obligation to take proper steps to discover any harmful characteristic of the drug is an exacting one, but the manufacturer will not automatically be liable if he fails to isolate that harmful characteristic, provided that he exercised reasonable care. He is not liable for unforeseeable effects, as by definition no amount of care can guard against injuries arising from the unforeseeable.

More straightforwardly, the manufacturer may be vulnerable if he has failed to supply adequate information on the preclinical testing of the drug to the investigator so that the investigator can satisfy himself that it is safe to proceed and rule out subjects who may be particularly at risk from the drug in question. Dukes and Swartz[32] have emphasized the degree to which "investigators" carrying out studies for the pharmaceutical industry are reliant upon the planning and expertise of the sponsor's own medical department. For this reason they prefer the use of the expression "clinician in charge" as indicating their more limited role in practice. The manufacturer undoubtedly has a crucial obligation to apprise the investigator of the research that has been done with the drug under trial and explain the results (and also to provide information in relation to knowledge acquired later), but equally this does not remove entirely the responsibility of the investigator in law to make an independent judgment, and indeed it is he who must be conversant with the perceived risks and benefits (if any) of the medicine and prepared to discuss them. The CPMP Guidelines require the sponsor to inform the investigator in detail of the scientific information said to justify the nature, scale, and duration of the study (see paragraph 2.3(b)). The same guidelines emphasize (see paragraph 2.5) that the investigator has a responsibility to be "thoroughly familiar" with the properties of the product under trial.

The manufacturer is not likely, as a matter of English law, to be found legally liable for injuries arising solely through the negligence of his investigator, where that person is not his employee. The manufacturer who delegates responsibility for carrying out the study to an outside investigator or contract research company must exercise reasonable care in the choice of his investigator. However, provided that he makes reasonable inquiries to establish the competence and experience of that person and the adequacy of the facilities for conducting the research, he should not be liable for his investigator's negligence in the performance of any procedure contemplated by the protocol.[33] Arguments to the contrary, based upon the concept of nondelegable duties whenever hazardous operations are involved, have been canvassed but find little support in English law.

5.2.2 Strict Liability

The legal exposure of the manufacturer might have been expected to change as a result of the imposition of strict liability upon "producers" under domestic legislation implementing the EEC Directive of 1985 on Liability for Defective Products.[34] In fact, this is not the case, and indeed doubt has been expressed as to whether the supply of research products is covered by the directive at all.

In the U.K. the directive is implemented by the Consumer Protection Act 1987,[35] and at the consultation stage the Department of Trade suggested that strict liability only applied to freely marketed products because research products were not "put into circulation" in the normal sense of this phrase.[36] Early drafts of the Consumer Protection Bill actually provided a defense to producers if a product found to be defective was put into circulation solely for the purpose of a test to be conducted with or upon it. In the event, the matter was clearly reconsidered, as such an exemption did not appear in the Act itself. Most commentators agree that the directive is applicable to research products, but there is continued uncertainty in some Member States. However, the particular form of strict liability it introduces will probably have limited impact for research in any event.

The new law impacts primarily on producers and the manufacturer of a medicinal product is a producer under the Act. However, a product is treated as defective only if its safety is not such as persons generally are entitled to expect, having regard to all the circumstances, including the manner in which, and the purposes for which, the product has been marketed and any instructions or warnings given in relation to it. It would appear to follow that the very status of research products would mean that any volunteer, aware that he was participating in research, would have difficulty in getting over the first hurdle, namely establishing that he was entitled to expect the product to be safe. In the case of processing defects such as contamination, this may not be a problem, but even if on the facts of a particular case a product's defective nature is established, the producer may still be able to avoid liability by proving that the development risk defense (otherwise known as "the state-of-the-art defense") applies. Under the directive, Member States are allowed to grant the producer this defense in their implementing legislation if they so wish, and where incorporated in the implementing legislation, it protects the producer if: "the state of scientific and technical knowledge at the time when he put the product into circulation was not such as to enable the existence of the defect to be discovered."[37] In the absence of the defense, the position on liability for injury arising in clinical trials is more exposed although the test of the safety that a person is entitled to expect "in all the circumstances" would seemingly allow knowledge of the research content to be taken into account in determining whether the plaintiff can prove the defective nature of the product on the facts of the case.

So far all members of the EU that have implemented the directive have incorporated the defense except Finland and Luxembourg. Spain has excluded it for pharmaceuticals and France (which is still to implement the directive) is thought likely to incorporate it. Several countries outside the EU have introduced liability laws that mirror the directive's provisions and Switzerland has provided for a development risk defense, but Norway has not. However, interpretation of the defense itself has also been the subject of much controversy. Even while the directive was under negotiation, somewhat different attitudes were adopted by Member States. In the U.K., after much discussion in Parliament, the Act was passed with the defense applying where: "the state of scientific and technical knowledge at the relevant time [essentially the time of supply of the product to another] was not such that a producer of products of the same description as the product in question might be expected to have discovered the defect if it had existed in his products while they were under his control."[38]

On the fact of it, therefore, discoverability in its purest sense — without regard to the practicability of discovery — is not made the test but rather whether a producer could be expected, by reference *inter alia* to prevailing industry standards, to have discovered the defect. This notion, while arguably more consistent with the directive's practical objective of balancing the need for better consumer protection against the need not to stifle innovation, varies little from the traditional negligence standard and indirectly allows the question of the economic feasibility of discovering the defective nature of the product to be considered.

This is particularly relevant to clinical research, given that preclinical testing tends to focus upon a limited number of experiments, in a limited number of laboratory species, using a limited number of animals in the treatment and control groups. Primate testing, while technically feasible and often more likely to reveal potential hazards in man, is still not routinely performed and ethical pressures are increasingly operating somewhat differently in that area. If the harmful characteristics of a drug could have been established in one particular species used in animal experiments but not habitually used, any manufacturer faced with the allegation that a harmful characteristic of the drug would have been revealed by a sufficiently large study in that species would hardly be able to say that the defect was not discoverable in a technical sense.

This controversy is yet to be settled and will not be resolved finally until the issue is argued before the European Court. Attempts by consumer associations in the U.K. to make the European Commission bring proceedings under the Treaty of Rome, challenging H.M. Government's interpretation, finally bore fruit in December 1988, when the commission announced that proceedings would be commenced against the U.K. and Italy for failing to implement the defense correctly. Pending the decision in those proceedings, it is reasonable to draw the conclusion that strict liability in the U.K. barely changes the legal obligations of the pharmaceutical manufacturer in relation to research, except that the manufacturer, rather than the injured volunteer, has the burden of establishing nondiscoverability. In other Member States that have not allowed the defense, or have adopted language more consistent with a narrow interpretation of the defense, the change might turn out to be more significant.

5.2.3 Criminal Liability

Setting aside criminal sanctions under any national regulatory requirements providing for notification or approval of clinical research proposals, suppliers of products for clinical trials must now have regard to general safety requirements arising out of the Product Safety Directive which was adopted by the EU in 1992[39] and must be implemented in Member States with effect from June 29, 1994. However, its application in practice to sectors such as pharmaceuticals where there is existing European law aimed specifically at ensuring supply of "safe" products remains controversial. The general aim is to ensure a high level of protection for the safety and health of consumers by making it an offense to place unsafe products on the market, but the additional provisions in the directive only apply to the extent that existing Community law governing safety does not cover the same ground. Where the same aspect of product safety or risk is addressed in both sets of provisions, the sector's specific rules take priority.

As research products are "used" by consumers and supplied in the course of a commercial activity, the directive would appear to apply to medicinal products supplied and administered in the context of clinical trials. That conclusion may be more easily challenged in relation to phase I studies where, arguably, healthy volunteers, receiving payment for participation in studies, are themselves engaged in commercial activity. Implementation of the directive will normally involve the imposition of criminal sanctions for breach impacting upon manufacturers, importers into the community, and any professional in the chain of supply whose activity may affect the "safety properties" of their products. The basic obligations in the research context would appear to be to provide consumers with information to enable them to assess the risks and confront and avoid the hazards of use as far as is practicable, but also to investigate adverse experiences and adopt measures to discontinue supply and withdraw products from use, as appropriate. In the absence of harmonized rules in the Community relating to clinical research, compliance with national law requirements applicable to the supply of research products for use in clinical trials (and with GCP) ought to be good evidence of compliance with these broader safety obligations. The obligation imposed on Member States to notify the European Commission if they decide to take action to prevent supply of a particular product and the power of the Commission to prompt action on a community basis in such circumstances, could be relevant to the field of clinical research, pending harmonization of controls by specific European pharmaceutical directives. For the present, the making of regulations in Member States to implement the directive will simply add a further and overlapping area of regulatory control for companies and the industry has a legitimate complaint that there is so much uncertainty as to how these regulations are to be interpreted, particularly given the fact that criminal penalties may be imposed upon those who transgress them.

6 THE LEGAL OBLIGATIONS OF THE INVESTIGATOR

Under English law, in the absence of a contractual relationship between investigator and volunteer, which is only likely to arise where a patient is treated privately or in the case of arrangements for healthy volunteer research, the investigator's obligations are primarily determined by the law of negligence —

the duty to exercise reasonable care. The standard of care required of a physician is in this respect the same as would apply in relation to conventional treatment, although in practice the investigator arguably has a stricter responsibility to supervise the actions of other health professionals assisting him. In nonexperimental contexts the duty has been well defined in a series of decisions,[40] and if the investigator acts in accordance with the professional norm and adopts the practice that a body of opinion skilled in his field would have adopted in similar circumstances, he is most unlikely to be found negligent. There is inevitably, therefore, a wide band in English law between what is the prevailing consensus on any given issue and what is indefensible in law. In other countries the duty to disclose is more comprehensive and onerous. This is discussed further in relation to the doctrine of informed consent.

All research involves risks and the exercise of reasonable care in practice obliges the investigator to make a careful judgment that these are proportionate to the possible benefits. Where no benefit for the individual is envisaged because he is a healthy volunteer, the risks must be kept to the minimum independent of any issue of consent. The same principle applies where phase I research is conducted in patient volunteers, but the administration is not related to the condition being treated, except that the investigator must also be alert to the issue of drug interactions between the trial compound and the patient's own treatment drug. In the case of therapeutic research where the patient is being treated with a new drug because established treatments have failed to provide an acceptable level of efficacy or produced unacceptable side effects for the patient, the prospect of benefit enables the investigator reasonably to advise the patient to embrace the somewhat greater risks. It is of interest that in the light of the more complicated balancing exercise to be conducted in research, German law requires[41] that a physician must have at least two years of experience in clinical research of drugs before he may conduct a study as principal investigator. The fact of approval by an ethics committee may assist the investigator if his conduct is challenged. The extent to which, in each case, the investigator must advise the volunteer of the nature and seriousness of those risks that cannot be excluded raises the wider issues of consent discussed in detail below.

Depending upon the manner and circumstances of recruitment of healthy volunteers, including, perhaps, whether payment is made in return for participation, a contractual relationship may arise between the investigator and the volunteer. Today it is common to see consent forms extended into documents that in truth amount to written contracts under which each party expressly accepts certain obligations. Obligations concerning confidentiality, compensation, etc. may be accepted by the investigator and obligations to disclose details of existing or recent medication and report promptly any deterioration of health during participation may be accepted by the volunteer. Breach of such obligations by one party may in theory give rise to a claim for damages by the other party, although in practice breach of the volunteer's obligations is, at most, likely to prejudice his right to full payment or, on grounds of contributory fault, his position under compensation arrangements. Independent of these express terms, where an investigator contracts with a volunteer, English law will also imply a warranty on the part of the investigator that reasonable care and skill will be exercised in relation to the study. This obligation is broadly comparable with that which arises under the law of negligence, independent of a contract.

The introduction of strict liability for product defects should not have major repercussions for the investigator, for, as explained above, strict liability invariably only attaches to the producer and primarily it is the manufacturer who is to be treated as the producer. However, if investigators prepare their own research products, they will be strictly liable for defects in them on the same basis as manufacturers. Furthermore, the liability of a producer is imposed upon any person supplying a defective product, if he is unable within a reasonable time to inform the injured person of the identity of the actual producer/importer into the EU or, at the very least, the person who supplied him with the product.[42] Given the discrete nature of clinical research, investigators should not be troubled by issues of identification and their liability will continue to rest firmly in negligence.

In practice, this means that the investigator will only be vulnerable to claims for compensation if he has negligently failed to consider carefully the preclinical and other information supplied by the sponsor and therefore has allowed an unsafe proposal to go forward, or if he has not passed material information to the volunteer or if he has failed to screen out volunteers unsuitable for participation in the light of the advised contraindications of the drug, or has failed to perform ancillary procedures carefully or supervise the study and response of subjects adequately. In this regard, it must be noted that if a patient is improperly removed from treatment that is required, the injury may arise out of the absence of the existing treatment following randomization to placebo or an ineffective new drug under trial. Patient selection and monitoring is, therefore, vital.

Finally, it should be noted that fraud in clinical trials has been an issue in recent years and in the U.K., for instance, reporting doctors found to have behaved improperly are now more frequent. This can result in loss of professional registration and ability to practice. The ABPI issued guidelines on this matter in 1992 and an initiative is underway to develop guidelines for the EU as a whole.[43]

6.1 Consent

The legal effect of consent under English law is embodied in the maxim *volenti non fit injuria*, meaning "to one who is willing no harm is done." In law this has been reframed as the proposition that one who expressly, or by implication, consents to the commission of a wrong against him (or an act that would have been wrongful apart from the consent) cannot thereafter claim damages for any harm suffered. However, the nature of the defense has been confused by the fact that it may arise in two distinct circumstances. The first of these is where the patient consents to an invasion of this physical integrity that would otherwise be actionable as a trespass to person. The second is where, having consented to that medical intervention, he also agrees to assume the risk of a specific injury to which he is exposed by the study in circumstances where, if inadequate information about that risk has been provided, the investigator would have been exposed to a claim in negligence for failure to take proper care in counseling the volunteer.

6.1.1 Consent and Trespass to Person

Through the concept of trespass to person, the English common law reflects the fundamental ethical principle that we should respect each other's physical integrity. An act which intentionally leads to some physical contact amounts, in the absence of consent, to a battery.[44] However, the law does allow a person to consent to the use of a reasonable degree of force on his person and so no wrong is committed where consent is freely given. Therefore, it has long been understood that if a doctor touches or examines a person in his care or adopts any invasive procedure, provided that he has obtained consent, the patient cannot thereafter claim compensation for any resulting injury on the grounds of trespass to person. The exceptions to obtaining consent, such as acting out of "necessity" to preserve life, are most unlikely to arise in clinical research.

Consent may be expressly given or inferred from conduct. Accordingly, a volunteer offering himself for participation in a research study and proffering his arm for an injection required by the protocol to the study will almost certainly be found to have consented to the physical contact involved. To operate as a defense, the consent must be real in the sense that the volunteer must be informed in broad terms of the nature and general purpose of the study and the consent must not be procured by fraud or misrepresentation.[45] In 1970 the ABPI noted in its guidelines relating to research in healthy volunteers[46] that a volunteer, suffering an ill effect which he believed should have been made the subject of a warning, might be expected to put forward a claim at law based on the combined allegation of trespass to person and negligence. One advantage of a claim in trespass is that damage need not be proved to have resulted from the wrongful act. In contrast, liability in negligence depends upon the claimant showing not only a breach of the duty of care, but also that the injury complained of is causally related to the breach of duty.

However, it is doubtful whether claims based on trespass will, in practice, feature greatly in the context of research. The Court of Appeal in England has suggested[47] that to succeed in trespass the plaintiff must prove that the physical contact not only was deliberate, but also was made with an element of hostility. On this basis, actions for battery against physicians would normally be completely untenable, but the meaning of "hostility" is somewhat unclear in this context and subsequent decisions have followed the traditional distinction, which recognizes deemed consent only in respect of physical contact falling within the reasonable and generally acceptable band of conduct which may occur in the ordinary course of daily life but requires express consent for contact falling outside the ordinary course. For the present, therefore, it would perhaps be unwise to treat trespass to person as a dead letter in the field of clinical research on this basis alone. Indeed, in a recent case the need for any element of malice or hostility was suggested to be wrong in law.[48]

However, the English courts have also made it tolerably clear that failure to disclose the risks of the procedure does not vitiate consent that is real in all other respects.[49] Such failure will not, therefore, expose the investigator to an action in damages for trespass to person, although it may provide grounds for an action in negligence based on failure to disclose material information. This is a more significant reason why a claim in trespass is now unlikely in practice unless it can be argued that any sort of consent is lacking.

6.1.2 Consent in Children and the Mentally Handicapped

Having regard to the matters to be explained to volunteers, there arises the issue of competence to understand that explanation. The law in relation to consent competency — the legal capacity to give consent — is very unclear, as regards both children and those suffering from mental disability. The Nuremberg Code does not expressly cover either group, but the Declaration of Helsinki states in relation to nontherapeutic research that, where the subject is "legally incompetent," the consent "of the legal guardian" should be procured.[50] As the ethical and legal legitimacy of research which offers no direct benefit to the individual is based firmly on obtaining valid consent, the implication is obvious; essential research is less likely to be performed, to the longer-term disadvantage of these classes of person. Indeed, the phrase "therapeutic orphans" has been coined in relation to children. The key to this issue is, therefore, ultimately the validity of proxy consent.

6.1.2.1 Children

In relation to children, the position in English law appears to be that in relation to clinical research as part of treatment, a child over 16 may validly consent to treatment without regard to the wishes of his parents. Below that age, a minor's capacity to consent depends upon his having sufficient understanding to make a reasonably informed decision and is not to be determined by reference to any judicially fixed age limit.[51] Where he does not have such understanding, the parents have a legal right to give consent on his behalf. Nevertheless, most ethical guidelines advise that even if an investigator believes that a child is capable of giving valid consent, the approval of a parent or guardian should still be obtained. The Medical Research Council (MRC) in their 1991 guidance[52] entitled "The Ethical Conduct of Research on Children" notes that a "principled case can be made on ethical grounds for research on children" subject to three safeguards. These are first, that research should only take place if the relevant knowledge cannot be gained by research in adults, secondly that all studies must be approved by an ethics committee, and thirdly, that the children participating must give their consent or consent must be given on their behalf by their parents.

There is no direct authority on the issue of consent in relation to nontherapeutic research, but the general principle that one should focus upon the particular child's capacity to make a rational decision would seem to apply. In the case of children unable to give a valid consent themselves, the more difficult question arises as to whether a parent can properly consent in law to a child being subjected to a procedure which carries no prospect of direct personal benefit but only risk. There is no English law authority on this point. Some commentators have argued that the duty of a parent to act in the best interests of a child can equally be termed an obligation not to do anything clearly against the interests of the child.[53] As Dworkin[54] has argued, this would allow consideration of wider issues than direct medical benefit, including social responsibility, and on this basis, provided that approval of an ethics committee has been obtained (which will only be forthcoming if a study involves minimal risk and considerable benefit to children as a group), it is unlikely that English courts would declare ineffective a fully informed parental consent. This would appear to be ethically sound, but in practical terms the uncertainty that hinders research will only be resolved by a clear decision of the courts.

In this regard, the reluctance of physicians to adopt the above approach has undoubtedly been fueled in the past by statements from the MRC to the effect that a strict view of the law would prohibit proxy consents by parents in respect of nontherapeutic research.[55] This view was later underwritten by a Department of Health circular,[56] despite the fact that no authorities could be cited to support the MRCs statement and it appeared to be based on one legal opinion only. The MRC has now qualified its original statements and their guidelines sanction nontherapeutic research where there is negligible risk which includes noninvasive monitoring and obtaining blood and urine samples. Neither the MRC nor the British Pediatric Association[57] (BPA) contemplate any study of medicinal products as being acceptable. The Department of Health in the U.K., in its circular of 1991,[58] contemplated the possibility of studies involving "no more than minimal risk," but did not address clinical trials directly. The department suggests that parents responsible for allowing a child to be subjected to any risk (unless *de minimus)*, without the prospect of benefit for that child, could be said to be acting illegally. The question may, in any event, be somewhat academic where medicines are involved, as most bodies — including the Medicines commission in the U.K.[59] — have recommended that no approach should be made to recruit children as healthy volunteers in studies of medicinal products.

6.1.2.2 The Mentally Handicapped

The position in relation to clinical research into mental illness, using the mentally handicapped as subjects, is equally unclear. The traditional legal analysis was that the law protects the physical integrity of all persons, and therefore any intervention may only take place when, in a lucid moment, the mentally handicapped subject can give consent. On this basis, in relation to an adult not subject to any lucid moment, it was said that the proxy consent of a relative would not suffice and the physician could not proceed.[60] Indeed, even where the subject is a child (and a parent might be viewed as capable of giving a valid consent), doubt over the legal position of those concerned with care of a mentally retarded child was sufficient to prompt an application to make the child a ward of court so that the court could be asked to approve sterilization, applying the traditional test of what was in the best interests of the child.[61]

Likewise, in a case involving a mentally handicapped adult (where wardship is not an option) the physicians involved in the patient's care refused to terminate pregnancy and sterilize the patient without the protection of the court. The mother therefore applied for a declaration that the intervention envisaged did not constitute a trespass to person. The declaration was granted on the basis that the only consideration was what was in the best interests of the patient and consistent with good medical practice. That decision was upheld on appeal with a finding that a doctor could lawfully treat an adult incapable of consenting provided it was in the patient's best interests. However, although not strictly necessary, it was suggested good practice in the case of sterilization to involve the courts.[62]

Such an approach might reasonably be adopted in relation to clinical research, for the recent case law lends support to the view that if the treating physician believes that there is a prospect of benefit if the patient participates in a trial of a new treatment for his mental illness, and in this sense it is good medical practice to enroll him in the study, an extended principle of necessity will protect the investigator from legal sanction. In all cases, however, it would still obviously be important on ethical grounds to obtain the approval of the responsible relative and ethics committee approval before proceeding. The MRC in its 1991 guidelines[63] entitled "The Ethical Conduct of Research on the Mentally Incapacitated" supports therapeutic research provided four safeguards are observed. First, it must be clear that the relevant knowledge cannot be gained by research upon those able to consent; secondly ethics committee approval should be obtained; thirdly the participation of a person who through mental incapacity cannot provide a valid consent must be agreed as of benefit to that person by an "informed and independent" person and fourthly, the participant should not appear by words or action to object to his involvement. The CPMP Guidelines contemplate therapeutic research in the mentally incapacitated (see paragraph 1.13) provided the research is in the interests of the subject and a "legally valid representative" has confirmed this fact. The guidelines do not appear to contemplate circumstances where a proxy consent on behalf of an adult is not legally effective, as in England.

However, the case law does not suggest that the doctor can dispense with consent in the case of nontherapeutic research and indeed, the decisions of the English courts suggest the contrary. The MRC guidelines condone such research (not specifically with medicines) "provided the risk of harm is minimal and the welfare of the individual is considered by the ethics committee and an informed independent person ..." However, the general consensus is that testing of medicinal products can never be justified in mentally handicapped subjects who cannot expect personal benefit. This is implied by paragraph 1.13 of the CPMP Guidelines and the U.K. Department of Health Circular of 1991 appears to exclude nontherapeutic research on mentally disordered people unless their mental state still allows "freely given" consent.

Legislation in the Republic of Ireland has seemingly ruled out proxy consents except in relation to the participation of patients in research for their direct therapeutic benefit.[64] Likewise, in the U.K. the Medicines Commission has advised that the recruitment of healthy volunteers unable personally to give a valid consent should not take place in relation to studies involving medicinal products.[65]

6.1.3 Consent and Negligence

One element of the general duty of care owed by the investigator to the patient or healthy volunteer is the duty to disclose and counsel the volunteer in relation to any material risks to his health and well-being that might result from participation in the study. The duty flows from the ethical requirement that one should respect the autonomy of others, i.e., the right of self-determination. The investigator must under English law provide sufficient information to give meaning to that right.[66] In English law, where a person volunteering for research is warned of the nature and extent of a specific risk and freely and voluntarily agrees to run that risk knowing that if he is injured because the risk materializes he will have no legal right of redress, that person has assumed the risk himself and his consent to do so acts as a defense to any claim in negligence based upon the existence of the risk.

However, the assumption of a specific risk prior to participating does not imply acceptance of the consequences of any unrelated failure by the investigator to take reasonable care in supervising the research or in treating him should he suffer an adverse reaction. Furthermore, any attempt by the investigator, in a consent form or otherwise, to exclude or restrict his liability generally for death or bodily injury resulting from the investigator's negligence will in English law be void.[67]

6.1.4 The Doctrine of Informed Consent

From these principles, it is often suggested that for the investigator to avoid an action in negligence all the possible risks must have been fully explained and understood, i.e., fully "informed consent" must be obtained. However, a series of cases show that this proposition is not correct as a matter of English law. All of these cases dealt with consent in the context of treatment but in the absence of any cases concerned with research they are a proper starting point. Indeed, there is little reason to argue that the principles ought to be different purely because in research personal benefit is more speculative (or indeed entirely lacking). However, this is a much discussed area of law where from the outset policy decisions appear to have distorted the logical progression from ethical principle to legal decision.

In England, the traditional view in relation to medical treatment has been that the issue of information on risks is a matter of clinical judgment and not of legal doctrine. Early cases suggested that the physician must decide what risks were material and should be communicated to the patient. At its most extreme this approach was used to justify misrepresenting the facts to the patient.[68] In contrast, in many jurisdictions in the U.S. there has been a trend toward a general rule of law — based in part on the proposition that a fiduciary relationship exists between physician and patient — requiring full disclosure, so that all risks must be disclosed which the patient might consider material to the decision as to whether to accept treatment or not.[69] The physician is invited to presume that he is dealing with a rational person and disclose all relevant risks, even if he believes that the risks are remote. In this regard, the right to know is treated as taking precedence over the need to know. The notable exception to this rule is where the physician has good reason to believe that proper disclosure will be detrimental to the physical or mental well-being of the patient, in which case it is the "therapeutic privilege" of the physician to limit his counseling accordingly. The rule has come to be called the "doctrine of informed consent."

In cases in England[70] patients injured during conventional therapy have invited the courts to adopt the North American approach, but the courts have declined to do so. It has been unequivocally stated that there is no difference between the standard of care required in giving advice on risks and that required in diagnosis and treatment. The primary obligation to disclose risks with a view to allowing the patient to make a rational choice has been re-emphasized, but the obligation has been limited to making such disclosure as is reasonable in the light of all the circumstances, so that the physician will normally have discharged his duty if he acts in accordance with practice accepted as proper by a body of physicians skilled in the relevant field. In cases where the question is whether the reasonable physician should have disclosed a particular risk, the courts will hear expert evidence before determining whether it should have been disclosed. This falls some way short of the North American approach, although the courts have warned the medical profession to be on its guard against being overpaternalistic and "playing at God," specifically declaring that the court has an inherent right to intervene and declare that a risk must be disclosed, even if evidence of medical practice to the contrary is shown to exist. As an illustration of this it has been suggested that no court would sanction the failure of a physician to disclose a 10% chance of serious harm.[71]

Thus, both in North America and in England, while the legal criterion for disclosure is the materiality of the risk, the determination in law of what risks are material, and should therefore be disclosed, varies. Whereas in some jurisdictions of North America and elsewhere a risk is treated as material where a reasonable person in the patient's position would be likely to attach significance to it when deciding whether or not to accept the medical intervention, the English courts have only wavered slightly from a standard under which materiality is judged by reference to the professional norm in any given case. In recent years the English law approach has been heavily qualified in some countries that typically have based their jurisprudence on English common law principles. The High Court of Australia recently applied a patient standard rather than professional standard requiring a doctor to warn a patient of any risk that a reasonable person in the patient's position, would, if warned of it, be likely to treat as significant.[72]

6.1.5 Disclosure of Risks and Research

In the U.S. the central features of the "doctrine of informed consent" have been reproduced in FDA requirements for all clinical research.[73] Investigators must state the immediate purpose of the research and the significance of the data to be generated, and must explain the procedures envisaged, how often they will be carried out, and the overall length of time each will take. In addition, a full description of any "reasonably foreseeable risks or discomfort" to the subject is required and the subject must also be told specifically of the possibility of "unforeseeable risks." Such a standard of disclosure, requiring notification of what is "reasonably foreseeable," is perhaps more onerous than the Nuremberg standard of disclosing what is "reasonably to be expected" or the Declaration of Helsinki requirement that subjects should be "adequately informed." Certainly, what is in theory foreseeable might still not be expected. Indeed, some researchers have drawn attention to the potential risk of overdisclosure and confusion as the essential features of the study's safety profile become blurred by a sea of detail and ill-defined possibilities.

The present approach of English law to disclosure of risks has been widely criticized as being out of line with the aspirations of modern society, which is more informed and questioning on matters relating to health. Inevitably, it has been suggested that a different test for judging materiality might apply outside the field of conventional treatment. However, it is difficult to see that this would be consistent with the overall approach of the English courts and above all the apparent concern of the judges to avoid defensive medicine — a concern that is all too obvious in their decisions. There is no logical basis for adopting an entirely different approach to patients simply because one form of treatment happens to take place in an experimental context, although one would expect the application of a "reasonable physician" test to materiality to focus more closely on the possible risks and particularly the risk of the unknown. For the time being, there is certainly no English case law relating to therapeutic research that would support the approach of the Canadian courts that "there can be no exceptions to the ordinary requirements of disclosure in the case of research as there may well be in ordinary medical practice."[74]

Although it is tempting to try to place research using healthy volunteers in an entirely different category, logically there is, again, no compelling reason why a different test should be applied. However, in nontherapeutic research, whichever standard is applied to judge materiality, the outcome should be the same. When dealing with healthy volunteers, there is no question of disclosure not being in the best interests of the subject on the grounds that it might dissuade him from accepting appropriate treatment. Accordingly, the reasonable physician will surely decide what is material by reference to what the "reasonable person" in the position of the healthy volunteer would want to know and, moreover, would attempt to learn whether the subject might indeed wish to know more. It is unlikely that the courts, no longer affected by the dangers of promoting defensive medicine, would find that any reasonable physician could properly adopt a practice that did not involve warning of all foreseeable risks, including a suspicion of risk where the outcome would be serious if the risk materialized. In short, because the volunteer is not being treated for illness, any foreseeable risk must be material when it is set against the absence of any prospect of compensating personal benefit.

This is not to say that the physician must teach volunteers the essence of clinical pharmacology, but he must ensure that the volunteer knows enough to make a rational decision. Even with healthy volunteers, irrelevant information which may distort the picture may justifiably be ignored. Equally, any request by the subject to limit the amount of information he is given must be taken into account, because real respect for autonomy dictates that it should, although failure to request information that the reasonable person would seek should raise a question mark in the investigator's mind as to the suitability of the volunteer for participation in the study. It is, therefore, difficult to justify anything less than comprehensive disclosure with healthy volunteers, and whether the courts choose to explain the result as arising from the application of a "reasonable physician" or "reasonable healthy volunteer" standard of materiality is of little practical significance.

Some indication that a consistent approach will be adopted by the English courts arises from two cases, the first[75] where the duty to inform was considered in the context of advice about the risks of failure associated with female sterilization. The judge at first instance suggested that a distinction could be made between advice in the therapeutic and "nontherapeutic" context, by which he meant where the "patient" was psychologically and medically normal, so that in the context of female sterilization the duty of disclosure need not be determined exclusively by reference to the practice of competent professionals. The Appeal Court overruled the decision. Likewise, in a case concerning a warning of the risks of the long-term contraceptive Depo-Provera to a perfectly healthy patient, a similar professional standard was applied to disclosure.[76]

This is not to say that the approach of English law is to be preferred or is likely to be adopted elsewhere. In one of the very few reported cases on research, a Canadian court recently emphasized the divergence of approach on these matters and perhaps a tendency to give plaintiffs the benefit of the doubt in a research context. The case of Weiss v. Solomon[77] involved healthy volunteer research. The trial studied the ability of indomethacin to reduce retinal edema after cataract surgery. It included fluorescein angiograms after administration. Information for the subject referred to the possibility of allergic reactions but was generally reassuring as to the level of risk that the trial would involve. Such information had been approved after incorporation of certain changes by the research committee for the hospital where the study was taking place. The subject gave a written consent. It turned out that he had a history of hypertrophic cardiomyopathy. There was no mention of a risk of cardiac arrest in the information sheet. The subject suffered a cardiac arrest and died immediately following an angiogram. His next of kin brought a claim both against the investigator and the hospital alleging inadequate screening and exclusion of unsuitable volunteers and alternatively inadequate advice and failure to ensure that there was adequate resuscitation equipment available.

The court found against the investigator and the hospital on all counts. Despite conflicting medical evidence as to what would have been considered an appropriate contraindication, the court found that the screening was inadequate. It also found that, if properly advised, the subject would not have participated because of his medical history. It was concluded that there was an obligation in healthy volunteer research to advise of known risks however remote they were. The protocol for the study required adherence to the Declaration of Helsinki and the court found that, properly interpreted, the declaration required full disclosure of risks. The court also found that the ethics committee should have known of the increased risk with conditions of the type present in this subject but, even if suitable exclusion criteria had not been demanded, the committee should have required the giving of a warning in the subject information sheet. The court relied upon the existing Canadian jurisprudence (referred to above) that relates disclosure to "materiality to the reasonable patient." Certain aspects of this judgment are unclear and the conclusions appear to conflict with certain of the evidence given but it does support the growing trend within the medical profession itself to be less paternalistic. It is noteworthy that guidelines being developed for ethics committees and professional codes of practice are now definitely more consistent with the North American doctrine than the approach of the English courts.

The original European guidelines of 1987[78] recommended informing patients and healthy volunteers verbally, and if possible also in writing, about "the possible risks and discomforts involved." The CPMP Guidelines (1990) provide[79] (at paragraph 1.12) that the patient must be given "a full and comprehensive explanation of the study (including its aims, expected benefits for subjects and/or others, reference treatments/placebos, risks, and inconveniences, e.g., invasive procedures, and, where appropriate, an explanation of alternative recognized standard medical therapy). This appears to go beyond the thrust of the Declaration of Helsinki, principle of which requires the patient to be "adequately informed." The guidelines require that oral and written information be given to volunteers, wherever practicable, and that volunteers must be told that they can withdraw from the trial at any stage. Consent must be documented either by the volunteer's signature or that of any independent witness verifying the volunteer's consent. The volunteer must have access to information about the procedures for obtaining compensation for injury.

Significantly, one of the first direct legislative interventions in the EU — the Control of Clinical Trials Act in the Republic of Ireland — has also enshrined an approach to clinical research of all types that would appear to involve full disclosure. The "person conducting the clinical trial" is obliged by Section 9 to ensure that the subject is made aware of, *inter alia,* "the risks and any discomfort involved in, and the possible side effects of, the trial." It may be argued that this leaves open the definition of "risks" but, on the face of it, the intention appears to be that the obligation is unqualified. The Irish Department of Health guidelines on the act go further and recommend that the consent form itself include "details of any foreseeable risks which may arise." Furthermore, under the Irish legislation, after the explanation of the objectives, risks, and other features of the trial, the subject must be allowed a period of 6 days within which to consider whether to participate and, except with the agreement of the Minister of Health, the trial cannot begin in the interim. New legislation in Spain and Norway expressly requires informed consent without defining the concept, although the Declaration of Helsinki is referred to in the Spanish law and Norwegian law in practice requires compliance with the Nordic guidelines.

Whatever the present state of English law — and it suggested that the approach adopted is only likely to be altered by legislation — if clinical research and, in particular, research in healthy volunteers is to be accepted by society as a whole, those supervising it must be seen to have made careful disclosure of all relevant information. This is one area where the ethical and legal requirements should certainly coincide. Properly informed consent has been described as "an obstacle to research,"[80] but the trend of professional ethical guidelines is toward more comprehensive counseling on risks and alternative treatments, and it will become less easy for physicians seeking to justify nondisclosure to find expert evidence to support their case.

6.2 Randomization and Placebo Controls

Studies that are methodologically unsound are incapable of providing valid data and thereby lose their ethical underpinning. The randomized controlled clinical trial conducted under "blind conditions" has been developed as the optimal design for experimental purposes. However, the physician responsible for the patients, though partly in search of new knowledge, must also not lose sight of the fact that he has an overriding duty in law to act reasonably and in the best interests of the patient. On this basis, it is difficult to see how he can advise a patient to enter a study unless it appears to him that the patient's health will not be prejudiced by his being part of either the case or control group. After taking account of the risks attending the treatment, and the benefits of the current treatment options, participation of his patients must hold out the chance of "saving lives, re-establishing health, or alleviating suffering," to use the Helsinki phraseology.

Where the design of the trial involves two therapeutic groups, problems in practice are seldom of great medicolegal significance, although the fact of randomization is so fundamental to the trial method that ethically and legally it should, except where "therapeutic privilege" is involved, be disclosed to the patient as part of the consent procedure. It has been persuasively argued, and would seem correct, that since the patient's assumption is that the physician will choose what he considers is the best treatment for the patient, any failure to explain the facts of randomization may involve the physician in "straying outside the terms of his patient's consent." The fact that many patients are not aware that they have been enrolled in a trial has given rise to considerable adverse publicity in the U.K., to the detriment of the research community.[81]

Where the control group is intended to receive a placebo, the medicolegal difficulties may be greater. It has been suggested by some that placebo controls are always unethical.[82] However, placebo groups are often considered essential, especially where the endpoint of treatment is difficult to assess and observer bias is a potential problem. Feinstein sums it up as follows: "If the question is worth asking, if its answer requires the use of placebo, and if the answer is worth getting, then the plan to use a placebo is justified."[83] He argues strongly that the ethical question boils down to one of consent. Patients must be informed of the plan and they are then free to refuse to participate. Certainly, the more commonly held view is that placebo controls are acceptable ethically and legally, notably where there is no alternative to the treatment under trial (or serious doubt as to efficacy of that treatment) or when the effect of adding a new treatment to an established one is under study. Such a position is adopted by the MRC in the U.K. As a matter of English law, it is suggested that provided that a patient is made fully aware of the possibility and risks to health of being randomized to placebo, and the risks are minimal, it is doubtful that the courts would rule that the patient's consent was invalid or that the investigator was negligent.

The view that the problem is essentially one of consent is supported by the new Irish legislation, which requires that any subject asked for consent must be made aware, where appropriate, of the possibility of receiving a placebo.[84] The CPMP Guidelines[85] make a similar recommendation. There has always been a degree of discomfort about placebo trials, but, as Gilbert has pointed out,[86] an absolute requirement for fully informed consent in all randomized controlled clinical trials may have a significant effect on trials comparing transparently different types of treatment (e.g., surgery vs. drug therapy) where patients are likely to have marked personal preferences, but will have a limited effect on the viability of drug trials which compare active treatment with placebo or new drugs with standard drugs.

6.3 Consent Forms

Under German law the consent of a patient volunteering to participate in trials of unlicensed drugs must be in writing or, if made orally, must be independently witnessed.[87] The requirement for written consent (with certain exceptions) also applies in the Republic of Ireland and France. Spain requires[88] consent "preferably in writing" or alternatively witnessed for patient volunteers and in writing for healthy volunteers. Hungary requires written consent.[89] Japanese guidelines[90] require informed consent and although there is no need for written consent and it is widely accepted that the traditional approach of physicians is to give limited information, if consent is oral that fact must be recorded. The trend is therefore very clear. However, all that is required under English law for consent to be effective is an actual statement from which it is reasonable to deduce that a volunteer has freely given his consent. An effective consent may be given orally, although as a matter of evidence it is desirable for it to be witnessed by someone other than the investigator himself. The U.K. Department of Health in its 1991 circular has advised that written consent be required except for the most trivial procedures.[91] It is now the case that most ethical guidelines advise that the subject's consent and the nature of the information disclosed as the basis for that consent should be recorded in writing. The CPMP Guidelines adopt this approach. Where consent forms are employed (and Dukes and Swartz have suggested that this is less frequent in countries where there is "no tradition of patient litigation") it is sometimes recommended, particularly in relation to healthy volunteers, that the investigator confirm in writing on the same form that he has advised the volunteer of the relevant features of the study. Increasingly, investigators cross-reference this statement to a volunteer information sheet, which contains written confirmation of the nature, purpose, and risks of the research.

However, a signed consent form is not decisive evidence that the consent was validly obtained or that proper care was exercised in counseling the subject. Consent issues essentially focus upon the volunteer's state of mind in deciding whether to participate and the true nature of the counseling received, rather than upon a signature on a document. Indeed, it is right that a volunteer should be able to withdraw consent at any time; no volunteer should feel contractually bound by having signed a consent form. This right is, in fact, enshrined in the Irish legislation. There is, however, a presumption under English law that the document has been read before signature and, at the very least, the preparation of consent forms directs the minds of those performing the research to the various ethical considerations, and provides a record that an attempt has been made to address them.

7 THE LIABILITY OF OTHER PARTIES TO RESEARCH

There are, of course, other parties to most research whose lack of care can cause injury. The hospital or other establishment in which the research takes place has a legal obligation to ensure, as with conventional therapy, that their facilities and the medical products and equipment made available for research are in proper order and are sterile and safe for normal use. In the U.K., the Royal Pharmaceutical Society has issued guidelines[92] relating to the obligation of pharmacists involved in the conduct of clinical trials in hospitals. The vicarious liability of the hospital for its own ethics committee has been noted above. However, the potential liability of hospitals and health authorities does not raise issues specific to clinical research. Equally, it must also be remembered that the volunteer, too, has certain obligations, breach of which in law may have implications — principally by reducing or extinguishing the volunteer's ability to claim compensation for any injury suffered by virtue of his own contributory negligence. The position of ethics committee and regulatory authorities requires special mention.

7.1 Ethics Committees

In 1964 the Declaration of Helsinki clearly established the need for all research protocols to be considered by an independent committee for guidance and, implicitly, approval. Ethics committee approval has now, in practice, become a necessary step in the performance of most research in Europe, although submission to ethics committees is not legally required in all Member States of the EU. Furthermore, in the absence of statutory intervention, progress in formalizing the status of ethics committees has been slow.

In the U.K. the Royal College of Physicians recommended in 1967 that all research projects performed in medical institutions should be approved by an independent group of doctors, and in 1973 the college made further recommendations concerning the composition and functions of such committees. In a circular in 1975[93] the Department of Health endorsed the college's proposals and required that they be implemented by health authorities. However, it was not until 1984 that the college issued detailed guidelines on the constitution and functions of ethics committees, but the practices of ethics committees remain far from uniform.[94]

The sole reference to ethics committees in the U.K. Medicines Act legislation appears in an order relating to notification of clinical trial proposals.[95] This order requires any refusal by an ethics committee to sanction a trial to be reported by the sponsor to the Licensing Authority. More recently, the Medicines commission was called upon to advise the Minister of Health on whether healthy volunteer studies should be brought under statutory control. While reporting that there is "inadequate reason on the basis of presently available information to recommend this course of action," the commission made various proposals[96] for a better system of self-regulation and notably recommended that "the role and constitution of ethics committees should be codified and elaborated by those concerned" and that the Department of Health should communicate guidance after consultation with interested bodies. The Department of Health guidelines of 1991[97] supersede the 1975 circular and provide detailed guidance on the constitution of ethics committees and their functions and procedures. In some respects the guidance conflicts with that provided by the Royal College of Physicians of London, who have published their own ethics committee guidelines and detailed guidelines for research in patients.[98] In 1994 detailed standards[99] for ethics committees were issued by the U.K. Department of Health, together with a full commentary on Standard Operating Procedures prepared by a member of this author's firm.

In contrast, in the U.S. Food and Drug Administration regulations[100] define the constitution and purpose of "institutional review boards" to which all clinical investigations requiring the consent of the FDA must be submitted for approval, and in the Republic of Ireland the Control of Clinical Trials Act now requires all clinical research to be submitted to an ethics committee, whose constitution is subject to review by the Minister of Health. The approval of a study by the Committee must be reported to the Minister, and the act also lays down the ethical issues to be considered by the committee.[101] Legislation in France[102] requires research to be submitted to ethics committees. Ethics committee approval is also required under statute in many other countries including Hungary,[103] Sweden,[104] Spain,[105] Switzerland,[106] Norway,[107] Finland, and Denmark.[108]

In the U.K., even without the existence of legislation to focus attention upon their role, ethics committees, and particularly the lay members, have become more concerned about their own legal position in the face of an increasingly litigious environment. As a matter of English law, 10 years ago few would have doubted that such a body, which holds itself out as there to protect the interests and health of research volunteers, does not owe a duty of care in law to those volunteers, breach of which could make the members vulnerable to claims for compensation on the grounds of negligence. The trend in English law, in recent years,[109] has been away from making bodies carrying out public functions liable in negligence, but on balance it is suggested that an ethics committee does owe volunteers a duty of care as a matter of private law. The claim would have to be made against the individual members for failure to exercise reasonable care in approving the trial, as committees are informal bodies and have no legal personality in their own right. This theoretical risk has certainly led some ethics committees to seek and obtain full indemnities from the authority appointing them in respect of any claim that might be advanced by an injured volunteer. In Canada it has been noted above that the risk is far from theoretical. The Department of Health in the U.K. advises National Health Service bodies to provide indemnity in terms described in its 1991 guidelines[110] for local research ethics committees.

7.2 Regulatory Authorities

Where a government regulatory authority reviews a proposal for research and consents to its performance, it may be exposed to claims if its review can be said to have been performed negligently. Under English law, although there is no direct authority on this matter, the Licensing Authority and the Committee on Safety of Medicines have been sued in relation to the approval of drugs for marketing,[111] and the principle ought to be the same. However, as mentioned above in relation to the status of ethics committees, recent decisions of the appeal courts in other areas of activity have raised question marks as to whether a public body, such as the Licensing Authority or its expert advisory committees, owe private law duties to individuals who might be affected by their actions. The issue remains uncertain, but even if a right of action does exist, the likelihood of such an action succeeding is comparatively small. The Licensing Authority would no doubt argue that in acting on the advice of its expert committee it was acting reasonably. In turn, the expert committee might reasonably be expected to defend a claim on the basis that the decision of a distinguished body of medical experts by definition could not be challenged as inconsistent with the opinion or practice of a reasonable body of professional opinion and therefore negligently reached. As regards clinical trial exemptions, it would be particularly difficult to show negligence, as neither the Licensing Authority nor its expert committees are in a position to consider the preclinical data fully and the system of negative clearance rests on the certification of the company's medical advisor or of the consultant engaged by the company.

8 COMPENSATION FOR INJURY

In Germany legislation relating to clinical trials provides for compulsory insurance, which must respond in relation to injury caused by participation.[112] Cover must amount to DM 500,000 per subject at least, but the cover must be proportionate to the risks involved. The insurance must be with an insurer based in Germany.

Standard policy wording has been negotiated by manufacturer interests. Only trials in Germany are covered and only injuries occurring within three years of the completion of the study are compensated. The volunteer may claim direct from the insurer. The maximum cover in aggregate is DM 30 million for over 3000 persons involved in a trial of one compound. If an injured subject claims compensation in law through the courts, the insurance proceeds are set off against the claim for damages. The insurer may thereafter seek contribution from the sponsor if he or the investigator were negligent and this caused the injury.

In France, decrees in 1990 and 1991 brought into force all the provisions of the laws[113] on biomedical research and this provided for compensation, backed by insurance, to be paid on a strict liability basis for injury due to participation in healthy volunteer and patient volunteer studies. SNIP, the French pharmaceutical industry trade association, negotiated a model contract with insurance companies with set premiums according to the phase and size of trials.

In Spain, under Article 62 of the 1990 law[114] no-fault insurance must be taken out by the sponsor to cover compensation for injury, but to the extent that this is not sufficient to compensate the subject adequately, the parties to the research are severally liable to meet the difference, independent of any fault on their part. Without insurance, ethics committee and regulatory approval will not be forthcoming. This law is widely interpreted as applying to phase I-IV. Under Article 62, unless otherwise established, injury during the trial and for one year after its termination is presumed to be due to the trial unless the defendant establishes the contrary; after that time the subject has the burden of proof again.

Italy has made[115] the provisions of the CPMP Guidelines part of its law and requires "appropriate" compensation. The vagueness of the provisions is reflected in uncertainty as to the extent to which (if at all) insurance is required to benefit subjects in the event of injury but the Ministry of Health treat the law as requiring the sponsor to arrange compensation by establishing insurance on a no-fault basis (including the fault of the investigator).

In Sweden injury arising in clinical trials should be compensated under the pharmaceutical insurance-based scheme (although there has not been a case thus far). In response to a requirement for insurance a no-fault compensation scheme was set up to cover injuries arising with marketed products or clinical trial products, unless the injury was covered by the parallel patient insurance scheme which responds to injury caused by physician negligence. However, not all injuries are compensated if they have been the subject of a warning and, having regard to risk/benefit, the patient must reasonably accept the risk. The Swedish Product Liability Act of 1993 excludes clinical trial products from coverage but if a research subject is dissatisfied with the outcome of a claim against the insurance scheme, a claim in negligence could be pursued under general law.

In the Republic of Ireland by law the person conducting the research must satisfy the ethics committee that adequate funds are available to provide compensation for any injury resulting from the trial, independent of negligence.[116] Insurance is not a requirement but is a way of providing such security.

In Finland[117] adherence to the Nordic guidelines is required but these are unclear on the issue of compensation. A circular under the Medicines Act does, however, recommend that sponsors establish insurance for compensation and a voluntary industry scheme has been established for research and marketed drugs. It is administered by the Finnish Pharmaceutical Insurance Pool which consists of the major Finnish insurance companies. This responds on proof of causation only but it does not cover known side effects unless these are more severe than expected. Investigators too have compulsory insurance requirements for performance of healthy volunteer and patient volunteer studies.

In Norway, the 1981 regulations[118] provide that all volunteers must be insured against injury but this obligation is now met by compliance with the provisions of the Norwegian Product Liability Act of 1988 and the insurance requirements thereunder. A no-fault compensation scheme was established under this Act for pharmaceuticals and sponsors of trials must be members of the Drug Liability Association which arranges insurance cover for company sponsors. The patient may proceed directly against the insurer. There are maximum levels of compensation allowed.

In Switzerland, the recent regulations[119] advise payment of compensation on a no-fault basis and insurance cover provided by the sponsor.

In Belgium, there is no legal requirement for insurance but ethics committees may seek it, although it appears to be standard practice for this to respond to the legal liabilities of the sponsor only and not to be on a completely no-fault basis.

In Denmark, there is no specific legal requirement to take out insurance but it is an obligation of the investigator to make sure that adequate insurance exists and in practice the sponsor takes out insurance but not on a no-fault basis. In Portugal, there are no compulsory insurance requirements and sponsor's liability appears to depend upon the general law. In Hungary, the requirement for ethics committee approval results in a requirement for compensation on injury and insurance for both the sponsor and the investigator's activities. In The Netherlands, requirements are being implemented for strict liability for the parties to research with insurance to cover that liability on a no-fault basis. In Japan, compensation is still not addressed by their GCP guidelines.

In the U.K. however, where a patient volunteer is injured in the course of research, his right in law to compensation will be determined solely by application of the principles of negligence and strict liability described earlier. It follows from what has been said about the nature of these remedies that the fact of even a serious injury occurring in research does not automatically imply a right to compensation. As a matter of English law the volunteer will be hard pressed to establish a right to compensation in negligence provided that the investigator ensured that the volunteer consented to participate in the study, and in all other respects both the manufacturer of the drug and the investigator exercised reasonable care in the planning and performance of the study. The nature of research is such that injury can arise however much care is taken by the participants and in all cases negligence will not be easy to prove for a private individual operating outside his field of knowledge with the burden of proof lying firmly with him. In terms of strict liability, whatever interpretation of the "state-of-the-art defense" is adopted, certain "development risks" will remain with the volunteer.

There has been considerable criticism in the U.K. of the fact that such risks should be left with individuals seemingly less able to bear the burden of the unexpected than the manufacturer or the institution under whose auspices the research is conducted. Once a product has completed its main research phase and is freely marketed, the arguments for leaving some risk with the consumer are more finely balanced, but a fundamental ethical principle of research is the requirement for fairness and this translates into the need to ensure that the burden and benefits of research are properly shared. The argument to compensate those injured in research through no fault of their own is therefore formidable, although interestingly the Declaration of Helsinki does not raise the issue. In the U.K. both the MRC and the Department of Health have represented[120] that they would consider making *ex gratia* payments in appropriate cases. However, the Royal Commission on compensation for personal injury (Pearson Commission) commented:[121]

> "We think that it is wrong that a person who exposes himself to some medical risk in the interests of the community, should have to rely on *ex gratia* compensation in the event of injury. We recommend that any volunteer for medical research...who suffers severe damage as a result should have a cause of action on the basis of strict liability, against the authority to whom he has consented to make himself available. Even with the increasing tendency of some healthy volunteers to treat participation in research as merely another form of 'work,' where it is questionable whether the desire to serve society is uppermost in the mind, the greater commercialization of such research arguably makes the case for compensation even stronger."

However, not all groups that have looked at this question felt able to support the idea of a strict liability remedy in law — a remedy that the Pearson Commission appeared to believe should be against the investigator's employer or perhaps the sponsor of the research. A group convened by the Ciba Foundation came out against the concept of claimants still having to seek redress through the courts against a named defendant, at least in relation to injuries other than those arising from processing or labeling defects.[122] In their view the objective of providing volunteers "with the sure knowledge that they would receive a quick and just response to their quest for compensation" required the introduction of a "no-fault compensation scheme" operating outside the system and financed jointly by those promoting and involved in research on an insurance-orientated basis.

Contrary to the intentions of the Pearson Commission, strict liability as established by the EEC directive does not provide volunteers with a much improved prospect of compensation, especially in those jurisdictions such as the U.K., where a "development risk defense" has been made available to the producer. However, the ethical imperative has long been recognized by the ABPI, first in 1970 in relation to healthy volunteers from its own staff[123] and later in 1988 for all healthy volunteers[124] and in 1983 for clinical trial patients.[125] The patient guidelines were amended and broadened in 1991.[126] Through separate contractual or quasi-contractual arrangements with volunteers the right to compensation is based solely on proof of a causal connection between the administration of the drug and the injury complained of. A study-based approach of this type avoids some of the significant problems of funding and administering a national no-fault scheme of the type envisaged by the Ciba Working Group.

8.1 Healthy Volunteers

In the case of healthy volunteers the present ABPI compensation guidelines recommend that a specific contractually binding undertaking is given to volunteers to compensate them (or their dependants) in the event of "any significant deterioration in health or well-being" caused by "participation" in the study, with compensation calculated by reference to the level of damages that would be awarded by the English courts for similar injuries had legal liability in negligence been established. The undertaking goes on to provide that any dispute as to the application of the compensation provisions is to be referred to an arbitrator. The guidelines provide that this undertaking should not seek to exclude compensation where there is an issue as to whether the negligence of the investigator may have caused the injury. The overriding consideration is to provide prompt compensation for the volunteer and it is suggested that the sponsoring company merely preserves its rights of recourse against third parties so that indemnity in respect of, or contribution toward, compensation paid to a volunteer can be recovered from third parties where they have been negligent. In England such a right of recourse will normally arise by operation of law but separate indemnities can be sought, as appropriate, and are freely given by the major commercial contract research companies. The guidelines do not preclude a volunteer from pursuing a claim in negligence or strict liability if he so desires. The Medicines commission has recommended[127] not only that companies should give an undertaking to provide compensation, but also that they should "provide evidence of their ability to fulfill it." The Department of Health endorsed that suggestion in its 1991 guidelines.[128]

8.2 Patient Volunteers

In the case of patient volunteers, somewhat different arrangements apply to research sponsored by members of the ABPI. Some patients entering clinical trials suffer from minor disorders but others from life-threatening diseases where discussion of compensation arrangements in the event of injury may well cause unnecessary alarm and not be in their best interests. For these reasons many doctors are reluctant to expose their patients to elaborate consent forms or the separate paperwork required to establish a binding contractual obligation to compensate. Instead, member companies are asked by the 1991 Guidelines[129] to give an "undertaking" to the investigator, to compensate for injuries which, while not legally binding, is unquestionably binding as a matter of commercial reality. Clearly, in the event of injury an ethics committee would monitor the fact that the undertaking was honored and a company that did not might find sponsoring future research very much more difficult for it, not to mention the adverse media comment that the failure would generate. The undertaking to pay compensation under the guidelines ends with the trial, so that patients continued on the trial drug thereafter are not covered.[130] The 1991 Guidelines apply to phases II-IV but while compensation is to be paid for injuries arising from participation for phases I-III, it is only offered at phase IV where injury arises from a procedure (not the trial drug) that would not have arisen except for the participation in the study.

In practice, therefore, the interests of volunteers are protected in industry-sponsored research, although some commentators have argued in favor of binding contracts with patients at phases I and II, and criticized the right to exclude payment under the 1991 Patient Guidelines where negligence of the investigator may have caused the injury. The fact that compensation is denied where the drug has failed to produce the desired effect — as might happen in an oral contraceptive trial — has also been criticized.[131] However, the infinite variety of clinical trials presents difficulties when drafting simple guidelines and in appropriate cases experience shows that companies are prepared to vary them to accommodate particular concerns. The text of the guidelines appears at Appendix 1.

The arrangements made by the industry have yet to be followed by government and academic interests initiating research, whose volunteers still must rely, at best, upon vague representations about *ex gratia* payments. This double standard has been criticized by the Royal College of Physicians of London,[132] which in relation to healthy volunteer studies has recommended that the concept of contractual undertakings developed by industry be extended in principle to universities and other institutions performing research. Ethics committees are advised by the Royal College to check carefully to see that arrangements have been made for compensating volunteers where the study is sponsored by industry, but the college appears to accept that the funding of academic research (or rather the lack of it) makes this impracticable for the moment in relation to research not industry sponsored. The Medicines Commission has advised that government should formally indicate "that sympathetic and comparable consideration" would be given to healthy volunteers injured in studies performed by publicly funded bodies.[133]

The 1991 Guidelines from the Department of Health[134] note that ethics committees should ensure that the sponsor, if a private sector company, accepts responsibility for compensation and provides details of the basis on which it will be provided and evidence of an ability to meet this undertaking. The department does not expressly state that it should be on a no-fault basis. For public body sponsors an injured volunteer would be "entitled to enter a claim for ex gratia payment," but each case will be considered on its merits as NHS bodies are not empowered to offer advance indemnity. The CPMP Guidelines require the sponsor (see para 2.3(i)) to provide "adequate compensation/treatment for subjects in the event of trial-related injury or death, and provide indemnity (legal and financial cover) for the investigator, except for claims resulting from malpractice and/or negligence." What is "adequate" compensation is not defined and the Annex to the Guidelines, which seeks to explain the practical implications of the provisions, uses different and somewhat confusing language (see paragraph 9) by saying that volunteers should be "satisfactorily insured" against any injury caused by the trial and the liabilities of all concerned in the conduct of the trial must be clearly understood before the trial starts. The reference to insurance is frequently used to suggest that sponsors should provide evidence of the existence of an insurance policy, but the better view is that this merely requires the sponsor to have proper arrangements in place to provide volunteers with compensation and treatment for injury caused. As a result, the ABPI Guidelines are generally viewed by ethics committees in the U.K. as sensible and fair in this regard, although it is arguable that the exclusion of medicine-induced injury in phase IV trials is inconsistent with the CPMP Guidelines. Many companies apply their principles to trials outside the U.K.

One can speculate whether the absence of a formal arrangement, now so commonly available, should be treated as a material fact to be disclosed by the investigator to the volunteer. One can envisage some volunteers, after sustaining injury, arguing that had they known compensation was not available they would not have volunteered. Certainly, DHHS regulations in the U.S. state that nonavailability of such compensation must be disclosed on the basis that it is a reasonable presumption for a volunteer to make that in the event of injury he will be provided for.[135] Surprisingly, however, special compensation arrangements do not appear to be a common feature of research in the U.S.

9 PROOF OF CAUSATION

Whether claims in respect of injury are made in negligence or strict liability or pursuant to a special contractual arrangement or under a centrally funded no-fault scheme, the common feature of all of these approaches is that the claimant must prove causation. In English law causation is a matter to be determined by the court as a reasonable inference to draw from admissible evidence and must be established on the balance of probability. Although tribunals of the type envisaged by the supporters of "no-fault" schemes might well be encouraged in practice to set aside the strict rules of evidence applied by courts in assessing what is reliable evidence of the facts alleged (this appears to be the case with the Swedish schemes), the burden of proving causation inevitably still normally rests with the claimant. The burden will sometimes be difficult to discharge, particularly in clinical trials where deterioration in health may simply reflect the progression of the underlying disease or the effect of a concomitant therapy. The Ciba Working Party concluded in relation to healthy volunteer studies that, because injuries during research are rare, the problems of establishing causation are unlikely to be substantial, it being "...reasonable to assume that any deterioration in health which occurs within a short time of the experiment, in the absence of any other evident explanation, is attributable to the experiment and should be compensated." In contrast, as regards clinical research with patients, the Working Party recognized[136] that "detailed consideration of the probability of a causal relationship between therapy and event would...be unavoidable particularly when larger scale and prolonged studies are carried out." In Spain, it has been seen that the law provides that where injury occurs during or within one year of the trial, causation will be assumed and need not be proven by the subject. The sponsor must seek to prove the assumption incorrect.

Difficult cases will arise but in practice, where corporate sponsors are involved, because of the commercial setting within which the injury has arisen, the pressure will be to give the benefit of the doubt to the volunteer. This was apparent in the case of a student who died after the administration of midazolam in a healthy volunteer study sponsored by Roche Products, where a payment was made despite the fact that there was little scientific evidence to suggest that the compound could have caused the aplastic anemia from which the volunteer died. Likewise, in its evidence to the Pearson commission the MRC noted that it had recommended an *ex gratia* payment in a case where a volunteer taking part in a trial of live attenuated influenza vaccine developed a neurological lesion shortly after administration, despite the fact that such a lesion had not previously been reported in association with vaccination. In the U.K., special insurance policies have been developed in the Lloyd's market[137] to provide indemnity to companies sponsoring research that responds in circumstances where the ABPI Guidelines would provide for the payment of compensation. These can be applied to trials taking place in most countries, but the U.S. is an express exception.

10 INDEMNITIES FOR INVESTIGATORS AND OTHERS CONNECTED WITH RESEARCH

The concern of ethics committees that they might be drawn into litigation if a volunteer is injured in clinical research has been mirrored in the U.K. by the concern of investigators and also the health authorities in whose hospitals research takes place to see that they are adequately protected from claims. In part the concern of the investigators has been heightened by discussions as to whether medical protection societies, faced with an increasing number of claims and the need to demand much higher premiums, will automatically continue to defend and indemnify their members in respect of activities that arguably fall outside their normal professional duties. Acting as investigators for the pharmaceutical industry not only might be viewed as more commercially motivated, but also is widely thought to increase the physician's potential exposure to claims. The protection societies in the U.K. have considered changing the basis upon which members' benefits are granted; acting as an investigator (unless as an employee of a pharmaceutical company) was traditionally treated as part of professional practice. However, the fact that the right to be indemnified is discretionary (membership does not amount to an insurance contract in the strict sense) has encouraged physicians to investigate whether further protection can be gained from those requesting their services as investigators. The Medical Defense Union now states that it will not provide indemnity if separate insurance exists through the employing pharmaceutical company.

As a result, it is now standard practice for an investigator to request a person who has instituted and sponsored the research to provide an indemnity for his benefit and that of his co-workers against any liability and expenses that the investigator may suffer as a result of claims in respect to personal injury made by volunteers involved in the study. As the majority of clinical research is today sponsored by the pharmaceutical industry, it is the individual company that is asked for such an indemnity. Typically, this will be drafted only to extend to injury which was not caused by the negligence of the investigator or the failure of the investigator to adhere to the protocol to a material extent. In the event that a claim is made, but is unsuccessful, the investigator not covered by a protection society can reasonably anticipate a significant loss in terms of irrecoverability of legal fees and other expenses, and the principal advantage of an indemnity of this type is that such costs will be paid for him. A corollary of the indemnity, however, is that the sponsor will make the indemnity conditional upon his receiving proper notice of any claim or circumstances likely to give rise to a claim, coupled with a right to take over the defense of the claim in the name of the investigator. Such provisions often concern investigators but are normal commercial practice in relation to indemnities which otherwise expose the person granting them to significant exposure, as there is no obligation in English law to mitigate loss in such circumstances and all costs and expenses arising from the event to which the indemnity relates are prima facie recoverable. Where entered into, the sponsor cannot assume his own liability insurance will respond to the increased liability he has voluntarily accepted.

Occasionally, as the price for agreeing to act as an investigator, some investigators will ask that the indemnity cover them against the consequences of their own negligence. The rationale of this appears to be that the opportunity for negligence only arises because the investigator is assisting the company and because of the limited practicability of the investigator obtaining separate professional indemnity insurance. The ABPI has advised that such indemnities should normally not be given, no doubt partly on the basis that the giving of the indemnity by the sponsoring company is too easy to characterize as an encouragement to the investigator to exercise less care than he might otherwise do. It seems very doubtful that this concern is valid, but when the relationship between physicians and the industry is so frequently the subject of criticism, it is entirely understandable.

More recently, health authorities in the U.K. have taken the initiative in seeking to establish a standard form of indemnity for all studies which will cover not only investigators but also the health authority against claims arising other than as result of their own negligence. An agreed form was issued in 1993 by the Department of Health after consultation with industry and the text appears as Appendix 2. Paragraph 3(b) of this indemnity extends to cover circumstances where declarations are sought from the court to enable doctors to cease treating patients who have suffered such injury that they are in a persistent vegetative state. The author is not aware of any such case in a trial of medicinal products to date and the inclusion of this provision merely reflected the topicality of the issue of obtaining such "consent" in the field of conventional medicine at the time the text was under negotiation.

Some health authorities request evidence of security for such an indemnity in the form of a parent company guarantee. These would seem to be matters of a commercial nature which must be negotiated in the light of particular circumstances. Of concern, however, is the fact that it is understood that some ethics committees have been asked to make approval of protocols conditional on the provision of such indemnities. This arguably requires the ethics committees to participate in commercial arrangements which fall outside their proper remit and the Royal College of Physicians has advised:[138] "Such indemnities relate to protecting investigators and employees rather than to protecting research subjects in the event that a claim arises. Such indemnities are not a necessary concern of RECs; they should be left to the parties to negotiate as they see fit." Such an approach would, in any event, be in marked contrast to the lack of initiative taken by most health authorities in the U.K. to ensure that unequivocal commitments to pay compensation may be made to volunteers who may be injured in studies that are not initiated by industry interests. It is suggested that over time as the direct no-fault compensation arrangements for research subjects become better understood and more widespread, the need for such indemnities will recede. They are not normally legal requirements even now. But like so much else in this field, law and practice often diverge and both remain in a state of flux.

REFERENCES

Appendix 1: ABPI Compensation Guidelines of 1991
Appendix 2: ABPI/Department of Health, Form of Indemnity

1. *The Nuremberg Code; Trials of War Criminals before the Nuremberg Tribunals* (1949). No. 10. Vol. 2, pp. 181-2, Washington D.C., U.S. Government Printing Office.
2. Regan, L.J. (1956). *Doctor and Patient and the Law,* 3rd ed, Mosby, St. Louis.
3. Principally 65/65/EEC (as amended), OJ No. 22, 09.02.65, p. 369 and 75/318/EEC OJ No. L 147, 9.6.75, p. 1 as amended by 91/507/EEC, OJ No. L 270/32, 26.9.91.
4. Medicines Act (1968). Chapter 67, HMSO, London.
5. European Commission Discussion Paper on the need for a directive on Clinical Trials III/304/91 of 23.1.91.
6. See English and Scottish Standing Medical Advisory Committee and Hansard, 15 February 1968, at p. 1608.
7. See HM(68)33 and Supervision of the Ethics of Clinical Research Investigations and Fetal Research, HSC (IS) 153, Department of Health, 1975.
8. Draft Guidelines for Local Research Ethics Committees. Department of Health, October 1989.
9. *Nature,* 307, 09.02.84, and *Daily Telegraph,* 31.05.84.
10. Department of Health Guidelines for Local Research Ethics Committees (HSG991)5.
11. Orme, M. et al. (1989). Healthy volunteer studies in Great Britain. *Br. J. Clin. Pharmacol.,* 27, 125-33; and Spiers, C. J. and Griffin, J. P. (1983), A survey of the first year of the operation of the new procedure affecting the conduct of clinical trials in the U.K., *Br. J. Clin. Pharmacol.,* 15, 649-55; Wells, F. Clinical Trial Compensation, *The Lancet,* Vol. 346, Oct. 28, 1995, p. 1164.
12. Federal German Pharmaceutical Law, dated 24.08.76, BGBle.1.1976, p. 2445; see Sections 40-42.
13. Control of Clinical Trials Act, Number 28 of 1987 and Number 24 of 1990. The Stationery Office, Dublin.
14. French law on the protection of persons undergoing biochemical research. No. 88, 1138 1988, Dec 20, and *Arpaillange,* et al. (1985). Proposal for ethical standards in therapeutic trials, *Br. Med. J.,* 291, 887.
15. Medicines Law 25/1990 of December 20, 1990.
16. Portaria No. 321/92 and decree on clinical trials of 9.4.94.
17. Decree of 27.4.92.
18. Medicines Act No. 1930 of 1987, S.86-88.
19. Clinical Trial Regulations of 1st January 1995.
20. Japanese Guidelines for GCP. Notification No. 874 of 1989 by Director of Pharmaceutical Affairs Bureau, Ministry of Health and Welfare and General Guidelines on clinical evaluation of new drugs issued 29.6.92.
21. EEC/CPMP. Working Party on Efficacy of Drugs, July 3, 1987, III/411/87/EN-Rev.
22. Hvidberg, E. F. (1988). Presentation to Interscience Conference on Conduct of Clinical Trials, Copenhagen.
23. Good Clinical Practice for Trials on Medicinal Products in the European Community. European Commission, III/3976/88-EN Final dated 4 May 1990.
24. World Medical Association. Declaration of Helsinki: Recommendations Guiding Medical Doctors in Biomedical Research Involving Human Subjects. Adopted 1964 and revised in Tokyo (1975) and Venice (1983).
25. Good Clinical (Research) Practice, Association of the British Pharmaceutical Industry, December 1992.
26. Guidelines for Phase IV Clinical Trials. Association of the British Pharmaceutical Industry, Sept 1993.
27. Supply of Goods and Services Act (1982). Chapter 29, HMSO, London.

28. The Unfair Contract Terms Act (1977). Chapter 50, HMSO, London (amended by Unfair Contract Terms and Consumer Contracts Regulations 1994 No. 3159).
29. E.C. Directive on Unfair Contract Terms in Consumer Contracts.
30. Association of British Pharmaceutical Industry, Guidelines on the Structure of a Formal Agreement to Conduct Sponsored Clinical Research; June, 1996.
31. For an explanation of the general principles see Donoghue v. Stevenson (1932), A.C. 562 H.L.; and Vacwell Engineering Co Ltd v BDH Chemicals Ltd (1971), IQB 88.
32. Dukes, M. N. G. and Swartz, B. (1988). *Responsibility for Drug-Induced Injury*, Elsevier, p. 299.
33. Cynat Products Ltd v. Landbuild (Investment & Property) Ltd (1984), 3 All ER 513.
34. Directive 85/374/EEC, OJ No. L 210/29.
35. Consumer Protection Act (1987). Chapter 43, HMSO, London.
36. Implementation of the E.C. Directive on Product Liability. An Explanatory and Consultative Note, Department of Trade, Nov. 1985, at 56, p. 14.
37. Directive 85/374/EEC, Supra at 23, Article 7(e).
38. Consumer Protection Act, Supra at 24, Section 4(l)(e).
39. Directive 92/59/EEC. OJ No. L 228/24.
40. *Sidaway v. Bethlem Royal Hospital Governors* (1985), AC 871, applying *Bolam -v- Friern Hospital Management Committee* (1957), 2 All ER 118.
41. Federal German Pharmaceutical Law, Supra at 9, Section 40(1.4).
42. Consumer Protection Act, Supra at 24, Section 3(3).
43. Fraud and Malpractice in the Context of Clinical Research; Report of the Medical Committee of the Association of the British Pharmaceutical Industry, May 1992.
44. *Collins -v- Wilcock* (1984), 1 W.L.R. 1172.
45. *Freeman -v- Home Office* (No. 2) (1984), QB 524.
46. The Report of the Committee to Investigate Medical Experiments on Staff Volunteers (1970). Association of the British Pharmaceutical Industry, 3.3. (Updated as Guidelines for Medical Experiments on Non-patient Volunteers, 1984.)
47. *Wilson -v- Pringle* (1987), QB 237, 253.
48. Re F. (1989) 2 WLR 1025.
49. *Freeman -v- Home Office* (No. 2), Supra at 45.
50. Declaration of Helsinki, Supra at 24 see Section I(ii).
51. Family Law Reform Act (1969), S.8(l), Chapter 36; and Gillick v. West Norfolk and Wisbech Area Health Authority and the Department of Health (1985), 2 All ER 402.
52. Medical Research Council "The Ethical Conduct of Research on Children" December 1991.
53. Kennedy, L. *The Patient on the Clapham Omnibus*, MLR, Vol. 47, 454.
54. Dworkin, G. (1978). *Arch. Dis. Child.*, 53, 443.
55. Report of the Medical Research Council of 1962-63 entitled *Responsibility in Investigations on Human Subjects*, Cmnd 2382, HMSO, London.
56. HSC (15) 153, Department of Health, Supra at 6.
57. Guidelines for the Ethical Conduct of Medical Research involving children of British Paediatric Association, August 1992.
58. Department of Health Circular HS9(91)5.
59. *Medicines Commission Advice to Health Ministers on Healthy Volunteer Studies* (1987), HMSO, London.
60. See Report of the Medical Research Council, Supra at 52 and TvT 1988 Fam. 62.
61. In Re B. (a minor) (wardship: sterilisation) 1988, AC199.
62. In Re F., Supra at 48.
63. Medical Research Council. The Ethical Conduct of Research on the Mentally Incapacitated, December 1991.
64. Control of Clinical Trials Act (1987), Supra at 13, see S.9(7).
65. Medicines Commission, Supra at 59.
66. Sidaway, Supra at 40.
67. Unfair Contract Terms Act (1977), Chapter 50, Supra at 28.
68. *Hatcher -v- Black* (1954) *The Times*, July 2nd.
69. *Canterbury -v- Spence* (1972), 464. F 2d 772; and Reibl v. Hughes (1981), 114 DLR (3d)1.
70. Sidaway, Supra at 40; *Gold -v- Haringey Health Authority* (1987), 2 All ER at 888; *Blyth v. Bloomsbury Health Authority* (1987), *The Times*, Feb 11, CA. See also the Scots law case of *Moyes -v- Lothian Health Board* (1990) SLT 444.
71. Sidaway, Supra at 40.
72. *Rogers -v- Whittaker* (1992) 109 ALR 625.
73. Food and Drug Administration Rules and Regulations Part 56 (1981). *Fed. Rep.*, 46 (17), Jan 27th.
74. *Halsuska -v- University of Saskatchewan et al.*, 1965, 52 WWR 616.
75. *Gold -v- Haringey Health Authority*, Supra at 70.
76. *Blyth -v- Bloomsbury Health Authority*, Supra at 70.
77. *Weiss -v- Solomon* 1989 RJQ 731 Quebec Superior Court.

78. EEC/CPMP Working Party Guidelines, Supra at 13.
79. GCP in the European Community. Supra at 23.
80. Frost, N. (1979). Sounding board. Consent as a barrier to research. *N. Engl. J. Med.*, 300, 1272-2.
81. See, for instance, *The Observer*, Editorial of 09.10.88.
82. For a general discussion see Vere, D. (1981). Editorial, *J. R. Soc. Med.*, 74 Feb; and Report of Cancer Research Campaign Working Party (1983). *Br. Med. J.*, 286, April 2nd.
83. Feinstein, A. R. (1980). *Eur. J. Clin. Pharmacol.*, 17, 1-4.
84. Control of Clinical Trials Act, Supra at 14, see S9(4)(d).
85. GCP in the European Community Supra at 23.
86. Gilbert, J. (1988). Letter, *IME Bull.*, Oct, p. 10.
87. Sections 40(2) and 41(6) Federation German Pharmaceutical Law, Supra at 12.
88. Medicines Act of 1990, Supra at 15.
89. Ordinance No. 11 of 19 August 1987 of Minister of Health on biomedical research.
90. GCP guidelines, Supra at 20.
91. Department of Health Guidelines, Supra at 10.
92. Medicines, Ethics and Practice. Royal Pharmaceutical Society: Council Statements at p. 103.
93. HSE (15) 153, Supra at 6.
94. *Guidelines on the Practice of Ethics Committees in Medical Research,* August, 1996. Royal College of Physicians of London.
95. The Medicines (Exemption from Licences) (Clinical Trials) Order SI 1995, No. 2808.
96. Medicines Commission, Supra at 44.
97. Department of Health Guidelines, Supra at 10.
98. Research Involving Patients. Royal College of Physicians 1990 of London.
99. Standards for Local Research Ethics Committees. A Framework for Ethical Review and SOP's for Local Research Ethics Committee — Comments and Examples by Christine Bendall of McKenna & Co; Department of Health (Sept 1994).
100. FDA Rules, Supra at 56.
101. S8(4) Control of Clinical Trials Act, Supra at 13. In contrast, in Denmark until March 1989, trials could begin before ethics committees had completed their review, which sometimes took place after trials were completed! (See *Scrip*, No. 1389, 24.02.89).
102. 1988 Act on the Protection of Persons Undergoing Biomedical Research: Title III.
103. Ordinance of 1987, Supra at 89.
104. Drug Ordinance No. 701 of 1962, amended 1983 by Ordinance No. 867 and Article 14 of Proclamation (1963: 439 amended 1983: 867) on the application of the Drug Ordinance.
105. Medicines Law 1990, Supra at 15.
106. Regulations of 1995, Supra at 19.
107. Norwegian Medicines Act of 20.6.64 (S.10) and Regulations concerning clinical trials of 21.8.81.
108. Medicines Act 1987, Supra at 18 (Finland) and Law on Research Ethics Committee System and the handling of biomedical research projects No. 503, 24.6.92 (Denmark).
109. See for instance Peabody Donation Fund v. Sir Lindsay Parkinson & Co Ltd (1985), Ac 210, and Rowling v. Takaro Properties Ltd (1988) AC 473.
110. Department of Health Guidance, Supra at 10.
111. See for instance the Opren (benoxaprofen) litigation settled before trial — Davies v. Eli Lilly and Others (1988), unreported.
112. S.40(3) Federal German Pharmaceutical Law, Supra at 12.
113. 1988 Act, Supra at 102.
114. Law 25/1990 Supra at 15.
115. Decree of 1992. Supra at 17.
116. S10 Control of Clinical Trials Act, Supra at 13.
117. Medicines Act 1987. Supra at 18.
118. Regulations of 1981, Supra at 107.
119. Regulations of 1995, Supra at 19.
120. See 1339 of Royal commission on Civil Liability and Compensation for Personal Injury, March, 1978, Cmnd 7054, HMSO, London; and letter (unpublished) of October, 1973 from Chief Medical Officers of Department of Health to President of Royal College of Physicians, London.
121. Royal Commission, Supra at 120.
122. *Medical Research: Civil Liability and Compensation for Personal Injury* (1980). The Ciba Foundation.
123. Association of the British Pharmaceutical Industry Report, Supra at 46.
124. Association of the British Pharmaceutical Industry Guidelines for Medical Experiments in Non-patient Human Volunteers. March 1988.
125. Association of British Pharmaceutical Industry Guidelines. Clinical Trials — Compensation for Medicine-induced Injury, August 1983.
126. Association of British Pharmaceutical Industry Clinical Trial Compensation, March 1991.

127. Medicines Commission, Supra at 59.
128. Department of Health Guidelines, Supra at 10.
129. Association of British Pharmaceutical Industry Guidelines, Supra 1t 126.
130. *Legal Liability and the Supply of Investigational Drugs* (1986). ABPI Circular No. 494/86.
131. Diamond, A. L. and Laurence, D. R. (1983). *Br. Med. J.*, Sept 3rd, p. 676.
132. Research on Healthy Volunteers (1986). A Report of the Royal College of Physicians, London.
133. Medicines Commissions, Supra at 59, see 6.16.
134. Department of Health Guidelines, Supra at 10.
135. FDA Rules Supra at 73. S50.25(a) and (b).
136. Ciba Foundation, Supra at a22 pp. 9 and 11.
137. The Fenchurch No-Fault Compensation Insurance Scheme for Clinical Trials/Volunteer Studies; available from Fenchurch Insurance Brokers Ltd, 136 Minories, London EC3N 1QN.
138. Royal College of Physicians Guidelines, Supra at 94, para 16.25.

APPENDIX 1

ABPI CLINICAL TRIAL COMPENSATION GUIDELINES

Preamble

The Association of the British Pharmaceutical Industry favours a simple and expeditious procedure in relation to the provision of compensation for injury caused by participation in clinical trials. The Association therefore recommends that a member company sponsoring a clinical trial should provide without legal commitment a written assurance to the investigator — and through him to the relevant research ethics committee — that the following Guidelines will be adhered to in the event of injury caused to a patient attributable to participation in the trial in question.

1. Basic Principles

1.1 Notwithstanding the absence of legal commitment, the company should pay compensation to patient-volunteers suffering bodily injury (including death) in accordance with these Guidelines.

1.2 Compensation should be paid when, on the balance of probabilities, the injury was attributable to the administration of a medicinal product under trial or any clinical intervention or procedure provided for by the protocol that would not have occurred but for the inclusion of the patient in the trial.

1.3 Compensation should be paid to a child injured *in utero* through the participation of the subject's mother in a clinical trial as if the child were a patient-volunteer with the full benefit of these Guidelines.

1.4 Compensation should only be paid for the more serious injury of an enduring and disabling character (including exacerbation of an existing condition) and not for temporary pain or discomfort or less serious or curable complaints.

1.5 Where there is an adverse reaction to a medicinal product under trial and injury is caused by a procedure adopted to deal with that adverse reaction, compensation should be paid for such injury as if it were caused directly by the medicinal product under trial.

1.6 Neither the fact that the adverse reaction causing the injury was foreseeable to predictable, nor the fact that the patient has freely consented (whether in writing or otherwise) to participate in the trial should exclude a patient from consideration for compensation under these Guidelines, although compensation may be abated or excluded in the light of the factors described in paragraph 4.2 below.

1.7 For the avoidance of doubt, compensation should be paid regardless of whether the patient is able to prove that the company has been negligent in relation to research or development of the medicinal product under trial or that the product is defective and therefore, as the producer, the company is subject to strict liability in respect of injuries caused by it.

2. Type of Clinical Research Covered

2.1 These Guidelines apply to injury caused to patients involved in Phase II and Phase III trials, that is to say, patients under treatment and surveillance (usually in hospital) and suffering from the ailment which the medicinal product under trial is intended to treat but for which a product license does not exist or does not authorize supply for administration under the conditions of the trial.

2.2 These Guidelines do not apply to injuries arising from studies in non-patient volunteers (Phase I), whether or not they are in hospital, for which separate Guidelines for compensation already exist.[1]

2.3 These Guidelines do not apply to injury arising from clinical trials on marketed products (Phase IV), where a product license exists authorizing supply for administration under the conditions of the trial, except to the extent that the injury is caused to a patient as a direct result of procedures undertaken in accordance with the protocol (but not any product administered) to which the patient would not have been exposed had treatment been other than in the course of the trial.

2.4 These Guidelines do not apply to clinical trials which have not been initiated or directly sponsored by the company providing the product for research. Where trials of products are initiated independently by doctors under the appropriate Medicines Act 1968 exemptions, responsibility for the health and welfare of patients rests with the doctor alone (see also paragraph 5.2 below).

3. Limitations

3.1 No compensation should be paid for the failure of a medicinal product to have its intended effect or to provide any other benefits to the patient.

3.2 No compensation should be paid for injury caused by other licensed medicinal products administered to the patient for the purpose of comparison with the product under trail.

3.3 No compensation should be paid to patients receiving placebo in consideration of its failure to provide a therapeutic benefit.

3.4 No compensation should be paid (or it should be abated as the case may be) to the extent that the injury has arisen:

3.4.1 through a significant departure from the agreed protocol;

3.4.2 through the wrongful act or default of a third party, including a doctor's failure to deal adequately with an adverse reaction;

3.4.3 through contributory negligence by the patient.

4. Assessment of Compensation

4.1 The amount of compensation paid should be appropriate to the nature, severity and persistence of the injury and should in general terms be consistent with the quantum of damages commonly awarded for similar injuries by an English Court in cases where legal liability is admitted.

4.2 Compensation may be abated, or in certain circumstances excluded, in the light of the following factors (on which will depend the level of risk the patient can reasonably be expected to accept):

4.2.1 the seriousness of the disease being treated, the degree of probability that adverse reactions will occur and any warnings given;

4.2.2 the risks and benefits of established treatments relative to those known or suspected of the trial medicine.

This reflects the fact that flexibility is required given the particular patient's circumstances. As an extreme example, there may be a patient suffering from a serious of life-threatening disease who is warned of a certain defined risk of adverse reaction. Participation in the trial is then based on an expectation that the benefit/risk ratio associated with participation may be better than that associated with alternative treatment. It is, therefore, reasonable that the patient accepts the high risk and should not expect compensation for the occurrence of the adverse reaction of which he or she was told.

4.3 In any case where the company concedes that a payment should be made to a patient but there exists a difference of opinion between company and patient as to the appropriate level of compensation, it is recommended that the company agrees to seek at its own cost (and make available to the patient) the opinion of a mutually acceptable independent expert, and that his opinion should be given substantial weight by the company in reaching its decision on the appropriate payment to be made.

5. Miscellaneous

5.1 Claims pursuant to the Guidelines should be made by the patient to the company, preferably via the investigator, setting out details of the nature and background of the claim and, subject to the patient providing on request an authority for the company to review any medical records relevant to the claim, the company should consider the claim expeditiously.

5.2 The undertaking given by a company extends to injury arising (at whatever time) from all administration, clinical interventions or procedures coccurring during the course of the trial but not to treatment extended beyond the end of the trial at the instigation of the investigator. The use of unlicensed products beyond the trial period is wholly the responsibility of the treating doctor and in this regard attention is drawn to the advice provided to doctors in MAL 30[2] concerning the desirability of doctors notifying their protection society of their use of unlicensed products.

5.3 The fact that a copmpany has agreed to abide by these Guidelines in respect of a trial does not affect the right of a patient to pursue a legal remedy in respect of injury alleged to have been suffered as a result of participation. Nevertheless, patients will normally be asked to accept that any payment made under the Guidelines will be in full settlement of their claims.

5.4 A company sponsoring a trial should encourage the investigator to make clear to participating patients that the trial is being conducted subject to the ABPI Guidelines relating to compensation for injury arising in the course of clinical trials and have available copies of the Guidelines should they be requested.

REFERENCES

1. Guidelines for Medical Experiments in Non-patient Human Volunteers, ABPI March, 1988, as amended May 1990.
2. MAL 30 - A Guide to the Provisions Affecting Doctors and Dentists, DHSS, (Revised June 1985).

APPENDIX 2

ABPI/DEPARTMENT OF HEALTH FORM OF INDEMNITY FOR CLINICAL STUDIES

From: [Name and address of sponsoring company] ("the Sponsor")

To: [Name and address of health authority/health board/NHS Trust] ("the Authority")

Re: Clinical Study No ( ) with [name of product]

1. It is proposed that the Authority should agree to participate in the above sponsored study ("the Study") involving [patients of the Authority] [non-patient volunteers] ("the subject") to be conducted

by [name of investigator(s)] ("the Investigator") in accordance with the protocol annexed as amended from time to time with the agreement of the Sponsor and the Investigator ("the Protocol"). The Sponsor confirms that it is a term of its agreement with the Investigator that the Investigator shall obtain all necessary approvals of the applicable Local Research Ethics Committee and shall resolve with the Authority any issues of a revenue nature.

2. The Authority agrees to participate by allowing the Study to be undertaken on its premises utilizing such facilities, personnel and equipment as the Investigator may reasonably need for the purpose of the Study.

3. In consideration of such participation by the Authority, and subject to paragraph 4 below, the Sponsor indemnifies and holds harmless the Authority and its employees and agents against all claims and proceedings (to include any settlements or *ex gratia* payments made with the consent of the parties hereto and reasonable legal and expert costs and expenses) made or brought (whether successfully or otherwise).
   (a) by or on behalf of Subjects taking part in the Study (or their dependents) against the Authority or any of its employees or agents for personal injury (including death) to Subjects arising out of or relating to the administration of the product(s) under investigation or any clinical intervention or procedure provided for or required by the Protocol to which the Subjects would not have been exposed but for their participation in the study.
   (b) by the Authority, its employees or agents or by or on behalf of a Subject for a declaration concerning the treatment of a Subject who has suffered such personal injury.

4. The above indemnity by the Sponsor shall not apply to any such claim or proceeding:

4.1 to the extent that such personal injury (including death) is caused by the negligent or wrongful acts or omissions or breach of statutory duty of the Authority, its employees or agents,

4.2 to the extent that such personal injury (including death) is caused by the failure of the Authority, its employees, or agents to conduct the study in accordance with the Protocol,

4.3 unless as soon as reasonably practicable following receipt of notice of such claim or proceeding, the Authority shall have notified the Sponsor in writing of it and shall, upon the Sponsor's request, and at the Sponsor's cost, have permitted the Sponsor to have full care and control of the claim or proceeding using legal representation of its own choosing,

4.4 if the Authority, its employees, or agents shall have made any admission in respect of such claim or proceeding or taken any action relating to such claim or proceeding prejudicial to the defense of it without the written consent of the Sponsor such consent not to be unreasonably withheld provided that this condition shall not be treated as breached by any statement properly made by the Authority, its employees or agents in connection with the operation of the Authority's internal complaint procedures, accident reporting procedures or disciplinary procedures or where such statement is required by law.

5. The Sponsor shall keep the Authority and its legal advisers fully informed of the progress of any such claim or proceeding, will consult fully with the Authority on the nature of any defense to be advanced and will not settle any such claim or proceeding without the written approval of the Authority (such approval not to be unreasonably withheld).

6. Without prejudice to the provisions of paragraph 4.3 above, the Authority will use its reasonable endeavours to inform the Sponsor promptly of any circumstances reasonably thought likely to give rise to any such claim or proceeding of which it is directly aware and shall keep the Sponsor reasonably informed of developments in relation to any such claim or proceeding even where the Authority decides not to make a claim under this indemnity. Likewise, the Sponsor shall use its

reasonable endeavours to inform the Authority of any such circumstances and shall keep the Authority reasonably informed of developments in relation to any such claim or proceeding made or brought against the Sponsor alone.

7. The Authority and the Sponsor will each give to the other such help as may reasonably be required for the efficient conduct and prompt handling of any claim or proceeding by or on behalf of Subjects (or their dependents) or concerning such a declaration as is referred to in paragraph 3(b) above.

8. Without prejudice to the foregoing if injury is suffered by a Subject while participating in the Study, the Sponsor agrees to operate in good faith the Guidelines published in 1991 by The Association of the British Pharmaceutical Industry and entitled "Clinical Trial Compensation Guidelines" (where the Subject is a patient) and the Guidelines published in 1988 by the same Association and entitled "Guidelines for Medical Experiments in non-patient Human Volunteers" (where the Subject is not a patient) and shall request the Investigator to make clear to the Subjects that the Study is being conducted subject to the applicable Association Guidelines.

9. For the purpose of this indemnity, the expression "agents" shall be deemed to include without limitation any nurse or other health professional providing services to the Authority under a contract for services or otherwise and any person carrying out work for the Authority under such a contract connected with such of the Authority's facilities and equipment as are made available for the Study under paragraph 2 above.

10. This indemnity shall be governed by and construed in accordance with English/Scots* law.

SIGNED on behalf of the Health Authority/Health Board/NHS Trust

....
Chief Executive/District General Manager

SIGNED on behalf of the Company

....

Dated..

*Delete as appropriate

(Published with permission of The Association of the British Pharmaceutical Industry, London, U.K.)

Part IV. Measuring Drug Activity in Humans

Chapter 12

Study Design and Assessment of Wanted and Unwanted Drug Effects In Phase I/II Trials

M. Thomas

CONTENTS

1 Introduction 157
2 Objectives 158
3 Study Design 158
  3.1 General Considerations 158
  3.2 Inclusion/Exclusion Criteria 159
  3.3 Study Restrictions 159
  3.4 Dosing Regimens 159
  3.5 Number of Subjects 160
  3.6 Route of Administration Phase I 160
4 Choice of Study Design 161
  4.1 Phase I Studies 161
    4.1.1 First Administration — Single Dose 161
    4.1.2 First Administration — Repeat Dose 163
  4.2 Phase II Studies 164
5 Measurements 165
  5.1 Plasma Drug Concentrations 165
  5.2 Assessment of Wanted Drug Effects 166
  5.3 Assessment of Unwanted Drug Effects 167
References 167

1 INTRODUCTION

The clinical development of a potential new medicine passes through three well-defined, if arbitrary phases, on its way to a Product License Application (PLA). Typically phase I studies which are usually undertaken in healthy (non-patient) volunteers span the whole of the development process from early studies where the main emphasis is on safety and tolerability, to a range of late studies with primarily pharmacokinetic objectives (Table 1). The latter, which are required to support the PLA, include bioequivalency studies with new and final pharmaceutical formulations, studies with radiolabeled drug to determine metabolic disposition, drug interaction studies, and studies to define subpopulations (e.g., the young, elderly and patients with hepatic or renal disease). However, good arguments can sometimes be mounted for bringing studies forward in the clinical program. For example, if there is evidence from animal studies to suppose that food affects absorption of drug from the GI tract, then it would be prudent to undertake a food interaction study in man before starting repeat dosing. One could also argue that radiolabeled studies to determine the metabolic disposition of the drug should be done earlier than is usually the case. Such data would not only help to predict the potential for interactions with other drugs metabolized by the same route, but would also help the toxicologists when selecting animal species for long-term safety evaluation studies.

Phase II studies involve first administration to patients with the target disease for which the new drug is intended, using dose defining study designs to evaluate therapeutic effects. Phase III studies are larger scale studies undertaken to confirm initial impressions gained on safety, tolerability, and efficacy seen during phases I and II (exploratory development). As results from phases I and II studies form the basis of the decision whether or not to proceed into phase III (full development), it is imperative that the right questions be addressed and the appropriate studies be undertaken during the period that the drug is in exploratory development. Failure to do so could result in a good drug being rejected, a poor drug being

0-8493-9230-6/97/$0.00+$.50
© 1997 by CRC Press, Inc.

Table 1 Early and Late Phase I Studies

Early	Late
First administration	Definitive pharmacokinetics/pharmacodynamics
First repeat dose	Bioavailability
Pilot pharmacokinetics/ pharmacodynamics	New formulations
	Interaction studies
	Drug/food
	Drug/drug
	Metabolic disposition
	Hepatic impairment
	Renal impairment
	Pharmacokinetics in the young and elderly

taken forward, or as is more often the case, a drug being taken forward with the wrong (usually too high) dose. With these points in mind, time spent upfront, i.e., during exploratory development establishing full and complete dose or plasma concentration effect curves for wanted and unwanted drug effects, will prove to be a good investment for the drug's future. It will not only help to ensure that the drug is marketed at the right dose, or dose range, but will also facilitate the approval of the PLA and thus help to contain the spiraling costs of drug development programs.

Quite apart from the fact that phase I and II studies involve dose-ranging with safety as a major consideration, they have other features in common which influence study design, e.g., they are undertaken using small numbers of healthy volunteers or patients, are intensively monitored, and are usually conducted in special centres.

2 OBJECTIVES

Before going on to discuss choice of study design, it will be useful to review briefly the main aims of phase I and II studies and their limitations.

Initial studies in healthy volunteers and patients are the start of the process by which the utility of a new drug in terms of its safety profile and therapeutic potential is assessed. The primary aim of phase I or II studies is not to *establish* human safety; this asks too much of studies where exposure to the drug in terms of number of subjects is extremely limited. All that one can achieve in phases I and II is to monitor carefully for adverse events and attempt to attribute causality, either to the drug or to some other factor. Of course, one may well come up with findings, e.g., changes in liver enzymes or in the case of parenteral administration, irritation at the injection site which contraindicates progressing the drug further, but as a rule this is the best one can hope to achieve when pronouncing on safety at this stage. The fact that progressing from phase I to II involves a number of extrapolations, i.e., health to disease (always), male to female (often), and young to elderly (sometimes) is a further limiting factor. With the latter in mind, it is now common practice to undertake phase I studies in elderly healthy subjects when the drug is likely to be used in elderly patients, while the American College of Clinical Pharmacy[1] has recommended that women be included in early drug development programs. This recommendation to involve women at an earlier stage in studies has been endorsed by the FDA.[2]

Traditionally, decisions relating to giving new drugs to patients have been based upon safety and pharmacodynamic and pharmacokinetic considerations using results from healthy volunteer studies. Basically, this remains so today but whenever possible studies should be designed so as to make full and better use of pharmacodynamic/pharmacokinetic modeling plus tools such as test models and clinical or laboratory markers (surrogate endpoints) of the target disease to help define appropriate dosage schedules for patient studies. Surrogate endpoints are also being used increasingly in early patient studies in a variety of therapeutic areas (e.g., hypertension, cancer, and AIDS) in an attempt to obtain early and reliable feedback on the effectiveness of drug interventions.

3 STUDY DESIGN

3.1 General Considerations

Ill-conceived experimental designs often result in the study ending in failure, and this applies to overelaborate as well as to inadequate designs. Obviously no single design can meet the needs of all early studies, so they have to be customized to comply with, not only the objectives of the study, but with the pharmacodynamic and/or pharmacokinetic profiles of the drug and in the case of phase II studies, the nature of the target disease. However, whichever design is eventually selected, it should be kept as simple as possible and this is made easier if the study tests a single hypothesis. One should avoid the temptation to list too many objectives in case none of them is adequately addressed. The investigator must also ensure that the design is suitable for the study population. Thus, a design which is acceptable for a study involving young healthy subjects may be totally inappropriate for a study in elderly subjects or patients. For example, the latter may well be intolerant of, or unable to, undertake studies involving repeat visits to the clinic, intensive monitoring, or multiple or late night blood sampling which young volunteers may readily accept. It is far better to opt for a design at the start which will not deter subjects be they young, elderly, or sick from participating in and completing the study, even if the design is less than optimal, rather than having to go back and redesign it when underway because of a failure to recruit adequate numbers.

3.2 Inclusion/Exclusion Criteria

Subject selection for a study, whether in healthy volunteers or patients, is usually decided by using a predefined set of inclusion/exclusion criteria. The reasons for this are twofold. First and most importantly in healthy volunteer studies, to exclude those in whom any risk is more than minimal and in patient studies, to minimize risk, and second, to achieve as homogenous a study group(s) as possible which will aid interpretation of results. In the case of early volunteer studies, the criteria for admission to the study are fairly standard, i.e., healthy males (based on the results of a medical history and physical examination, plus routine laboratory safety screens) of a given age range (18 to 40/50 years), and body weight range (e.g., ± 15% of ideal weight) who have not taken part in a drug study within the previous 3 to 4 months. Commonly used exclusion criteria include a history of alcohol or drug abuse, regular courses of medication and depending upon the type of study, volunteers who have donated blood to a blood transfusion service within the previous 3 months, and cigarette smokers or those who smoke more than a certain number of cigarettes or equivalent a day. In the case of patient studies, gender and age are often recruitment criteria as are the severity and duration of the disease to be treated. In early patient studies, patients on certain types of medication may also be excluded from a study, at least until more is known about the likelihood of interaction with the drug under test. However, even though volunteer and patient selection criteria serve important purposes, they will invariably lead to a proportion of subjects being rejected from the study. Of course, if the criteria are too rigid too few subjects may be recruited to make the study a viable proposition. When this happens, the investigator may need to consider relaxing the conditions which lead to entry to the study without putting subjects at risk or the aims of the study in jeopardy.

3.3 Study Restrictions

In volunteer studies, in particular, conditions are imposed on the subjects when they are in the study. These may relate to the time they are expected to spend in the clinic, including overnight stays, or to restrictions with respect to intake of food and drink including alcohol, exercise, cigarette consumption, driving, and operating machinery. The protocol usually states that restrictions will apply during the study day and for a period before and after its completion, but the time frames are often arbitrary. The need for the restrictions themselves are sometimes debatable, particularly when they are included as part of a checklist. If the study restrictions are too severe, particularly if there is no good reason for them or the subject has not been told why they must be adhered to, they could result in protocol violations. This point is worth bearing in mind when drawing up a list of study "dos" and "don'ts".

3.4 Dosing Regimens

The selection of the initial and top dose for a first administration study in healthy volunteers is an exercise in extrapolation using the results from animal pharmacology and safety evaluation studies. The latter include acute studies in which exaggerated pharmacological responses are sought in anesthetized and conscious animals using doses between 30- and 100-times, the anticipated therapeutic dose, as well as general toxicological studies in which animals are dosed for 2 to 4 weeks. Decisions on dosing are made on a case-by-case basis, but the first human dose is often between $^1/_{10}$ and $^1/_{100}$th of the ED_{50} or some other quantifiable measure of drug effect in the animal species most sensitive to the actions of the drug. Once the first dose in humans has been safely administered, life becomes a little easier for the investigator as he has experience in man to use as a guide for further dose escalations. However, although the prime determinants of the actual top dose given are the effects of previous doses in man, it is usual to define the anticipated top dose in the protocol. The latter is usually decided by considering the no-effect dose seen in animal safety evaluation studies, and possibly by the anticipated therapeutic dose. It is customary to take the top dose in volunteers to a level which is two- to fourfold higher than the anticipated therapeutic dose to provide an adequate ceiling for dosing in patients. In the absence of side effects or pharmacodynamic effects, the dose is progressed by doubling the previous dose, but whatever the magnitude of the increase between doses, unless there are sound reasons for dosing otherwise, it should remain constant throughout the dose range. In other words, having started off by say doubling doses, there is little justification for switching to smaller increments with higher doses, unless there are sound reasons for doing so, such as nonlinearity between dose and plasma drug concentrations or evidence to support an exaggerated dose response.

3.5 Number of Subjects

Whether it is phase I or II, a sufficient number of subjects must be included in a study if valid conclusions are to be drawn from the results. Studies in healthy volunteers and patients are inherently flawed when it comes to assessing safety and tolerability because of the small numbers of subjects involved and only the most guarded of conclusions are possible. It is easier to draw valid conclusions in respect to drug action involving pharmacodynamic, surrogate, or clinical endpoints because one is able to specify beforehand the magnitude of the difference which constitutes a useful drug effect and thus calculate the number of subjects needed to give the study adequate statistical power. The same is true of bioequivalency studies, except that regulatory authorities rather than the investigator specify the criteria which have to be met to enable different formulations to be judged bioequivalent.

3.6 Route of Administration Phase I

Just as new drugs must be tested in animals by the route to be used in man, so must they be tested in volunteers using the intended route for patients. But there are clear benefits in testing all drugs when going into man for the first time using intravenous infusions, even if systemic exposure in patients will be achieved by another route. These benefits relate primarily to the fact that intravenous infusion allows for precise control of drug administration.

- In the event of a serious or otherwise distressing adverse event during the infusion, drug delivery can be halted.
- As the drug is delivered directly into the blood stream this ensures 100% exposure and overcomes problems relating to bioavailability which may occur with other routes but in particular, dosing by the oral route when the drug may be destroyed in the GI tract or metabolized presystemically in the gut wall or in the liver.
- Delivery of the full dose into the blood stream, coupled with a uniform delivery rate, results in less variability in plasma or tissue concentrations of drug than is possible using oral dosing where, not only the extent but also the rate of absorption from the GI tract can vary considerably between subjects. Less intersubject variability in plasma concentrations of drug in turn enables the study to be done using smaller numbers of subjects and also offers advantages for drugs it is anticipated might have narrow therapeutic ratios.
- Intravenous dosing allows the true disposition kinetics of the drug to be evaluated and makes the assessment of PK/PD relationships easier to perform.
- Pharmacokinetic scaling between species, i.e., animals to man, is made simpler as fewer assumptions need be made about extent and rate of exposure in man. This in turn helps in dose selection for human studies.
- Blinding of studies is made easier when intravenous dosing is used, i.e., there is no need to produce matching placebos while intravenous dosing overcomes any problems relating to taste which can make it difficult in blind studies involving oral dosing.

The primary disadvantage of using intravenous dosing for first time in human studies is that additional resource will be needed to be spent in toxicology and pharmacy on a drug which might fail at the first hurdle in man, as indeed many do. For this reason investigators often prefer to administer drugs for the first time in healthy volunteers using the route to be used in patients and dose intravenously to establish the drug's pharmacokinetic profile only when they feel reasonably certain that it is likely to be a candidate for further development.

4 CHOICE OF STUDY DESIGN

4.1 Phase I Studies

4.1.1 First Administration — Single Dose

First-time administration of single doses of new drugs are undertaken using a wide range of study design, but in essence there are several basic designs available which are modified to meet the needs of a given study. Fundamental to all designs is that in the interests of safety, successive subjects are exposed to increasing doses of the drug. The fact that doses are titrated upward, either in the same subject or groups of subjects and not randomized to remove the potential for bias, can be argued is a design weakness but there is no alternative. Nevertheless, an ordered dose response can be taken as reasonable evidence of a drug-related effect. In addition, the use of placebo which enables studies to be conducted on either a single- or a double-blind basis will help to minimize bias. For this reason, placebo control is an integral part of a phase I study. Unwanted feelings or sensations are common occurrences in every day life, hence it is to be expected that adverse events will be encountered during phase I studies. Adverse events may be drug-related, study-related, or result from something which has nothing to do with the drug or the study. They may act singly or in combination. For example, headache which is one of the commonest, if not the commonest symptom reported by volunteers taking part in phase I studies, can result from any one of the following: fasting, caeffine withdrawal, feeling anxious about the study, an impending attack of influenza, or a combination of all four factors. Thus without placebo control it becomes difficult to differentiate between headache which is drug related and headache which is non-drug related. But placebo is not only of value in helping to distinguish between drug- and non-drug-related subjective effects, it also plays a role in the interpretation of results from laboratory and other safety tests and pharmacological tests which maybe influenced by diverse factors such as diet, physical activity, mental state, circadian or other biological rhythms, and asymptomatic illnesses, e.g., subclinical viral infections.

The different designs available for a first-time into man study all have their own advantages and disadvantages. At the end of the day it is down to the investigator to weigh up the pros and cons of each and then to choose the design which best meets the aims of the study. In an attempt to examine their strengths and weaknesses, let us consider some designs open to an investigator who wishes to undertake a single rising dose safety and tolerability study with a new drug. A typical protocol might require:

- Placebo control
- The dose be increased from x (first dose) to 64x (top dose)
- Twofold increases in successive doses (within or between subjects)
- A 7-day within subject washout period
- A minimum of four subjects to receive each dose level

Some design options are shown in Tables 2 to 6, while the implications for going with one or other in terms of subject numbers, number of clinic visits, highest first dose given to a subject, biggest increment in dose, and time to complete the study are given in Table 7.

Table 2 Phase I Study – Design A

No. Visits*	Volunteer No.	Treatment			
4	1-4	x	2x	4x	(P)
4	5-8	4x	8x	16x	(P)
4	9-12	16x	32x	64x	(P)

Note: x — first dose; (P) — randomized placebo; and * — volunteers receive a single dose of drug on each of three visits and placebo on one visit.

Designs D and E require more than threefold, the number of volunteers needed for the other designs. This requirement is compounded by the fact that one third of the volunteers will receive placebo. I elected to have two volunteers on placebo in each group — some might have opted for a single volunteer and others for 3 to 6. Whichever way, designs D and E require large numbers of subjects which could present problems when recruiting suitable subjects. The situation is made more difficult when numbers on the volunteer panel are limited (which is often the case) and when one is attempting to recruit "A1" volunteers who also satisfy the inclusion/exclusion criteria for a first-time into man

Table 3 Phase I Study — Design B

Visit	Volunteer No.		Volunteer No.		Volunteer No.	
1	1	P	5	x	9	2x
	2	x	6	P	10	2x
	3	x	7	2x	11	P
	4	x	8	2x	12	4x
2	1	4x	5	P	9	4x
	2	4x	6	4x	10	P
	3	4x	7	4x	11	8x
	4	P	8	4x	12	8x
3	1	8x	5	16x	9	P
	2	8x	6	16x	10	16x
	3	P	7	16x	11	16x
	4	16x	8	P	12	16x
4	1	16x	5	32x	9	64x
	2	P	6	32x	10	64x
	3	32x	7	P	11	64x
	4	32x	8	64x	12	P

Note: x — first dose and P — placebo.

Table 4 Phase I Study — Design C

No. Visits	Volunteer No.	Treatment			
2	1-4	x	2x	4x	(P)
2	5-8	4x	8x	16x	(P)
2	9-12	16x	32x	64x	(P)

Note: x — first dose; (P) — randomized placebo; and * — volunteers receive three doses of drug on one visit and placebo on the other visit.

Table 5 Phase I Study — Design D

Group	Number of Subjects Who Received Each Treatment							
	Placebo	x	2x	4x	8x	16x	32x	64x
1	2	4						
2	2		4					
3	2			4				
4	2				4			
5	2					4		
6	2						4	
7	2							4

Note: x — first dose.

study. It can also be argued that if the drug under test proved to be toxic, then more subjects would be exposed to its harmful effects. On the other hand, if the drug turns out to be well-tolerated it can be argued equally well that exposing a larger number of subjects is a better basis on which to proceed to the next study.

Designs D and E, however, have two clear advantages over the other designs. First, as only one visit to the clinic is required, this will encourage the volunteer to take part in and complete the study. Second, they are ideal designs for drugs with long pharmacological, clinical, or chemical half-lives when a 7-day washout period is an inadequate time for the drug effects to disappear or for it to be cleared from the body.

In the interests of safety, the lower the dose the volunteer is given on first exposure to the drug, the better. However as it is impractical to start everyone off with dose x, the next best thing one can do is

Table 6 Phase I Study — Design E

Group	Placebo	Number of Subjects Who Received Each Treatment						
		x	2x	4x	8x	16x	32x	64x
1	2	4	1					
2	2		3	1				
3	2			3	1			
4	2				3	1		
5	2					3	1	
6	2						3	1
7	2							3

Note: x — first dose.

Table 7 Comparisons of Study Designs A–E

	A	B	C	D	E
No. of volunteers	12	12	12	42	42
No. of clinic visits	4	4	2	1	1
Highest first dose to a subject	16x	8x	16x	64x	64x
Largest within subject increment in dose	x2	x16	x2	—	—
Times to do study	9 weeks	4 weeks	3 weeks	3–6 weeks[a]	3–6 weeks[a]

[a] Dependent upon whether dosing takes place once or twice weekly.

to keep the first dose given to a volunteer in each group as low as possible within the confines of the design of the study. In this respect, design B scores best and designs D and E do badly.

With designs A and C, twofold increments in dose are uniformily made throughout the whole dose range. This is in contrast to design B in which the size of dosage increments over the dose range within subjects varies between 2- and 16-fold. Thus design B might be an unwise choice for a drug anticipated to have a narrow therapeutic index or a steep dose response.

Assuming the study goes according to plan (which is often not the case in first-administration studies) and depending upon the study design used, it will take between 3 and 9 weeks to complete. However, although design C (in which the dose is increased stepwise on the same study day) offers the advantage of speed, the fact that it can only really be used for drugs given by the intravenous route and for drugs with rapid onsets and offsets of action limits its usefulness in practice.

4.1.2 First Administration — Repeat Dose

In clinical practice, drugs are often prescribed for illnesses which require regular treatment for days, weeks, months, or years. For drugs used in this way, testing on a repeat dose basis in volunteers is required to evaluate safety and tolerability before treating patients. As with first-time single dose studies, first-time repeat dose studies can be undertaken using different designs but with the emphasis again on safety and tolerability. The cornerstone design is a randomized, rising dose, placebo-controlled group comparative evaluation. Whichever design is used, the investigator has to decide upon an appropriate dosing schedule. The choice of a unit dose and dosing interval depends primarily upon the results from the single-dose study. To illustrate this point, if we assume that the top dose (i.e., 64x) given in the previously described single-dose study proved to be well-tolerated, then we might opt for the dosing schedule given in Table 8. Of course, the frequency of dosing will depend upon the pharmacodynamic and/or pharmacokinetic profile of the drug. Ideally, dosing should be continued until steady-state plasma concentrations of drug have been achieved, but this may not be practical for drugs with long half-lives. More often than not volunteers are dosed for 7 to 10 days but in certain circumstances, if toxicological cover is available and there is a definite need to do so, volunteers may be dosed for 4 weeks. Even if the intent is to dose more than once daily (as in Table 8 where twice-daily [bd] dosing is required), giving single doses on the mornings of day 1 and the last day of dosing (i.e., day 7) offers certain advantages. For example, it allows for a longer period to assess tolerability before the second dose of drug is given to a volunteer who more than likely will not have been exposed to the drug previously. It also enables comparisons to be made between drug plasma concentration time profiles over 24 h and the elimination kinetics of the drug at the start and end of dosing.

Table 8 Design and Dosing Schedule for a First Repeat-Dose Phase I Study

Group	Day 1	Days 2-6	Day 7
1	8x	8x bd	8x
2	16x	16x bd	16x
3	32x	32x bd	32x

Note: bd — twice a day.

In the interests of safety, doses are increased between groups sequentially and as a rule dosing is completed in the previous group before dosing is started in the next group. However, if groups are to be dosed for more than 7 to 10 days or a large number of increments in dose is planned, particularly if more than one dosing frequency is under test, the investigator might choose to overlap dosing between one group and the next thus enabling the study to be completed in a reasonable time frame. Within each group, volunteers are randomly allocated to receive drug or placebo. The size of the groups usually varies between 6 and 12 with the numbers of subjects receiving drug and placebo in a group being subject to investigator preference.

4.2 Phase II Studies

In terms of safety evaluation, early patient studies are an extension of volunteer studies, but they also provide the first opportunity to evaluate the drug in terms of clinical efficacy. Study designs governing the conduct of patient studies, both in terms of evaluating efficacy and safety, have attracted a great deal of attention over the past 30 years or so; testimony to this fact being the wide literature in this area. They vary from the simple to the complex which leaves the investigator to decide upon the design of choice. Uncontrolled (noncomparative) studies are of little or no value in assessing the therapeutic utility of a drug, except possibly as a pilot to help define a dose range for a randomized, double-blind comparative investigation. The latter may involve a between-patient (group) comparison in which patients in two or more treatment groups are treated in parallel or a within-patient (cross-over) comparison, where patients take two or more treatments in sequence or random order. The fact that between-patient designs are simple and associated with fewer problems than within-patient designs makes them universally accepted, although as with phase I studies between-patient comparisons require larger numbers of patients than do between-patient designs. The principal limitations of within-patient designs relate to the fact that they cannot be used in conditions which respond fully to the first treatment lest there be nothing left to treat, that allowances may have to be made for carry-over or period effects (which might complicate the interpretation of the results) and that they generally require greater cooperation on the part of the patients which may lead to unacceptably high drop-out rates. Depending upon the amount of information being sought from a single study, relatively simple designs can be made more complex by adopting in the case of between-subject comparisons the use of stratified randomizations in an attempt to balance between treatment groups for possible prognostic factors such as sex, age, severity, or duration of the disease and in the case of within-subject comparisons, incomplete block designs (e.g., five treatments in a three-period cross-over design), or latin-square designs for a multiperiod cross-over comparison.

On the basis that controlled studies only are acceptable in the eyes of regulatory authorities to show clinical efficacy, the test drug will need to be compared with placebo or a standard treatment of proven value. If the latter does not exist then the matter is straightforward in that the new drug can be tested against a placebo control on the basis that the patients are not being deprived of the best available treatment. When there were few effective treatments or at least treatments which had not been shown to be of clear value, the use of placebo was easy to justify, but its use becomes more difficult to support as effective treatments become available for a wide variety of illnesses. However, there is ample evidence in the literature to show that new drugs are still being tested against placebo, rather than a drug of proven benefit in a number of conditions. This issue has been highlighted by Rothman and Michels[3] who state that placebo-controlled studies have been conducted in onchocerciasis, rheumatoid arthritis, depression, chemotherapy-induced emesis, congestive heart failure, and mild-to-moderate hypertension, despite the availability of effective treatments in all of these conditions. To show clinical superiority over placebo as opposed to an established drug requires fewer patients because the treatment difference should be greater, hence one can readily see the attractions of using placebo controls in phase II studies which by their very nature employ relatively small numbers of patients. But even if an investigator elects for placebo control, it can only be used in conditions which are self-limiting, e.g., mild-to-moderate pain, nausea, or insomnia where there are unlikely to be serious clinical sequelae and where provision is made for rescue medication in the event of symptoms becoming more severe. Quite apart from the fact that placebo-controlled studies offer quicker feedback on comparative efficacy because smaller numbers of patients are needed, they are also undertaken because they are accepted by regulatory authorities. However, evidence of good efficacy against an effective therapy is needed during phase II to help ensure that a drug which is inferior to existing treatments is not taken forward into full development.

The safe and effective use of new drugs requires that the relationships between dose or even better drug concentration in blood and clinical response be investigated. The FDA has published a draft guideline to this effect which is based upon recommendations put forward by the Efficacy Expert Working Group of the International Conference on Harmonization for Registration of Pharmaceuticals for Human Use. Ideally, the doses selected for an initial dose-finding exercise in patients should incorporate the no-effect dose and maximum effective doses with the aim of selecting an optimum dose or dose range to take forward into phase III clinical trials. Often the start dose is a "best estimate" so the chances are the investigator will need to titrate the dose upward or downward against a surrogate or clinical endpoint. What constitutes an optimum dose is often a matter of opinion. For a drug with a good separation between the doses producing wanted and unwanted effects, the temptation is to go with the highest tolerated dose on the basis that the maximum number of patients are likely to derive benefit. At best, this is an inefficient way (in terms of costs) and at worst, a potentially dangerous way of selecting a dose because the higher the dose the more likely the chances of side effects, possibly serious side effects which may only become apparent when larger numbers of patients are exposed to the drug. In terms of tolerability and safety, the lower the dose the better but this approach could result in an appreciable number of patients being underdosed and ending up as treatment failures. Realistically for most drugs a universal ideal dose probably does not exist, as what might be optimal for one patient may be unsuitable for another patient. The best one can hope to achieve is to select a dosage schedule which will benefit the majority of patients without causing too many side effects.

5 MEASUREMENTS

When designing a protocol for a phase I or II study the means by which drug action is going to be assessed must be given consideration. This not only involves ensuring that the appropriate measurements or assessments are made but that they are made at the right times. Thus thought will need to be given to the timings of measurements relative to dosing, as well as to the frequency and duration of measurements. To help ensure that measurements are made at optimum times it might be necessary to undertake a pilot study beforehand. The same applies to the taking of blood samples for pharmacokinetic or other purposes. The relationship of one measurement to another or to the time a blood sample is taken may also need to be taken into account. If it is likely that the procedures involved in making one measurement are likely to disturb another measurement then the latter should be made first. To give a simple example, cadiovascular measurements should be made before lung function measurements when the latter require forced respiratory effort. If the intention is to investigate the relationship between drug action and plasma concentration of drug then the timings of the blood sample and the measure of drug effect assume particular importance.

5.1 Plasma Drug Concentrations

Monitoring plasma concentrations of drugs offers considerable advantages and should be undertaken whenever feasible during the course of phase I and II studies.

Plasma concentrations are a better guide to levels of systemic drug exposure than are doses of drug administered. This point is well illustrated by the example given below in which plasma drug concentrations were disproportionately higher in man than would have been anticipated based on comparisons of doses administered to the rat, dog and man.

This information resulted in the level of toxicological cover which was initially based on dose/body weight having to be revised downward.

	Dose (mg/kg)	C_{max} (μg/mL)	AUC (μg.h/mL)
Rat	100	165	850
Dog	100	155	460
Man	2	25	300

Level of drug exposure may also provide an explanation for either a lack of effect or an exaggerated response in a given individual or in a group of individuals, for example, as a result of poor or excessive absorption from the GI tract following oral dosing.

Doses are often progressed on the assumption that a doubling of dose will provide a corresponding increase in plasma concentrations, but on occasions this is not the case with the result that inappropriately high plasma concentrations can result from modest increases in dose. An early warning of nonlinearity between dose and plasma concentrations is obtained when plasma concentrations are monitored in dose escalation studies. The investigator is then able to modify the proposed dosing schedule accordingly.

Monitoring of plasma concentrations also enables the investigator to obtain information on plasma concentration time relationships and to ally this information to dynamic, surrogate, or clinical endpoints in attempts to gain a better understanding of mechanisms of drug action and of relationships between dose and drug effects.

The early use of plasma drug concentrations will also enable important subgroups of patients to be identified before the drug passes into large-scale clinical trials.

Measurement of plasma drug concentrations requires a reliable, specific, and sensitive assay which takes time to develop so such an assay may not be available early on in the drug development process. In the first instance the assay used for animal studies may also have to suffice for initial studies in man, even though such an assay may lack the sensitivity to measure plasma concentrations after low doses of the drug or to follow plasma concentrations for long enough to measure the drugs terminal elimination half-life.

5.2 Assessment of Wanted Drug Effects

Specific aspects concerning the measurement of drug action in different therapeutic areas will be discussed in following chapters so I shall restrict my comments to issues of a general nature.

Conclusions with regard to efficacy of a drug in a particular illness or disease may be based upon evidence of clinical (symptomatic) improvement, or changes in biological or biochemical markers. Investigators are always on the look out for outcome measures from phase I studies which translate into therapeutic effect and can be used to make predictions about what will happen in patients. This is the prime motivation behind the development of pharmacodynamic models and the increasing use of surrogate markers in healthy volunteers, but whether the endpoint be pharmacodynamic, pharmacokinetic, or a surrogate the same fundamental questions must be answered before they are incorporated into the protocol:

- Can I measure it?
- Need I measure it?
- Can I put the result into a clinical context?

The answer to the first question involves making an assessment of the precision, accuracy, and repeatability of the technique, as well as how easy it is to perform.

The second question brings into consideration the reason for including the measurement in the study. The investigator must be able to justify all data items. Will its inclusion help to take the drug forward, i.e., produce pivotal data or "nice to have data." This differentiation becomes more important when the measurement is complex to undertake or expensive in terms of resource and cost, but quite apart from anything else the more variables that are measured in a study the greater the amount of data to be analyzed and interpreted. If the study includes several quite separate and diverse endpoints, e.g., clinical, biochemical, and histological, the investigator will need to decide at the study design stage which are pivotal to achieving the objectives of the study. If the outcome measures are not given priority, the investigator may end up with a number of conflicting results and find himself unable to reach a conclusion.

The last question pertains to the value and limitations of study endpoints in respect of their ability to reflect the therapeutic action of a drug. This issue can only be addressed by testing for correlations between endpoints and clinical benefit.

5.3 Assessment of Unwanted Drug Effects

Because of the relatively small numbers of volunteers and patients involved only the most common of drug-related adverse events are likely to be detected during early studies. For example, to have a 95% chance of picking up three subjects who have experienced an adverse reaction (with no background incidence) which occurs in 1 in every 100 subjects treated with the drug, it would need to be given to 650 subjects.[5] Matters are made worse when the adverse event in question also occurs in the general population, which is usually the case with the kind of symptoms reported by volunteers and patients taking part in drug studies. No matter how good the study design nothing can compensate for this problem of inadequate numbers. In this respect all of the study designs described earlier are more or less equally adequate or inadequate as the case may be.

Monitoring for drug-related adverse events employs the same or similar methods in both volunteers and patients. In both cases assessments of tolerability and safety are based upon symptom reports, routine laboratory safety screens, ECG monitoring, and on occasions special tests designed to detect unwanted effects associated with a particular class of drug. The chances of obtaining reliable information on a drug's safety profile are enhanced by detailed and careful monitoring. Symptoms may be reported spontaneously or elicited in reply to standard questions. Open questions such as "how are you feeling" are to be preferred to leading questions on the basis that they result in fewer reports of adverse events. If leading questions are used they need to be carefully worded. A certain amount of basic information is required on all adverse events, i.e., type, severity, time of onset in relation to time of dosing, duration, and causality. Attributing the cause of an unwanted effect to the drug or some other factor can be difficult particularly when little is known about the drug, as is often the case at the stage of initial studies in volunteers or patients. Rechallenge with the drug ideally using the same dose or if need be (because the event caused a degree of discomfort) a reduced dose is probably the single best way of proving or disproving a causal relationship; but if done the rechallenge procedure must be designed using placebo as comparator under double-blind conditions. Obviously rechallenges can be done only if the adverse event was reversible, did not cause excessive discomfort, and most importantly was not life threatening.

REFERENCES

1. Women as Research Subjects, *Pharmacotherapy,* 13(5), 534, 1993.
2. Merkatz, R. B., Temple, R., Sobel, S., Feiden, K., Kessler, D. A. Women in clinical trials of new drugs. A change in Food and Drug Administration policy. *N. Engl. J. Med.,* 329, 292, 1993.
3. Rothman, K. J., Michels, K. B. The continuing unethical use of placebo controls. *N. Engl. J. Med.,* 331, 394, 1994.
4. International Conference on Harmonisation; Dose-response Information to Support Drug Registration; Notice of Availability of Draft Guideline, *Fed. Reg.,* Friday, July 9, 1993.
5. Lewis, J. A. Postmarketing surveillance: How many patients?, *Trends Pharmacol. Sci.,* 2(4), 93, 1981.

Chapter 13

The Assessment of Pharmacokinetics in Early Phase Drug Evaluation

P. E. Rolan

CONTENTS

1 Introduction 169
2 Absorption and Bioavailability 169
3 Relating Plasma Concentrations to Effects 170
3.1 Relating the Time-Course of Plasma Concentrations to the Time-Course of Effect 170
3.2 Pharmacokinetic/Pharmacodynamic Modeling 171
4 Understanding Human Metabolism of the Drug 173
5 The Effect of Food 174
6 Special Patient Groups 174
7 Summary: The Role of the Clinical Pharmacokineticist in Early Phase Drug Development 175
References 175

1 INTRODUCTION

In modern drug development, companies wish to make rational decisions whether to proceed with or abandon further development based on the likelihood of the compound meeting its target profile. This likelihood changes most rapidly in early phase development and most compounds abandoned during clinical development are abandoned in this phase, with the most common reason being unsuitable pharmacokinetics (Prentis et al., 1988). Hence the assessment of pharmacokinetics in early phase drug development is strategically important. Some of the drug development issues which are likely to be answered at least in part by a thoughtful interpretation of pharmacokinetic data include the following:

1. Is the compound adequately absorbed to be likely to have a therapeutic effect?
2. Is the compound absorbed with a speed consistent with the desired clinical response?
3. Does the compound stay in the body long enough to be consistent with the desired duration of action?
4. Is the within- or between-subject variability acceptable given the likely therapeutic index of the compound?
5. Is there evidence of a formulation problem?
6. Is there a dose range which produces plasma (or tissue) concentrations which are likely to be associated with a desired clinical response, or which gives rise to safety concerns?
7. Is there a relationship between plasma concentrations and a relevant measure of drug effect?
8. Are metabolites produced which may confound the therapeutic response or safety profile?
9. From the absorption, metabolism, and excretion profile, are there subsets of the target population which may behave differently from expected?
10. Considering the above issues, what is a suitable dosing regimen for clinical efficacy trials?

This chapter will discuss these and related issues further. However, for details of pharmacokinetic theory and analysis, the reader is referred elsewhere (Rowland and Tozer, 1989).

2 ABSORPTION AND BIOAVAILABILITY

As most drugs are given orally, absorption which is complete, consistent, and predictable is desirable. Although it may be possible from solubility, lipophilicity, pKa, molecular size, and animal data to make some prediction about likely absorption, only a study in humans will give quantitative data as the

0-8493-9230-6/97/$0.00+$.50
© 1997 by CRC Press, Inc.

mechanisms of drug absorption are complex and still incompletely understood (see Rowland and Tozer, 1989). It may be helpful here to distinguish between the terms "absorption" and "bioavailability."

"Absorption" refers to the fraction of the administered dose which is taken into the body. If a drug is taken up into intestinal cells but then extensively metabolized, it is still regarded as having been absorbed. However, for drug to be "bioavailable," unchanged drug must reach the systemic circulation. Hence a drug with very high first-pass metabolism might be well absorbed but poorly bioavailable. Although in therapeutic terms poor absorption and poor bioavailability pose similar problems, it is important to distinguish between them, because there are likely to be different possible solutions. Poor absorption might be approached by reformulation, change in the route of administration, or the development of a prodrug; extensive presystemic metabolism might only be avoided by change in the route of administration or chemical modification. Poor absorption is still frequently encountered in modern drug development, because the rational drug discovery process often puts more emphasis on potency and selectivity (because these programs are run by biochemists and pharmacologists) than factors likely to be associated with good absorption. This can result in lead compounds which perform very well *in vitro* but which may present major bioavailability and/or formulation problems (see discussion of this by Taylor (1993) and example by Rolan et al. (1994).

Quantitative assessment of the extent of absorption (absolute bioavailability) is most rigorously obtained by comparison of the areas under the plasma concentration-time curves (after adjusting for dose) following i.v. and oral administration. However, even after oral administration alone some idea of absorption or bioavailability can be obtained in the following ways:

1. If a drug is not substantially metabolized, urinary excretion of unchanged drug may be a useful measure of absorption and bioavailability.
2. If a drug is substantially metabolized but it is reasonable to assume that metabolites are not produced in the gut lumen, urinary recovery of drug and metabolites might be a useful measure of absorption.
3. If the "apparent" plasma clearance (dose/area under the plasma concentration-time curve; equivalent to true clearance/fraction of dose absorbed) gives an implausibly high value of clearance (e.g., greater than hepatic and renal plasma flow), it is likely the bioavailability is low. However, this could be due to presystemic metabolism in addition to low absorption.
4. If there is very large within- or between-subject variability in "apparent" clearance this might indicate variable absorption or bioavailability, which in turn is often seen when absorption or bioavailability is low.

Determining whether absorption is related to the formulation or to an intrinsic property of the molecule can be obtained by comparing absorption from a solid formulation and an oral solution, ideally with an i.v. solution as a reference.

Some idea of the rate of absorption can be obtained from examination of the plasma concentration-time profile. It should be remembered, however, that the time to maximum plasma concentration (t_{max}) is not when absorption is complete but when the rates of drug absorption and elimination are equal. Thus two drugs with the same absorption rate will differ in t_{max} if elimination rates differ. Assessment of the rate of absorption can also be confounded by complex or slow drug distribution. For example, the calcium-channel blocker amlodipine has a much later t_{max} than other similar drugs. This is not due to slow absorption but to partitioning in the liver membrane with slow redistribution (Walker et al., 1994). A quantitative assessment of the rate of absorption can be obtained by deconvolution of plasma profiles following i.v. and oral administration.

3 RELATING PLASMA CONCENTRATIONS TO EFFECTS

3.1 Relating the Time-Course of Plasma Concentrations to the Time-Course of Effect

A critical decision to be made after the first human study is whether the compound's speed of onset and duration of action are likely to be consistent with the desired clinical response. Speed of onset is clearly of interest for treatments which are taken intermittently for symptoms relief, e.g., acute treatments for migraine, analgesics, or antihistamines for hay fever. Duration of action is particularly important when the therapeutic effect needs to be sustained continuously, e.g., anticonvulsants. The first information on the probable time course of action often comes from the plasma pharmacokinetic profile. However, it has become increasingly evident that the kinetic profile alone may be misleading, with the concentration-time and effect-time curves being substantially different. Some reasons for this, including examples, include:

1. The effect may be delayed with respect to plasma concentration because of slow uptake into the target tissue from the plasma. A well-known example is digoxin, where there is a delay of several hours between peak plasma concentration and peak effect.
2. The effect may wane faster than the plasma elimination curve due to tolerance, e.g., benzodiazepines and nitrates.
3. The effect may persist despite apparent elimination from plasma. This can occur with an irreversible effect of the drug (e.g., acetylation of platelet cyclooxygenase by aspirin). Another reason is very tight binding of the drug near the receptor (e.g., salmeterol) or concentration and trapping in the target tissue (omeprazole).
4. The formation of active metabolites may also contribute to a delay in onset and/or prolongation of action.

Some of these mechanisms may become apparent during animal pharmacology studies, but the clinical pharmacologist must always be aware of the possible discrepancy between concentration and effect-time curves. Clearly, if a relevant drug effect can also be measured in early human studies, establishing a relationship between plasma concentration and effect may be possible. If the desired clinical effect can be measured directly (e.g., blood pressure for an antihypertensive drug), the pharmacokinetic profile may not contribute greatly to the assessment of time course of action, but these circumstances are the exception rather than the rule. Because of the many causes of discrepancies between the time course of drug concentrations and effect, and often the difficulty in measuring the clinical effects directly, a potentially useful approach comes from the use of *surrogate markers* of drug effect (discussed elsewhere in this book) combined with pharmacokinetic-pharmacodynamic modeling to explore the relationships between dose, plasma concentrations, and effects.

3.2 Pharmacokinetic/Pharmacodynamic Modeling

As has been mentioned above, there are several reasons why the time course of drug effect may differ from the plasma concentration-time curve. However, some relationship between plasma drug concentration often is still present even when this may not immediately be apparent because of confounding factors. Elucidating the underlying concentration-response relationship can be a powerful technique as it may enable the prediction of an effect-time-course with a given dosage regimen in a special patient group or to suggest the release characteristics of a novel formulation in order to achieve a desired effect-time profile. It may also be possible to determine whether confounding factors are present and allow deductions about possible mechanisms responsible.

The basic approach is as follows. A study is performed in which drug effect is measured frequently with simultaneous plasma (and if appropriate, metabolite) concentrations. The effect may be the desired effect or a surrogate of a desired or undesired effect. Individual plots are made of simultaneous plasma concentration and effect. In the absence of confounding factors such as those listed above, the underlying concentration-effect relationship may be revealed. This may be linear or sigmoid depending on the pharmacology and the part of the concentration-response curve covered in the human study. However, frequently the underlying relationship may not be immediately apparent, such as in Figure 1. A clearer relationship emerges when the individual points are joined with a line in the order of time, (Figure 2). It can now be seen that the same concentration is associated with different effect, depending on the time during the experiment the observation was made. This phenomenon of the concentration-effect relationship being time-dependent is referred to as *hysteresis*. In the example it is now apparent that at the early time points high plasma concentrations are associated with little drug effect but later the reverse is true. Because the line joining points goes counter clockwise, this is called *counter clockwise hysteresis*. The commonest mechanisms underlying this would be a delay in distribution of drug from plasma to the receptor, but other theoretically possible mechanisms include the formation of an active agonist metabolite or increasing sensitivity of the receptor *upregulation*. If we assume *stationarity*, (i.e., the same concentration at the receptor produces the same concentration independent of time) then it is possible to estimate the time delay between concentrations in the plasma and at the receptor *effect site concentration*. It is then possible to produce a plot of estimated effect-site concentrations against effect which may reveal the underlying relationship which can be described quantitatively (Figure 3). As the basic plasma pharmacokinetic properties, the time-course of distribution and efflux of drug from the plasma to the effect site, and the effect-site concentration-effect relationship are all known it is now possible to estimate the effect-time curve for different dosing regimens. Similarly, if the reason for the hysteresis is the formation of an active metabolite or upregulation this approach may give quantitative information on the metabolite or the time-course of upregulation.

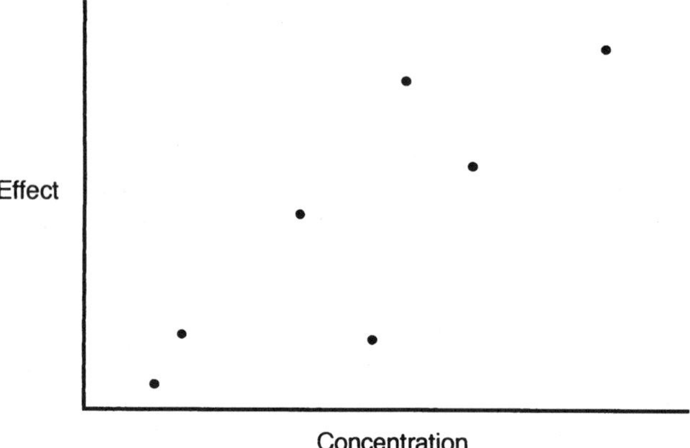

Figure 1 Raw plot of measurements of drug effect against simultaneous plasma concentrations showing no clear relationship.

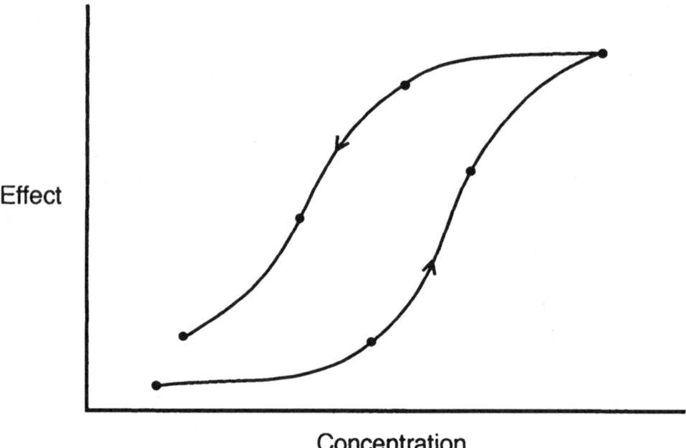

Figure 2 As in Figure 1 but with the points connected in the direction of time showing counterclockwise hysteresis.

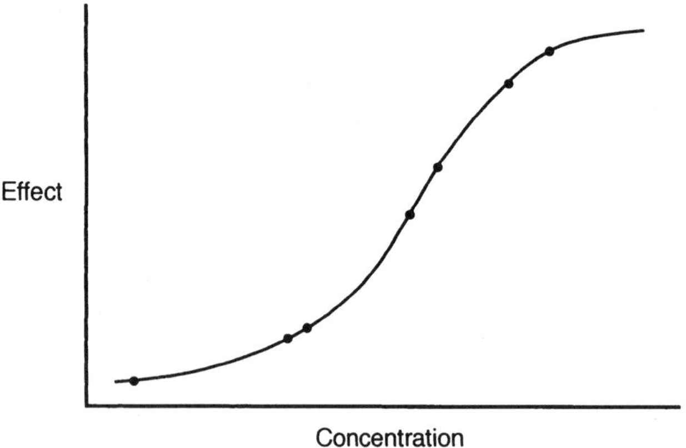

Figure 3 Same data as in Figures 1 and 2 but using estimated effect-site concentrations instead of plasma concentrations by correcting for the time delay between plasma and effect-site concentrations. Note that a clear concentration-effect relationship is evident.

Plots of effect against plasma concentration may also show clockwise hysteresis. Possible mechanisms include the development of pharmacological tolerance or downregulation, or the formation of an inhibitory active metabolite. However, the same approach to data analysis can be used. For a review of this approach, see Holford and Sheiner (1981).

This approach of pharmacokinetic/pharmacodynamic modeling has recently become popular with several international symposia dedicated to it. The FDA has also expressed interest in seeing this form of data analysis as a tool to rationally select dosing regimens. For some drug classes where drug effect can be easily measured accurately (e.g., neuromuscular blockers) this technique has been useful. However, this form of data analysis should not be used uncritically, as it has some weaknesses. First, the analysis is dependent on a measurer of drug effect or surrogate which can be measured repeatedly with accuracy comparable to that of plasma drug assays. This is often not possible. To cope with error in measuring drug effect, the analysis has sometimes been performed on naively pooled data. This has the weakness of assuming the same concentration-effect relationship for the whole study population. A population approach using nonlinear mixed-effect modeling (Sheiner, 1984) is probably superior. When using an effect variable with a non-zero baseline value (e.g., blood pressure) another problem is whether to use raw values or change from baseline as the marker of drug effect. The latter approach assumes that in the absence of drug there is no change in the effect value and this is not always true, e.g., the diurnal variation in FEV_1 in asthmatics. If change from baseline is used but individual baselines vary, whether absolute or relative changes from baseline are used as the measure of drug effect needs consideration. However, despite these concerns, it is likely that pharmacokinetic/pharmacodynamic modeling will continue to be used increasingly in early and later phase drug development to select and justify dosage regimens.

4 UNDERSTANDING HUMAN METABOLISM OF THE DRUG

There are three important reasons for understanding the metabolic fate of a new compound in man as early as possible. First, an active metabolite may be formed which may alter the clinical profile in a desired (e.g., prolongation of action) or undesired manner (different side effect profile) manner. Even though *in vitro* work with human microsomes and comparison with animal data may allow some prediction of whether active metabolites are likely, only *in vivo* data in humans will confirm or refute this and more importantly quantitate the circulating concentrations. Secondly, new metabolites may be produced in humans which were not observed in the animal toxicology studies, or in quantities which approach or exceed those associated with toxicity in the animal studies despite concentrations of parent drug unassociated with toxicity. In these circumstances, further toxicology studies with the metabolite(s) may be required, or toxicology studies may need to be repeated with another animal species which more closely resembles the human metabolic profile. Given the delays and costs of such extra work, it may be appropriate to discontinue further development of the compound and proceed with a follow-up compound which has a more favorable metabolic profile.

If the metabolic fate is confined to a small number of chemical species and particularly if the major method of elimination of drug and metabolites is via the urine, characterizing the metabolic fate of a compound can be performed using standard assay techniques. Under other circumstances it is necessary to ensure labeling of the molecule in some way so that all drug-derived material can be universally detected. Conventionally this is achieved by incorporating one or more radioactive atoms into the molecule, usually ^{14}C. However, with the growing public sensitivity to radiation issues, the approval required and adequate recruitment are increasingly difficult. An alternative approach is to use a stable isotope labeled drug. Although this avoids radiation concerns, clear results depend on highly sophisticated mass spectrometry equipment and specialized staff, compared to the simpler methods which are adequate for radiolabeled drugs. Another possible approach using unmodified drug is using magnetic resonance spectroscopy, but sensitivity is only likely be adequate with fluorine-containing molecules present in high concentrations.

Third, with the large increase in our understanding of the substrate specificities of different metabolic processes (in particular, cytochrome P-450 isozymes), identification of the enzymes responsible for metabolism may help predict important drug interactions, or, more helpfully, identify classes of drugs with which the new compound is unlikely to interact. This makes selection of human drug interaction studies a little more rational. As this work can be performed *in vitro* requiring modest resources, and can increase the potential pool of patients in efficacy studies by allowing more concomitant medications, this approach is recommended as being resource-efficient.

5 THE EFFECT OF FOOD

Food is one of the most important factors under patient control which may affect absorption and bioavailability (Welling, 1989). Food can dramatically increase absorption, have no effect, or may decrease absorption. Even when the extent of absorption is unaffected, the rate is often delayed due to the inhibition of gastric emptying. In addition to affecting absorption, postprandial changes in hepatic blood flow can also affect hepatic extraction and hence bioavailability of some high first-pass drugs. First-time administration studies in man are usually performed in the fasting state to avoid the possible confounding effects of food. However, as absorption will have only been demonstrated in studies where the volunteers were fasted, patients in clinical trials would need a similar restriction which is often impractical and may affect compliance. Hence, in order to expedite early clinical trials it is advisable to have some idea of the effect of food on absorption. Often some idea of the likely effect of food can be estimated from the physical characteristics of a drug; for example, a poorly absorbed lipophilic drug can reasonably be expected to have improved absorption after food. For such a drug a separate study of the effect of a high-fat meal may be appropriate. However, when it is thought that the effect of food is unlikely to be clinically important, including a single fed limb in the first ascending dose study may be an efficient way of screening for an important effect. A more formal and adequately powered study may still be required later for registration purposes.

6 SPECIAL PATIENT GROUPS

Another important issue in early phase development is whether to perform kinetic studies in special patients groups (elderly, patients with renal or hepatic disease) and if so when and how. As the elderly are the majority users of many medicines, the subject of evaluating new drugs in the elderly is a major issue which is discussed in detail elsewhere. Unless a medication is unlikely to be used in the elderly some data will be required by regulators for registration. However, an important issue in early phase development is whether to perform a separate elderly volunteer kinetic/tolerability study before elderly patients are included in later phase clinical trials. The major argument for doing so includes the possible reluctance of clinical investigators to enroll elderly patients without such data being available because of safety concerns, however, the utility of such studies has been questioned. The subjects in elderly volunteer studies are usually in much better health than the general population they are intended to represent. Also, the elderly may differ from the young not so much in terms of mean kinetic parameters but the variability in the elderly may be much greater. The relatively small sample size (typically 12–18) may not allow a good estimation of the variability within the elderly population. For these reasons the FDA have recommended that information about the kinetics of a drug in the elderly should come from a larger group representative of the target population and this can be done in the efficacy clinical trials. Although these data are useful, it is not always an acceptable substitute for a specific elderly volunteer pharmacokinetic study because the information is only available after many patients have been exposed rather than before and clinical investigators may be reluctant to enroll patients without such data in advance. In practice, for a drug likely to be given to the elderly, an elderly volunteer study should be performed soon after a young healthy volunteer study to expand the potential population for efficacy studies as much as possible. If elderly patients are then included in the main efficacy/safety studies, the population approach can then be used to explore the pharmacokinetic variability in this subset of the population and whether this is associated with an altered clinical outcome.

A similar rationale can be used to decide whether special kinetic (and possibly, dynamic) studies should be performed in patients with renal or hepatic disease. For example, if the compound is largely metabolized to inactive metabolites, renal function can reasonably be expected not to have a major effect on kinetics. However, regulators usually will want some information as some exceptions do exist to the above assumption. An example is the "futile cycle" involving some NSAIDS — where prolonged residence of inactive acyl glucuronide metabolites in the plasma in patients with renal disease allows breakdown back to the parent molecule resulting in accumulation (Sallustio et al., 1989). As outlined above, a population approach could be used to screen for an effect of disease on drug kinetics, but some investigators may need reassurance before enrolling patients in trials. A small study in patients with advanced renal disease may be able to provide this reassurance. Liver disease can be handled similarly for drugs which are primarily eliminated renally.

7 SUMMARY: THE ROLE OF THE CLINICAL PHARMACOKINETICIST IN EARLY PHASE DRUG DEVELOPMENT

The clinical pharmacokineticist can contribute to early phase drug development in many ways. The most important contributions relate to examining the relationship between dose, plasma concentrations, and drug effects so that an estimate of whether the compound and formulation meet the target profile can be made and if so, what may be the best dosing regimen or whether a different formulation may improve the clinical profile. Additional important contributions include early examination of factors likely to affect drug handling so that the widest possible range of patients with the fewest restraints can be enrolled into efficacy trials so that these can be completed rapidly and are representative of the target population.

REFERENCES

Holford NH and Sheiner LB. Understanding the dose-effect relationship — clinical applications of pharmacokinetic–pharmacodynamic models. *Clin. Pharmacokinet.* 1981; 6:429-453.

Prentis RA, Lis Y and Walker SR. Pharmaceutical innovation by the seven UK-owned pharmaceutical companies (1964-1985). *Br. J. Clin. Pharmacol.* 1988; 25:387-396.

Rolan PE, Mercer AJ, Weatherley BC, Holdich T, Meire H, Peck RW, Ridout G and Posner J. Examination of some factors responsible for a food-induced increase in absorption of atovaquone. *Br. J. Clin. Pharmacol.* 1994; 37:13-20.

Rowland M and Tozer T. *Clinical Pharmacokinetics*, 2nd edition. Lea & Febiger, Philadelphia, 1989.

Sallustio BC, Purdie YJ, Birkett DJ and Meffin PJ. Effect of renal dysfunction on the individual components of the acyl-glucuronide futile cycle. *J. Pharmacol. Exp. Ther.* 1989; 25:288-294.

Sheiner LB. The population approach to pharmacokinetic data analysis: rationale and data analysis methods. *Drug Metab. Rev.* 1984; 15:153-171.

Taylor JB. Discovery of new medicines. In *The Textbook of Pharmaceutical Medicine,* eds. Griffin JP, O'Grady J and Wells FO. Greystone Books, Belfast, 1993.

Walker DK, Humphrey MJ and Smith DA. Importance of metabolic stability and hepatic distribution to the pharmacokinetic profile of amlodipine. *Xenobiotica* 1994; 24:243-250.

Welling PG. Effects of food on drug absorption. *Pharm. Ther.* 1989; 43:425-441.

Part V. Assessment of Drug Effects on the Cardiovascular System

Chapter 14

Noninvasive Measurement of Cardiovascular Response

Kirsteen M. Donaldson and John D. Harry

CONTENTS

1 Introduction 179
2 General Considerations 180
  2.1 Repeatability 180
  2.2 Validity 181
  2.3 Sensitivity 182
3 Interpretation of Measurements Obtained with Noninvasive Techniques 182
4 Noninvasive Methods Available to Study the Effects of Drugs on the Cardiovascular System in Early Development Studies 183
  4.1 Measurement of Cardiac Output 183
    4.1.1 Impedance Cardiography 183
    4.1.2 Doppler or Echo-Doppler Cardiography 184
    4.1.3 CO_2 Rebreathing Techniques 185
    4.1.4 Choice of Method 186
  4.2 Other Measures of Cardiac Performance 187
    4.2.1 Systolic Time-Intervals 187
    4.2.2 Echocardiography 187
    4.2.3 Displacement Cardiography 188
  4.3 Noninvasive Methods of Measuring Blood Pressure and Heart Rate 188
    4.3.1 Blood Pressure 189
      4.3.1.1 Noninvasive Continuous (Beat-By-Beat) Blood Pressure Measurement 189
      4.3.1.2 Ambulatory Blood Pressure Monitoring 190
    4.3.2 Heart Rate Variability 191
5 Conclusions 192
References 192

1 INTRODUCTION

While clearly understood by research workers, particularly those involved with assessing the effects of drugs on cardiac function, the term noninvasive technique lacks a clear definition. A working definition could be: "noninvasive techniques, when applied to studies involving measurements of cardiac function, are those which do not employ direct entry into the circulation such as occurs when measuring cardiovascular parameters from cardiac catheterization." Measurements using such techniques, therefore, will be made from the surface of the body and will not involve breaking the skin (other than perhaps venepuncture). Noninvasive measurements of cardiovascular function are attractive when assessing whether a new untested chemical entity (NCE) affects the activity of the heart or other parts of the cardiovascular system. Little discomfort or risk is experienced by the subject and repeated measurements can be made over a period of time after dosing with the NCE, allowing the assessment of both short- and long-term affects of the intervention and the comparison of the effects of the novel compound with placebo and other comparator drugs.

Few new techniques for measuring cardiac performance using noninvasive methods have been developed over the 7 years since the subject was reviewed in the first edition of this book.[1] However, research has continued to evaluate and employ different aspects of the techniques that were discussed in that chapter, allowing an update with this more recent information. At the same time, a new edition gives the opportunity to offer a more detailed review of these techniques. Both have been incorporated into this review. It is hoped to provide the reader with sufficient information regarding the noninvasive

0-8493-9230-6/97/$0.00+$.50
© 1997 by CRC Press, Inc.

methods that have been employed in the early development of drugs to examine their cardiovascular actions to enable the investigator to identify a method that may be suitable for solving a particular problem and to direct the researcher as to where further information may be found regarding those methods that might be of interest.

In this chapter, particular emphasis will be directed to those methods which are applicable to early development (phase I and early phase II) studies of the effects of new drugs on the cardiovascular system. These methods should be suitable for use in the typical clinical pharmacology unit with a reasonable capital equipment cost and no requirement for a dedicated department. Hence, radionuclide techniques and magnetic resonance imaging and spectroscopy will not be considered further, although both techniques may have a role in the noninvasive evaluation of cardiac function in volunteers and patients in the hospital setting and the role of radionuclide techniques might be extended by recent advances in the development of portable nonimaging nuclear probes.[2-6] The parameters which the clinical pharmacologist has greatest interest in measuring are those that reflect global cardiovascular function and that allow description of the effects of an intervention. Measurements of other parameters such as left ventricular function may help in determining the mode of action of a putative cardiovascular drug. This chapter will deal specifically with measures of left ventricular performance, blood pressure, and heart rate, and will not attempt to consider other noninvasive measures of cardiovascular activity such as those which measure peripheral blood flow, effects on electrocardiographic measurements, etc.

2 GENERAL CONSIDERATIONS

Two types of questions are asked of new compounds with respect to their effects on the cardiovascular system when they are investigated in early trials in volunteer subjects. First, if the compound is a putative cardiovascular agent or an agent that, while not primarily cardiovascular, is believed on the basis of preclinical or early clinical studies to possess significant cardiovascular activity, then specific studies of its effect on the heart or peripheral circulation may be required. Second, if the compound is other than a cardiovascular compound, all that may be required is to determine any general effects that the compound may have on the circulation. A number of noninvasive techniques are now available to assess the effects of drugs on cardiac function but, clearly, more sophisticated tests would be applicable in the former situation than in the latter. Some techniques are easier and cheaper to set up than others. Whatever method of assessment is selected, it should fulfill certain important criteria before it can be accepted as yielding results that are sufficiently meaningful to permit decisions to be made about the effects of untested compounds. Some of these criteria are considered below.

In later sections, different noninvasive methods of evaluating cardiovascular performance will be discussed, with particular attention to how well each method meets these criteria. Several other factors will influence the usefulness of a test in the routine evaluation of cardiovascular function. These include the ease of use: how much training of the staff and volunteer are required? Is the technique operator-dependent? How well tolerated is it by the volunteer? Is the method tolerant of postural change and motion artifact, e.g., during exercise? Is it able to detect transient changes, e.g., during the shift from lying to standing or during a Valsalva maneuver? Does the method yield quantitative results? Many of these factors will also be considered in these later sections.

2.1 Repeatability

The ability of noninvasive techniques to detect changes in cardiovascular function as a consequence of the administration of a novel chemical entity depends upon the precision of the technique, i.e., the extent to which repeated measurements agree with each other. This in turn depends upon measuring errors specific to the technique and on physiological changes in cardiovascular function. A number of external variables such as room temperature, time of day, posture, activity, and food intake are known to exert profound effects on the cardiovascular system. These variables should be standardized throughout all study periods. Subjects should be familiarized with the techniques to be employed to minimize anxiety.

In order to compare different noninvasive techniques, it is useful to be able to quantify the repeatability of each technique. Statistical techniques for doing this are described in more detail by Healy[7] and by Altman and Bland.[8] Repeatability is determined by taking a number of measurements in each of a series of subjects. It is best expressed as the repeatability coefficient, defined in accordance with the British Standards Institute and described by Altman and Bland.[8] This measure provides an estimate of the greatest difference that would be expected between two single test results made in the same individuals under the same circumstances using the same technique; the smaller the repeatability coefficient, the more reproducible the test. It is calculated most easily when duplicate measurements have been performed in an adequately large series of subjects. However, in practice, in many methodology studies intended to evaluate the repeatability of a technique, the measurements are repeated a number of times in a relatively small number of subjects. Calculation of the repeatability coefficient is then more complex and the coefficient of variation is often used as a measure of reproducibility. This produces a range of values (one in each subject) which may be difficult to interpret. In this chapter, the repeatability coefficient has been employed in evaluating noninvasive methods where possible, but it may not be available for some of the older techniques that are used in clinical research. The coefficient of variation is therefore also quoted to permit some comparison of the repeatability of the different techniques. Any such comparison should, however, be interpreted with caution.

It is well recognized that even when established invasive techniques for evaluating cardiovascular function are employed and external factors are standardized as far as possible, substantial variation may be seen between repeat measurements. For example, the repeatability coefficient for cardiac output determination using the indicator dye dilution technique has been reported to be 0.88 $L.min^{-1}$; the same study reported that the repeatability coefficient using the thermodilution technique was 2.2 $L.min^{-1}$.[9] It is probably unrealistic to require that the noninvasive techniques perform better than this. However, unless the repeatability of a noninvasive technique is comparable to that of the invasive techniques, it is unlikely to be sufficiently sensitive to detect changes in cardiovascular function as a consequence of intervention.

2.2 Validity

As any technique for measuring biological activity, noninvasive techniques for assessing cardiovascular function must be validated: does the technique measure what it claims? This depends both on any assumptions implicit in the technique (are they justified?) and on its repeatability. If a method has poor repeatability, i.e., there is considerable variation in repeated measurements in the same subject, the agreement between the test results obtained and the "true" measure will be poor. The validation may take various forms but should include comparison with an established technique. In this context, the direct invasive techniques for determining cardiovascular function such as the indicator dye dilution, direct Fick, or thermodilution techniques of measuring cardiac output are regarded as the "gold standards." However, all these invasive methods make several assumptions that may not be met *in vivo* (including nonpulsatile flow, no injectate recirculation, no loss of indicator substance, thorough mixing of the indicator substance with blood). Comparisons of novel techniques with such established techniques can only give an indication of whether the new method yields results that are comparable with the old. Agreement is limited by deficiencies in both techniques; it is not possible to determine if either method gives the true value. There may be subtle differences in what is being measured, for example Doppler techniques for determining cardiac output measure aortic flow; flow into the coronary arteries is not included. In view of the nature of the invasive assessments, comparisons with noninvasive techniques are generally performed in patients rather than in volunteers; in some cases the underlying disease or condition (hemodynamic shock, valvular heart disease, dysrhythmia, pulmonary disease) may affect the accuracy of the noninvasive technique. Further, it is difficult to compare methods during exercise. However, despite these problems, to be of use in determining the effects of drugs on the heart, results obtained using a noninvasive assessment of cardiovascular function should show some relationship to those obtained using invasive assessments. Ideally, the noninvasive technique should be compared with more than one invasive technique, including those which employ independent measurements and different assumptions.

Historically, the correlation coefficient has been employed to compare values obtained by two methods of determining the same variable. However, this is more correctly a measure of the strength of a relation between results obtained using the two techniques rather than a measure of agreement. Provided that test results obtained using the two methods are linearly related, the correlation coefficient will be high, but the results will only show good agreement if the slope of the relationship is 1 and the intercept 0. The correlation will also be high if the variation between individuals is large compared with the measurement error, although there may be substantial disagreement between test results obtained using the two techniques in the same individual.[8] A more acceptable approach has been described by Bland and Altman.[8] At its simplest, the variable of interest is determined once using each of the two techniques under evaluation in a series of study subjects. The mean difference between the results obtained using the different techniques is calculated: is there a systematic bias; does one technique consistently over- or underestimate the value compared with the other? The limits of agreement are then calculated to provide an estimate of the greatest difference that might be expected between results obtained using the two techniques. In clinical studies intended to compare different methodologies, several data points are often collected from each of a small number of subjects. The correct analysis of these data is complex; usually a simpler, but less correct, analysis is performed.[10,11]

When different invasive techniques of determining cardiac output are compared, the agreement between results obtained with the two techniques appears to be variable and may be quite poor. For example, in a comparison of the direct Fick and thermodilution methods of determining cardiac output, no significant bias was observed and the limits of agreement were found to be –0.64 to +0.48 $L.min^{-1}$, i.e., the result obtained using the thermodilution method could be between 0.64 $L.min^{-1}$, less than and 0.48 $L.min^{-1}$ greater than the result obtained using the direct Fick technique.[12] However, a similar comparison between the thermodilution and indicator dye dilution methods revealed both a systematic bias, the cardiac output measured by the thermodilution technique being a mean of 1.85 $L.min^{-1}$ greater than that measured by the indicator dye dilution technique, and poor agreement, the limits of agreement being –0.63 to 4.33 $L.min^{-1}$.[9] Such wide limits of agreement are likely to be due both to poor precision (repeatability) and to inaccuracies in these established invasive techniques. These factors will also influence the agreement when noninvasive techniques are compared with these techniques and similarly wide limits of agreement are likely to be described. When a noninvasive technique such as the CO_2 rebreathing technique for determining cardiac output has been compared simultaneously with two different invasive techniques, the limits of agreement between the noninvasisve and invasive techniques have been similar to[9] or slightly wider than[12] those between the two invasive techniques.

In clinical pharmacology, the ability to measure change in a parameter of interest is critical but the ability to record absolute values is less important; this is in contrast to clinical practice. Some bias in the technique may not invalidate results obtained using it, provided that any bias is consistent over the measurement range of interest so that the measurement of change is valid.

2.3 Sensitivity

To be useful in determining the effects of drugs on cardiac function, noninvasive techniques need to be sensitive enough to detect any changes that may occur. This is a function of both the repeatability and the validity of the technique. It should be demonstrated that a noninvasive test is able to detect the expected changes in cardiovascular function as a consequence of stimuli such as postural change, exercise, food, or drugs with known cardiovascular effects, e.g., the effect of dobutamine on cardiac output. The response to different perturbations should be examined to determine the validity of the measured changes, i.e., is the test really measuring the expected change or merely a related change such as in heart rate or ventilation?

3 INTERPRETATION OF MEASUREMENTS OBTAINED WITH NONINVASIVE TECHNIQUES

The interpretation of measurements of cardiac function must be carried out with care. There are two considerations that need to be addressed, the first practical, the second conceptual.

The practical consideration relates to the handling of data. Noninvasive techniques permit measurements to be repeated over prolonged periods of time. Some methods record data on a beat-by-beat basis. With these techniques, it is possible to generate immense amounts of information very rapidly. Data management and statistical analysis plans need to be developed to handle these data. Should they be averaged over predetermined periods? Should the maximum or minimum values be recorded? Is the short term variability of the data important, for example, in evaluating any effect of a novel drug on the autonomic control of heart rate.[13,14] Is a bespoke data logging system available or is it necessary to commission one? How will the data be stored.

The conceptual consideration relates to the interpretation of the cause and effect of any changes that are observed. Changes induced in the inotropic state of the heart by a drug or other intervention may be secondary to changes elsewhere within or outside of the circulation rather than a consequence of direct action on the heart itself. For example, changes in preload (venous pressure and venous return) and afterload (arterial blood pressure) are known to affect the inotropic state of the heart. Control of heart rate, blood pressure, and cardiac function is under the regulation of the autonomic nervous system. Thus, these parameters could be altered as a consequence of either a direct action on the cardiovascular system, e.g., a direct acting vasodilator, or indirectly via an effect on the central nervous system; some drugs such as methyldopa may have both actions. This does not invalidate the description of the effects of a drug on the cardiovascular system. It does, however, make an analysis of the mechanism of action on the drug difficult. So, if a new compound is tested in early phase I studies using noninvasive techniques, any effect that the compound produces can be recorded. If only one of the parameters changes and the preclinical pharmacology of the compound is consistent with this change then the mechanism of action is obvious. If, however, heart rate, blood pressure, or other cardiovascular parameters change (and these are not always being measured, e.g., venous pressure), then other approaches may prove necessary to establish the mechanism of action of the drug in man. For example, the effect of the dihydropyridine calcium antagonist, nifedipine, on myocardial contractility differs according to whether it is administered directly into a coronary artery (where it exhibits a negative inotropic action) or intravenously (where its vasodilator activity provokes a compensatory reflex positive inotropic effect).[15]

4 NONINVASIVE METHODS AVAILABLE TO STUDY THE EFFECTS OF DRUGS ON THE CARDIOVASCULAR SYSTEM IN EARLY DEVELOPMENT STUDIES

4.1 Measurement of Cardiac Output

4.1.1 Impedance Cardiography

The bioimpedance method of determining cardiac output uses changes in the transthoracic electrical impedance during cardiac ejection to calculate stroke volume. Thoracic bioimpedance consists of a steady-state component and a variable component. The steady state component (thoracic fluid index, TFI, previously known as base impedance Z_0) represents the total impedance of the thorax. It is dependent on the thoracic cross-section and on the volume of fluid within the thorax (which in turn depends on posture, etc.). The variable component is derived from physical motion (artifact), respiration, and blood pumping activity (which is associated with pulsatile changes in the volume of blood in the thorax and alignment of the erythrocytes). During impedance cardiography, electrodes are placed at the root of the neck and the level of the xiphisternum to sense changes in thoracic impedance during the application of a sinusoidal current through additional electrodes situated immediately outside the first. Stroke volume is calculated from the total thoracic bioimpedance, the maximum velocity of the impedance changes related to the cardiac cycle (dZ/dt_{max}), and the ventricular ejection time (VET). There are essentially two methodological approaches to this calculation. The traditional approach employs circular tape electrodes (which may be uncomfortable), a phonocardiogram to detect aortic valve closure, graphical signal analysis, and Kubicek's equation to estimate stroke volume.[16] Kubicek used a model in which the chest is considered to be a column to devise a plethysmographic formula for estimating stroke volume from the magnitude of the systolic thoracic impedance change. Acceptance of the graphical signal analysis and measurement of thoracic length requires operator intervention. The result may be corrected for packed cell volume.[17] More recently, an alternative approach has been developed using point electrodes, a "black-box" which performs automated signal analysis, and a different equation, the Sramek equation.[18] The thorax is regarded as a truncated cone. The volume of electrically participating tissue is calculated automatically from a nomogram employing the subject's sex, height, and weight. This system provides a very simple beat-by-beat, operator-independent, patient- and clinician-friendly method of determining stroke volume. However, this method has been criticized since the automated signal analysis does not permit direct inspection of the signal quality, although the box can reject inadequate signals. In addition, the ventricular ejection time is determined only from the electrocardiogram and dZ/dt; this may not be as reliable as employing a phonocardiogram. The use of a nomogram to calculate thoracic length is also a potential source of error in the determination of absolute cardiac output (although this would not influence the sensitivity of the method of detecting change as a consequence of pharmacological intervention).

Both methodological approaches are reported to give excellent reproducibility at rest. Thus, the coefficient of variation for repeated measures of cardiac output made on the same occasion is consistently less than 5%.[19-22] Accurate electrode emplacement is critical to the repeatability of stroke volume determination.[23] Between-day variability is greater (coefficient of variation 12.4%).[19] The primary parameter calculated during impedance cardiography is stroke volume. This shows greater variability than does cardiac output.[20,22] Thus, the within-day coefficient of variation is up to 13.7%. When reproducibility is examined by determining the (within-day) repeatability coefficient for the measurement of stroke volume, this is found to be similar for the two methodological approaches: 23.4 mL (mean stroke volume 108 mL) using the Kubicek approach and 29.0 mL (mean stroke volume 136 mL) using the Sramek approach.[24] The repeatability of the technique does not appear to be affected significantly by posture. However, recordings are more difficult to obtain and less repeatable during strenuous exercise, the repeatability coefficient deteriorating from 28.6 to 47.2 mL with little change in mean stroke volume.[20,25,26] Repeatability can be improved if exercise is stopped briefly during the recording period.[22]

The impedance method of determining cardiac output has been validated by comparison with invasive methods. At rest, the limits of agreement between results obtained using the Sramek approach and the thermodilution and indicator dye dilution techniques, although wide,[21,23,27] appear to be comparable with some of those reported when different invasive techniques are compared.[9,12] Good correlation has also been reported between results obtained using the Kubicek method and the invasive techniques (direct Fick and indicator dye dilution).[22,26] A number of concerns have been expressed regarding the validity of the bioimpedance technique for determining cardiac output.[28] Both the Kubicek and Sramek formulae use a measure related to body size in the numerator and the thoracic base impedance, which is inversely related to body size, in the denominator (in the first or second power). The measured stroke volume is thus strongly related to body size and likely to be highly correlated with stroke volume determined by an independent method. Heart rate is an important determinant of cardiac output, particularly on exercise, and this could produce spuriously high correlation with cardiac output determined by other methods. The pulsatile changes in thoracic bioimpedance are likely to be small compared with the total impedance of the thorax and the system (electrode-skin contact, etc.). The agreement between measures of stroke volume obtained using the two different methodologies is poor.[24] In view of these concerns it is important to establish whether the technique is able to measure changes in stroke volume as a consequence of intervention.

The expected changes in stroke volume as a consequence of postural change or medication have been detected using either methodology.[24,27,29-32] Using the beat-by-beat capability of the Sramek method, transient changes in stroke volume occurring during a Valsalva maneuver can also be recorded.[33] However, Thomas noted that while the magnitude of the drug-induced changes detected by the impedance technique (Sramek method) were similar to those detected by the indicator dye dilution technique, the exercise-induced changes in stroke volume were significantly smaller.[27] Other groups have reported changes similar to those expected from the literature, i.e., stroke volume increases early in exercise. With greater amounts of exercise, increases in cardiac output are achieved by increasing heart rate. However, there has been no independent validation of the magnitude of the changes in stroke volume observed during exercise.[20,22,34] Although the relationship between cardiac output determined by the impedance technique and oxygen consumption has been reported to be linear,[17,19,26] this has been disputed,[28] which raises doubts regarding the validity of the method.

Other factors which may influence signal quality and the agreement between the bioimpedance and invasive techniques of determining cardiac output are unlikely to apply in volunteer studies.[35,36]

4.1.2 Doppler or Echo-Doppler Cardiography

The apparent increase (or decrease) in the frequency of sound waves when the source and observer become closer (or more distant) is referred to as the Doppler effect. This principle is employed in Doppler cardiography by measuring the shift in frequency of incident sound waves reflected off the cellular elements of blood (principally erythrocytes) to determine blood velocity ultrasonically. Two Doppler ultrasound methodologies are employed. In pulsed Doppler, a single transducer emits a short pulse of ultrasound and then switches into receive mode; it is then activated by the reflected signal. The delay between the time of pulse emission and the reception of its reflection determines the depth at which the Doppler shift is recorded; this can be adjusted. This method is unsuitable for recording high velocities. Continuous wave Doppler employs separate transducers for emitting the signal and receiving the reflected wave. Both emission and reception occur continuously. The depth from which the signal is received cannot be controlled.

Blood flow velocity may be determined in any blood vessel which is accessible through a suitable physiological window. In determining cardiac function, the most common approaches are via the suprasternal notch to the ascending aorta, the apical approach to the mitral valve orifice, or left ventricular outflow tract. The shift in frequency is in the audible range; both the audiosignal and the visual display may be used to guide the position of the probe and depth of field to obtain the best signal strength.

A number of parameters that may be influenced by change in cardiac function are determined from the blood velocity profile; these are usually averaged over several beats. These include the peak velocity and the pulsatility index (a measure of the range of Doppler frequency shift over the cardiac cycle). Integration (by triangulation or curve following) of the aortic blood velocity over the ejection time yields the stroke distance (stroke velocity integral). Multiplying stroke distance by heart rate gives the minute distance. These latter two parameters are analogous to stroke volume and cardiac output but are relative measures. They are useful for comparative purposes, but are not easily related to conventional cardiac performance indices.[37,38] Volume flow, i.e., stroke volume and cardiac output, may be estimated by multiplying stroke distance and minute distance, respectively, by the cross-sectional area of the vessel measured by an independent technique (usually echocardiography) at the same level as the flow velocity or estimated from a nomogram.[21,35] The accuracy of this determination is limited by the resolution of the technique employed to measure the cross-sectional area. The vessel is generally assumed to be circular and not to vary in size during the cardiac cycle.

Traditionally, measurement of blood volume flow, e.g., cardiac output using Doppler technology requires the determination of the angle between the Doppler beam and the direction of blood flow (Doppler angle). This is difficult to measure in clinical practice and is often assumed to be zero. Other assumptions are that flow is laminar (nonturbulent) and that it has a flat velocity profile ("plug flow").

More recently, the need to measure the Doppler angle and vessel area has been avoided by employing the Hottinger principle.[39,40] A specially designed transducer produces two pulsed ultrasonic beams. A wide beam uniformly insonates a large area encompassing the whole of the vessel lumen. The intensity of each Doppler shifted frequency in this beam is proportional to the number of cells moving in the beam at a specific velocity. This area must be well defined and limited in extent with zero sensitivity outside this area; partial illumination of a second vessel may cause error in the estimate of flow through the vessel of interest. A second narrow beam lying entirely within the area formed by the first and the vessel lumen provides a reference for detecting the effects of blood scattering efficiency and round-trip attenuation.

The reproducibility of the Doppler cardiography techniques during supine rest is good when performed by a trained and experienced operator, the short-term coefficient of variation for peak velocity, peak acceleration, stroke distance, stroke volume, and cardiac output being of the order of 3-9%.[20,41-45] Day-to-day variability is slightly greater (coefficient of variation 6-13%).[44,45] Variability between operator is greater than intraoperator variability (even in analyzing the same recording); it is preferable for research purposes if the same operator performs all procedures.[45,46]

Doppler measurement of cardiac output has been validated by comparison with invasive techniques. There has been moderate agreement between cardiac output determined using the thermodilution technique and using traditional Doppler technology with echocardiographic measurement of aortic cross-sectional area[21] and using equipment employing the Hottinger principle.[43] Less good agreement has been reported in another study in which a nomogram was employed to determine aortic diameter.[35] Other factors that may influence agreement have also been considered.[35]

Doppler techniques have proved sensitive to the expected changes in cardiac function following postural change (although in some subjects the suprasternal notch may be poorly defined in the upright posture and it is difficult to obtain an adequate signal) and treatment with dobutamine or the calcium antagonist, nicardipine.[20,43,45] They are widely used to evaluate the hemodynamic effects of novel compounds.[41,47-49] However, they are less satisfactory on exercise when movement artifact makes the procedure technically difficult.[20,46] This problem may be minimized by asking the subject to stop exercising briefly while recordings are made and, if necessary, hold their breath in end-expiration. However, these maneuvers will alter the parameter of interest. Although measures of left ventricle contractility such as ascending aorta peak velocity, are reported to increase,[44] the expected increase in stroke volume does not appear to be detected consistently by these techniques.[20,46,48]

4.1.3 CO_2 Rebreathing Techniques

Carbon dioxide (CO_2) rebreathing techniques for measuring cardiac output were first described in the early years of this century.[50] Technical improvements in rapid CO_2 analyzers, increasing automation, and on-line computerized data handling have made possible the production of mobile, free-standing systems which are easier to use after short periods of training and have increased the popularity of the techniques. The method employs an adaptation of the Fick principle using CO_2 as the indicator. CO_2 production (V_{CO_2}) is measured directly from expired air. The partial pressure of CO_2 (P_{CO_2}) in arterial blood is determined from end-tidal CO_2.[50] Mixed venous P_{CO_2} is estimated from a rebreathing procedure using one of two approaches.[50-52] In the equilibrium method, the subject rebreathes air from a bag with an initially high P_{CO_2} until a plateau in expired P_{CO_2} is reached; the plateau bag P_{CO_2} provides an estimate of mixed venous P_{CO_2}. The time for the P_{CO_2} to reach a plateau depends on the volume of the rebreathing bag and the initial P_{CO_2} in the bag. If it takes too long, "recirculation" occurs which could result in overestimation of mixed venous P_{CO_2}; guidelines have been established to estimate the appropriate initial P_{CO_2} to minimize the likelihood of this occurring.[53] However, rebreathing air with a relatively high P_{CO_2}

is uncomfortable for the subject. In the exponential method, subjects rebreathe from a bag containing air with an initially low P_{CO_2}. Mixed venous P_{CO_2} is determined from the exponential rate of rise of bag P_{CO_2}. This is less uncomfortable. In some systems, corrections are applied to allow for the small differences between the measured end-tidal and rebreathing P_{CO_2} and arterial and mixed venous P_{CO_2}, respectively. The accuracy of determining arterial and mixed venous P_{CO_2} could also be affected by areas of ventilation-perfusion mismatch.[50] This mismatch is likely to be greater in an upright than in a supine position and might theoretically be a greater concern when the exponential method is used since the equilibrium method allows a contribution to be made from areas of lung that equilibrate more slowly with expired air. Other diseases may also affect the relation between end-tidal and arterial P_{CO_2}.[54] Both methods of determining mixed venous P_{CO_2} yield similar results.[51]

Arterial and mixed venous CO_2 contents (Ca_{CO_2} and Cv_{CO_2}) are calculated from the respective P_{CO_2} using standard CO_2 dissociation curves.[55] These require assumptions to be made regarding hemoglobin concentration, oxygen saturation, pH, and temperature. Clearly these parameters may vary during the course of a study, for example, on exercise.

Cardiac output (CO) is calculated by solving the equation:

$$CO = V_{CO_2}/(Cv_{CO_2} - Ca_{CO_2}) \tag{1}$$

Since the three measures (CO_2 production, arterial P_{CO_2} and mixed venous P_{CO_2}) are determined sequentially, cardiac output can only be estimated at steady state and the method is not suitable for use at maximal exercise, although methods have been described for using the technique during progressive exercise.[56,57] This technique is generally well accepted by subjects, although some patients may be intolerant of its use.[58]

Determination of cardiac output by the CO_2 rebreathing method has been reported to have moderate short-term and day-to-day reproducibility, the coefficient of variation between duplicate measurements being approximately 10% at rest[12,54] and the repeatability coefficient at rest (2.7 $L.min^{-1}$) being a little greater than that of the thermodilution technique (although rather worse than the indicator dye dilution technique).[9] The CO_2 rebreathing method of determining cardiac output is unusual in that it is more reproducible on exercise than at rest since the arteriovenous CO_2 difference is larger and equilibration occurs more rapidly.[12,59] In comparison with invasive methods, the CO_2 rebreathing technique has been reported to give values which are comparable with those obtained using the indicator dye dilution technique and to underestimate cardiac output in comparison with the thermodilution technique at rest.[9,12] Reports of its comparison with the direct Fick technique have been inconsistent.[12,59] The limits of agreement between all the techniques have been comparable. The CO_2 rebreathing technique is able to detect the expected changes in cardiac output following eating and on exercise.[12,58,60] The linear relation between cardiac output determined by this technique and oxygen consumption on exercise has been used to validate this method.[19] However, since both values are dependent on the measurement of ventilation, the two measures are not strictly independent.

4.1.4 Choice of Method

The fact that several noninvasive methods of estimating cardiac output remain in regular use might be expected to indicate that none of them is ideal. That this is the case is confirmed by the studies in which the different techniques have been compared.

The bioimpedance technique for estimating cardiac output using the Sramek approach has proved, in comparison with the Doppler techniques and the CO_2 rebreathing techniques, to be the simplest method to use.[20,21,28,35] It enables continuous beat-by-beat monitoring of stroke volume to be performed and results are available instantly. In contrast, estimation of stroke volume using the Doppler techniques must be performed by a trained and experienced operator. The equipment employed when using the CO_2 rebreathing techniques is also more difficult to use. Neither the Doppler nor rebreathing techniques permit continuous monitoring of cardiac output or provide an instant result. At rest, the bioimpedance technique provides the most repeatable results. However, during exercise, both the bioimpedance and Doppler techniques provide less repeatable measures with a proportion of data points missing due to inadequate recordings. In contrast, the rebreathing techniques provide more reliable measures during exercise. Further, although estimations of cardiac output made using the bioimpedance and Doppler techniques appear to agree equally well with determinations made by the thermodilution technique, the accuracy of the bioimpedance technique in comparison with oxygen uptake is reported to be poor even at rest and deteriorate on exercise. The doubts regarding the validity of this technique have been considered above. Both the bioimpedance and Doppler techniques have been widely used in the evaluation of drug action.

4.2 Other Measures of Cardiac Performance

The previous sections have considered the noninvasive methods available to estimate stroke volume and cardiac output. When evaluating the actions of novel drugs on cardiac function other markers that are thought to be related to the inotropic state of the heart may also prove useful, although they are less clearly related to easily recognized physiological parameters such as cardiac output. Some of these (stroke distance, minute distance, etc.) were discussed briefly in the section on Doppler cardiography. Others are considered further below.

4.2.1 Systolic Time-Intervals

Systolic time-intervals (STIs) represent the duration of left ventricular electromechanical systole. This technique is well established.[61,62] Three principal measures are recorded: the total duration of electromechanical systole (QS_2, from the onset of ventricular depolarization until aortic valve closure); left ventricular ejection time (LVET, the phase of systole during which blood is ejected from the ventricle to the arterial system); and pre-ejection period (PEP, the interval between the beginning of ventricular depolarization and the beginning of left ventricular ejection, i.e., isovolemic contraction). The ratio of PEP/LVET may also be calculated. Conventionally, these measures were made from high quality simultaneous recordings of the electrocardiogram (ECG), phonocardiogram (PCG), and external carotid arterial pulse. More recently, STIs have also been determined using impedance cardiography by measuring the intervals between the impedance inflections and the ECG in place of the external carotid pulse. The phonocardiogram may be determined simultaneously, although it has been claimed that this may not be necessary.[24,27,61,63,64]

STIs, particularly LVET and QS_2, are known to vary with heart rate and a number of regression equations have been developed to correct for this in different groups of subjects. Unfortunately, there is no general agreement regarding the best way to derive these equations. In spite of this, it is usual to employ one of these equations to correct the measured parameters for changes in heart rate.[61,62]

Under controlled conditions, the technique has proved to be reproducible. Noninvasive measurement of STIs has been validated by comparison with invasive measurement of the corresponding intervals, both at steady state and during acute interventions. STIs have also been shown by their correlation and with other invasively determined measures of cardiac function such as ejection fraction and peak dP/dt, under different conditions to be physiologically relevant.[27,62]

The ability of STIs to detect the expected changes in ventricular function as a consequence of food, posture, and drugs with established cardiovascular actions has been studied extensively. Food is associated with shortening of the PEP and QS_2 and reduction in PEP/LVET ratio. Changes in LVET were inconsistent.[62,63] Tilting, which reduces preload, is associated with an increase in PEP and increased LVET.[64] A relatively pure positive inotrope such as dobutamine causes dose-dependent reductions in PEP, LVET, and QS_2.[65] The beta-adenoceptor antagonist, atenolol, causes a prolongation of the PEP and LVET.[63,64] The effects of other drugs such as frusemide, angiotension II, dihydralazine, nitrates, isoprenaline, and prostaglandins, with more complex actions on preload and afterload in addition to direct cardiac effects, have also been well described.[61,62] In general, a reduction in preload is associated with increases in PEP and the PEP/LVET ratio, a decrease in LVET, and no consistent change in QS_2. Reduction in afterload results in shortening of PEP, lengthening of LVET, and reduction in the PEP/LVET ratio. Positive inotropism is associated with reductions in PEP, LVET, QS_2, and the PEP/LVET ratio, while these measures are increased by negative inotropic agents. STIs are commonly used to evaluate the cardiovascular effects of novel compounds.[64-67]

Attempts have been made to evaluate STIs during exercise, particularly using the impedance methods which may avoid the need for a separate phonocardiogram. Exercise may be stopped briefly in order to make measurements or measurements may be made during breath-holding to avoid excessive motion. Controversy persists regarding the appropriate heart rate correction to make during exercise. In general, PEP and LVET are reduced and PEP/LVET ratio is increased by exercise.[27,61,64]

4.2.2 Echocardiography

The principle of echocardiography is similar to that of sonar.[68] A high frequency sound wave is generated by the passage of an electric current through a piezoelectric crystal. This signal is targeted at the heart via a physiological window, usually using the left parasternal or apical approaches. A proportion of the sound energy is reflected at the interfaces between tissues of different acoustic impedance such as between the pericardium and myocardium. These reflected pulses are detected by a receiving crystal. The density and position of the spot on the display screen are determined by the time difference between the transmission and return of the pulse and the magnitude of the received signal.

An M-mode image is constructed by transmitting and recording along one line only, displaying the returning signal as a graph of depth against time. Direct measurements that can be made include the thickness of the interventricular septum and the posterior wall of the left ventricle. The distance between the endocardial surfaces of the septum and the posterior wall is a measure of the size of the left ventricle. The direction of scanning must be perpendicular to the walls of the left ventricle, since if these are transected at an angle all dimensions will be overestimated. The difference between the cubed left ventricle dimension in diastole and systole can be used to estimate stroke volume. This is likely to be inaccurate as an absolute measure since only one level of the left ventricle is evaluated in this way and the proportional change in left ventricle dimension changes at different levels of the ventricle; however, it may be useful as a relative measure.

Sector scans are produced by transmitting pulses along a number of scan lines over an arc. The reflected signal is analyzed to give a two-dimensional motion picture. This is best suited to the qualitative detection of abnormalities in morphology, motion, and acoustic density, especially in regions that are poorly accessible to M-mode echocardiography such as the apex of the left ventricle. Quantitative measurement of cardiac function can be made by defining the internal borders of the ventricle using either a light pen and digitizing techniques or an automated border detection algorithm and hence calculating the cross-sectional area at end systole and end diastole. These techniques have been validated by comparison with established techniques (ejection fraction determined by invasive or radionuclide techniques, left ventricular end-diastolic pressure).[69-72]

The place of echocardiography in clinical practice is now well established. However, it has a number of limitations and has found little role in the evaluation of cardiac function in clinical pharmacology. The ribs and lungs mask the heart from ultrasound except at small physiological windows in the parasternal area and over the apex. In a significant proportion of patients adequate pictures cannot be obtained despite optimum positioning. Image quality is improved by using the transesophageal approach which allows the transducer to be placed closer to the heart. However, this technique is more invasive and is associated with some risk.[73] It has a role in monitoring changes in global and regional left ventricular function in intensive care units or operating theaters and could be employed in the early evaluation of drugs intended for these patient populations.[74-76] It is not suitable for use in volunteer studies.

Echocardiography has been used to evaluate left ventricular function during stress. However, because of the difficulties in obtaining adequate images during exercise, it has become routine to record echocardiographic images as soon as possible after exercise interruption instead of at peak exercise, although even this may not be possible. The principal indication for this procedure is to detect reversible abnormalities of regional wall motion in patients with coronary artery disease; in view of the technical difficulties, pharmacological stress tests are increasingly performed.[77,78] It seems unlikely that this technique would prove suitable for evaluating exercise-induced changes in cardiac function in healthy volunteer subjects.

4.2.3 Displacement Cardiography

Displacement cardiography is a general term used to describe methods that measure the movement of the body in response to the movement of the heart. A number of these techniques have been described including apexcardiography, kinetocardiography, ballistocardiography, and cardiokymography; however, these have not found widespread use because of technical difficulty and uncertain clinical applicability.[79] More recently, seismocardiography has been developed using methodology derived from the study of seismic phenomena to record low frequency vibrations detected at the precordium. The technique is easy to perform and recordings are reproducible over periods of at least 3 months. They are sensitive to changes in cardiac function as a consequence of coronary angioplasty and ventricular pacing.[79] The principal limitation is that the technique is largely descriptive. However, quantitative measures are being developed and it has been employed to demonstrate changes induced by medication.[80]

4.3 Noninvasive Methods of Measuring Blood Pressure and Heart Rate

Measurement of blood pressure and heart rate form the "cornerstone" of the cardiovascular assessment of new chemical entities in man, being global assessments of any drug action on the physiological system. Probably because of their usage, these measurements are not normally considered in a review of noninvasive assessment of cardiovascular function. However, some newer developments that have been made in the methods of measuring heart rate and blood pressure are beginning to be used to assess the actions of compounds on the cardiovascular system. Some of these aspects will be considered in this review.

4.3.1 Blood Pressure

Only two aspects will be covered in this review; namely continuous noninvasive blood pressure monitoring and ambulatory monitoring. For further discussion of established methods of measuring blood pressure, the reader is directed to other reviews.[81-83]

4.3.1.1 Noninvasive Continuous (Beat-By-Beat) Blood Pressure Measurement

In the early 1970s a Czech physiologist, Peñáz, described a new approach to continuous noninvasive recording of blood pressure at the finger level based on a volume clamp method. Technical improvements have been made subsequently by Wesseling and co-workers; the method and factors affecting its reliability have recently been reviewed by this group.[84] A finger cuff containing a photoplethysmographic volume transducer and an inflatable air bladder connected to a fast response servo control system are employed to regulate the pressure applied to the finger through the bladder and thus the pressure applied to the wall of the arteries. Pulsatile changes in blood pressure are associated with corresponding changes in the volume of the finger. These volume differentials are measured by the plethysmographic transducer. The servo control responds to the changing volume by adjusting cuff pressure until the original arterial size and blood volume are again reached. The cuff pressure closely follows the intra-arterial pressure within the finger, allowing measurement of the cuff pressure itself as a function of the arterial blood pressure. This system permits the short-term continuous monitoring of arterial blood pressure on a beat-by-beat basis with an instant response and both digital and graphical output. Two principal factors can affect the validity of the measured values. First, there is a gradually increasing distortion of the intra-arterial pressure waveform toward the periphery as a consequence of reflections of the pulse wave, the taper of the arterial cross-section, and changes in the elastic modulus of the arterial wall. These changes are more significant in younger and normotensive subjects than older and hypertensive subjects. They are associated with an overshoot in systolic blood pressure and an increase in the pulse pressure. Secondly, there must be a pressure gradient between central and peripheral arteries; the true blood pressure in the finger will be lower than that in the aorta or brachial artery. Adequate recordings can be obtained in the majority of subjects, including those with peripheral vascular disease. However, recordings may not be possible in those with severe deformity of the finger or poor general condition (low cardiac output, cool peripheries).[85,86]

Within-subject variability of resting blood pressure determined using this technique and a commercially available device has been reported to be low and similar to that of intra-arterial pressure recordings.[87-90]

The accuracy and precision of this method of estimating blood pressure may be examined by comparison with simultaneously recorded intra-arterial pressure. There is no optimal way to compare these two techniques: if the same arm is employed for both techniques the presence of a cannula may interfere with the arterial pressure waveform more distally while if contralateral arms are employed, systematic pressure differences between the two arms may interfere. Good agreement has generally been reported between mean and diastolic arterial pressures determined simultaneously using the commercially available photoplethysmographic device and intra-arterial monitoring in both normal subjects and patients with hypertension or peripheral vascular disease; the limits of agreement being approximately ±14 mmHg. This is comparable to the level of agreement between an oscillometric device and intra-arterial measurements. However, systolic blood pressure appears to be consistently overestimated by this technique, the average difference between measurements being 7-14 mmHg with wide limits of agreement.[85,86,88-90] Agreement between measures obtained using the two methods may be improved by using adapted finger cuffs on the thumb. Our own experience suggests that absolute values are very sensitive to change in the relative position of the finger and heart.

The ability to record rapid changes in blood pressure during physiological or pharmacological maneuvers using this technique has been examined. The beat-to-beat changes in blood pressure were on average similar to those measured intra-arterially during tests that induced a pressor or depressor response (hand grip, cold pressor test, diving test, Valsalva maneuver, intravenous injections of phenylephrine and glyceryl trinitrate) as well as tests that caused vasomotor changes without major variations in blood pressure (lower body negative pressure, passive leg raising). The average between method discrepancy (SD) was never greater than 4.3 (4.6) and 2.0 (1.6) mmHg for systolic and diastolic blood pressure, respectively, (mean (standard deviation)).[90,91] The pressure differences between determinations made with the two techniques appear to vary with flow during a Valsalva maneuver; however, this variation is a small fraction of the absolute change in blood pressure during this manuever.[92] The technique has been employed to estimate blood pressure during exercise.[88,93] In comparison with measurements made using a random zero sphygmomanometer, the photoplethysmographic technique appears to overestimate systolic pressure by a greater amount on exercise than at rest; estimates of diastolic blood pressure by the two techniques were observed to change in opposite directions.

The ability of the photoplethysmographic technique to monitor rapid changes in blood pressure during a Valsalva maneuver and during a brief period of orthostatic fainting is illustrated in Figure 1.

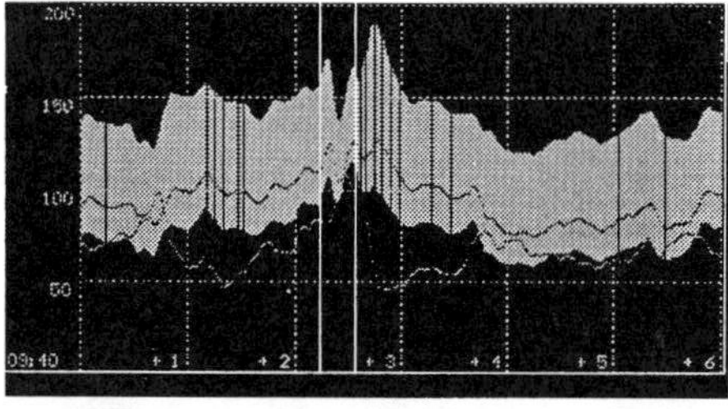

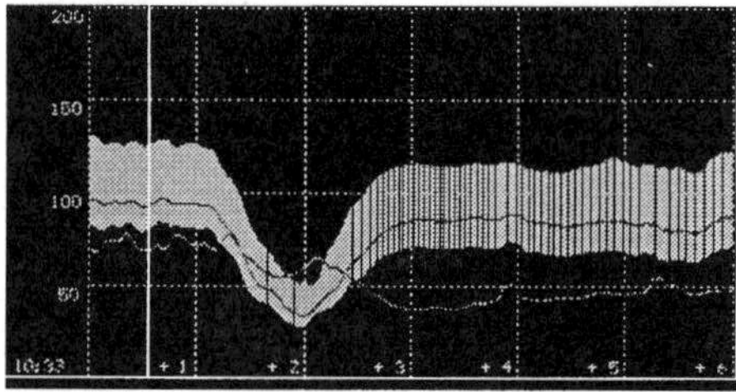

Figure 1 Continuous recordings of blood pressure made using the photoplethysmographic technique. The upper limit of shading indicates systolic blood pressure; the lower limit indicates diastolic. Mean arterial pressure is indicated by the upper continuous line and heart rate by the lower dotted line. A typical Valsalva maneuver is illustrated in the upper figure. The two solid vertical lines indicate the beginning and end of the period of strain. The four phases of the normal hemodynamic response are clearly seen. A period of orthostatic fainting is illustrated in the lower figure. The solid white line indicates the time when the subject was tilted. The subject was placed in a supine position as soon as symptoms developed. A rapid fall and subsequent recovery in blood pressure is illustrated. This could not be detected using a conventional oscillometric technique.

During periods of blood pressure measurement using this technique, the finger cuff remains inflated to between systolic and diastolic pressure. This is associated with a minor degree of hypoxia and desaturation of hemoglobin in the finger distal to the cuff. Although some cyanosis is apparent, this would not be expected to have any adverse effects in healthy volunteers but theoretically could in patients with sickle cell disease. Some swelling and numbness of the finger distal to the cuff are also noted following prolonged application. These changes resolve very rapidly following release of the cuff.[94]

4.3.1.2 Ambulatory Blood Pressure Monitoring

Noninvasive ambulatory techniques have been developed to obtain monitoring of blood pressure over more prolonged periods of time during normal activities of daily life.[81-83,94-98] These devices all use the occlusion/detection technique of blood pressure measurement, employing the same detection methods as other automatic blood pressure monitors (oscillometric or Korotkoff sound technique). Technological advances have led to the development of monitors that are small and may be carried either by a shoulder strap or attached to a belt, reasonably quiet, automatic, and capable of making and storing up to 100 readings in a 24-h period. At the end of the recording period, measurements are down-loaded into a computer for subsequent data handling. Most ambulatory blood pressure software packages provide some editing of physiologically improbable readings. However, the extent to which suspected artifacts in the data should be eliminated is one question that needs to be addressed. Information provided by these devices may be useful in evaluating the efficacy and duration of action of hypotensive medication.

However, like other automatic blood pressure monitors, they require calibration, provide intermittent measures, and are unreliable during periods of activity. Measures will obviously be affected by posture, mood, etc. at the time of the measurement. In addition, measures made during the first 2 h after commencing monitoring are higher than those made subsequently, and cuff inflation does disturb sleep and therefore blood pressure.

As with all noninvasive techniques, ambulatory blood pressure monitoring requires validation by comparison with invasive techniques. A number of ambulatory systems have been evaluated in this way. Important differences have been reported between different systems. Thus, some systems show similar or better agreement with simultaneously recorded intra-arterial pressure both at rest and during exercise than clinicians using a conventional sphygmomanometer. However, others show significantly poorer agreement at rest and/or reject an unacceptable number of measurements during activity.[91,100]

4.3.2 Heart Rate Variability

In health, heart rate is not constant but varies continuously in response to external factors such as changing posture, exertion or stress, and internal factors including respiration, blood pressure regulation, circadian rhythm, etc. This heart rate variation is regulated by the autonomic nervous system. The use of measures of heart rate variability to examine the autonomic regulation of heart rate and the effects of autonomic denervation (either pathological or pharmacological) is well established, for example, in References 101-104; normal ranges for responses have been defined. However, a number of recent developments have led to a resurgence of interest in their use as research tools. These include improvements in the rapid computerized analysis of heart rate variability, accumulating evidence that decreased heart rate variability is predictive of increased mortality following myocardial infarction and in cardiac failure, and the observation that heart rate variability can be modified in both healthy volunteers and patients by pharmacological intervention.[13,14,105,106] A number of measures of heart rate variability are available.

1. **Cardiovascular reflexes**
   Several physiological maneuvers can be employed to provoke changes in heart rate. The magnitude of the observed changes may then provide an indication of the autonomic regulation of the heart beat. The measures employed most commonly are[107,108]
   - **Respiratory ratio** — the ratio of the shortest to the longest R-R interval during forced expiration and deep inspiration.
   - **Valsalva ratio** — the ratio of the longest R-R interval following completion of the strain to the shortest R-R interval during a standardized Valsalva maneuver.
   - **30:15 ratio** — the ratio of the 30th to the 15th R-R interval immediately after assuming a standing position.
2. **Derived from continuous recordings of the R-R interval**
   Beat-by-beat measures of the R-R interval can be determined from continuous recordings of the electrocardiogram (e.g., 24-h tapes) or blood pressure.[87] A high quality recording is required; it must be critically evaluated for the presence of artefacts and arrhythmias. Two types of measures of heart rate variability can be made from these recordings. Time domain variables provide an estimate of the total heart rate variability. These are based on either the interbeat interval (e.g., SDNN, the standard deviation of all normal R-R intervals) or on comparisons of the lengths of adjacent cycles (e.g., pNN50, the percent of differences between adjacent normal R-R intervals that are greater than 50 ms). Interbeat measures are influenced by both short- (e.g., respiration) and long-term factors (e.g., circadian rhythm). Adjacent cycle measures are relatively independent of long-term trends. Measures made in the frequency domain employ spectral analysis to provide information regarding the amount of the overall variance in heart rate resulting from periodic oscillations in heart rate at different frequencies. Oscillations are divided into high and low frequency components; other very low frequency components may also be described. Such spectral analysis requires more complex calculation than analysis in the time domain and is of limited value when the total heart rate variability is restricted. Measurement of the ultra low frequency components requires a full 24-h recording; other measures may be made from shorter recording periods (approximately 5 min). All these measures have been reviewed recently.[13,14]

In interpreting changes in all these measures of heart rate variability, it is necessary to consider possible confounding variables including changes in mean heart rate, age (associated with a decrease in all measures of heart rate variability), and circadian rhythm (heart rate variability increasing at night).[101,104,105,108]

The sensitivity of these measures to changes in the autonomic innervation of the heart has been evaluated. In healthy volunteers, atropine is associated with a marked reduction in the respiratory ratio and the 30:15 ratio and a smaller (nonsignificant) reduction in the Valsalva ratio. Propranolol causes a slight increase in the rebound bradycardia observed on standing.[102,107] However, measures of total heart rate variability derived from continuous recordings of heart beat have in general proved more sensitive to the effects of pharmacological or pathological intervention. Thus Ewing et al. described a reduction in NN50 in a proportion of diabetic patients who had normal cardiovascular reflexes in addition to those diabetics with clinical evidence of autonomic neuropathy and transplant patients.[101] Our experience also suggests that it is more sensitive to the action of drugs than the cardiovascular reflexes. Resting supine heart rate variability is widely used as a marker of parasympathetic activity since it is substantially reduced by atropine but unaffected by propranolol. However, it may also be reduced by the β-adrenoceptor agonist isoprenaline.[108] Other drugs have been reported to increase (e.g., digoxin, angiotensin-converting enzyme inhibitors, atenolol) or decrease (e.g., class 1C antiarrhythmic drugs, tricyclic antidepressants) heart rate variability in healthy volunteers or in patients.

Studies such as these have encouraged the use of measures of total heart rate variability in describing some cardiovascular actions of novel compounds. It has been suggested that spectral analysis provides more information regarding the autonomic input to the heart; the high frequency component being a reliable marker of vagal activity. However, the relative roles of the parasympathetic and sympathetic nervous systems in regulating the low frequency component are less well established.[13,14]

5 CONCLUSIONS

Various noninvasive methods are now available to assess the effects of drugs on cardiovascular function in man. Each of the methods outlined in this chapter allows a description of some of the effects of drugs in early development on cardiac function in volunteers and patients at rest; some also on exercise. However, each method relies on some assumptions that may not be valid under all circumstances and the use of sophisticated technology. Persons making the assessments must be trained in the technique and then validate and assess reproducibility, etc. in their own setting before meaningful results on which decisions regarding pharmacological actions of new chemical entities may be based can be achieved. Some comments made by Pickering 40 years ago in consideration of an invasive method of estimating cardiac output apply equally to the indirect methods considered above:

> ...discussion on cardiac output illustrates with great clarity the difficulty of considering any single characteristic of the circulation except in relationship to the circulation as a whole and with the proviso, which is very rarely justified, that all other factors remain unaltered... the frustrated investigator all too often finds that his arguments closely imitate the behavior of the blood in following a similar circular course (Pickering, 1955).[109]

REFERENCES

1. Harry, J. D., Noninvasive measurement of cardiovascular response, in *Early Phase Drug Evaluation in Man,* O'Grady, J. and Linet, O. I., McMillan Press, London, 1990, chap. 21.
2. Rebergen, S. A., van der Wall, E. E., Doornbos, J., and de Roos, A., Magnetic resonance measurement of velocity and flow: technique, validation, and cardiovascular applications, *Am. Heart J.,* 126, 1439, 1993.
3. Conway, M. A., Bristow, J. D., Blackledge, M. J., Rajagopalan, B., and Radda, G. K., Cardiac metabolism during exercise in healthy volunteers measured by ^{31}P magnetic resonance spectroscopy, *Br. Heart J.,* 65, 25, 1991.
4. Auffermann, W., Wagner, S., Holt, W. W., Buser, P. T., Kircher, B., Schiller, N. B., Lim, T. H., Wolfe, C. L., and Higgins, C. B., Noninvasive determination of left ventricular output and wall stress in volume overload and in myocardial disease by cine magnetic resonance imaging, *Am. Heart J.,* 121, 1750, 1991.
5. Breisblatt, W. M., Schulman, D. S., and Follansbee, W. P., Continuous on-line monitoring of left ventricular function with a new nonimaging detector: validation and clinical use in the evaluation of patients post angioplasty, *Am. Heart J.,* 121, 1609, 1991.
6. Newman, G. E., Rerych, S. K., Jones, R. H., and Sabiston, D. C., Noninvasive assessment of the effects of aorta-coronary bypass grafting on ventricular function during rest and exercise, *J. Thorac. Cardiovasc. Surg.,* 79, 617, 1980.
7. Healy, M. J. R., Measuring measuring errors, *Stat. Med.,* 8, 893, 1989.
8. Altman, D. G. and Bland, J. M., Measurement in medicine: the analysis of method comparison studies, *Statistician,* 32, 307, 1983.

9. Russell, A. E., Smith, S. A., West, M. J., Aylward, P. E., McRitchie, R. J., Hassam, R. M., Minson, R. B., Wing, L. M. H., and Chalmers, J. P., Automated noninvasive measurement of cardiac output by the carbon dioxide rebreathing method: comparisons with dye dilution and thermodilution, *Br. Heart J.*, 63, 195, 1990.
10. Ng. H. W. K. and Walley, T., Impedance cardiology, *Br. J. Clin. Pharmacol.*, 36, 88, 1993.
11. Thomas, S. H. L., Reply, *Br. J. Clin. Pharmacol.*, 36, 89, 1993.
12. Nugent, A. M., McParland, J., McEneaney, D. J., Steele, I., Campbell, N. P. S., Stanford, C. F., and Nicholls, D. P., Noninvasive measurement of cardiac output by a carbon dioxide rebreathing method at rest and during exercise, *Eur. Heart J.*, 15, 361, 1994.
13. Malliani, A., Lombardi, F., and Pagani, M., Power spectrum analysis of heart rate variability: a tool to explore neural regulatory mechanisms, *Br. Heart J.*, 71, 1, 1994.
14. Stein, P. K., Bosner, M. S., Kleiger, R. E., and Conger, B. M., Heart rate variability: a measure of cardiac autonomic tone, *Am. Heart J.*, 127, 1376, 1994.
15. Schanzenbächer, P., Liebau, G., Deeg, P., and Kochsiek, K., Effect of intravenous and intracoronary nifedipine on coronary blood flow and myocardial oxygen consumption, *Am. J. Cardiol.*, 51, 712, 1983.
16. Kubicek, W. G., Karnegis, J. N., Patterson, R. P., Witsoe, D. A., and Mattson, R. H., Development and evaluation of an impedance cardiac output system, *Aerospace Med.*, 37, 1208, 1966.
17. Edmunds, A. T., Godfrey, S., and Tooley, M., Cardiac output measured by transthoracic impedance cardiography at rest, during exercise and at various lung volumes, *Clin. Sci.*, 63, 107, 1982.
18. Sramek, B. B., Hemodynamic and pump-performance monitoring in electrical bioimpedance: new concepts, in *Problems in Respiratory Care*, MacIntyre, N. and Branson, R., Eds., J. B. Lippincott, 2, 274, 1989.
19. Moore, R., Sansores, R., Guimond, V., and Abboud, R., Evaluation of cardiac output by thoracic electrical bioimpedance during exercise in normal subjects, *Chest*, 102, 448, 1992.
20. Ng. H. W. K., Walley, T., Tsao, Y., and Breckenridge, A. M., Comparison and reproducibility of transthoracic bioimpedance and dual beam Doppler ultrasound measurement of cardiac function in healthy volunteers, *Br. J. Clin. Pharmacol.*, 32, 275, 1991.
21. Northridge, D. B., Findlay, I. N., Wilson, J., Henderson, E., and Dargie, H. J., Non-invasive determination of cardiac output by Doppler echocardiography and electrical bioimpedance, *Br. Heart J.*, 63, 93, 1990.
22. Teo, K.-K., Hetherington, M. D., Haennel, R. G., Greenwood, P. V., Rossall, R. E., and Kappagoda, T., Cardiac output measured by impedance cardiography during maximal exercise tests, *Cardiovasc. Res.*,19, 737, 1985.
23. Jewkes, C., Verhoeff, F., Sear, J. W., and Foëx, P., Noninvasive cardiac output measurement by bioimpedance: is it reliable, *Br. J. Anaesth.*, 63, 619P, 1989.
24. de Mey, C. and Enterling, D., Disagreement between standard transthoracic impedance cardiography and the automated transthoracic electrical bioimpedance method in estimating the cardiovascular responses to phenylephrine and isoprenaline in healthy man, *Br. J. Clin. Pharmacol.*, 35, 349, 1993.
25. Cox, C., Millson, D. S., Hobson, S., and Harry, J., Continuous measurement of cardiac output by impedance cardiography during submaximal exercise, *Br. J. Clin. Pharmacol.*, 28, 227P, 1989.
26. Denniston, J. C., Maher, J. T., Reeves, J. T., Cruz, J. C., Cymerman, A., and Grover, R. F., Measurement of cardiac output by electrical impedance at rest and during exercise, *J. Appl. Physiol.*, 40, 91, 1976.
27. Thomas, S. H. L., Impedance cardiography using the Sramek-Bernstein method: accuracy and variability at rest and during exercise, *Br. J. Clin. Pharmacol.*, 34, 467, 1992.
28. Smith, S. A., Russell, A. E., West, M. J., and Chalmers, J., Automated noninvasive measurement of cardiac output: comparison of electrical bioimpedance and carbon dioxide rebreathing techniques, *Br. Heart J.*, 59, 292, 1988.
29. Dixon, R. M., Meire, H. B., Posner, J., and Rolan, P. E., Evaluation of noninvasive techniques to assess vasoconstriction by methoxamine in healthy volunteers, *Br. J. Clin. Pharmacol.*, 37, 473P, 1994.
30. Frey, M. A. B., Lathers, C., Davis, J., Fortney, S., and Charles, J. B., Cardiovascular responses to standing: effect of hydration, *J. Clin. Pharmacol.*, 34, 387, 1994.
31. Frey, M. A. B., Tomaselli, C. M., and Hoffler, W. G., Cardiovascular responses to postural changes: differences with age for women and men, *J. Clin. Pharmacol.*, 34, 394, 1994.
32. Johnson, M. A., McDowall, J. E., and Keene, O. N., The repeatability of change in cardiac function after salmeterol using electrical bioimpedance cardiography, *Br. J. Clin. Pharmacol.*, 34, 177P, 1992.
33. Smith, S. A., Salih, M. M., and Littler, W. A., Assessment of beat to beat changes in cardiac output during the Valsalva manoeuver using electrical bioimpedance cardiography, *Clin. Sci.*, 72, 423, 1987.
34. Veigl, V. L. and Judy, W. V., Reproducibility of hemodynamic measurements by impedance cardiography, *Cardiovasc. Res.*, 17, 728, 1983.
35. Wong, D. H., Tremper, K. K., Stemmer, E. A., O'Connor, D., Wilber, S., Zaccari, J., Reeves, C., Weidoff, P., and Trujillo, R. J., Noninvasive cardiac output: simultaneous comparison of two different methods with thermodilution, *Anesthesiology*, 72, 784, 1990.
36. Appel, P. L., Kram, H. B., Mackabee, J., Fleming, A. W., and Shoemaker, W. C., Comparison of measurements of cardiac output by bioimpedance and thermodilution in severely ill surgical patients, *Crit. Care Med.*, 14, 933, 1986.
37. Haites, N. E., McLennan, F. M., Mowat, D. H. R., and Rawles, J. M., Assessment of cardiac output by the Doppler ultrasound technique alone, *Br. Heart J.*, 53, 123, 1985.
38. Gibson, D. G., Stroke distance — an improved measure of cardiovascular function? *Br. Heart J.*, 53, 121, 1985.

39. Evans, J. M., Skidmore, R., Luckman, N. P., and Wells, P. N. T., A new approach to the noninvasive measurement of cardiac output using an annular array doppler technique. I. Theoretical considerations and ultrasonic fields, *Ultrasound Med. Biol.,* 15, 169, 1989.
40. Hottinger, C. F. and Meindl, J. D., Blood flow measurement using the attenuation-compensated volume flowmeter, *Ultrasonic Imaging,* 1, 1, 1979.
41. Lipworth, B. J. and Dagg, K. D., Comparative effects of angiotension II on Doppler parameters of left and right heart systolic and diastolic blood flow, *Br. J. Clin. Pharmacol.,* 37, 273, 1994.
42. Jassal, V., Harris, C. M., and Silke, B., Reproducibility of a new continuous echo-Doppler method (ExerDop) in man, *Br. J. Clin. Pharmacol.,* 35, 87, 1993.
43. Silke, B., Evans, J. M., and Taylor, S. H., A critical assessment of a new computerized non-imaging echo-Doppler method, *Automedica,* 13, 149, 1991.
44. Rimoy, G. H., Bhaskar, N. K., and Rubin, P. C., Reproducibility of Doppler blood flow velocity waveform measurements: study on variability within and between day and during haemodynamic intervention in normal subjects, *Eur. J. Clin. Pharmacol.,* 41, 125, 1991.
45. Harry, J. D., Millson, D. S., and Morton, P. B., Use of Doppler echocardiography to determine the cardiac effects of dobutamine in volunteers, *Pharmaceut. Med.,* 3, 173, 1988.
46. Moscarelli, E., Reisenhofer, B., Levantest, D., Michelassi, C., Distante, A., and L'Abbate, A., Monitoring of cardiac output during exercise in cornonary patients: a Doppler study, *Eur. Heart J.,* 12, 338, 1991.
47. Clifton, G. D., Harrison, M. R., Wermeling, D. P., Long, R. A., Fleck, R. J., Rolleri, R. L., Weller, S., Brown, A. R., and Welch, R. M., Pharmacokinetics and pharmacodynamics of a new cardiotonic vasodilator agent, 349U85, in normal subjects, *Clin. Pharmacol. Ther.,* 55, 55, 1994.
48. Silke, B. and Spiers, P., Exercise cardiac output actions of elgodipine assessed with the quantascope, *Br. J. Clin. Pharmacol.,* 37, 483P, 1994.
49. Wheeldon, N. M., McDevitt, D. G., and Lipworth, B. J., Cardiac effects of the β_3-adrenoceptor agonist BRL35135 in man, *Br. J. Clin. Pharmacol.,* 37, 363, 1994.
50. Collier, C. R., Determination of mixed venous CO_2 tensions by rebreathing, *J. Appl. Physiol.,* 9, 25, 1956.
51. Muiesan, G., Sorbini, C. A., Solinas, E., Grassi, V., Casucci, G., and Petz, E., Comparison of CO_2-rebreathing and direct Fick methods for determining cardiac output, *J. Appl. Physiol.,* 24, 424, 1968.
52. Defares, J. G., Determination of $PvCO_2$ from the exponential CO_2 rise during rebreathing, *J. Appl. Physiol.,* 13, 159, 1958.
53. Jones, N. L. and Campbell, E. J. M., *Clinical Exercise Testing,* W. B. Saunders, Philadelphia, 2nd. edition, 1981, chap. 8.
54. Hargreaves, M. and Jennings, G., Evaluation of the CO_2 rebreathing method for the non-invasive measurement of resting cardiac output in man, *Clin. Exp. Pharmacol. Physiol.,* 10, 609, 1983.
55. Reybrouck, T., Amery, A., Billiet, L., Fagard, R., and Stijns, H., Comparison of cardiac output determined by a carbon dioxide-rebreathing and direct Fick method at rest and during exercise, *Clin. Sci. Mol. Med.,* 55, 445, 1978.
56. Auchincloss, J. H., Gilbert, R., Morales, R., and Peppi, D., The effect of progressive exercise on the equilibrium rebreathing cardiac output method, *Med. Sci. Sports Exer.* 23, 1111, 1991.
57. McKelvie, R. S., Heigenhauser, G. J. F., and Jones, N. L., Measurement of cardiac output by CO_2 rebreathing in unsteady state exercise, *Chest,* 92, 777, 1987.
58. Cowley, A. J., Stainer, K., Murphy, D. T., Murphy, J., and Hampton, J. R., A noninvasive method for measuring cardiac output: the effect of Christmas lunch, *Lancet,* ii, 1422, 1986.
59. Reybrouck, T. and Fagard, R., Assessment of cardiac output at rest and during exercise by a carbon dioxide rebreathing method, *Eur. Heart J.,* 11, 21, 1990.
60. Yi, J. J., Fullwood, L., Stainer, K., Cowley, A. J., and Hampton, J. R., Effects of food on the central and peripheral haemodynamic response to upright exercise in normal volunteers, *Br. Heart J.,* 63, 22, 1990.
61. Li, Q. and Belz, G. G., Systolic time intervals in clinical pharmacology, *Eur. J. Clin. Pharmacol.,* 44, 415, 1993.
62. Hassan, S. and Turner, P., Systolic time intervals: a review of the method in non-invasive investigation of cardiac function in health, disease and clinical pharmacology, *Postgrad. Med. J.,* 59, 423, 1983.
63. de Mey, C., Enterling, D., and Meineke, I., Cardiovascular effects of eating, atenolol and their interaction: β_1-adrenergic modulation does not play a predominant role in the genesis of postprandial effects, *Br. J. Clin. Pharmacol.,* 36, 427, 1993.
64. Thomas, S. H. L., Comparison of the cardiovascular effects of nifedipine and nicardipine in the presence of atenolol, *Eur. J. Clin. Pharmacol.,* 41, 201, 1991.
65. Harry, J. D., Norris, S. C., Percival, G. C., and Young, J., The dose in humans at which ICI 118,551 (a selective β_2-adrenoceptor blocking agent) demonstrates blockade of β_1-adrenoceptors, *Clin. Pharmacol. Ther.,* 43, 492, 1988.
66. de Mey, C., Breithaupt, K., Schloos, J., Neugebauer, G., Palm, D., and Belz, G. G., Dose-effect and pharmacokinetic-pharmacodynamic relationships of the β_1-adrenergic receptor blocking properties of various doses of carvedilol in healthy humans, *Clin. Pharmacol. Ther.,* 55, 329, 1994.
67. Walley, T. J., Heagerty, A. M., Woods, K. L., Bing, R. F., Pohl, J. E. F., and Barnett, D. B., Acute inotropic effects of intravenous nifedipine and its vehicle compared with saline: a double-blind study of systolic time intervals in normal subjects, *Br. J. Clin. Pharmacol.,* 25, 187, 1988.
68. Chambers, J. B., Monaghan, M. J., and Jackson, G., Echocardiography, *Br. Med. J.,* 297, 1071, 1988.

69. Thomas, M. R., Pruvulovich, L., Jewitt, D. E., and Monaghan, M. J., Assessment of ejection fraction by echocardiographic automatic boundary detection following myocardial infarction: comparison with radionuclide angiography, *Br. Heart J. Suppl.*, 71, 33, 1994.
70. Michalis, L., Thomas, M. R., Jewitt, D. E., and Monaghan, M. J., On-line echocardiographic automatic boundary detection assessment of left ventricular cardiac contractility, *Br. Heart J. Suppl.*, 71, 33, 1994.
71. Gorscan, J., Lazar, J. M., and Schulman, D. S., and Follansbee, W. P., Comparison of left ventricular function by echocardiographic automated border detection and by radionuclide ejection fraction, *Am. J. Cardiol.*, 72, 810, 1993.
72. Clements, F. M. and de Bruijn, N. P., Perioperative evaluation of regional wall motion by transesophageal two-dimensional echocardiography, *Anesth. Analg.*, 66, 249, 1987.
73. Pearlman, A. S., Transesophageal echocardiography — sound diagnostic technique or two-edged sword? *N. Engl. J. Med.*, 324, 841, 1991.
74. O'Kelley, B. F., Tubau, J. F., Knight, A. A., London, M. J., Verrier, E. D., Mangano, D. T., and the Study of Perioperative Ischemia Research Group, Measurement of left ventricular contractility using transesophageal echocardiography in patients undergoing coronary artery bypass grafting, *Am. Heart J.*, 122, 1041, 1991.
75. Urbanowicz, J. H., Shaaban, M. J., Cohen, N. H., Cahalan, M. K., Botvinick, E. H., Chatterjee, K., Schiller, N. B., Dae, M. W., and Matthay, M. A., Comparison of transesophageal echocardiographic and scintigraphic estimates of left ventricular end-diastolic volume index and ejection fraction in patients following coronary artery bypass grafting, *Anesthesiology*, 72, 607, 1990.
76. Konstadt, S. N., Thys, D., Mindich, B. P., Kaplan, J. A., and Goldman, M., Validation of quantitative intraoperative transesophageal echocardiography, *Anesthesiology*, 65, 418, 1986.
77. Iliceto, S., Galiuto, L., Marangelli, V., and Rizzon, P., Clinical use of stress echocardiography: factors affecting diagnostic accuracy, *Eur. Heart J.*, 15, 672, 1994.
78. Iliceto, S. and Rizzon, P., Stress echocardiography: ready for routine clinical use? *Eur. Heart J.*, 12, 262, 1991.
79. Salerno, D. M. and Zanetti, J., Seismocardiography: a new technique for recording cardiac vibrations. Concept, method, and initial observations, *J. Cardiovasc. Tech.*, 9, 111, 1990.
80. Silke, B., Spiers, P., Herity, N., and Drake, M., Seismocardiography during therapeutic intervention, *Br. J. Clin. Pharmacol.*, 37, 418P, 1994.
81. Pickering, T. G., Blood pressure measurement and detection of hypertension, *Lancet*, 344, 31, 1994.
82. Pickering, T. G., *Modern Approaches to Blood Pressure Measurement*, Science Press Ltd., London, 1992, chaps. 4 and 22.
83. Harry, J. D., The monitoring of arterial pressure, in *First I.C.R. Symposium, Clinical Measurement in Drug Evaluation*, Nimmo, U. S. and Tucker, G., Eds., Wolfe Publishing Ltd., London, 1991, chap. 4.
84. Wesseling, K. H., Finapres, continuous noninvasive finger arterial pressure based on the method of Peñáz, in *Blood Pressure Measurement*, Meyer-Sabellek, W., Anlauf, M., Gotzen, R., and Steinfeld, L., Eds., Stenkopff-Verlag, Darnstadt, 1990, 161.
85. East, T. D., Pace, N. L., Sorensen, R. M., East, K. A., and Westenskow, D. R., Effect of peripheral vascular disease on accuracy of noninvasive, continuous, blood pressure measurement from the finger (Finapres), *Anesthesiology*, 67, No 3A, A186, 1987.
86. Kurki, T., Smith, N. T., Head, N., Dec-Silver, H., and Quinn, A., Noninvasive continuous blood pressure measurement from the finger: optimal measurement conditions and factors affecting reliability, *J. Clin. Monit.*, 3, 6, 1987.
87. Dimier-David, L. A., Billion, N., Costagliola, D., Jaillon, P., and Funck-Brentano, C., Reproducibility of noninvasive measurement and of short-term variability of blood pressure and heart rate in healthy volunteers, *Br. J. Clin. Pharmacol.*, 38, 109, 1994.
88. Silke, B., McParland, G., Whyte, P., Young, S., Wylie, S., Anderson, V., Sheik, V., and Scott, M. E., Accuracy and reproducibility of continuous noninvasive blood pressure determination (Finapres) during pharmacodynamic intervention, *Br. J. Clin. Pharmacol.*, 33, 540P, 1991.
89. Imholz, B. P. M., Wieling W., Langewouters, G. J., and Van Montfrans, G. A., Continuous finger arterial pressure: utility in the cardiovascular laboratory, *Clin. Autonomic Res.*, 1, 45, 1991.
90. Parati, G. and Mancia, G., Continuous non-invasive finger blood pressure recording by the Finapres device: a new approach to beat-to-beat blood pressure monitoring, *J. Nephrol.*, 1, 73, 1989.
91. Parati, G., Casadei, R., Groppelli, A., de Rienzo, M., and Mancia, G., Comparison of finger and intra-arterial blood pressure monitoring at rest and during laboratory testing, *Hypertension*, 13, 647, 1989.
92. Imholz, B. P. M., van Montfrans, G. A., Settels, J. J., Van der Hoeven, G. M. A., Karemeker, J. M., and Wieling, W., Continuous noninvasive blood presssure monitoring: reliability of Finapres device during the Valsalva manoeuver, *Cardiovasc. Res.*, 22, 390, 1988.
93. Silke, B., Boyd, S., McParland, G., and Scott, M. E., Validation of a continuous noninvasive blood pressure method (Finapres), *Br. J. Clin. Pharmacol.*, 35, 88P, 1993.
94. Gravenstein, J. S., Paulus, D. A., Feldman, J., and McLaughlin, G., Tissue hypoxia distal to Penaz finger pressure cuff, *J. Clin. Monit.*, 1, 120, 1985.
95. Davies, R. J. O., Jenkins, N. E., and Stradling, J. R., Effect of measuring ambulatory blood pressure on sleep and on blood pressure during sleep, *Br. Med. J.*, 308, 820, 1994.
96. Prasad, N., McDonnell, S. J., Ogsten, S. A., Peebles, L., and MacDonald, T. M., Ambulatory blood pressure monitoring for 24 or 48 hours? *Br. Heart J. Suppl.*, 71, 60, 1994.

97. Whelton, A. and Tresznewsky, O. N., Ambulatory blood pressure monitoring: a new window to clinical therapeutic decisions in hypertension, *J. Clin. Pharmacol.*, 30, 1061, 1990.
98. Duggan, J., Ambulatory blood pressure monitoring, *Pharma. Ther.*, 63, 313, 1994.
99. Barthélémy, J. C., Geyssant, A., Auboyer, C., Antoniadis, A., Berruyer, J., and Lacour, J. R., Accuracy of ambulatory blood pressure determination: a comparative study, *Scand. J. Clin. Invest.*, 51, 461, 1991.
100. White, W. B., Lund-Johansen, P., and Omvik, P., Assessment of four ambulatory blood pressure monitors and measurements by clinicians versus intraarterial blood pressure at rest and during exercise, *Am. J. Cardiol.*, 65, 60, 1990.
101. Ewing, D. J., Neilson, J. M. M., and Travis, P., New method for assessing cardiac parasympathetic activity using 24 hour electrocardiograms, *Br. Heart J.*, 52, 396, 1984.
102. Ewing, D. J., Hume, L., Campbell, I. W., Murray, A., Neilson, J. M. M., and Clarke, B. F., Autonomic mechanisms in the initial heart rate response to standing, *J. Appl. Physiol.*, 49, 809, 1980.
103. Taylor, A. A., Davies, A. O., Mares, A., Raschko, J., Pool, J. L., Nelson, E. B., and Mitchell, J. R., Spectrum of dysautomania in mitral valve prolapse, *Am. J. Med.*, 86, 267, 1989.
104. O'Brien, I. A. D., O'Hare, P., and Corrall, R. J. M., Heart rate variability in healthy subjects: effect of age and the derivation of normal ranges for tests of autonomic function, *Br. Heart J.*, 55, 348, 1986.
105. Malik, M. and Camm, A. J., Heart rate variability and clinical cardiology, *Br. Heart J.*, 71, 3, 1994.
106. Butler, G. C., Yamamoto, Y., and Hughson, R. L., Heart rate variability to monitor autonomic nervous system activity during orthostatic stress, *J. Clin. Pharmacol.*, 34, 558, 1994.
107. Julu, P. O. O. and Hondo, R. G., Effects of atropine on autonomic indices based on electrocardiographic R-R intervals in healthy volunteers, *J. Neurol. Neurosurg. Psych.*, 55, 31, 1992.
108. Broadstone, V. L., Roy, T., Self, M., and Pfeifer, M. A., Cardiovascular autonomic dysfunction: diagnosis and prognosis, *Diab. Med.*, 8 (Symp.), S88, 1991.
109. Pickering, G. W., *High Blood Pressure,* Churchill, London, 1955, chap. 4.

Chapter 15

Antianginal Drugs

Nancy Pauly and Edmond Roland

CONTENTS

1 Introduction 197
2 Pathophysiology of Coronary and Myocardial Function in Angina Pectoris:Critical Aspects for Drug Evaluation 198
3 Methods for Early Evaluation of Antianginal Drugs 199
3.1 Pharmacodynamic Profile in Man 199
3.1.1 Hemodynamic Studies: Right and Left Catheterization Protocols 199
3.1.2 Quantitative Coronary Angiography 201
3.1.3 Atrial Pacing 201
3.1.4 Assessment of Coronary Blood Flow 202
3.1.5 Radionuclide Methods 202
3.1.5.1 Radionuclide Procedures for Myocardial Perfusion 203
3.1.5.2 Assessment of Left Ventricular Performance with Radionuclide Angiography 203
3.1.6 Pharmacological Stress Test 204
3.2 Direct Evidence of Efficacy: Exercise Tests 204
3.2.1 Exercise Test Modalities 204
3.2.2 Test Protocols 205
3.2.3 Interpretation of Exercise Test 206
3.2.4 Evaluation of ECG Data 206
3.2.5 Heart Rate and Blood Pressure 207
3.2.6 Maximal Work Capacity 207
3.2.7 Respiratory Gas Exchange Techniques 207
3.2.8 Effort Angina 207
3.2.9 Measured Variables for Evaluation of Anti-Ischemic Interventions and Testing Endpoints 208
4 Methodological Issues in the Early Evaluation of Antianginal Drugs 208
4.1 Patient Selection 208
4.2 Protocol Design 209
5 Conclusion 210
References 210

1 INTRODUCTION

The purpose of this chapter is to give practical information to people confronted with the need to design initial trials of antianginal drugs and who have little previous experience in this field. The description of the various methods is detailed enough to serve as preparatory reading before drafting a protocol or approaching the expert in the specific field. In addition some pathophysiologic considerations are first presented to better understand the scope of application of various methods and their limitations. The preferred subjects for assessment of an antianginal effect is obviously patients with ischemic heart disease. Information derived from healthy volunteers are only for safety and the present chapter will only deal with early phase II protocols.

0-8493-9230-6/97/$0.00+$.50
© 1997 by CRC Press, Inc.

2 PATHOPHYSIOLOGY OF CORONARY AND MYOCARDIAL FUNCTION IN ANGINA PECTORIS: CRITICAL ASPECTS FOR DRUG EVALUATION

Under physiological conditions, a close correlation is observed between the increase in myocardial oxygen consumption and coronary blood flow over a wide range.[1] Coronary flow is regulated by oxygen demand (momentary oxygen consumption) and by oxygen delivery. The main factors which determine myocardial oxygen consumption (MVO_2) are those using most of the available energy: heart rate, contractility, and wall tension. In wall tension, it is mainly pressure development and left ventricular volume. In contractility, it is the velocity of fiber shortening. Unlike the situation in skeletal muscle, oxygen extraction by the myocardium is almost at a maximum level at rest; this results in a wide and constant arteriovenous oxygen difference between coronary arteries and coronary sinus in man. The normal coronary system consists of large epicardial vessels, which normally function as passive conduits and offer little intrinsic resistance to flow.[1,2] The intramyocardial arterioles, on the other hand, alter their intrinsic tone in response to the demands of the myocardium of oxygen. Because of their small diameter and well-developed media, they have the capacity to alter profoundly resistance to flow.[1,2] Through the autoregulatory system provided by these arterioles, myocardial oxygen delivery and myocardial oxygen consumption are closely linked; when MVO_2 increases the resistance vessels dilate thereby permitting myocardial flow to increase in proportion to the increased oxygen demands.[2,3] Ischemia is induced when the capacity of oxygen delivery cannot meet oxygen demand any longer, owing to increasing proximal resistance in the coronary system. This situation is provoked by either excessive increase in MVO_2 beyond a certain threshold or a primary critical reduction in the coronary lumen.[3]

When a large epicardial vessel is narrowed by a fixed atherosclerotic lesion, its conductance function is compromised and it now offers considerable resistance to flow. If no other alteration occurs, the increased resistance leads to a decrease in flow and thereby causes ischemia. However, ischemia-induced metabolic derangements activate autoregulatory mechanisms, resulting in arteriolar dilatation and decrease in arteriolar resistance.[1] Although this compensatory mechanism may prevent the appearence of ischemia under resting conditions, it is not adequate to prevent ischemia when large increments in flow are required, as with exercise. When this maximal flow threshold is exceeded, myocardial ischemia and angina appear. Although the concept of fixed obstruction provides a ready explanation for the onset of angina with exercise when MVO_2 increases considerably, it cannot explain the onset of angina occurring at rest without obvious increase in MVO_2 or why anginal threshold should vary markedly in individual patients.[3-5] The finding that dynamic increases in either large- or small-vessel coronary resistance can also precipitate ischemia or reduce the threshold of MVO_2 at which it occurs has important implications for the therapy of angina pectoris.[2] This dynamic coronary obstruction may occur within or outside a stenotic segment. The product of systolic pressure and heart rate (double product) at angina onset is a reflection of the maximal rate at which the obstructed coronary artery is capable of delivering oxygen. By examining the effect of antianginal agents on the double product as indirect index of myocardial oxygen demand, two types of pharmacological interventions could be considered. If an intervention improves exercise capacity, but the double product at angina is no higher than control levels, it implies that the intervention causes the beneficial effect by decreasing oxygen demand at any level of external stress and this type of pharmacological action would be more effective against fixed coronary obstruction. If exercise capacity is improved and double product at angina increases, the implication is that the myocardium can attain a higher workload before ischemia occurs, most probably because myocardial flow has increased and such intervention is designed more against dynamic coronary obstruction. Of course, a single antianginal agent can combine both types of response.

The onset of myocardial ischemia is followed by left ventricular dysfuntion, electrocardiographic changes, and angina, in that order. In the presence of ischemia, the absence of angina does not signify the absence of ventricular dysfunction.[1-3] The first hemodynamic changes observed during exercise-induced ischemia are the slowing of isovolumic relaxation and contraction. This is followed by an abnormal increase in end-diastolic pressure due to the loss on contraction and increased wall stiffness in the ischemic left ventricular wall segment. Of special importance is the relation between diastolic pressure and volume, i.e., diastolic compliance during ischemia. Several studies have clearly shown that during ischemia the immediate hemodynamic alterations may result primarily from a change in left ventricular diastolic compliance rather than left ventricular systolic pressure.[1] Thus, the increase in left ventricular end-diastolic pressure is a very early sign of ischemia. In addition, it has been shown that abnormalities of the level of the small coronary arteries (endocardial layers) can contribute to precipitation of myocardial ischemia, either by dynamically increasing coronary resistance in response to vasoconstrictor influences profound enough to cause ischemia at rest or by restricting vasodilator reserve and thus the potential to augment flow, which would predispose to the development of ischemia during interventions that increase myocardial oxygen requirements.[4] Although the abnormal coronary vasodilator reserve can be ascribed to vasoconstrictor influences modulating the tone of small coronary arteries, it is also possible that the inadequate vasodilator reserve could be due to abnormal myocardial compressive force, i.e., increased left ventricular diastolic pressure might increase myocardial wall tension during diastole and thereby interfere with coronary flow.[1,3,6] This fact emphasizes the complex relationship between left ventricular function and coronary flow, particularly in the endocardial layers.[6] Furthermore, subendocardial blood flow rather than oxygen demand may be the major determinant of exercise-induced myocardial ischemia.[7] Because the majority of coronary blood flow occurs during diastole, the diastolic perfusion time may be an excellent measure of myocardial oxygen supply.[7,8]

In summary, pharmacodynamic effects which reduce myocardial oxygen consumption are: (1) a decrease in preload (left ventricular diastolic pressure), (2) a decrease in heart rate, (3) a decrease in contractility, and (4) a decrease in afterload through a decrease in arterial impedance. Pharmacodynamic effects aiming at reducing the dynamic coronary obstruction are: (1) spasmolytic action on coronary arteries and (2) reduction of preload through a decrease in diastolic pressure.

3 METHODS FOR EARLY EVALUATION OF ANTIANGINAL DRUGS

By definition, angina pectoris is a clinical symptom which implies acute transient myocardial ischemia. The goal of therapy will be to alleviate ischemia pain through a reduction of the imbalance between oxygen suppply and consumption. This chapter is mainly devoted to the evaluation of drugs for exertional angina. Methods for early evaluation of antianginal agents can be divided into two categories: (1) measurements which give the pharmacodynamic profile in man and indirect evidence for efficacy and (2) methods which determine direct evidence of drug efficacy.

3.1 Pharmacodynamic Profile in Man

From the pathophysiology of angina pectoris, it is obvious that it is important to consider the mode of action in man of a potential antianginal drug, which may predict its clinical efficacy.[9] However, such studies, in general, do not provide direct evidence for antianginal efficacy of the drug. Many antianginal agents act, at least in part, by causing dilatation of the peripheral vessels.[9] Therefore, when animal studies indicate that the experimental drug has vasoactive effects at concentrations at all comparable with the therapeutic level, initial studies in man should include an assessment of the effects of the compound on resistance in arteries and veins. While the symptoms of angina pectoris and their relief by antianginal agents can be assessed only with reference to the sufferer, a full understanding of the mechanisms of action of antianginal drugs requires objective assessment of their circulatory effects, including those on the peripheral circulation. Such drugs can relieve anginal pain through myocardial oxygen consumption by either cardiac or extracardiac effects.[9] The cardiac effects may include contractility, heart rate, coronary flow, left ventricular function, and direct myocardial cell protection. The extracardiac effects involve the peripheral circulation by reducing preload or afterload. Preload is reduced when venous capacity rises as a result of venous dilatation and, hence, venous return and cardiac filling are decreased. In fact, reduction of preload and afterload is also a possible means of treating heart failure, so that the same vasodilator drug may be of benefit in both angina and heart failure. This convergence of interests strengthens the case for adequate assessment of the peripheral actions of antianginal drugs and the major role played by hemodynamic studies at this stage.

3.1.1 Hemodynamic Studies: Right and Left Catheterization Protocols

The purpose of such study is to gain information on the effects of the antianginal agent on basic hemodynamic parameters, and more precisely on cardiac loading condition. The adequate population would be at the beginning patients undergoing routine right or left catheterization for chest pain and with normal left ventricular function of patients who need a close monitoring of their hemodynamic state, for example, after an acute myocardial infarction with signs of heart failure.

Right heart catheterization — With the technique of flow-directed right heart catheterization the effects of antianginal medication on cardiac output and left ventricular filling pressure can readily be quantified and even monitored at the bedside throughout the medical intervention. Pressures measured by flotation catheters must be referred to an appropriate zero point (related to the level of the tricuspid valve, which is usually located in the supine position at the upper border of two thirds of the tranverse diameter of the thorax, measured from the table surface). Different types of catheters are available, ranging from the 4F end-hole latex system for single pressure recordings to the 7F double-lumen flotation catheter (Swan-Ganz type) used for double-chamber diameter pressure recordings and evaluation of cardiac output by thermodilution. With careful maintenance of the zero reference point and exact calibration, pressure may be recorded with an accuracy of ±2 mmHg under clinical conditions. Left ventricular end-diastolic pressure is reflected by the pulmonary end-diastolic pressure in wedge position (PWP), if both mitral stenosis and pulmonary hypertension are absent. Thus, PWP is a good assessment of cardiac preload and the normal value is less than 12 mmHg.

Thermodilution is the most common technique for the determination of cardiac output because of its convenience. Ice cold water is injected into the right atrium and the change in temperature is detected by a thermistor located 4 cm from the catheter tip, which is positioned in the main stem of the pulmonary artery. The blood need not be withdrawn, in contrast with other indicator techniques, i.e., indocyanine green. The procedure is easily carried out at the bedside by one person. The thermodilution technique meets the assumptions of Fick's law of diffusion if homogeneous temperature mixing is present. Portable computer devices providing rapid data display are commonly used for uniform sampling and calculation of the transient changes in blood temperature. To improve precision, repeated (at least three consecutive) measurements of the same conditions are advisable and the mean value should be taken.

Left heart catheterization — This is only acceptable if patients have an indication for coronary angiography. Left heart catheterization from the right femoral sheath may be performed with a variety of catheters. Manometer-tipped catheters, with which the transducer is placed in the cardiac chamber, are usually used to achieve the most accurate recording of pressures. The principal advantage of left heart catheterization is the facility to assess left ventricular contractility or performance through measurements of left ventricular pressures, stroke volume, and ventricular volume.

Pressure measurements — The accuracy of the assessment of cardiac performance can be increased by adding a measurement of left ventricular end-diastolic pressure to that of stroke volume. Thus, when the ventricular end-diastolic pressure is elevated and the stroke index is reduced, myocardial contractility is probably impaired. Since changes in the maximum rate of rise of ventricular pressure (peak dp/dt) are known to be highly sensitive to acute changes in contractility, measurement of ventricular dp/dt may be employed along with filling pressure in the assessment of contractility. High-fidelity catheter-tip micromanometers should be employed to obtain a reliable assessment of peak dp/dt. Peak dp/dt is largely independent of afterload and appears to be more markedly affected by changes in contractility than by preload. However, the latter influence cannot be disregarded.

Quantitative angiography — Measurements of the volumes of cardiac chambers can be made utilizing cineangiograms with contrast material injected into the left ventricle. The hyperosmolarity produced by the contrast agent increases blood volume, which begins to raise preload and heart rate within 30 s of the injection, an effect which may persist for as long as 2 h. Therefore, when multiple observations in a comparable state are desired, it is essential to monitor the hemodynamics, to ensure that they have returned to control levels, before the angiogram is repeated. Selective injection of contrast material is essential to obtain the image of the opacified left ventricular cavity in either monoplane or biplane views. The ejection fraction (EF) is derived from planimetric measurements with the assumption that the ventricle is ellipsoidal in shape. The definition of the ejection fraction is:

$$\text{EF}\ (\%) = \frac{\text{end - diastolic volume} - \text{end - systolic volume}}{\text{end - diastolic}} \times 100$$

In addition to the measurement of the global EF of the left ventricle, the ventriculogram can also assess regional EF to detect segmental wall motion abnormalities.[10] The wall motion may be normal or may show decreased inward movement (hypokinesis) or absent movement (akinesis). The presence of a hypokinetic or akinetic segment on the resting ventriculogram may not necessarily indicate fibrous scarring after infarction, but can also be caused by severe underperfusion of still-viable myocardium. The regional wall motion can be readily improved after acute reduction of preload by vasodilating drugs. Pharmacologically induced venous pooling has beneficial effects on both myocardial oxygen supply and demand, especially when ventricular diastolic pressures are elevated. Moreover, when coronary vessels are narrowed by atherosclerotic lesions or by spasm, relaxation of normal or increased smooth muscle tone at the site of the stenosis by a vasodilating agent may increase native and collateral flow,[6] enabling critically underperfused territories to reestablish contractile function.[10] Depressed regional left ventricular

EF due to regional ischemia will normalize if the oxygen supply/demand ratio is normalized by any pharmacological intervention.

3.1.2 Quantitative Coronary Angiography

Quantitative measurement of stenosis severity could become a useful tool in the evaluation of vasoactive drugs.[10-12] Adequate geometric analysis by quantitative coronary arteriography includes dimensions of percentage narrowing, absolute diameter, and length combined into fluid dynamic equations to provide a single integrated measure of severity, i.e., flow reserve.[12] This anatomic-geometric method has been validated experimentally, completely automated and tested for routine clinical use.[11] Both the area of stenosis and the cross-sectional area of a normal segment can dilate with infusion of vasodilators. In the presence of coronary stenosis involving primarily a single vessel, downstream flow may be maintained through collateral channels arising from neighboring relatively normal coronary arteries.[6] Thus, in the presence of coronary obstruction localized to a territory with collateral development, vasoactive agents may increase collateral flow through vasodilation of collateral vessels or by relaxation of normal smooth muscle tone at the site of the stenosis.

There are four different mechanisms for altered severity of coronary artery stenosis during changing vasomotor states of the distal vascular bed: (1) arterial smooth muscle relaxation and vasodilation of the stenotic segment; (2) vasodilatation of the coronary artery adjacent to the stenotic segment; (3) the appearance of fully developed turbulence in the stenotic segment; and (4) narrowing of the stenotic segment due to decreasing intraluminal pressure caused by arteriolar vasodilatation and decreasing distending pressure.

When performing pharmacological interventions during coronary angiography, two different approaches may be used: either repeated angiography in the same single view without altering the X-ray setting, or use of multiple angiographic views.[11] In the first case, if the coronary segment is nonaxisymmetric, induced vasodilatation may accentuate asymmetry of the lumen by preferentially relaxing the nonatherosclerotic part of the arterial wall. Consequently, the use of a single angiographic view will be misleading.[11] Thus, the effects of vasodilators are better quantified if multiple projections are obtained. This will increase the accuracy of diameter measurements and will better reflect the true luminal cross-sectional area.

The attempt to visualize the vasodilation action of drugs with antianginal potency by quantitative evaluation of coronary arteriograms is often difficult, since relief of angina depends on several mechanisms.

3.1.3 Atrial Pacing

Left ventricular catheterization and left ventricular angiography provide further functional information if performed under stress, such as atrial pacing.

Rapid atrial pacing has been used in the catheterization laboratory as a controlled and reproducible method of producing myocardial ischemia in patients with coronary artery disease. In this condition, pacing has been shown to induce angina-like chest pain, electrocardiographic S-T segment depression, myocardial lactate production, increases in left ventricular filling pressure, decreases in left ventricular EF, and segmental wall motion abnormalities.[13] Usually the right atrial pacing test is performed 30 min after the completion of coronary arteriography; using the percutaneous femoral approach, a bipolar flared pacing catheter is placed within the right atrium. When a satisfactory pacing threshold has been achieved, the pacing rate is increased by increments of 10 or 20 beats per min rapidly until anginal or atrioventricular block occurs. If atrioventricular block develops at a rate that is less than 85% of the age-predicted maximal heart rate, 1 mg atropine is administered intravenously. Pacing is initiated at a rate of 80 beats/min. At each pacing rate, the presence, intensity and character of chest discomfort are recorded. Pacing is discontinued either when typical chest symptoms with significant ECG changes have developed or when a pacing rate has been achieved that is a least 85% of the age-predicted maximal rate. Three-channel ECG monitoring is continued during pacing and a 12-lead ECG is obtained before, during each pacing level, immediately after cessation of pacing, and until chest pain and ECG changes resolve. The usual ECG criteria for myocardial ischemia are 1 mm or more of horizontal or downsloping segment depression from 0.08 s or longer beyond the J point, in any lead using the PR segment as the baseline. The changes must be observed on at least three consecutive beats with a steady baseline. Hemodynamic measurements are performed at baseline, peak pacing rate, and 30 s after abrupt termination of pacing.

Although atrial pacing seems to be a very simple method to produce myocardial ischemia, the electrocardiographic, metabolic, and hemodynamic alterations that may accompany pacing-induced ischemia are specific but relatively insensitive markers of ischemia.[13] Chest pain during atrial pacing is a nonspecific occurrence, appearing with similar frequency in normal subjects and patients with coronary artery disease and pacing-induced ischemia. Post-pacing ECG S-T segment depression >0.1 mV occurs in slightly more than half of those with pacing-induced ischemia, but it also occurs on occasion in normal subjects.[13] Both peak-pacing myocardial lactate production and post-pacing elevation of left ventricular end-diastolic pressure are highly specific but relatively insensitive reflectors of pacing-induced ischemia. This relative insensitivity might improve if atrial pacing were performed more rapidly (>140 beats/min) or for a longer period of time (>4 min).

3.1.4 Assessment of Coronary Blood Flow

Following the discovery that the coronary sinus could safely be catheterized in man, a variety of techniques have been developed using coronary sinus intubation and sampling.[14]

Continuous thermodilution — Coronary sinus thermodilution is an inexpensive, widely available technique for the measurement of coronary flow and is the most frequently applied approach to studying coronary flow in patients. This technique needs a preformed triple-function Webster catheter. Cold saline or dextrose is infused continuously down the catheter into the coronary sinus at a high flow rate of 35–55 ml/min, to ensure adequate mixing. The resistance of the infused saline and the saline-blood mixture is recorded by two thermistors, from which sinus flow is calculated. There are several advantages to this technique. It requires only right heart catheterization to cannulate the coronary sinus and is therefore remarkably safe. This method can be repeated on several occasions during cardiac catheterization and is ideal for drug studies on myocardial metabolism, as coronary sinus samples can be obtained at constant heart rates by use of the pacing facilities of the catheter and the lumen of the catheter. The equipment is cheap compared with the cost of radioisotope methods, but X-ray screening is required. Despite these attractive features, the method has severe limitations. Phasic coronary flood or rapid changes in mean flow cannot be assessed, because the time constant of the technique is slow. Perfusion in specific transmural layers cannot be estimated, and regional left ventricular flow measurements are confined to crude separation of anterior vein flow (left ventricular anterior wall and septum) and perfusion to a large but indeterminate area of the left ventricle (distal coronary sinus). Convincing validation studies, coronary sinus thermodilution employed under clinically relevant conditions vs. an accepted standard, have never been presented.[14] In spite of its limitations, the technique of continuous thermodilution remains one of the fundamental methods available for the study of the effects of drugs on coronary flow with facilities for simultaneous study of myocardial metabolism and oxygen consumption.

Gas clearance methods — Several nonradioactive gases (nitrous oxide, hydrogen, helium, argon) and radioactive ^{133}Xe have been used in such studies.[14] This approach requires obtaining simultaneous arterial and coronary sinus blood for measurements of gas concentration during the saturation or desaturation phase of gas administration. All the limitations of thermodilution methods are equally applicable to gas clearance methods. Several test curves are necessary to construct reliable arterial and coronary sinus curves with heterogeneous flow. Overall, the method takes time and is not the most suitable for studies of changes of flow following drug intervention.

Electromagnetic flow probes and Doppler techniques — These have been used mainly to assess flow in vein bypass grafts and rarely to measure flow in native coronary vessels.[14] Although the intraoperative Doppler technique is useful for research applications, the clinical applicability is minimal because the measurement can only be obtained during open heart surgery. Recently, a small 3F Doppler catheter has been developed which can measure flow in major coronary vessels. However, because the Doppler catheters require intracoronary cannulation, there will always be some risk associated with this approach, which does not seem attractive for drug evaluation.

Positron-emission tomography — This could in theory be used for precise noninvasive measurement of regional myocardial perfusion. In practice, this goal has not yet been achieved in drug development, because the radionuclides available for positron-emission tomography are not ideal and many imaging artifacts continue to plague this method. On the horizon, a new generation of techniques, magnetic resonance imaging, ultrafast computed tomography, and contrast echocardiography, may permit precise measurement of perfusion in different layers of the left ventricle without cardiac catheterization. Although very promising, these new techniques are not yet validated for drug development.

3.1.5 Radionuclide Methods

Radionuclide methods have demonstrated value in the diagnosis and prognosis evaluation of patients with coronary artery disease.[15,16] The experience in drug evaluation with these techniques is still limited.

However, they may be useful since radionuclide methods have demonstrated utility in the evaluation of patients with coronary artery revascularization, either percutaneous coronary angioplasty or coronary artery bypass surgery.[15,16]

Radionuclide methods are performed at rest and when myocardial ischemia occurs under stress conditions i.e., most often exercise test and more recently under pharmacological stress. Two types of information could be gathered with radionuclide methods: myocardial perfusion and myocardial function.

3.1.5.1 Radionuclide Procedures for Myocardial Perfusion

Myocardial perfusion imaging can be performed with thallium 201, which is still the agent of choice at the present time, or with the newer ^{99m}Tc agents sestamibi.[15-17] Clinical imaging can be performed using either planar or single-photon emission computerized tomography (SPECT) techniques. SPECT imaging offers the potential for improved resolution and regional localization of perfusion abnormalities, though its advantage over planar imaging has not yet been fully demonstrated.[16] Following an intravenous injection, ^{201}Tl accumulates in the myocardium very rapidly and myocardial concentration is proportional to flow. The initial extraction fraction is 85-88%. Because of this high extraction efficiency during the first pass, thallium concentration in the blood is low, approximately 10% of the initial concentration 2 min after injection and less than 1% after 2 h.[16] In clincial use, 1.5-2 mCi of ^{201}Tl is injected intravenously with the patient at rest or while exercising.[15] The exercise images are of better quality because of a higher myocardial concentration of thallium (a result of inward coronary blood flow) and lower background activity. In exercise studies, the patient should continue to exercise an additional 1 min after thallium injection, to ensure the distribution of ^{201}Tl at peak exercise. The presence of a perfusion defect on the initial image may represent either ischemia or scar or both. The distinction can be made by comparing the initial images with delayed images obtained 4 h after injection. The persistence of a defect in the delayed images denotes a fixed defect.[15,16] The advantages of ^{201}Tl over exercise ECG are higher sensitivity (80-90%) and specificity (85-95%) and ability to localize the disease vessels and to assess the viability of the myocardium.[15,16] However, the sensitivity and specificity of exercise thallium image depend, to a certain extent, on the observer's interpretative ability and experience. The variability of observers in interpretation as to the presence or absence of a defect is 10-15%, and even higher variations are noted when the anatomical location of the defect is examined.[18] Thallium scintigraphy is difficult to use for evaluating antianginal drugs, mainly because an acute test (control and drug intervention study in one session) is not feasible. After the control examination, a relativery long time has to elapse until radioactivity can be applied again. Repositioning of the patient and gamma camera is necessary, which affects reproducibility. More important, the patient has to be exposed to another dose of radiation. In addition, quantification is difficult.

3.1.5.2 Assessment of Left Ventricular Performance with Radionuclide Angiography

The approach of nuclear cardiology is based on the assumption that cyclic motion of each myocardial region can be described as a set of time-dependent count rates. After radiolabeling the blood pool (with 20 mCi ^{99m}TC), the myocardial count rate depends on the volume changes of the heart. This technique involves external imaging of the cardiac blood with an external imaging device, such as a probe or gamma scintillation camera. The simplest procedure is to show the scans in rapid sequence, so that the heart motion becomes visible. Two methods of radionuclide analysis of left ventricular function have been utilized.[15,19] In the first method, the transit of a bolus of radionuclide material as it passes through the central circulation is observed (first-pass technique). In the second method, the left ventricle is visualized using radioactive substances that circulate in the blood in a steady state. This equilibrium technique requires gating of multiple R-R intervals to produce a summed, composite cardiac cycle (gated blood-pool technique). The latter is preferred for pharmacological intervention, since after one injection serial studies of EF and volume can be performed for several hours. Regional wall motion abnormalities can be detected immediately. This is of special interest for drug administration, because after injection of ^{99m}TC-labeled erythrocytes, the heart motion can be observed for about 5-7 h. Thus, improvement of regional wall motion after administration of antianginal drugs can be closely monitored.[20]

Rest and exercise radionuclide angiography is a useful technique to study the cardiac adaptation during exercise in patients with coronary artery disease. Most patients with coronary artery disease have an abnormal EF response to exercise.[15,19] Radionuclide angiography permits evaluation of the regional and global systolic function and the pressure-volume relationship during both systole and diastole.[15] Reproducibility and variabiltiy in these measurements should be considered. In good laboratories, the inter- and intraindividual variability is less than 5%; but each laboratory should establish its own reproducibility results.[20] A more important point, however, is the reproducibility of results when measurements are separated by days or weeks. Sequential studies in normal individuals and patients with coronary artery disease have shown up to 10% differences in EF, especially in subjects with normal resting EF. While such variation may reflect technical limitations, it could also be due to variation in sympathetic tone.[20] Similar variations in EF have been observed when contrast angiography is used instead of radionuclide angiography. In addition, the drug-induced changes in EF may depend on baseline EF and the presence or absence of myocardial ischemia. The latter is especially important in interpreting changes in exercise EF.

3.1.6 Pharmacological Stress Test

Pharmacological stress tests can be categorized into two groups, those that produce coronary vasodilatation as a mean of assessing coronary vasodilator reserve (dipyridamole and adenosine) and those that produce ischemia by increasing myocardial oxygen demand (dobutamine). This alternative form of stress is used either in conjunction with radionuclide myocardial perfusion imaging or with two-dimensional echocardiography.[21-23] Similar to radionuclide images, echocardiographic images are now often acquired on dedicated software, for analysis of regional wall motion. Because of technical difficulties with physical exercise on bicycle,[24] stress two-dimensional echocardiography is increasingly performed in conjunction with pharmacological stress test. In view of the different mechanisms of action of adenosine and dobutamine, it is not clear which pharmacological stress is best suited for which imaging modality.[21,22] If two-dimensional echocardiography is used, dobutamine pharmacological stress is the stress agent of choice, whereas if myocardial perfusion imaging is used, either adenosine or dobutamine is an appropirate agent.[21,22] Pharmacological stress test does not reproduce the physiological condition of physical exercise and therefore should be considered as a surrogate or second choice stress test. Pharmacological stress test has not been widely used in the assessment of antianginal drug efficacy, although some publications have shown interesting results.[23]

3.2 Direct Evidence of Efficacy: Exercise Tests

Exercise testing is an established method for detecting coronary artery disease and evaluating the severity of disease and prognosis.[25,26] In addition, exercise tolerance testing is considered the primary method for establishing prophylactic antianginal efficacy[27] and is widely used to evaluate anti-ischemic interventions.[26]

3.2.1 Exercise Test Modalities

Two types of exercise tests can be used: isometric or dynamic. Isometric exercise, defined as constant muscular contraction without movement (i.e., handgrip), imposes a disproportionate pressure load on the left ventricle relative to the body's ability to supply oxygen. Dynamic exercise, defined as rhythmic muscular activity resulting in movement, initiates a more appropriate increase in cardiac output and oxygen exchange.[25,28] Because a delivered workload can be accurately calibrated and the physiological response easily measured, dynamic exercise is preferred for clinical testing.[25,26,28] Using progressive workloads of dynamic exercise, patients with coronary disease can be protected from rapidly increasing myocardial oxygen demand. A maximal exercise test brings an individual to a level of intensity where fatigue or symptoms prohibit further exercise or when maximal oxygen consumption (VO_2 max) is achieved and no further increase in heart rate occurs. Estimates of predicted maximal heart rate may be used as a guide for test termination, but these estimates should not be used as predetermined termination points in maximal testing.[25,29]

When measurement of maximal exercise capacity is intended, possibilities include the treadmill and the upright bicycle ergometer.[28] Cycle ergometer tests provide for stable ECG and blood pressure recording. Intravascular catheters may be kept in place, expired air may be collected easily, and both echocardiographic and scintigraphic observations may be made. Their main disadvantages are that individuals who are not accustomed to cycling will often be unable to reach maximal heart rates owing to leg fatigue, and results depend upon complete subject cooperation in order to maintain a constant work rate in following a specific protocol.

Treadmill testing permits the highest oxygen consumption rate of any common exercise device, usually 10-15% higher than cycle exercise.[29] Both speed and elevation can be varied over a wide range of exercise intensities with excellent reproducibility.[25,26,28,29] External control of the work rate is attained with a minimum of subject cooperation. It may be more difficult to obtain exact recording of the blood pressure and ECG at near-maximal workloads. In addition, treadmill exercise is not suitable for studies requiring a relatively immobile thorax, such as those involving indwelling vascular catheters or sensitive precordial detectors such as echocardiographs or scintillation cameras.

3.2.2 Test Protocols

For each subject an appropriate cardiovascular history and examination shoud be performed prior to the exercise test. The subject should be tested either after an overnight fast or no earlier than 2 h after a light meal. Patients should abstain from tobacco, alcohol, and caffeine for at least 3 h prior to testing.[25,28,29] The subject should be informed of the indications for the test, the details of its procedure, and the potential hazards of testing, and should then provide written informed consent.[25,28] A 12-lead conventional resting electrocardiogram must be recorded and examined for possible contraindications (Table 1)[25] and the interpretation should be recorded prior to exercise. A number of different treadmill and cycle ergometer protocols are widely used (Table 2).[25,26,28,29] Cycle ergometer protocols use an increased external work of 25–30 W per stage. The duration of each stage should be 2-3 min. For drug evaluation, generally, protocols with small increments in work, with work rates set to yield a test duration of approximately 10 min, are recommended.[29] A new protocol in which the work rate increases progressively and continuously is the ramp test. This protocol may offer some advantages but is not yet widely used for drug assessment.[29]

Table 1 Contraindications to Exercise Testing

(1)	Recent acute myocardial infarction (less than 3 months)
(2)	Unstable angina pectoris
(3)	Severe aortic stenosis
(4)	Uncontrolled cardiac dysrhythmia
(5)	Acute myocarditis or pericarditis
(6)	Severe hypertension
(7)	Congestive heart failure
(8)	Intracardiac conduction block greater than first-degree
(9)	Suspected or known dissecting aneurysm
(10)	Thrombophlebitis or pulmonary embolus
(11)	Acute systemic illness

Table 2

	Stage	Speed (mile/h)	Elevation (%-grade)	Duration
Bruce test	1	1.7	10.0	3
	2	2.5	12.0	3
	3	3.4	14.0	3
	4	4.2	16.0	3
	5	5.0	18.0	3
	6	5.5	20.0	3
	7	6.0	22.0	3
Naughton test	1	2.0	0.0	3
	2	2.0	3.5	3
	3	2.0	7.0	3
	4	2.0	10.5	3
	5	2.0	14.0	3
	6	2.0	17.5	3
	7	2.0	21.0	3

ECG tracing should be continuously displayed on a scope and then recorded on paper at least once per exercise stage and at each minute post exercise. Blood pressure should be measured before exercise, at least once during each exercise stage and every 2 min post exercise until stable. Exercise is continued by the subject until termination points are reached (Table 3). In the post-exercise period a complete 12-lead ECG should be recorded immediately and at 2 and 4 min post exercise in addition to any other leads. Post-exercise observation should continue for 6 min or until all exercise-induced abnormalities

Table 3 Indications for Stopping an Exercise Test

(1)	Angina-like pain that is progressive during exercise (stop at 3+ level or earlier on as scale of from 1+ to 4+)
(2)	Excessive degree (≥0.4mV) of ischemic type of ST-segment depression or elevation
(3)	Ventricular tachycardia, multifocal premature ventricular contractions or frequent (>30%) premature ventricular contractions aggravated or precipitated by exercise
(4	Ectopic supraventricular tachycardia
(5)	Exercise-induced intracardiac block
(6)	Signs of severe peripheral circulatory insufficiency: pallor, confusion, ataxia, diminished pulse
(7)	Any significant drop (10 mmHg) of systolic blood pressure or failure of the systolic blood pressure to rise with an increase in exercise load
(8)	Excessive blood pressure rise: systolic greater than 250 mmHg, diastolic greater than 120 mmHg
(9)	Unexplained inappropriate bradycardia
(10)	Excessive fatigue or dyspnea
(11)	Failure of monitoring system
(12)	Subject requests to stop

have disappeared. Exercise testing should be supervised by a physician trained in the procedure, and the exercise laboratory should be equipped and organized for patient safety measures.[25,28]

The risk of exercise testing is approximately 10 myocardial infarctions or deaths or both per 10,000 tests.[25] The more common risk can be detected by careful search for contraindications to exercise testing (Table 1).

3.2.3 Interpretation of Exercise Test

Exercise testing in clinical practice has two main objectives. First, to provoke an identifiable clinical response which may be a symptom such as angina pain, a change in some physiological variables including heart rate or blood pressure, or the appearance of a specific ECG abnormality, most commonly ST segment shift. Secondly, to determine the workload achieved at the time of the response or at the maximum effort. Some criteria for stopping a test are listed in Table 3. Some criteria constitute an abnormal response to exercise testing. These abnormal responses may or may not be a result of ischemia.

3.2.4 Evaluation of ECG Data

Many different leads systems have been used for exercise testing.[25,26,28] Since the question of how many leads need to be recorded during an exercise test has not been resolved, it seems advisable to record as many as are economically and practically possible. As a minimal approach, it is advisable to record three leads — a V5 type lead, an anterior V2 type lead, and an inferior lead such as a VF — but a 12-lead system should usually be preferred (Mason-Likar system). The normal ST-segment vector response to tachycardia and to exercise is a shift to the right and upward. The most common manifestation of exercise-induced myocardial ischemia is ST-segment depression. The standard criterion for this type of abnormal response is horizontal or downsloping ST-segment depression of 0.1 mV (1 mm) or more for 80 ms.[25,30] The probability and severity of coronary artery disease are directly related to to the amount of J-junction depression and are inversely related to the slope of the ST-segment. Table 4 lists some of the conditions that can possibly result in false-positive responses. Digitalis, psychotropic drugs such as tricyclic agents, and other antidepressant drugs can cause exercise-induced repolarization abnormalities, especially in women. Anemia, electrolyte abnormalities, meals, and even glucose ingestion can alter the ST segment and T wave in the resting ECG and can potentially cause a false-positive response.[30] To avoid this problem, all ECG studies should be performed after at least a 2-3 h fast. This requirement is also important because of the hemodynamic stress put on the cardiovascular systems by eating. After a meal functional capacity is decreased and the ischemic threshold may vary. Left bundle branch block, left ventricular hypertrophy, and WPW syndrome may induce ST depression without coronary artery disease. Exercise electrocardiographic responses in men correspond more closely than in women with the presence or absence of coronary artery disease.[30]

Development of ST-segment criteria other than exactly one or two divisions of the chart paper and problems with exercise artifact distortion of the ECG have set the stage for computer enhancement of ECG evaluation.[31] By computerized averaging of ECG complexes, artifacts are reduced. Recognition algorithms identify the points on the ECG to be measured. This analysis made by comptuer has the capacity of much greater precision than is possible by visual measurement of conventional ECG. This

Table 4 Conditions that Cause a False-Positive Exercise Test

Drug administration (digitalis, psychotropic drugs)
Left ventricular hypertrophy
Bundle branch block
Wolff-Parkinson-White syndrome
Electrolyte abnormalities
Anemia
Pericardial disorders
Mitral valve prolapse syndrome
Valvular heart disease

is particularly crucial for some criteria such as determination of time to 1 mm ST-segment depression. Several computer systems have been developed and commercial adaptations are available.

3.2.5 Heart Rate and Blood Pressure

The normal blood pressure response to exercise is a progressive rise in systolic pressure with little change in the diastolic pressure. In most exercise protocols, the systolic blood pressure rises about 8-10 mmHg per stage. A pathological fall in blood pressure during exercise is encountered occasionally and although an insensitive sign, it is claimed to be highly specific for severe coronary artery disease.[25,32] During dynamic exercise, heart rate increases linearly with work load. The heart rate-pressure product is an accurate noninvasive index of myocardial oxygen demand.[29] Therefore a comparison of a given treatment at this point on a patient's rating of angina pain or ST-segment depression provides an efficacy parameter.[29] A close match of the rate-pressure product between treatment is more important than the rate-pressure product per se. A point as late in exercise as possible closer to the functional limits of the patient is of greater interest for evaluation of treatment effect.[29]

3.2.6 Maximal Work Capacity

During exercise oxygen uptake (VO_2) is directly related to the work performed. At rest, the VO_2 is approximately 3.5 $ml.kg^{-1}$, min^{-1} which is referred to as one metabolic equivalent or MET.[25,26,32] In practice, the average peak VO_2 of symptomatic patients taking part in clinical trials corresponds to approximately 6 METS.[26] It is usual to record effort capacity in terms of minutes for treadmill tests and watts for bicycle tests. However, these values vary considerably according to the exercise modality, creating confusion in the interpretation of the result when data from various exercise protocol are pooled.[26] Therefore, effort capacity should be expressed in METS.[25,26,32] Stages I and III of the Bruce protocol represent 3 and 10 METS, respectively. This conversion is more difficult for bicycle exercise, but standard tables are available based on workload and body max index. In the evaluation of drug efficacy, most often the same standard exercise protocol is used in a given clinical trial therefore expressing results in minutes or watts is still valid.

3.2.7 Respiratory Gas Exchange Techniques

In drug studies, maximal oxygen uptake (VO_2 max) is usually derived from treadmill time or bicycle work. Although VO_2 max and treadmill time are closely related with correlation coefficient to range between 0.80 and 0.90, a wide scatter around these regression lines has been observed.[33] Measured oxygen uptake seems to be more accurate and reproducible than treadmill time and may improve the quantification of the drug effect in clinical studies.[29] The use of gas-exchange techniques, however, is still limited due to the availability of exercise test laboratories with adequate expertise in this field.[26]

3.2.8 Effort Angina

For drug evaluations studies, it is preferable for patients to exhibit both subjective (angina) and objective (ST-segment shift) markers of ischemia during exercise.[26,29] Although a quantification of the patients perceived symptom during exercise is subjective, the Borg scale seems to be the most useful method.[25,26,29] Rating of a patient's symptoms at each minute and at peak exercise is better than rating only at the end of each stage.[29] The endpoint of exercise test should be the point of pain that would typically cause the patient to stop his activity or take nitroglycerin outside the laboratory setting.[29]

3.2.9 Measured Variables for Evaluation of Anti-Ischemic Interventions and Testing Endpoints

In angina studies, the effect of the intervention on the patient's perception of chest pain during the test is usually the primary efficacy parameter.[26,27,29] In addition to angina a number of measured variables during exercise, both maximal and submaximal, can provide important information regarding treatment effects.[26,29] These points are

- ST-segment depression during identical workloads, especially the highest workload reached pre- and post-intervention
- Maximal exercise tolerance (watts, exercise time, or METS)
- Rate-pressure product (RPP) matched at identical workload and maximal exertion
- Exercise tolerance (watts, exercise time, METS, RPP) without angina pectoris, i.e., angina free exercise tolerance
- Exercise tolerance (watts, exercise time, METS, RPP) at 0.1 mV (1 mm) ST-segment depression

Consistent endpoints for exercise testing are of paramount importance for drug evaluation protocols. This is particularly true for placebo-controlled multicenter studies and when patients are not limited by angina. A practical approach would be in the analysis to substitute the total exercise time for the time to angina or 0.1 mV (1 mm) ST-segment depression in those who do not develop these manifestations. These times are then said to be censored.[26] Other testing endpoints such as age-predicted maximal heart rate and gas exchange data (respiratory exchange ratio and oxygen uptake plateau) are inappropriate for pharmacological investigations.[29]

4 METHODOLOGICAL ISSUES IN THE EARLY EVALUATION OF ANTIANGINAL DRUGS

The objective of this early phase are twofold:

1. Exploratory clinical pharmacology to identify some surrogate evidence for drug efficacy in angina. The various methods described in the pharmacodynamic section are relevant to address this issue. These exploratory studies might be important when developing drugs with a completely new mechanism of action for which some clues for a beneficial effect are needed before embarking on a full phase II development program. These methods are, however, inadequate as endpoints for dose-ranging protocols.
2. Dose determination is indeed the most important objective at this stage and can only be addressed with exercise-test protocols. Exercise testing is the most clinically relevant technique to evaluate anti-ischemic interventions. In addition, exercise protocols are considered by regulatory agencies as the efficacy variable most closely related to clinical benefit.

This section will deal with key points for the design of adequate dose-ranging trials.

4.1 Patient Selection

The quality of studies using exercise test to evaluate drug efficacy in angina patients depends heavily on careful screening of patients.[26,27,29,34] Those patients should be suffering from stable angina of effort which should be well characterized from patients' histories. The main task is to recruit only patients with true ischemic heart disease. Therefore, ischemic heart disease should be diagnosed using an acceptable objective criterion: documented past history of myocardial infarction; significant stenosis (>50%) of at least one major coronary artery on the coronary angiogram; positive symptom-limited exercise test (patients should exhibit both markers of ischemia during exercise, i.e., angina pain and 0.1 mV ST-segment depression); and positive thallium stress test. A patient's condition should be stable, i.e., over a period of at least 1 month there should have been no clear deterioration or improvement. The resting electrocardiogram should be such as not to interfere with the interpretation of ST-segment changes during angina. For this reason it is advisable to recruit only male patients in early pilot trials and to exclude patients with left bundle branch block.

Suitable study subjects should be identifed by their response to exercise test. The primary efficacy criterion is the occurrence of anginal pain during exercise. An antianginal agent cannot be considered antianginal unless it increases the amount of exercise that a patient can perform prior to the development of angina after drug administration.[27]

In order to be able to demonstrate an improvement in exercise capacity, selected patients should have neither too severe a form of angina nor too mild a degree of coronary artery disease. In this respect, the best population is patients who experience chest pain within 3-7 min of beginning exercise with the Bruce protocol.[29] In addition, for purposes of being able to detect efficacy using small sample size, the reproducibility of the anginal pain in relationship to exercise becomes an important consideration. It has been reported that exercise capacity has a variability of 10-15% with serial testing on the same day and on different days.[29,30] Thus, prior to randomization, the reproducibility of exercise tolerance should be evaluated and the decision to randomize patients should incorporate one additional criterion: a reproducibility exercise test within the range of 10% with at least two exercise tests on separate days.[29] In contrast to a reasonably rigorous means of identifying patients with stable angina pectoris suitable for randomization for early efficacy trials, a patient population with vasospastic angina, unstable angina, or silent myocardial ischemia is more difficult to deal with. Owing to the high variability and often critical condition of those patients, it is not recommended to focus early trials on this specific population when rough information on drug efficacy, dose-response relationship, and duration of effect is not yet available. Therefore, evaluation of antianginal drugs in this specific setting is beyond the scope of this chapter.

In summary, the logic of the selection scheme for early efficacy trials with exercise protocols is to: select patients who have stable angina due to myocardial ischemia; demonstrate that such patients have a positive symptom-limited exercise test; and that spontaneous variation of exercise capacity to serial maximal exercise testing is less than 10%.

4.2 Protocol Design

Treating angina is particularly challenging, because the patient's symptoms are subjective and highly prone to amelioration through a placebo effect.[35,36] This placebo effect may cause a 30-80% reduction in angina frequency. Even objective improvement as assessed by exercise test has been reported with an increase in exercise performance of 14-49%.[37] Therefore, the most unambigous means of demonstrating efficacy at this early stage is to use a placebo control. However, such placebo-controlled trials are not always easy to implement in symptomatic patients with coronary artery disease. This difficulty could be overcome by careful selection of patients and rather short duration of treatment; from 2 days to 2 weeks. It has been shown that assignment to placebo group is not associated with increased adverse experience in short-term trials[38] or even in a long-term protocol[37] and should be considered quite ethical.[26]

For exercise efficacy protocols, a run-in period is essential. After carefully supervised withdrawal of prior antianginal drug therapy, the patient may be started on a single-blind placebo run-in period of 1 week which allows: (1) assessment of exercise capacity and variability and (2) accustoming of the patient to the experimental procedure.

Because maximal oxygen uptake is generally higher on the treadmill than bicycle tests for studies in which the efficacy parameters include the functional limits of the patient and objective signs of ischemia, the treadmill is preferable. An exercise protocol with small increments in work and with work rates set to yield a test duration of approximately 10 min is recommended.[29,34]

Titration studies can be useful for early dose finding. It is important to start with low doses since the noneffective dose or minimum effective dose should be determined. The most common titration design is one where each patient is titrated up to a certain point according to specified rules, either forced titration or according to efficacy/safety criteria. A minimum of four different dose levels should be explored. The advantage of this design is that few patients are required. Disadvantages are possible carry-over effects from one dose to another, confounding of dose and time, and problems with early withdrawals from study, thus incomplete data in some patients. The titration rules must be clearly defined in the protocol and carefully explained to investigators. Frequently investigators titrate patients according to different criteria and no firm conclusions can be drawn from the analysis. A control group preferably on placebo is mandatory.

The parallel-group design is in fact the most appropriate for confirmatory dose finding. The earlier tiration studies will have identified the range of a possible dose and the confirmatory placebo-controlled studies are then carried out on only 3 or 4 doses. Duration of studies should be long enough to detect tachyphylaxia, i.e., a minimum of 2-4 weeks. Careful assessment of differences between results from intention-to-treat and per protocol analysis is particularly important in dose-finding studies. For parallel design protocol using a placebo-controlled group, it is usual to recruit 40-80 patients per group. These dose-ranging studies should be performed with patients receiving no other antianginal agents except sublingual nitroglycerin for relief of anginal pain.

The exercise test should be performed under well-defined conditions as regards the time of the day, the period which has elapsed following administration of the drug or placebo, and the timing with respect to meals.[25,26,29] Exercise tolerance tests should be carried out, if possible, between 9:00 and 11:00 h in the fasting state or at least 2 h after a light breakfast. With frequent exercise testing, carried out on the same day or on successive days, a training effect may be observed.[29] This fact emphasizes the need for adequate randomization and for a control group.

In terms of analysis, the variables described for evaluation of exercise test are recommended. The main efficacy criteria are changes in exercise performance and were discussed earlier. Demonstration that an antianginal drug is active means that it is both antianginal and antiischemic.[27] This latter fact implies that the agent will delay the time to 1 mm ST-segment depression or for a given workload ST-segment depression will be reduced as compared with control state. Diary studies with counts of anginal attack rate or nitroglycerin consumption may provide supportive evidence of efficacy. However, such measurements cannot be the major data upon which a decision will rest at this early stage.

The time-effect relationship of single and multiple doses of drug is necessary to assess. This duration-of-effect evaluation should be performed with serial exercise tolerance tests. Such designs are usually flexible and do not raise safety issues. Every attempt should be made to study the relationship between blood concentrations and measures of efficacy. This can be performed during the dose-effect, time-effect studies. The correlation or lack of correlation between blood levels and effect or time-course of blood concentrations and time-course of effect should be considered a necessary description of the clinical pharmacology of the antianginal agent. Some "model" clinical trials are cited in the References 39-43.

5 CONCLUSION

In the early evaluation of antianginal drugs, exercise test protocols performed in a selected population of patients are the only means to accurately determine appropriate doses and dosing intervals. However, even with great attention to detail, the evaluation of drug effects during exercise testing could be imprecise. It is therefore important to follow recommendations that are made for optimizing exercise testing for pharmacological investigations. Other pharmacodynamic measurements may provide insights into the mechanism of drug action but cannot be selected as surrogates for dose-ranging or regulatory purposes.

REFERENCES

1. Schaper, W., Schaper, J., and Hoffmeister, H. M., Pathophysiology of coronary circulation and of acute coronary insufficiency, in *Clinical Pharmacology of Antianginal Drugs*, Abshagen, U., Ed., Springer-Verlag, Berlin, 1985, 47.
2. Epstein, S. E., Cannon, R. O., Watson, R. M., Leon, M. B., Bonow, R. O., and Rosing, D. R., Dynamic coronary obstruction as a cause of angina pectoris: implication regarding therapy, *Am. J. Cardiol.*, 55, 61B, 1985.
3. Collins, P., Fox, K. M., Pathophysiology of angina, *Lancet*, 335, 94, 1990.
4. Maseri, A., Role of coronary artery spasm in symptomatic and silent myocardial ischemia, *J. Am. Coll. Cardiol.*, 9, 249, 1987.
5. Gage, J. E., Hess, O. M., Murakami, T., Ritter, M., Grimm, J., and Krayenbuehl, H. P., Vasoconstriction of stenotic coronary arteries during dynamic exercise in patients with classic angina pectoris: reversibility by nitroglycerine, *Circulation*, 73, 865, 1986.
6. Klocke, F. J., Ellis, A. K., and Canty, J. M., Interpretation of changes in coronary flow that accompany pharmacologic interventions, *Circulation*, 75 (Suppl. V), V34, 1987.
7. Crawford, M. H., Exercise-induced myocardial ischemia, importance of coronary blood flow, *Circulation*, 84, 424, 1991.
8. Ferro, G., Spinelli, L., Duilio, C., Spadafora, M., Guarnaccia, F., and Condorelli, M., Diastolic perfusion time at ischemic threshold in patients with stress-induced ischemia, *Circulation*, 84, 49, 1991.
9. Kraupp, O., Pharmacodynamic principles of action of antianginal drugs, in *Clinical Pharmacology of Antianginal Drugs*, Abshagen, U., Ed., Springer-Verlag, Berlin, 1985, 97.
10. Nienaber, C. and Bleifeld, W., Assessment of coronary artery disease and myocardial ischemia by invasive methods, in *Clinical Pharmacology of Antianginal Drugs*, Abshagen, U., Ed., Springer-Verlag, Berlin, 1985, 239.
11. Reiber, J. H. C., Serruys, P. W., Kooijman, C. J., Wijns, W., Slager, C. J., Gerbrands, J. J., Schnurbiers, J. C. H., Den Boer, A., and Hugenholtz, P. G., Assessment of short, medium and long term variations in arterial dimensions from computer-assisted quantitation of coronary cineangiograms, *Circulation*, 71, 280, 1985.
12. Demer, L., Gould, K. L., and Kirkuide, R., Assessing stenosis severity: coronary flow reserve, collateral function, quantitative coronary angiography, positron imaging and digital substraction angiography: a review and analysis, *Prog. Cardiovasc. Dis.*, 30, 307, 1988.

13. Markham, R. V., Winniford, M. D., Firth, B. G., Nicod, P., Dehmen, G. J., Lewis, S. E. and Hillis, L. D., Symptomatic, electrocardiographic, metabolic and hemodynamic alterations during pacing-induced myocardial ischemia, *Am. J. Cardiol.*, 51, 1589, 1983.
14. Marcus, M. L., Wilson, R. F., and White, C. W., Methods of measurements of myocardial blood flow in patients: a critical review, *Circulation*, 76, 245, 1987.
15. Guidelines for clinical use of cardiac radionuclide imaging, December 1986, A report of the American College of Cardiology/American Heart Association task force on assessment of cardiovascular procedures (Subcommittee on Nuclear imaging), *J. Am. Coll. Cardiol.*, 8, 1471, 1986.
16. Froelicher, V. F., Myers, J., Follansbee, W. P., and Labovitz A. J., Stress radionuclide myocardial perfusion imaging, in *Exercise and the Heart*, Mosby, St. Louis, 1993, 252.
17. Chua, T., Kiat, H., Germano, G., Mauser, G., Van Train, K., Friedman, J and Berman, D., Gated technetium-99m sestamibi for simultaneous assessment of stress myocardial perfusion, post exercise regional ventricular function and myocardial viability-correlation with echocardiography and rest thallium-201 scintigraphy, *J. Am. Coll. Cardiol.*, 23, 1107, 1994.
18. Iskandrian, A. S. and Hakki, A. M., Thallium-201 myocardial scintigraphy, *Am. Heart J.*, 109, 113, 1985.
19. Froelicher, V. F., Myers, J., Follansbee, W. P., and Labovitz A. J., Exercise radionuclide ventricular function imaging, in *Exercise and the Heart*, Mosby, St. Louis, 1993, 294.
20. Nestico, P. F., Hakki, A. H., and Iskandrian, A. S., Effects of cardiac medications on ventricular performance: emphasis on evaluation with radionuclide angiography, *Am. Heart J.*, 109, 1070, 1985.
21. Marwick, T., Willemart B., D'Hondt, A. M., Baudhuin, T., Wijns W., Detry J. M., and Melin J., Selection of the optimal non exercise stress for the evaluation of ischemic regional myocardial dysfunction and malperfusion, *Circulation*, 87, 345, 1993.
22. Wackers, F. J. Th., Which pharmacological stress is optimal? A technique-dependent choice, *Circulation*, 87, 646, 1993.
23. Lattanzi, F., Picano, E., Bolognese, L., Piccinino, C., Sarasso, G., Orlandini, A., and L'Abbate, A., Inhibition of dipyridamole-induced ischemia by antianginal therapy in humans, *Circulation*, 83, 1256, 1991.
24. Iliceto, S., Galinto, L., Marangelli, V., and Rizzon P., Clinical use of stress echocardiography factors affecting diagnostic accuracy, *Eur. Heart J.*, 15, 672, 1994.
25. Fletcher, G. F., Balady, G., Froelicher, V. F., Hartley, L. H., Haskell, W. L., and Pollock, M. L., Exercise standards — a statement for Healthcare professionals from the American Heart Association, *Circulation*, 91, 580, 1995.
26. ESC working group on exercise physiology, physiopathology and electrocardiography, Guidelines for cardiac exercise testing, *Eur. Heart J.*, 14, 969, 1993.
27. Guidelines on the quality, safety and efficacy of medicinal products for human use. Antianginal drugs, in *The Rules Governing Medicinal Products in the European Community,* Vol III, 187, 1989.
28. Pina, I. L., Balady G. J., Hanson, P., Labovitz, A. J., Madonna, D. W., and Myers, J., Guidelines for Clinical Exercise testing laboratories. A statement for healthcare Professionals from the committee on Exercise and Cardiac Rehabilitation American Heart Association, *Circulation*, 91, 912, 1995.
29. Myers, J. and Froelicher, V. F., Optimizing the exercise test for pharmacological investigations, *Circulation*, 82, 1839, 1990.
30. Froelicher, V. F., Myers, J., Follansbee, W. P., and Labovitz, A. J., Interpretation of ECG responses, in *Exercise and the Heart,* Mosby, St. Louis, 1993, 99.
31. Froelicher, V. F., Myers, J., Follansbee, W. P., and Labovitz, A. J., Special methods — computerized exercise ECG analysis, in *Exercise and the Heart*, Mosby, St. Louis, 1993, 48.
32. Froelicher, V. F., Myers, J., Follansbee, W. P., and Labovitz, A. J., Interpretation of hemodynamic responses to exercise testing: exercise capacity, heart rate and blood pressure, in *Exercise and the Heart*, Mosby, St. Louis, 1993, 71.
33. Froelicher, V. F., Myers, J., Follansbee, W. P., and Labovitz, A. J., Special methods: ventilatory gas exchange, in *Exercise and the Heart*, Mosby, St. Louis, 1993, 32.
34. Webster, M. W. I. and Scharpe, D. N., Exercise testing in angina pectoris: the importance of protocol design in clinical trials, *Am. Heart J.*, 117, 505, 1989.
35. Benson, H. and McCallie, D. P., Angina pectoris and the placebo effect, *N. Engl. J. Med.*, 300, 1424, 1979.
36. Parisi, A. F., Strauss, W. E., McIntyre, K. M., and Sasahara, A. A., Considerations in evaluating new antianginal drugs, *Circulation*, 65 (Suppl. I), 138, 1982.
37. Boissel, J. P., Philippon, A. M., Gauthier, E., Schbath, J., Destors, J. M., and the B. I. S. Research Group, Time course of long-term placebo therapy effects in angina pectoris, *Eur. Heart J.*, 7, 1030, 1986.
38. Glasser, S. P., Clark, P. I., Lipicky, R. J., Hubbard, J. M., and Yusuf, S., Exposing patients with chronic, stable exertional angina to placebo periods in drug trials, *JAMA*, 265, 1550, 1991.
39. Scheidt, S., Le Winter, M. M., Hermanovith, J., Venkataraman, K., and Freedman, D., Efficacy and safety of nicardipine for chronic stable angina pectoris: a multicentre randomized trial, *Am. J. Cardiol.*, 58, 715, 1986.
40. Frishman, W., Chanlap, S., Kimmell, B., Teicher, M., Cinnamon, J., Allen, L., and Strom, J., Diltiazem, nifedipine and their combination in patients with stable angina pectoris: effects on anigna, exercise tolerance and the ambulatory electrocardiographic ST segment, *Circulation*, 77, 774, 1988.

41. Gheorghiade, M., Weiner, D. A., Chakko, S., Lessem, J. N., and Klein, M. D., Monotherapy of stable angina with nicardipine hydrochloride; double-blind, placebo-controlled, randomized study, *Eur. Heart J.*, 10, 695, 1989.
42. Thadani, U., Zellner, S. R., Glasser, S., Bittar, N., Montoro, R., Miller, A.B., Chaitman, B., Schulman, P., Stahl, A., DiBianco, R., Bray, J., Means, W. E., and Morledge, J., Double-blind, dose-response placebo-controlled multicenter study of nisoldipine: a new second-generation calcium channel blocker in angina pectoris, *Circulation*, 84, 2398, 1991.
43. Thadani, U., Ezecowitz, M., Fenney, L., and Chiang, Y. K., for the Ranolazine study group, Double-blind efficacy and safety of a novel anti-ischemic agent, ranolazine, versus placebo in patients with chronic stable angina pectoris, *Circulation*, 90, 726, 1994.

Chaper 16

Antiarrhythmic Agents

Pran K. Marrott

CONTENTS

1 Introduction......213
2 Ventricular Arrhythmias......213
3 Supraventricular Arrhythmias......215
4 Conclusion......215
References......215

1 INTRODUCTION

The 1990s have seen important developments in antiarrhythmic research. These developments have altered radically, physicians' perception of the benefits of antiarrhythmic drug therapy and have highlighted the potential dangers from using antiarrhythmic drugs. The current thinking has not only dampened the enthusiasm of the pharmaceutical industry for developing antiarrhythmic agents, but has also created confusion in the minds of pharmaceutical research physicians on the type of data that should be generated for approval. A discussion of the reasons for the current state of affairs and the principles that might be successfully adopted for future antiarrhythmic drug development will be discussed.

2 VENTRICULAR ARRHYTHMIAS

The first setback to conventional thinking of the role of antiarrhythmic therapy came when the interim results of the Cardiac Arrhythmia Suppression Trial (CAST) were announced.[1] This multicenter randomized placebo-controlled trial was undertaken to test the hypothesis that suppression of asymptomatic or mildly symptomatic ventricular arrhythmias with antiarrhythmic drug therapy after myocardial infarction would reduce the incidence of arrhythmia-related deaths. The rationale for undertaking CAST was based on the known risks relating to arrhythmic deaths in post-myocardial infarction patients with premature ventricular contractions (PVCs).[2] The drugs encainide, flecainide, and moricizine were chosen for CAST on the basis of the results of the Cardiac Arrhythmia Pilot Study (CAPS) which showed that the three drugs were effective in suppressing PVCs and were tolerated over a 12-month period.[3] CAPS showed that flecainide could cause congestive heart failure in patients with reduced left ventricular ejection fraction (LVEF) and therefore, in CAST, patients with LVEF <30% did not receive flecainide. In April 1989, The Data and Safety Monitoring Board of CAST recommended, after a review of interim unblinded data, that investigators withdraw all patients from encainide and flecainide because of a significant increase in total and arrhythmia-related mortality compared to placebo. Of note was the observation that the increased risk in patients receiving encainide or flecainide continued for the duration of long-term treatment. This new finding was contrary to popular belief that proarrhythmia from antiarrhythmic drugs was restricted to the first few days or weeks following the initiation of or a change in the dose of antiarrhythmic therapy. The board recommended the continuation of the trial (CAST II) with placebo and moricizine. Subsequently moricizine was also withdrawn because of lack of benefit. The interim results of CAST I (the earlier segment of CAST), the full results of CAST I, and results of CAST II (the later segment of CAST) have been published.[1,4,5]

The implications of the CAST data were widely debated. In an editorial published in the *New England Journal of Medicine,* August 10, 1989, Jeremy Ruskin, a member of the Data and Safety Monitoring Board wrote,

0-8493-9230-6/97/$0.00+$.50
© 1997 by CRC Press, Inc.

> "Sudden cardiac death remains a public health problem of major importance, and safe and effective prophylactic interventions are long overdue. CAST, despite its limitations and in part because of its surprises, is an important milestone in contemporary cardiology. Rather than serving as the definitive study of asymptomatic ventricular arrhythmias, CAST has instead upended old landmarks, challenged our perceptions, and set new standards for research on cardiac arrhythmias. It is hoped that the preliminary findings of CAST will provide the impetus for additional placebo-controlled mortality trials among patients who are at high risk for sudden death. The study should also catalyze renewed interest in the mechanisms of action and proarrhythmic effects of antiarrhythmic drugs and in the electrophysiology of sudden cardiac death."

The impact of CAST has been far reaching:

1. There has been a reduction in the development of antiarrhythmic drugs with class IC activity. Clinical trials of diprafenone hydrochloride an antiarrhythmic drug with class IC activity have been stopped. Indecainide, a drug with IC antiarrhythmic activity, was approved by the FDA, but has not been marketed by the company.
2. Most physicians believe that the increased risk extends also to the use of Class IA drugs. Supporting this belief are the results of a meta-analysis of data from trials where quinidine, a Class IA drug, was compared to class IB or IC drugs in patients with mostly benign ventricular arrhythmias.[6] The meta-analysis showed an excess of mortality over other class I drugs (mexiletine, flecainide, and encainide).
3. The consensus now is that antiarrhythmic drugs should not be routinely prescribed for treating PVCs or nonsustained ventricular tachycardia (NSVT) since the potential risk exceeds the clinical benefit.
4. The FDA is unlikely to approve antiarrhythmic drugs for suppressing PVCs or NSVT unless there is more favorable data on mortality.
5. A "warning" section in the labeling for all antiarrhythmic drugs used for the treatment of ventricular arrhythmias is required by the FDA to highlight the potential risks. In addition, a statement to the effect that the use of antiarrhythmic drugs in life-threatening ventricular arrhythmia is not associated with improved survival, is mandatory.
6. In the U.S., antiarrhythmic drugs will now be approved only for the treatment of life-threatening ventricular arrhythmias (ventricular tachycardia, VT or ventricular fibrillation, VF) and even for this limited indication, an improvement in survival or a lack of a deleterious effect on survival should be shown.

For the management of VT or VF most cardiac electrophysiologists in the U.S. base the predictability of long-term benefit of an antiarrhythmic drug on whether or not it is capable of preventing (or modifying favorably) induction of sustained monomorphic VT. It was shown previously that as a tool for assessing ability of a drug to prevent life-threatening ventricular arrhythmias long-term, an electrophysiologic (EP) study was superior to Holter monitoring. Most investigational drug studies in life-threatening ventricular arrhythmias were undertaken using EP as a tool for predicting benefit from the use of the drug long-term. Recently, however, the results of ESVEM an NIH-sponsored study, have shown that recurrences of VT or VF during long-term treatment with drugs selected on the basis of suppression of ventricular arrhythmias by Holter evaluation or prevention of inducibility of VT during EP, were similar.[7] The implication is that if patients with life-threatening ventricular arrhythmias have PVCs (≥10/h) Holter monitoring could be used instead of EP for selecting drugs and testing the long-term benefit from treating these patients.

Drug development for life-threatening ventricular arrhythmias should now include:

1. Early phase studies for selecting a range of doses and the dosing frequency. Such studies could be undertaken in patients with life-threatening ventricular arrhythmias (VT or VF). This holds true especially for class III drugs (the only class of investigational drugs now being evaluated for life-threatening ventricular arrhythmias). An acute drug response could be used as a surrogate measure of long-term efficacy.
2. A phase II study looking at safety (proarrhythmic response) and long-term efficacy of the drug in patients with VT or VF with the decision to proceed long-term with the drug, based either on Holter monitoring or on an EP study.

3. A placebo-controlled trial examining the effect of the drug on shock rate or on survival, in patients with VT or VF receiving ICD devices.
4. A possible fourth study in patients with NSVT and an EP-induced sustained VT. An NIH-sponsored study (MUSTT) to examine the role of antiarrhythmic drugs vs. no treatment in preventing arrhythmia recurrences or deaths and overall mortality, in this subpopulation, is ongoing. If results of drug therapy are favorable compared to placebo, NSVT could become an additional approvable indication.

3 SUPRAVENTRICULAR ARRHYTHMIAS

The perception that antiarrhythmic drugs may increase mortality has infiltrated to the supraventricular arrhythmia patient population. Concerns here are more serious since supraventricular arrhythmias are not life-threatening. A meta-analysis of data from six randomized trials in which quinidine was compared with placebo or no treatment showed an increased mortality (2.9%) from quinidine compared to placebo or no treatment (0.8%).[8] Drug studies for this indication may require the inclusion of data to examine whether the use of antiarrhythmic drug therapy is associated not only with a demonstratable clinical benefit, but also a better quality of life and no deleterious effect on mortality.

Pritchett and Wilkinson have listed the following possible claims for supraventricular arrhythmias:[9]

1. Prophylaxis of symptomatic arrhythmias in groups of patients with paroxysmal supraventricular tachycardia (PSVT) or with paroxysmal atrial fibrillation (PAF).
2. Maintenance of sinus rhythm after cardioversion in patients with PAF.
3. Restoration of sinus rhythm by antiarrhythmic drug given intravenously in patients with PSVT or PAF.
4. Slowing the ventricular rate during atrial fibrillation by antiarrhythmic drug given intravenously.
5. Slowing the ventricular rate in atrial fibrillation with antiarrhythmic drug given orally.
6. Restoring sinus rhythm in atrial fibrillation with oral antiarrhythmic therapy.

Flecainide was approved recently, in the U.S., for the prevention of symptomatic recurrences of PSVT or atrial fibrillation not associated with organic heart disease. A study design proposed by Pritchett and Lee[10] and used for studies with flecainide and recently for propafenone has found favor with the FDA. The reader should refer to this study and to publications related to studies with flecainide and propafenone in patients with supraventricular arrhythmias for guidance on the methodologies used.[11-13] The study design proposed can be adopted for a phase II dose-response study as well as for phase III studies. An intravenous formulation of an antiarrhythmic drug may also be studied for the conversion of atrial fibrillation or flutter to sinus rhythm or for the conversion of PSVT to sinus rhythm. Recently adenosine has been approved in the U.S. for the latter indication. In addition to two well-controlled studies, drug development for the former indication should include a placebo-controlled dose-response study with provisions for alternate treatment if the arrhythmia does not revert to sinus rhythm.

4 CONCLUSION

The results of antiarrhythmic research over the last 5 years have altered our perception of the benefit from antiarrhythmic therapy and highlighted the potential dangers from the use of these agents. In order to be approved for use in life-threatening ventricular arrhythmias, drugs have now to show an improvement in long-term survival. Antiarrhythmic drugs are not recommended for the treatment of benign ventricular arrhythmias. A novel approach has been recommended for the development of antiarrhythmic drugs for the treatment of PSVT or atrial fibrillation or flutter. Data generated based on this approach has led to approval of flecainide (in the U.S.) and is recommended for newer compounds. Scope exists for developing intravenous formulation of antiarrhythmic drugs for conversion of atrial fibrillation/flutter or PSVT although there is an abundance of suitable i.v. drugs for the latter, including the recently approved drug adenosine.

REFERENCES

1. (CAST) Investigators, The cardiac arrhythmia suppression trial, *N. Engl. J. Med.*, 321, 406, 1989.
2. Bigger, J. T., Identification of patients at high risk for sudden cardiac death, *Am. J. Cardiol.*, 54, 3D, 1984.

3. The Cardiac Arrhythmia Pilot Study (CAPS) Investigators, Effects of encainide, flecainide, imipramine and moricizine on ventricular arrhythmias during the year after acute myocardial infarction: the CAPS, *Am. J. Cardiol.*, 61, 501, 1988.
4. Echt, D. S., Liebson, P. R., Mitchell, L. B., Peters, R. W., Obias-Manno, D., Barker, A. H., Arensberg, D., Baker, A., Friedman, L., Greene, H. L., Huther, M. L., Richardson, D. W., and the CAST Investigators, Mortality and morbidity in patients receiving encainide, flecainide, or placebo, *N. Engl. J. Med.*, 324, 781, 1991.
5. The Cardiac Arrhythmia Suppression Trial II Investigators, *N. Engl. J. Med.*, 327, 227, 1992.
6. Morganroth, J. and Goin, J. E., Quinidine-related mortality in the short-to-medium-term treatment of ventricular arrhythmias, A meta-analysis, *Circulation*, 84, 1977, 1991.
7. Mason, J. W., for the Electrophysiologic Study Versus Electrocardiographic Monitoring Investigators, A comparison of electrophysiologic testing with holter monitoring to predict antiarrhythmic-drug efficacy for ventricular tachyarrhythmias, *N. Engl. J. Med.*, 329, 445, 1993.
8. Coplen, S. E., Antman, E. M., Berlin, J. A., Hewitt, P., and Chalmers, T. C., Efficacy and safety of quinidine therapy for maintenance of sinus rhythm after cardioversion, a meta-analysis of randomized control trials, *Circulation*, 82, 1106, 1990.
9. Pritchett, E. L. C. and Wilkinson, W. E., New drug application strategies for supraventricular arrhythmias, *Clin. Pharmcol. Ther.*, 49, 481, 1991.
10. Pritchett, E. L. C. and Lee, K. L., Designing clinical trials for paroxysmal atrial tachycardia and other paroxysmal arrhythmias, *J. Clin. Epidemiol.*, 41, 851, 1988.
11. Anderson, J., Gilbert, E., Alpert, B., Henthorn, R., Waldo, A., Bhandari, A., Hawkinson, R., and Pritchett, E., Prevention of symptomatic recurrences of paroxysmal atrial fibrillation in patients initially tolerating antiarrhythmic therapy. A multicenter, double-blind crossover study of flecainide and placebo with transtelephonic monitoring, *Circulation*, 8, 1557, 1989.
12. Henthorn, R., Waldo, A., Anderson, J., Gilbert, E., Albert, B., Bhandari, A., Hawkinson, R., Pritchett, E., and the Flecainide Supraventricular Tachycardia Study Group. Flecainide acetate prevents recurrence of paroxysmal supraventricular tachycardia, *Circulation*, 83, 119, 1991.
13. Pritchett, E. L. C., McCarthy, E. A., and Wilkinson, W. E., Propafenone treatment of symptomatic paroxysmal supraventricular arrhythmias, *Ann. Int. Med.*, 114, 539, 1991.

Chapter 17

Antihypertensive Drugs

Kevin P. J. O'Kane and David J. Webb

CONTENTS

1 Introduction ... 217
2 Healthy Volunteers ... 218
2.1 Selection Criteria ... 219
2.2 Safety Considerations ... 219
2.3 Methods ... 220
2.3.1 General Trial Design ... 220
2.3.2 Pharmacokinetic Issues ... 224
2.3.3 Pharmacodynamic Issues ... 226
3 Patient Studies ... 230
3.1 Selection Criteria ... 230
3.2 Safety Considerations ... 230
3.3 Methods ... 230
3.4 Surrogate Markers ... 231
4 Decision Making ... 231
References ... 232

1 INTRODUCTION

Hypertension is a major risk factor for stroke and heart attack[1,2] and current treatment of hypertension is successful in preventing stroke,[3] though perhaps less effective in preventing heart attack.[4-6] Cardiovascular disease accounts for about 1.5 million deaths (44% of all deaths) in the European Community each year.[7] Statistics are available in the U.S. which show that high blood pressure is the single most common cause of physician visits,[8] and cardiovascular disease costs the American economy in excess of $128 billion annually.[9] The range of drugs available for treating high blood pressure has increased substantially over the past 20 years with the addition of calcium antagonists, angiotensin converting enzyme (ACE) inhibitors, and very recently, angiotensin receptor antagonists, to the more traditional thiazide diuretics and alpha- and beta-adrenoceptor antagonists. Guidelines for the diagnosis and management of hypertension have recently been published by several national[10-13] and international groups.[14,15]

In spite of the wide availability of effective drugs, and the proliferation of guidelines, management of hypertension in the community remains poor. In the U.K., the so-called "rule of halves" was first described in the early 1970s. Community-based studies show that only half of all hypertensive patients are detected; of these, only half receive treatment, and in only half of these is blood pressure adequately controlled.[16-19] However, treating hypertension is cost effective, being cheaper than treating the cardiovascular events that may otherwise ensue.[20] Therefore, the large market for antihypertensive drugs is still sufficient to reward the pharmaceutical industry, which is spending ~$250 million for each licensed new drug.[21]

The purpose of phase I studies of antihypertensive drugs is principally to determine the safety and tolerability of new drugs or novel formulations of established drugs, and additionally to gather pharmacokinetic data to guide further development. Phase I studies of antihypertensive drugs may also provide valuable information about the efficacy of, and dose-response relationships for, the study compound, although these are investigated more fully in phase II.

0-8493-9230-6/97/$0.00+$.50
© 1997 by CRC Press, Inc.

2 HEALTHY VOLUNTEERS

Gender

Most phase I and II studies of antihypertensive drugs are performed in male subjects. This standardizes the conditions under which drugs are studied. Studies of antihypertensive drugs in premenopausal women can be complicated by cyclic changes in pharmacokinetics and pharmacodynamics associated with the menstrual cycle; by using males it is possible to avoid these confounding variables. Furthermore, by studying only men at this early stage, teratogenicity studies can be delayed until it is clear whether the drug has potential for further development.

It can be argued that this traditional approach, effectively excluding women from the early phases of clinical trials, is a weakness[22,23] because women may show significant pharmacokinetic and pharmacodynamic differences from men.[24-26] They also constitute a large proportion of the target population for new antihypertensive agents, although their major risks do not develop until after menopause. Drug absorption, metabolism, and excretion are all influenced by the menstrual cycle, by pregnancy and by the menopause,[24] and observations in men may not be directly relevant to women. For instance, propranolol is more slowly metabolized in women than in men, possibly because estrogens regulate enzymes responsible for metabolism of the drug.[27] Similarly, there may be differences in side effects between males and females; cough associated with ACE inhibitors is substantially more common in women than in men[28] and might have been detected early on if more women had been included in clinical trials. The use of treatments in women which clinical trials have shown only in men to be effective has been criticized.[29] Recent guidelines from the American Food and Drug Administration (FDA) recommend the inclusion of women in clinical trials at an early stage of drug development,[29] and, as a consequence of the National Institutes of Health (NIH) Revitalization Act (1993), federally funded researchers are now obliged to include women in clinical trials.[29,30] The Institute of Medicine has recently published a report[31] which condemns "...the protectionism previously accorded women of reproductive potential...," and suggests that information on safety and efficacy of new drugs in pregnancy and lactation should be gathered before a product license is awarded, even though it may put the offspring at some risk. The report argues women's right of access to clinical trials on an equity rather than an efficacy basis, though the extent to which it will be implemented remains to be seen.

Age

Studying young subjects in early phase trials, usually in the 18-40 years age range, minimizes the potential effects of covert disease processes, (such as subclinical ischemic heart disease), and of degenerative changes in the cardiovascular system, which might be found in older subjects.

However, given that hypertension in older adults is associated with increased risk of cardiovascular disease, particularly stroke,[32-36] and that the proportion of elderly individuals in the developed world is rising,[37] it is crucial to determine the effect of new antihypertensive agents in the elderly at an early stage, particularly as the physiological changes which accompany aging are known to influence pharmacokinetics in a nonuniform manner.[38-40] International agreement has recently been reached on the inclusion of elderly subjects in clinical trials;[41] the influence of age on the response to new antihypertensive agents should be studied at an early stage in drug development, ideally during phase I.[42]

Race

There may be important differences in drug efficacy and metabolism among the races.[43] For instance, hypertensive black subjects are often relatively insensitive to beta-adrenoceptor antagonists and ACE inhibitors,[44-46] but are relatively more sensitive to thiazide diuretics.[46,47] Drug acetylation is controlled by an autosomal recessive gene, and there is a higher proportion of slow metabolizers in Japanese than Western populations. Hence, they are more prone to accumulate drugs, such as hydralazine, which depend on acetylation for their excretion, leading to an increased potential for dose-related toxicity. Indeed, it has generally been maintained that in many disease areas the Japanese require smaller doses of medication than their Western counterparts.[48] For these reasons, it is important to exercise care in extrapolating clinical trial findings among different racial groups.[43] Such differences have sometimes been reflected in legislation; until recently, regulatory studies of all new pharmaceutical preparations intended for use in Japan had to be carried out in Japanese subjects. However, two recent studies, one of nonsteroidal anti-inflammatory drugs and one of antihypertensive drugs,[48] suggest that interethnic kinetic and dynamic differences are probably less important than intersubject variability. This has led to a joint European/American/Japanese consensus on ethnicity requirements in drug testing.[48]

2.1 Selection Criteria

The investigator in nontherapeutic research has an obligation to ensure the safety of all research subjects.[49] This encompasses not only protocol design, provision of adequate research facilities, and familiarity with the study drug, but also subject selection. The investigator must ensure that an adequate medical history is available, and, as far as possible, guard against the overenthusiastic subject who may be participating in studies without sufficient drug-free periods to safeguard his health and the validity of the study results.[50]

2.1.1 Drugs

In selecting healthy volunteers, one must ensure that they do not consume prescribed drugs on an excessive basis and do not consume substances of abuse. Excessive alcohol consumption is associated with a pressor effect in both normotensive[51,52] and hypertensive subjects.[53] Alcohol withdrawal, too, is associated with a pressor response[54] and its social effects may be disruptive in clinical trials. Finally, alcohol can induce mixed function oxidase, and thus increase the metabolism of drugs dependent on hepatic activation or inactivation. For these reasons, only moderate drinkers (≤21 units/week for men and ≤14 units/week for women) should be included in early phase studies, and alcohol should be avoided for at least 48 h before participation.

Smoking has an acute hypertensive effect, mediated, at least in part, by increased levels of circulating catecholamines.[55] This may have a confounding effect in studies of drugs acting through the adrenergic system.[56] However, ambulatory blood pressure measurements in smokers show greater variability than in nonsmokers, and this trend increases during abstention.[57] Ideally, only nonsmokers should participate in clinical trials, but when this is not possible, heavy smokers should be excluded.

Caffeine can produce an acute pressor effect,[56] but its withdrawal may be associated with headache, anxiety, and irritability.[58,59] There is no established consensus regarding caffeine intake in studies of antihypertensive medication, but abstinence for 24 h before studies and throughout their duration might seem a reasonable precaution.

Subjects who abuse nonlicensed drugs may present particular difficulties in clinical trials of antihypertensive agents. Problems may arise which are directly related to the pharmacological effects of the substance of abuse, such as the pressor effects of cocaine and amphetamine derivatives, or to the hemodynamic and social effects of its withdrawal, for instance with opiates. Marijuana causes reductions in blood pressure and impaired cerebral autoregulation which may lead to postural symptoms.[60] Acutely, marijuana increases heart rate and impairs human performance skills for up to 24 h after use.[61] One should consider that young male subjects may be illicitly using anabolic steroids; steroid abuse may increase blood pressure and cause hypokalemic alkalosis.

There are a number of simple commercially available screening kits which detect drugs of abuse and their metabolites in urine samples. These can be employed at the interview or pretrial medical stage to eliminate abusers. False-positive results can occur, but equivocal or contested positive results can be verified by high pressure liquid chromatography. We would also recommend random screening for drugs and alcohol on the first day of each phase of "in-house" studies, and on study days when volunteers are not resident within the research center. Although self-reporting of smoking habits is generally accurate when verified by biochemical assessment,[62] measurement of plasma or salivary cotinine is both sensitive and specific,[63,64] and can be used during pretrial screening to corroborate reported cigarette consumption. Illicit smoking during studies can be confirmed using an inexpensive user-friendly apparatus such as the "Smokelyzer" (Bedfont Technical Instruments, Upchurch, Kent, England) which measures the carbon monoxide concentration of expired air.

The use of over-the-counter pharmaceutical preparations must also be considered. For instance, sympathomimetics (commonly used as nasal decongestants) may exert a systemic pressor effect.[65] Nonsteroidal anti-inflammatory drugs may cause salt and water retention[66] and block prostaglandin production, and so should be avoided for a minimum of two weeks before studies of antihypertensive drugs. They may particularly interfere with the actions of diuretics and ACE inhibitors.

2.2 Safety Considerations

The physician performing clinical pharmacology studies is bound by the Hippocratic principle *primum non nocere* (first do no harm). This has been enshrined in local codes of practice[49,67] and in international guidelines.[68] Tolerability and safety data should be collected from the first drug administration to man onward. There are no requirements in terms of the minimum number of healthy volunteers who should be exposed to a drug for safety assessments but, by the end of the drug development program, data should eventually be available from in excess of 1500 hypertensive patients (see Table 1). Details of (postural) hypotensive episodes and their relation to drug dosage should be recorded, particularly stating if they have occurred on first exposure to drug or are associated with increasing dose. Changes in the electrocardiogram should be characterized. Evidence of changes in heart rate, vasodilatation, and fluid retention should be reported as well as more serious side effects such as the develoment of renal impairment or heart failure, as should central nervous effects, sexual dysfunction, and changes in serum lipids, glucose, or electrolytes. Subjects should be studied not only during periods of drug administration, but also following withdrawal, and withdrawal effects should be fully characterized unless the new drug is a member of a class known to be free from such effects. Any relationship between drug dose and side effects should be investigated. Adverse effects should be separated to distinguish those on monotherapy from those which occur during combination therapy. Subjective changes, for instance in mood or alertness, associated with drug treatment can be characterized using visual analogue scales.[69]

Table 1 Numbers of Healthy Volunteers and Patients Exposed to New Active Substances at the Time of Marketing (1987-1989)

	Median	(Range)
Healthy volunteers	67	(41-742)
Efficacy studies	1,120	(43-4,906)
Safety database	1,528	(43-15,962)

From Rawlins, M.D. (1995). *J. R. Coll. Phys.*, **29,** 41-49. With permission.

2.3 Methods

2.3.1 General Trial Design

2.3.1.1 Diet

Diet plays an important role in modifying the pharmacokinetics of many compounds and should be standardized during all clinical studies. The presence of food may impair the absorption of orally administered drugs. Gastric absorption is generally favored by an empty stomach, but the absorption of highly lipophilic drugs is aided by a fatty meal. Food has little effect on the absorption and bioavailability of captopril[70,71] or enalapril,[72] but the bioavailability of atenolol is reduced by about 20%.[73] However, food increases the bioavailability of propranolol and metoprolol by 30-80%,[73,74] and of labetalol by 40%,[75] by changing the extent of their first-pass metabolism through the liver. First-pass metabolism of felodipine and other dihydropyridine calcium antagonists is inhibited by grapefruit juice,[76] an effect which may be clinically important because (study) medication is often consumed at breakfast time. Citrus juices should not be part of the dietary regimen for dihydropyridine studies.

Dietary salt intake must be considered in all studies of antihypertensive agents. Salt depletion activates the renin-angiotensin system, and may sensitize subjects to the hypotensive effects of renin inhibitors,[77] ACE inhibitors,[78] and angiotensin receptor antagonists.[79] Indeed, salt depletion may be a valuable strategy to maximize the pharmacodynamic effects of such drugs in healthy subjects,[77] in whom the effects of hypotensive drugs are typically small. By increasing the magnitude of the hypotensive response, salt depletion can increase the power of a study to detect an effect of treatment. Conversely, subjects on high salt diets will have a reduced response to these drugs, but may be more sensitive to the effects of diuretics.

Detailed guidance on the regulatory requirements of food interaction studies is available from the FDA.[80]

2.3.1.2 First-into-Man Studies

Safety is the primary concern during the first administration of a new drug to man. The starting dose should be chosen on the basis of preclinical data, and is usually 100 to 1000-fold less than the minimum effective dose or the maximum nontoxic dose in animal studies. Initial studies are limited to single doses until a human dose-response relationship, pharmacokinetic profile and safety have been established. Blood pressure and heart rate should be monitored at regular intervals throughout the study; automated or semi-automated blood pressure monitoring may offer the advantage of eliminating observer bias (see Section 2.3.3). Continuous monitoring of the electrocardiogram should be mandatory in first-into-man studies, and regular noninvasive measurement of cardiac output, for example, by bioimpedance cardiography, to obtain a measure of peripheral vascular resistance, may add valuable information on efficacy of relevance to the design of subsequent studies (see Section 2.3.3). Indeed, this technique may be more sensitive than blood pressure in determining whether or not a drug is an effective vasodilator agent. For instance, bioimpedance measurements during the first human systemic studies of endothelin receptor antagonists[81] demonstrated that a small reduction in blood pressure was accompanied by a more marked reduction in peripheral vascular resistance; also, bioimpedance measurements during the first studies with the nitric oxide synthase inhibitor L-NMMA[82] showed that a rather small increase in blood pressure was associated with a large and highly significant increase in peripheral vascular resistance. In studies with drugs which block the renin-angiotensin system, salt depletion may be used to maximize the effects of the study drug and may reduce the number of volunteers needing to be studied.

In ascending-dose, single-dose studies, subjects are randomly allocated to placebo or to a fixed dose of drug. Doses rise logarithmically between phases (1x, 3x, 10x, 30x, etc.). Different subjects are usually used in each phase. The response of each group of subjects is compared. Typically around six volunteers might take part in any phase, four receiving active medication and two placebo. This study design allows placebo-controlled data to be collected relatively quickly and comparisons to be made between subjects, but it does not allow intrasubject comparisons to be made, such that variability tends to be large. This study design is relatively resistant to protocol violations (subject withdrawals), although the number of subjects required is generally larger than for cross-over studies.

In ascending-dose, multiple-dose cross-over studies, all subjects will receive all or some of the treatments in a predetermined ascending dose fashion. Fewer subjects are needed than with the single-dose design. Cross-over studies have distinct pharmacological advantages. Both inter- and intrasubject comparisons can be made, so reducing variability. Furthermore, the statistical power of cross-over studies is greater than that of parallel group studies. However, cross-over studies carry with them certain inherent design difficulties. They are most easily conducted when drug effects develop and stop quickly; carry-over effects from treatment are always possible, and the washout period between phases must take account of this to ensure comparability of baseline parameters between phases. Cross-over studies depend on subjects' baseline blood pressure remaining constant between phases, although, in the absence of carry-over effects, this will usually be the case. Inclusion of a placebo phase is essential to determine whether side effects are drug related in these early phase studies. Cross-over studies are often of relatively long duration, and may be complicated by subjects dropping out, for one reason or another, before the study is complete (although all data generated by defaulters can be included in the analysis as far as is statistically appropriate). When such defaulters have to be replaced, it can markedly impede progress with the study. If a subject in a "first-into-man" study experiences a clinically significant adverse event, it may become necessary to postpone the completion of the study. It may be decided to abandon further investigation of the drug in man, or to investigate the effects of a lower dose on a larger number of subjects before proceeding to higher doses. Finally, the number of phases in a cross-over study may be limited by the total blood loss, or by the volunteers' total exposure to study drug. Both of these study designs can be expanded by studying larger numbers of subjects at the maximum tolerated dose.

2.3.1.3 Early Phase Studies

There are no fixed guidelines with regard to the number of doses of drug which should be studied in phases I and II. The optimal dose in clinical practice is the lowest which produces the desired therapeutic effect. Although there will be individual variation in the magnitude of the response to any given drug, it is usually not feasible to investigate more than a few doses. It has been suggested[83] that at least three dose levels are assessed against placebo during the drug development program. Comparison of only one dose with placebo may allow the null hypothesis to be rejected, but will not allow the construction of a dose-response relationship. Although a linear relationship might be demonstrated with two doses of active drug and placebo, it is unlikely that studying only two doses at phase III will be sufficient for registration purposes.[83] Ideally, a dose near the bottom of the response curve, a dose near the top of the curve, a maximal dose, and a supramaximal dose would be studied early in the drug development program (Figure 1). By the end of phase II, one should know the minimum effective dose in man and the maximum tolerated dose. In addition, one should have an indication of the probable dose range in the patient population. Although dose-response data will be available from phase III and IV trials, it is prudent to carry out dose-ranging studies early in development (phase I or early phase II) to avoid performing phase III trials using doses which may be widely different from those which will subsequently be recommended for clinical use, or the need to revise the dosing schedules of the entire clinical program at phase III or IV, and the accumulation of a large database at subtherapeutic or excessive doses. This has been a common problem for antihypertensive drugs in the past, usually overestimating the required dose.

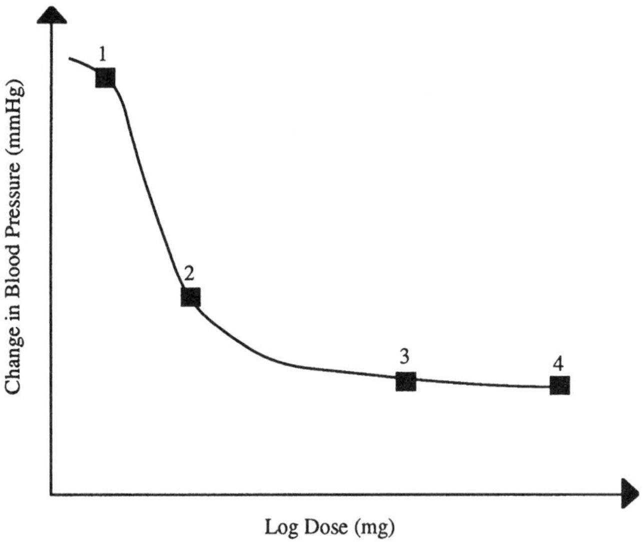

Figure 1 The effect of dose of antihypertensive agent on blood pressure. Ideally, during phase II, a minimum of four drug doses from the initial dose-ranging studies should be studied in detail. These should include a dose with threshold effects on blood pressure (1), a dose with near maximum effects (2), a maximal dose, (3) and a supra-maximal dose (4). The supra-maximal dose should be two to three times the lowest dose producing the maximum drug effect. (From FDA. (1988) Division of Cardio-Renal Products, *Proposed Guidelines for the Clinical Evaluation of Antihypertensive Drugs.* Washington, D.C., Government Printing Office.)

After the initial administration to man, dose-ranging trials in hypertension can follow a number of designs, including parallel group, cross-over, and titration models. Initial studies are performed with single drug doses, but when sufficient safety data are available, multiple dose studies are required. The initial dose for multiple dose studies will be determined by the pharmacokinetic, pharmacodynamic, and safety data generated during the preceding single dose studies. In order to ensure comparability of subject groups and to avoid investigator bias, studies should be of adequate power, well controlled, randomized, and, ideally, performed double-blind. The dose range in such studies should be as wide as is compatible with subject safety. This can avoid revision of dosing schedules during the later stages of the development program.

After phase I, dose-response relationships are probably most commonly examined using a parallel study design in which subjects are randomized to several fixed doses of active drug.[84] The possibility of a confounding change in blood pressure independent of treatment can be avoided by including a placebo group. Although in theory it is not always necessary to include a placebo, because higher doses reducing blood pressure more than lower doses can be interpreted as evidence of drug effect, the inclusion of a placebo also allows the magnitude of the drug effect to be defined, and is particularly important if all the doses administered lie at the top of the dose-response curve (cf. Figure 1). The reduction in blood pressure which occurs with repeated measurements can also be minimized by performing frequent measurements using an automated ambulatory blood pressure recording device. Parallel group studies allow information about a range of doses to be gathered over a short period of time but, because for the purpose of analysis each subject receives only one dose of drug, it is difficult to obtain information about individual dose-response relationships. Furthermore, relatively large numbers of subjects may be required to reach statistically significant conclusions. For these reasons, cross-over or dose titration designs in which subjects receive more than one dose of drug are preferable.[85] Cross-over designs facilitate the collection of individual dose-response information from all participants. They are discussed in detail in this section.

The investigation of new antihypertensive drugs often involves a period of dose titration or escalation, doses being increased at predetermined intervals until fixed efficacy endpoints are reached.

This study design is generally more common in phase III. However, it can be usefully employed in studies of new antihypertensive agents by including hypertensive subjects in phase II. This design ensures that subjects are initially exposed to only low doses of drug, and at the same time allows a dose sufficient to produce a predetermined effect to be reached, while providing dose-response information from all participants. In this way, by exposing subjects to a range of doses limited by response, dose titration studies resemble the situation in clinical practice. However, the usual design of dose titration studies allows drug and time-effects to become confused. These studies cannot distinguish a response to increased drug dose from a response associated with increased time on study medication, and so are unsatisfactory when the full response to a drug is delayed as is usually the case in hypertension. For instance, the hypotensive response to propranolol develops only slowly; administration is initially associated with a reduction in cardiac output and heart rate, but if prolonged, a decrease in blood pressure also occurs, reflecting a fall in peripheral resistance.[86] This can lead to overestimation of the dose of drug needed, and it is therefore important that early phase multiple dose studies are of sufficient duration to achieve steady-state pharmacodynamic effects. Similarly, the effective dose of a drug may be overestimated because nonresponders are included in the study population. Studies of antihypertensive drugs are particularly prone to errors of this kind, because patients often have a spontaneous fall in blood pressure during research studies. This was well illustrated in the Medical Research Council trial in mild-to-moderate hypertension, where there were substantial reductions in blood pressure during the first three months of placebo treatment.[5] The same phenomenon was also observed in early studies of captopril, and probably contributed to dose-related toxicity. Indeed, these drugs were almost withdrawn from investigation before reaching clinical practice because of their side effects at high doses.[87] Studies of a similar design led to inappropriately high doses of both atenolol and chlorthalidone being employed for many years in clinical practice.[84] Another difficulty with titration studies is that the dose-response relationship is often spuriously flattened because poor responders make up a substantial proportion of subjects receiving the highest dose of drug. Instead of a linear relationship between blood pressure and drug dose, a minority of subjects will be relatively resistant to the effects of any given drug, and increasing the dose in these subjects will not result in a further fall in blood pressure. It should be remembered, however, that an excessive first dose effect can occur, as with ACE inhibitors and alpha-adrenoceptor blocking drugs.

Titration studies are most successful when the duration of the drug effect and the number of withdrawals is small. Under these circumstances, they can provide a reasonable indication of the dose-response relationship, which can be elaborated upon in subsequent studies. They have the advantages that fewer subjects are needed than in parallel group designs, and they are generally shorter than cross-over studies, while still providing individual dose-response data. As with cross-over studies, data from subjects who default before titration studies are complete can be included in the final analysis.

Clinical trials must consider not only the dose-response relationship of the therapeutic effects of the drug, but also the relationship between overall exposure to the study drug and the incidence of adverse events; one must consider both the duration of treatment and the dose of drug administered. For instance, side effects which are time related may not be apparent during the relatively short duration of most early phase studies. Furthermore, side effects may occur across a different dose range from the therapeutic effect. For many years, what are now considered to be relatively high doses of thiazide diuretics were used both in clinical practice and in large scale outcome trials evaluating their effects on cardiovascular morbidity and mortality. After more than 20 years of clinical experience, it is now clear that the metabolic effects of the thiazide diuretics occur at higher doses than the hypotensive effects,[88-90] (Figure 2), and that higher doses produce more side effects without increased antihypertensive efficacy. Thus, single dose and chronic dosing studies must be performed early in the drug evaluation program to characterize the temporal nature of the drug response.

2.3.1.4 Statistical Considerations in Hemodynamic Studies

Studies should ideally be performed on the basis of power calculations including a sufficient number of subjects to allow a statistically meaningful conclusion to be drawn from the results. Analysis of cross-over studies should be of a nature which excludes carry-over effects, and analysis of titration trials should take account of the fact that all subjects may not have received the same dose of study drug. Specific maneuvers such as salt depletion (see Section 2.3.1) and ambulatory blood pressure monitoring (see Section 2.3.3) can be used to increase the power of early phase studies to detect hemodynamic effects.

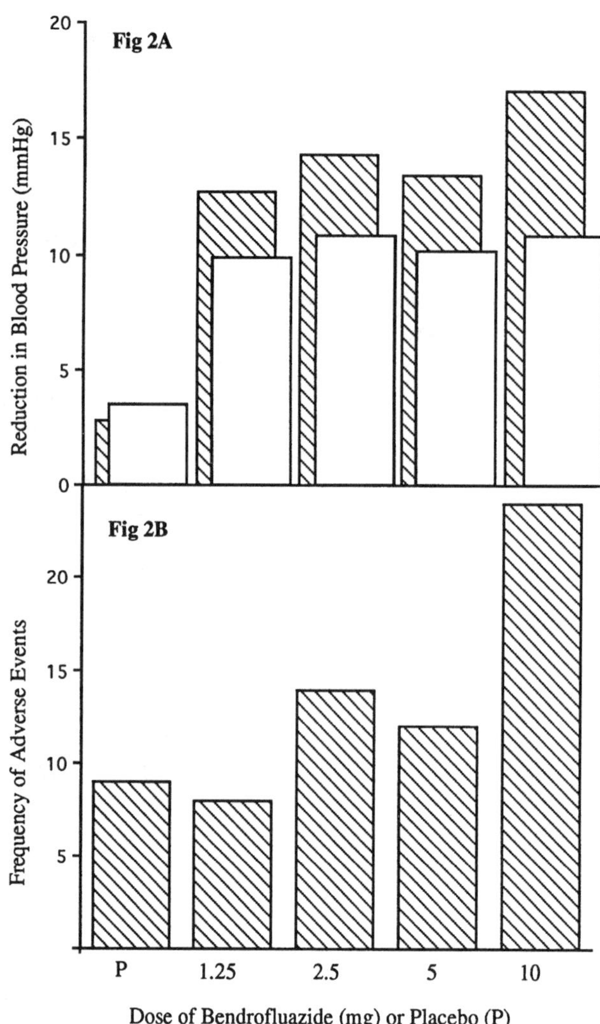

Figure 2 Relationships between bendrofluazide dose and diastolic blood pressure, plasma urate and plasma potassium. Figure 2A shows the reduction in systolic (striped) and diastolic (solid) blood pressure in response to 10-12 weeks' treatment with placebo or bendrofluazide. Figure 2B shows the overall numbers of adverse events for each treatment group, and Figures 2C and 2D show the change in plasma urate and potassium associated with each treatment. Although the effect on blood pressure is essentially maximal at 1.25 mg bendrofluazide daily, the effects on plasma urate and plasma potassium, and the incidence of adverse events are significantly higher with 5 and 10 mg bendrofluazide daily than with the lower doses. (Adapted from Carlsen, J.E. et al. (1990), *Br. Med. J.,* **300,** 975-978. With permission.)

2.3.2 Pharmacokinetic Issues

One of the main objectives of phase I studies is to obtain pharmacokinetic data. Pharmacokinetic studies may be usefully performed in normotensive and hypertensive subjects and, although studies in individuals who resemble the target population are encouraged,[91] pharmacokinetic measurements in normotensive subjects usually reflect the situation in hypertensive patients. However, the major demographic or pathophysiological characteristics of the target population, such as age, race, renal disease, and the use of common concomitant medication, should all be considered at an early stage in the drug development program, though further data will accrue during the course of phase III studies.

Where possible, oral and intravenous dosing regimens should be studied in order to generate a complete metabolic and pharmacodynamic profile of the drug. For instance, orally administered propranolol relies on first-pass metabolism to generate its active hydroxylated derivative, but this does not happen with intravenous dosing,[86,92] and many ACE inhibitors are prodrugs which are de-esterified by

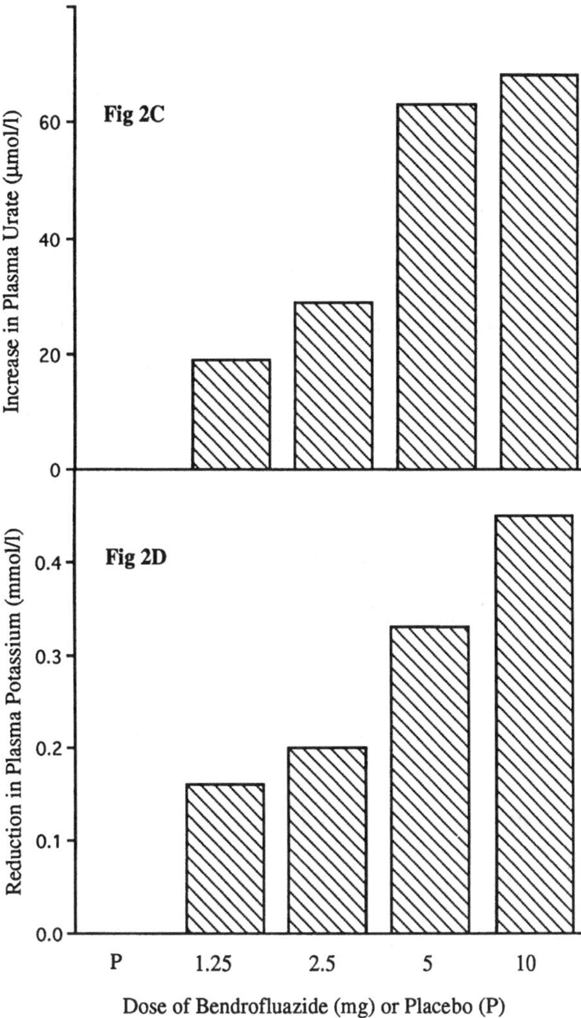

Figure 2 (continued)

the liver to yield the active compounds.[93] The availability of an intravenous preparation in phase II can facilitate the gathering of useful information on efficacy more quickly, by eliminating considerations of bioavailability, permitting acute hemodynamic studies, and allowing "proof of concept studies," for instance, using local infusions of subsystemic doses of drug (see Section 2.3.3). However, intravenous preparations of antihypertensive drugs usually have limited therapeutic potential, and so are not always included in the development program. This can prove to be a false economy.

Pharmacokinetic studies provide information not only about the general metabolic fate of a drug, but also about the relationship between plasma drug concentration and the therapeutic response. Pharmacokinetic/pharmacodynamic relationships for individual subjects can be examined in early phase studies.[94] There may be a relatively narrow dose range over which the drug is active, as with beta-blockers and thiazide diuretics, or else there may be a wider dose range, as with ACE inhibitors. Such pharmacokinetic studies may also yield important information concerning the mechanism of action of drugs. For instance, the hypotensive effect of ACE inhibitors correlates poorly with reduction of circulating ACE activity,[95] and the response is more closely related to inhibition of the tissue enzyme;[96] thus, the hemodynamic effect of an ACE inhibitor may be quite independent of its inhibition of the circulating enzyme, and its calculated circulating plasma half-life may have little bearing on its duration of action.[97]

Formulations of antihypertensive drugs which allow smooth blood pressure control with once daily dosing are a particular boon for the treatment of this asymptomatic condition and improve patient compliance. Beta-adrenoceptor blockers, calcium antagonists, thiazide diuretics, and the angiotensin receptor antagonist, losartan, can usually be prescribed once daily; many ACE inhibitors are also effective with once-daily dosing. For shorter acting agents, if the relationship between the plasma levels of an immediate release (IR) formulation of a drug and its clinical response is well established, a sustained release (SR) preparation of the drug may qualify for approval on the basis of bioequivalence studies. If a linear relationship exists for drug clearance, it will be necessary to demonstrate that the maximum plasma concentration (C_{MAX}) of the SR preparation is no greater, and the minimum plasma concentration (C_{MIN}) no less, than that of the IR formulation, in studies using doses within the projected therapeutic ranges of both preparations. For drugs with nonlinear elimination, a minimum of two doses of the SR preparation should be compared with doses at the top and bottom of the projected therapeutic range of the IR preparation; the C_{MIN} of the SR preparation should be no less, and the C_{MAX} and area under plasma concentration (AUC) should be no greater, than those of the IR formulation. If the plasma drug concentration/effect relationship, drug efficacy and time-effect relationships are not well established for the IR preparations, then they should be fully characterized for the SR preparation in studies of an appropriate design. There are now many effective, well-tolerated drugs which can be taken once or twice daily for the treatment of hypertension, such that it is unlikely that new compounds with short half-lives requiring more than twice daily dosing will be commercially successful. Indeed, once-daily drugs may soon prove to be the rule.

2.3.3 Pharmacodynamic Issues

The processes involved in the maintenance of blood pressure in hypertension may be different from those in health, and it might be argued that the response, or lack of it, in a healthy volunteer study would not reliably predict the situation in hypertensive patients. However, all the drugs which are currently used in the treatment of hypertension can be described as "hypotensive," rather than "antihypertensive" because they lower blood pressure to the same proportionate level in normotensive subjects as in hypertensive patients. A truly antihypertensive drug would need to have a blood pressure-lowering action specific to the pathology of the hypertensive process, and this seems unlikely in a polygenic condition also influenced by a wide range of environmental factors.[98,99]

One of the purposes of phase I pharmacodynamic studies is to establish that the hemodynamic responses and *in vitro* effects observed in preclinical studies are also present in man. The hypotensive dose range should be defined in placebo-controlled dose-ranging studies. At the end of these studies, data should be available from a range of doses which includes a dose near the start of the dose-response relationship, and either a dose near or at the upper end of the dose-response curve, or a dose which produces less than the maximum response, but beyond which side effects are unacceptable (see Figure 1). The FDA suggests that a dose can be demonstrated as producing a maximal response when doses two to threefold higher produce no greater effect.[91] It is not necessary to demonstrate significantly different responses between the doses studied to establish the useful dosing range of the drug, but only a significant difference from placebo. Hemodynamic and pharmacokinetic results should be correlated, and the hemodynamic response at trough and peak plasma levels examined in the same studies. An "all or nothing" relationship between drug dose and hypotensive effect may suggest that supramaximal doses of drug are being studied (cf. Figure 1), and indicates that lower doses should be investigated to establish the dose-response relationship. This phenomenon was originally observed with hydralazine,[100] but also explains the lack of relationship between hypotensive response and dose of beta-adrenoceptor antagonist in many studies.[101] The doses of many of the older antihypertensive drugs now commonly employed in clinical practice are much lower than in earlier years. Generally, antihypertensive drugs have been launched at doses which have subsequently been shown to be too high, and this may, to some extent, reflect poor study design; studies may have been of insufficient duration to allow the full hypotensive effect of the drug to develop, or else unnecessarily high doses have been selected on the basis of forced titration studies.

It has been suggested that the efficacy of antihypertensive drugs should be evaluated as a trough:peak ratio, which is calculated as the percentage of the maximum decrease in blood pressure which is still detectable at the end of the dose interval.[102] The FDA has adopted the trough:peak ratio as a criterion for the evaluation of new antihypertensive drugs,[91] and suggests that new antihypertensive agents or formulations should have 50-60% of their maximum efficacy at trough plasma concentrations. These guidelines set a new safety standard which should ensure that peak effects are not much more pronounced than trough effects, decreasing the risk of wide fluctuations in blood pressure between doses and consequent symptomatic hypotension. Furthermore, this parameter provides a method of assessing the appropriateness of the dosing interval to allow smooth control of blood pressure between doses; in particular, it should prevent the administration of unnecessarily high doses of short-acting agents in attempts at once-daily dosing. Frequent measurements of blood pressure by "ambulatory" methods may be particularly useful in determining trough:peak relationships. In reality, these usually comprise frequent automated, rather than truly ambulatory, measurements. Unfortunately, however, thus far there have been no guidelines for the methodology or equipment which should be used to determine this ratio.

Although the time-course of the dose-response relationship can be examined using ambulatory blood pressure monitoring equipment, at present there are no official guidelines for the interpretation of such data. However, ambulatory blood pressure monitoring has already proven a valuable research tool.[103] It eliminates observer bias during blood pressure measurements, and does not give rise to a "white coat effect."[104] Twenty-four hour ambulatory blood pressure recordings performed every 30 min correspond closely with simultaneous intra-arterial recordings,[105] and are highly reproducible.[106] Furthermore, no placebo response to ambulatory monitoring is seen in clinical trials,[107,108] such that it may provide valuable information even in studies which lack a placebo limb, and could simplify the conduct of trials of antihypertensive drugs.[109] It has been suggested that ambulatory blood pressure monitoring offers a precision which allows valid conclusions to be drawn using smaller numbers of subjects than are required in trials using manual blood pressure measurement,[107,110] and the routine use of ambulatory blood pressure recording in clinical trials of antihypertensive drugs has been strongly advocated.[111] However, this remains controversial, and a recent study suggests that this technique may not necessarily economize on cohort size.[112]

2.3.3.1 Systemic Hemodynamic Studies

Measurement of blood pressure represents the minimum investigation necessary to characterize the hemodynamic effects of new antihypertensive drugs. Although supine or sitting blood pressures are acceptable as evidence of efficacy,[91] postural effects should be characterized by erect and supine measurements as evidence of safety. It is important that early phase studies are designed to yield information about the systemic hemodynamics and mechanism of drug action. This can be achieved by measurement of cardiac output and total or local vascular resistance. In recent years, it has become possible to measure many hemodynamic parameters noninvasively.[36,113-115] For instance, cardiac output can be assessed quickly, simply, and noninvasively by measurement of transthoracic bioimpedance.[81,82,116] Transthoracic bioimpedance measurements allow good intrasubject assessment of drug effects on cardiac output and peripheral vascular resistance (see Section 2.3.1). Noninvasive measurement of large artery pulse wave reflection provides information about the arteriovenous selectivity of antihypertensive drugs, and may contribute to our understanding of the long-term structural changes associated with antihypertensive therapy.[117] Vasodilatation in medium-sized arteries can also be simply and noninvasively measured using wall-tracking devices.[118] Useful safety information can be obtained by recordings of the electrocardiogram at fixed time points, or continuously by Holter monitoring or telemetry.

2.3.3.2 Local Hemodynamic Studies

It is now possible to investigate the drug effects in human arteries, arterioles, veins, and capillaries *in vivo*. These techniques can replace, or at least complement, some animal experimentation, are safe (using only subsystemic doses of drug), and can easily be employed early in the clinical drug development program to provide useful mechanistic information. They can provide *in vivo* proof of concepts generated during experiments *in vitro*. For instance, enalapril had been shown *in vitro* to block vascular ACE. In forearm studies in man, the active metabolite, enalaprilat, antagonizes the vasoconstrictor effects of exogenous angiotensin I, but not angiotensin II, consistent with ACE inhibition as its mode of action,[119] (Figure 3A). Furthermore, the kinetics of subsystemic drug administration to the forearm confirm that angiotensin conversion occurs at the level of the vascular (rather than the circulating) enzyme. Additionally, such studies have shown that vascular ACE metabolizes bradykinin *in vivo*[119] and suggest that ACE inhibitors may affect endothelial function through inhibition of bradykinin metabolism,[120] with potential clinical benefits occurring through nitric oxide generation and independent of their well-recognized effect on angiotensin metabolism. Such studies depend on the availability of an intravenous formulation of drug, or, where appropriate, its active metabolite.

The vasoactive effects of antihypertensive agents can be studied in forearm resistance vessels,[81,115] and cutaneous capacitance vessels[115,121,122] using subsystemic, locally active doses of drug. This approach has several attractions. First, because these techniques employ only a hundredth to a thousandth of the dose of drug required to produce central or systemic effects, they are particularly safe, and can be utilized early in the clinical program. Second, because such doses are only locally active, they allow direct

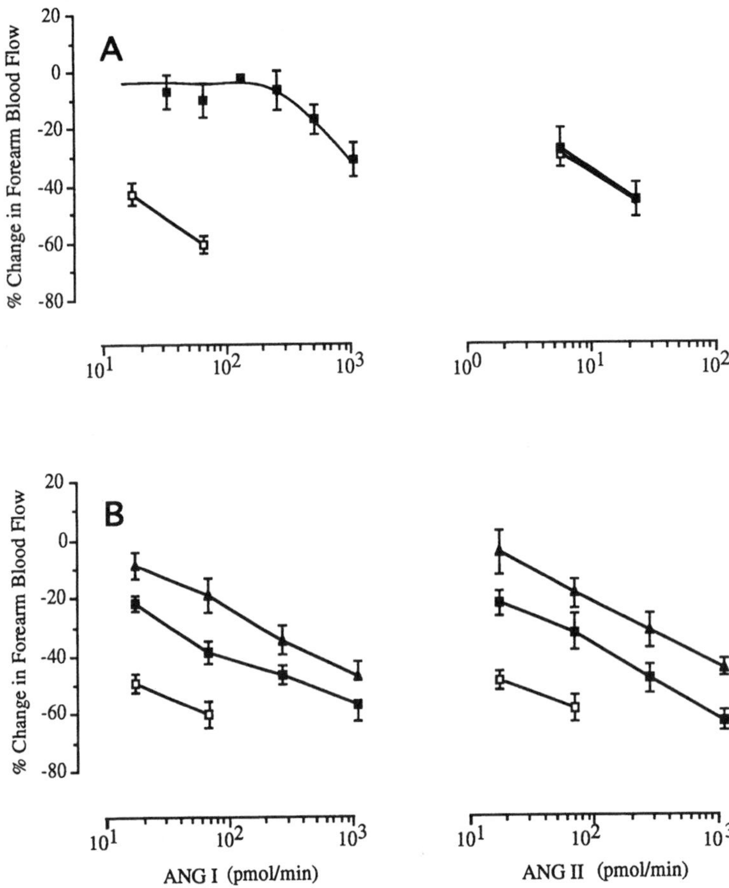

Figure 3 Effect of orally administered losartan on forearm blood flow response to subsystemic doses of angiotensin. Figure 3A shows the effect on forearm blood flow of subsystemic doses of angiotensin I (ANG I) and angiotensin II (ANG II) administered via the brachial artery in the presence ■ and absence □ of a subsystemic infusion of enalaprilat. Both angiotensin I and angiotensin II produce dose-dependent reductions in forearm blood flow. In the presence of enalaprilat, the dose-response relationship to angiotensin I, but not to angiotensin II, is markedly shifted to the right, consistent with vasoconstriction to angiotensin I occurring only after conversion to angiotensin II by ACE. Figure 3B shows the effect of subsystemic doses of angiotensin I and angiotensin II administered via the brachial artery after oral administration of placebo □, losartan 20 mg ■, or losartan 100 mg ▲. In contrast to enalaprilat, which has a selective effect on the response to angiotensin I, losartan causes a dose-dependent attenuation of the vasoconstriction in response to both angiotensin I and angiotensin II, consistent with angiotensin receptor antagonism as its mode of action. (Adapted from Benjamin, N. et al. (1989) *J. Physiol.*, **412,** 543-555 and Cockcroft, J.R. et al. (1993). *Cardiovasc. Pharmacol.*, **22,** 579-584. With permission.)

assessment of the effects of a drug on the resistance vessels without eliciting effects mediated through actions on other organs or by stimulation of neurohumoral reflexes. Third, the forearm responses obtained during local drug infusions tend to reflect those of the major resistance beds.[115] These techniques are potentially useful for "proof of concept" studies.

Forearm blood flow can be measured simply, using venous occlusion plethysmography together with drug administration at subsystemic doses via a fine-bore brachial artery cannula. The technique is of proven reproducibility,[123] and changes in blood flow at a fixed perfusion pressure provide a reliable measure of resistance vessel tone. Because the drug is effectively confined to the infused limb and perfusion pressure remains constant, the opposite forearm can serve as an untreated contemporaneous control.[119] The forearm vessels have endogenous tone, allowing the effects of both vasodilators and vasoconstrictors to be assessed. This technique has been used to study the vasodilation caused by ACE inhibitors,[119,124] potassium channel openers,[125] endothelin converting enzyme inhibitors (ECE; Figure 4),[126] and endothelin receptor antagonists,[81] confirming the mechanisms of action of these drugs predicted from *in vitro* studies. In addition to providing a proof of concept of previous *in vitro* work, these studies have provided new insights into vascular physiology. For instance, studies with the nitric oxide synthase inhibitor, L-NMMA, have shown that nitric oxide exerts a tonic vasodilator effect in resistance vessels[127] and studies with phosphoramidon, thiorphan, and the endothelin A-type receptor antagonist, BQ-123, indicate a tonic constrictor role for endothelin.[128] These studies predicted the pressor response to systemic L-NMMA[82] and the depressor response to systemic doses of endothelin antagonist in man.[81]

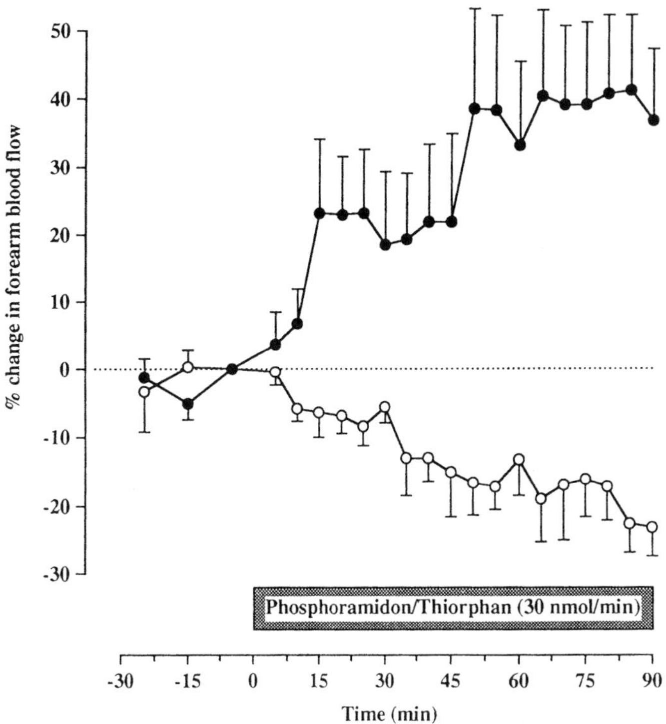

Figure 4 Effect of intra-arterial infusion of subsystemic doses of phosphoramidon and thiorphan on forearm blood flow. In separate experiments, the mixed ECE and NEP inhibitor, phosphoramidon •, and a relatively selective NEP inhibitor, thiorphan ○, were infused at a subsystemic concentration via the brachial artery. Phosphoramidon produces a progressive vasodilatation, whereas thiorphan causes vasoconstriction. The vasoconstrictor response to thiorphan was not predicted, and is consistent with the balance of the effects of NEP inhibition being to decrease degradation of vasoconstrictors, including angiotensin II and endothelin-1, more than to reduce degradation of the vasodilator natriuretic peptides. (Adapted from Haynes, W.G. and Webb, D.J. (1994). *Lancet,* **344,** 852-854. With permission.)

When the mixed ECE and neutral endopeptidase (NEP) inhibitor phosphoramidon is administered via the brachial artery, substantial forearm vasodilatation results.[128] Theoretically, this effect could be mediated by decreased generation of endothelin-1, or by decreased degradation of the vasodilator, atrial natriuretic peptide. In order to determine which of these mechanisms was responsible, the relatively selective NEP inhibitor thiorphan was separately infused by the brachial artery route. Perhaps surprisingly, thiorphan caused vasoconstriction, probably because the balance of its effects favors decreased metabolism of angiotensin II and/or endothelin-1, over decreased breakdown of natriuretic peptides. These observations confirm that ECE inhibition causes the vasodilatation associated with phosphoramidon. Vasoconstriction in response to NEP inhibition was not envisaged from the preclinical data, but is consonant with the failure of NEP inhibitors to lower blood pressure in hypertensive patients.[129] Early phase mechanistic studies in humans might have obviated the need for an extensive, and ultimately unsuccessful, development of these new drugs for the treatment of essential hypertension.

Changes in dorsal hand vein size can be measured by the Aellig technique. In warm, rested, healthy subjects the hand veins have no endogenous tone and can be used to directly assess the effects of vasoconstrictors on the cutaneous capacitance vessels.[130,131] Additionally, the vessels can be preconstricted by a local infusion of noradrenaline to allow studies of vasodilators.[125,131,132] The effects of drugs on human arteries and veins *in vivo* have been measured and compared using forearm plethysmography and the Aellig technique, leading to the concept of arteriovenous selectivity.[133] For instance, prazosin and the organic nitrates have been shown to exert their vascular effects mainly in the venous system, whereas cromakalim, hydralazine, and nifedipine are predominantly arterioselective.[125,132]

These techniques need not always be used with locally administered subsystemic doses of drug; they can also be employed in systemic dosing studies. For instance, forearm plethysmography has recently been employed to assess the vascular effects of orally administered ACE inhibitor (enalapril) and angiotensin receptor antagonist (losartan).[134] Both compounds produce a "right shift" of the dose-response curves to intra-arterial angiotensin I, but only losartan shifts the curve for angiotensin II, indicating that losartan is a selective antagonist of the angiotensin receptor and shows no ACE inhibitor activity (Figure 3). This study provides *in vivo* proof of the mechanism of action of losartan observed in earlier *in vitro* studies. Such studies may be valuable at a very early stage of clinical development.

These methods can be included safely in phase I and II clinical trials, permitting mechanistic studies of new vasoactive pharmaceutical agents to corroborate the results of earlier animal studies in man. They allow concepts to be more quickly transferred from the laboratory to the clinic, the objective of early phase trials, and through their application the divisions between basic and clinical research are steadily being broken down.

3 PATIENT STUDIES

The general considerations outlined above concerning subject selection, methods, trial design, and duration apply to studies with hypertensive as well as normotensive subjects. There are, however, some special considerations relating to the inclusion of hypertensive patients in clinical trials.

3.1 Selection Criteria

Before participation in studies, hypertensive patients should be characterized according to the severity of their hypertension (cf. Table 1) and the presence or absence of left ventricular hypertrophy. Assessment of the grade of hypertension is of particular importance in parallel group studies to guarantee equivalence between treatment groups. Furthermore, as cardiovascular risk is related to the severity of hypertension, there are important ethical considerations concerning withdrawal of treatment from patients with more severe hypertension. In this situation, an alternative approach is randomized placebo-controlled studies of withdrawal of one agent, where blood pressure has initially been adequately controlled on a combination of drugs. This study design allows the contribution of individual agents to be legitimately assessed by their withdrawal.

Secondary causes of hypertension should be excluded,[135] as the mechanisms underlying essential hypertension may be different, and this may be reflected in the response to a novel hypotensive drug. It would seem reasonable to specifically seek a secondary cause of high blood pressure in young patients (<30 years), those whose blood pressure remains uncontrolled on two drugs, and those with accelerated hypertension or hypertension of sudden onset.[135]

3.2 Safety Considerations

These have been discussed in detail above (Section 2.2). It should be remembered that the absolute reduction in blood pressure associated with drug administration in patients with high blood pressure may be substantially greater than that in healthy volunteers, such that it may be safer to perform first-into-man studies of novel antihypertensive agents in healthy subjects. In terms of recruitment of adequate numbers of untreated subjects, it would probably also be impractical to perform all early phase studies of antihypertensive drugs in patients.

3.3 Methods

The main study designs have been described above (Section 2.3.1). As with early phase studies in healthy volunteers, the parallel group design is probably the most common.[48] There are, however, a number of special considerations in early phase studies of hypertensive subjects.

Dose-ranging trials may be counted as efficacy studies for the purposes of registration, providing a sufficient number of patients is included. It may not always be ethical to include patients in a placebo-controlled trial, particularly in the situation, as with hypertension, where drugs of established efficacy are available. Under these circumstances, patients may usefully be included as part of a factorial trial, receiving study drug and an established therapy.[136] The reference drug in factorial trials should always be selected with respect to efficacy (superior to others) and safety (largest amount of clinical data available). Often in trials of antihypertensive drugs the reference drug is a thiazide diuretic and, given that nondiuretic antihypertensive agents are likely to be co-administered with diuretics in clinical practice, the interaction with thiazides should be considered at an early stage in the drug development program. The use of a reference drug can be particularly important in estimating the frequency of adverse effects in clinical trials. Many common symptoms, such as headache, lethargy, and cough can occur with placebo as well as with drugs of different classes. For instance, the frequency of cough in patients who had previously experienced cough with an ACE inhibitor is 29% with the angiotensin receptor blocker losartan, which is similar to that with hydrochlorothiazide (34%), and substantially lower than that is associated with re-exposure to ACE inhibitor (72%), but still not negligible;[137] the inclusion of hydrochlorthiazide as a comparator in this study suggests that cough with losartan is nonspecific. It can also be useful to include a reference drug of the same class as the trial drug to compare their antihypertensive effects; the inclusion of such a reference drug offers a measure of "assay sensitivity" in clinical studies, allowing the distinction to be made between an ineffective drug and an "ineffective" (i.e., null hypothesis) study. Another strategy is to perform placebo-controlled, randomized withdrawals from both arms of a study comparing the new drug to the standard agent from the same class; this is particularly useful in studies of patients with severe hypertension (see Section 3.1).

3.4 Surrogate Markers

Blood pressure reduction is commonly used as a surrogate endpoint for reduction of cardiovascular morbidity and mortality, serving as a better index in stroke than heart attack (see Section 1). However, in preliminary dose-ranging studies in man, reduction in diastolic and systolic blood pressure is a simple measure and serves as a primary endpoint for antihypertensive efficacy. The difficulties of using surrogate endpoints are discussed in detail elsewhere.[138,139]

In addition to surrogate endpoints, a number of parameters associated with blood pressure control, including effects on insulin sensitivity and endothelial function, and with cardiovascular prognosis, such as effects on plasma lipids, can be investigated early in the drug development program.

4 DECISION MAKING

Early phase clinical trials of new antihypertensive agents should be regarded as more than just preliminary exercises necessary to permit larger scale patient studies. Usually, they are performed in young normotensive men. However, studies in hypertensive subjects, and in population ranges which mirror the target population for the study drug with regard to sex, race, age, associated diseases (e.g., ischemic heart disease and peripheral vascular disease), and medications, can also be performed early in the development program. Choosing an appropriate study population and design allows the collection of high quality data which can be used in subsequent registration applications, and the inclusion of hypertensive subjects at this stage of the development program also yields valuable efficacy information.

Phase I and II studies should provide not only data on safety and tolerability, but also a pharmacokinetic profile, dose definition, and preliminary information about efficacy. Mechanistic studies using systemic or subsystemic doses of drug can be performed in phases I and II, and can offer proof of concepts observed during *in vitro* studies, and even some indication of possible extended therapeutic targets.

The quality and quantity of useful data generated in phase I and II studies will be governed by the quality of their design. Well-designed early phase studies have major implications in terms of both safety and cost for the drug development program: they can lead to the speedy withdrawal of ineffective or dangerous drugs from investigation, can characterize the target population most likely to benefit from the new therapy, and can facilitate the rapid progress of registration applications for more promising compounds. Well-designed, carefully conducted early phase studies are a prerequisite for good phase III and IV studies, and they can save time and money later in the drug development program.

REFERENCES

1. Framingham Study. (1971). Systolic versus diastolic blood pressure and risk of coronary heart disease. *Am. J. Cardiol.*, **27**, 355-346.
2. Kannel, W.B. (1975). Role of blood pressure in cardiovascular disease: the Framingham Study. *Angiology*, **26**, 1-14.
3. Dollery, C.T. (1987). Risk predictor, risk indicator and benefits in hypertension. *Am. J. Med.*, **82** (Suppl. 1A), 2-8.
4. Veterans Administration Cooperative Study Group. (1967). Veterans Administration Cooperative Study Group on Antihypertensive Agents. Effects of treatment on morbidity in hypertension: results in patients with diastolic blood pressures averaging 115 through 129 mmHg. *JAMA*, **202**, 1028-1034.
5. Medical Research Council Working Party. (1985). Medical Research Council trial of treatment of mild hypertension: principal results. *Br. Med. J.*, **291**, 97-104.
6. Collins, R. et al. (1990). Blood pressure, stroke and coronary disease. *Lancet*, **335**, 827-838.
7. World Health Organization. (1993). Health for all indicators. Copenhagen: Regional Office for Europe.
8. Alderman, M.H. (1994). The 1994 Model of Hypertension Management. *Curr. Opin. Nephrol. Hypertens.*, **3**, 241-244.
9. American Heart Association. (1990). American Heart Association. 1990 Heart and Stroke Facts. National Health Interview Survey, Vital Health Statistics, Series 10 (National Center for Health Statistics, Detroit, MI, 1983).
10. Joint National Committee on Detection, Evaluation and Treatment of High Blood Pressure. (1993). The Fifth Report of the Joint National Committee on Detection, Evaluation and Treatment of High Blood Pressure. *Arch. Intern. Med.*, **153**, 155-183.
11. Carruthers, S.G. et al. (1993). Report of the Canadian Hypertension Society Consensus Conference: I. Introduction. *Can. Med. Assoc. J.*, **149**, 289-293.
12. Jackson, R. et al. (1993). The management of raised blood pressure in New Zealand. *Br. Med. J.*, **307**, 107-110.
13. Sever, P. et al. Management guidelines in essential hypertension: report of the second working party of the British Hypertension Society. (1993). *Br. Med. J.*, **306**, 983-987.
14. World Health Organization/International Society for Hypertension. (1993). The Guidelines Subcommittee of the WHO/ISH Mild Hypertension Liaison Committee. 1993 Guidelines for the management of mild hypertension. *Hypertension*, **22**, 392-403.
15. Alderman, M.H. et al. (1993). International Roundtable Discussion of National Guidelines for the Detection, Evaluation, and Treatment of Patients with Hypertension. *Am. J. Hypertens.*, **6**, 974-981.
16. Hart, J.T. (1975). The management of hypertension in general practice. *J. R. Coll. Gen. Pract.*, **25**, 160-192.
17. Heller, R.F. (1976). Detection and treatment of hypertension in an inner London community. *Br. J. Prev. Soc. Med.*, **30**, 168-171.
18. Kurji, K.H. and Haines, A.P. (1984). Detection and management of hypertension in general practices in north west London. *Br. Med. J.*, **288**, 903-906.
19. Smith, W.C.S. et al. (1990). Control of blood pressure in Scotland: the rule of halves. *Br. Med. J.*, **300**, 981-983.
20. Bulpitt, C.J. and Fletcher, A.E. (1993). Cost-effectiveness of the treatment of hypertension. *Clin. Exp. Hypertens.*, **15**, 1131-1146.
21. Vagelos, P.R. (1991). Are prescription drug prices high? *Science*, **252**, 1080-1084.
22. Kinney, E.L. et al. (1981). Under-representation of women in new drug trials. *Ann. Intern. Med.*, **95**, 49-9.
23. Horton, R. (1994). Trials of women. *Lancet*, **343**, 745-746.
24. Guidicelli, J.F. and Tillement, J.P. (1977). Influence of sex on drug kinetics in man. *Clin. Pharmacol.*, **2**, 157-166.
25. Hamilton, J.A. and Parry, B. (1983). Sex-related differences in clinical drug response: implications for women's health. *J. Am. Med. Wom. Assoc.*, **38**, 126-132.
26. Hamilton, J.A. (1986). An overview of the clinical rationale for advancing gender-related psychopharmacology and drug abuse research. In Ray, B.A. and Braude, M.C. (Eds.), *Women and Drugs: A New Era for Research. National Institute on Drug Abuse Research Monograph 65*. National Institute on Drug Abuse, pp. 14-20.
27. Walle, T. et al. (1989). Pathway-selective sex differences in the metabolic clearance of propranolol in human subjects. *Clin. Pharmacol. Ther.*, **46**, 257-263.
28. Webb, D.J. et al. (1987). Cough associated with captopril and enalapril. *Br. Med. J.*, 1987; **295**, 272.
29. Merkatz, R. B. et al. (1993). Women in clinical trials of new drugs: a change in Food and Drug Administration Policy. *N. Engl. J. Med.*, **329**, 292-296.
30. Caschetta, M.B. et al. (1993). FDA policy on women in drug trials. *N. Engl. J. Med.*, **329**, 1815.
31. Mastroianni, A.C. et al, (Eds). (1994). *Women and Health Research: Ethical and Legal Issues of Including Women in Clinical Studies.* Institute of Medicine, Washington, D.C.
32. Amery, A. et al. (1981). Hypertension in the elderly. *Acta Med. Scand.*, **210**, 221-229.
33. Kannel, W.B. et al. (1981). Systolic blood pressure, arterial rigidity, and risk of stroke: the Framingham study. *JAMA*, **245**, 1225-1229.
34. Miall, W.E. and Brennan, P.J. (1981). Hypertension in the elderly: the South Wales study. In Onesti, G. and Kim, K., (Eds), *Hypertension in the Young and Old,* Grune & Stratton, New York, pp 277-283.
35. Miall, W.E. (1984). The epidemiology of hypertension in old age. In Stout, R.W. (Ed.), *Arterial Disease and the Elderly.* Churchill-Livingstone, Edinburgh, pp. 154-174.
36. Bennett, E.D. et al. (1984). Ascending aortic blood velocity and acceleration using Doppler ultrasound in the assessment of left ventricular function. *Cardiovasc. Res.*, **18**, 632-636.

37. Anderson, R. et al. (1992). The coming of age in Europe: older people in the European Community. Age Concern England, London.
38. Crooks, J. et al. (1970). Pharmacodynamics in the elderly. *Clin. Pharmacokin.*, **1**, 280-296.
39. Klotz, U. et al. (1975). The effects of age and liver disease on the disposition and elimination of diazepam in adult man. *J. Clin. Invest.*, **55**, 347-359.
40. Aiayi, A.A. et al. (1986). Age and the pharmacodynamics of the angiotensin converting enzyme inhibitors enalapril and enalaprilat. *Br. J. Clin. Pharmacol.*, **21**, 349-357.
41. ICH. (1993). International Conference on Harmonisation of Technical Requirements for the Registration of Pharmaceuticals for Human Use. Studies in support of special populations: geriatrics. *Fed. Reg.*, **58** (No: 72), 21082-21083.
42. FDA. (1989). *Guideline for the Study of Drugs Likely to be Used in the Elderly.* Washington D.C., Government Printing Office.
43. Kaplan, N.M. (1994). Ethnic aspects of hypertension. *Lancet,* **344**, 450-452.
44. Bühler, F.R. et al. (1975). Antihypertensive beta-blocking action as related to renin and age: a pharmacological tool to identify pathogenic mechanisms in essential hypertension. *Am. J. Cardiol.*, **36**, 653-9.
45. Cruickshank, J.K. and Beevers, D.G. (1985). Ethnic and geographical differences in blood pressure. In Bulpitt, C.J. (Ed.), *Epidemiology of Hypertension.* Elsevier, Cambridge, pp. 70-89.
46. Seedat, Y.K. (1989). Varying response to hypotensive agents in different racial groups: black versus white differences. *J. Hypertens.*, **7**, 515-518.
47. Materson, B.J. et al. (1993). Single-drug therapy for hypertension in men: a comparison of six antihypertensive agents with placebo. *N. Engl. J. Med.*, **328**, 914-921.
48. Baber, N. (1994). International conference on harmonisation of technical requirements for registration of pharmaceuticals for human use. *Br. J. Clin. Pharmacol.*, **37**, 401-404.
49. Association of the British Pharmaceutical Industry. (1988). *Guidelines on Good Clinical Research Practice.* ABPI, 1988.
50. Warot, D. (1991). Les essais de medicaments chez le volontaire sain: quelques aspects legislatifs et ethiques. *Encephale*, **17**, 93-95.
51. Klatsky, A.L. et al. (1977). Alcohol consumption and blood pressure: Kaiser Permanente multiphasic health examination data. *N. Engl. J. Med.*, **196**, 1194-200.
52. Potter, J.F. et al. (1986). The pressor and metabolic effects of alcohol in normotensives. *Hypertension,* **8**, 625-31.
53. Potter, J.F. et al. (1986). Alcohol raises blood pressure in hypertensive patients. *J. Hypertens.*, **4**, 435-41.
54. Bannon, L.T. et al. (1984). Effect of alcohol withdrawal on blood pressure, plasma renin activity, aldosterone, cortisol and dopamine beta-hydroxylase. *Clin. Sci.,* **66**, 659-63.
55. Cryer, P.E. et al. (1967). Norepinephrine and epinephrine release and adrenergic mediation of smoking associated hemodynamic and metabolic events. *N. Engl. J. Med.*, **295**, 573-7.
56. Freestone, S. and Ramsay, L.E. (1983). Effect of beta-blockade on the pressor response of coffee plus smoking in patients with mild hypertension. *Drugs*, **25**, 141-145.
57. Stewart, M.J. et al. (1994). Cardiovascular effects of cigarette smoking: ambulatory blood pressure and blood pressure variability. *J. Hum. Hypertens.*, **8**, 19-22.
58. Griffiths, R.R. et al. (1986). Human coffee drinking: reinforcing and physical dependence producing effects of caffeine. *J. Pharmacol. Exp. Ther.*, **239**, 416-425.
59. Galletly, D.C. et al. (1989). Does caffeine withdrawal contribute to post-operative headache? *Lancet,* **i**, 1335.
60. Matthew, R.J. et al. (1992). Middle cerebral artery velocity during upright posture after marijuana smoking. *Acta Psych. Scand.*, **86**, 173-178.
61. Heishman, S.J. et al. (1990). Acute and residual effects of marijuana: profiles of plasma THC levels, physiological, subjective, and performance measures. *Pharmacol. Biochem. Behav.*, **37**, 561-565.
62. Patrick, D.L. et al. (1994). The validity of self-reported smoking: a review and meta-analysis. *Am. J. Public Health,* **84**, 1086-1093.
63. Etzel, R.A. (1990). A review of the use of saliva cotinine as a marker of tobacco smoke exposure. *Prevent. Med.*, **19**, 190-197.
64. Pre, J. (1992). Les marqueurs du tabagisme. *Pathol. Biol.*, **40**, 1015-1021.
65. Bravo, E.L. (1988). Phenylpropanolamine and other over-the-counter vasoactive compounds. *Hypertension,* **11**, 4-6.
66. Oates, J.A. (1988). Antagonism of antihypertensive drug therapy by nonsteroidal anti-inflammatory drugs. *Hypertension*, **11**, 4-6.
67. Medical Research Council. (1964). Medical Research Council: responsibility in investigations on human subjects. *Br. Med. J.*, **2**, 178-180.
68. Declaration of Helsinki. (1964). Recommendations guiding doctors in clinical research. (Revised version, 1975), in Mason, J.K. and McCall-Smith, R.A. (Eds.), *Law and Medical Ethics,* (Third Edition, 1991), Butterworths, Edinburgh, pp. 446-449.
69. Bond, A. and Lader, M. (1974). The use of analogue scales in rating subjective feelings. *Br. J. Med. Psychol.*, **47**, 211-218.
70. Ohman, KP. et al. (1985). Pharmacokinetics of captopril and its effect on blood pressure during acute and chronic administation and in relation to food intake. *J. Cardiovasc. Pharmacol.*, **7**, S20-40.

71. Salvetti, A. et al. (1985). Influence of food on acute and chronic effects of captopril in essential hypertensive patients. *J. Cardiovasc. Pharmacol.*, **7**, S25-29.
72. Swanson, B.N. et al. (1984). Influence of food on the bioavailability of captopril in healthy subjects. *J. Pharm. Sci.*, **73**, 1655-1657.
73. Melander, A. et al. (1977). Enhancement of the bioavailability of propranolol and metoprolol by food. *Clin. Pharmacol. Ther.*, **2**, 108-112.
74. McLean, A.J. et al. (1981). Reduction of first pass hepatic clearance of propranolol by food. *Clin. Pharmacol. Ther.*, **30**, 31-34.
75. Daneshmend, T.K. and Roberts, C.J.C. (1982). The influence of food on the oral and intravenous pharmacokinetics of a high clearance drug: a study with labetalol. *Br. J. Clin. Pharmacol.*, **14**, 73-78.
76. Bailey, D.G. et al. (1994). Grapefruit juice and drugs: how significant is it? *Clin. Pharmacokinet.*, **26**, 91-98.
77. Webb, D.J. et al. (1983). Reduction of blood pressure in man with H142, a potent new renin inhibitor. *Lancet*, **2**, 1486-1487.
78. Hodsman, G.P. et al. (1983). Factors related to the first dose hypotensive effect of captopril: prediction and treatment. *Br. Med. J.*, **284**, 832-4.
79. Doig, J.K. et al. (1993). Dose-ranging study of angiotensin type 1 receptor antagonist losartan (DUP 753/82K954) in salt deplete man. *J. Cardiovasc. Pharmacol.*, **21**, 732-738.
80. FDA. (1984). Division guideline for the evaluation of controlled release products. Washington D.C., Government Printing Office.
81. Haynes, W.G. et al. (1995). Vasodilator effects of the $ET_{A/B}$ antagonist, TAK-044, in man. *J. Cardiovasc. Pharmacol.*, in press.
82. Haynes, W.G. et al. (1993). Inhibition of nitric oxide synthesis increases blood pressure in healthy humans. *J. Hypertens.*, **11**, 1375-1380.
83. ICH. (1993). International Conference on Harmonisation of Technical Requirements for the Registration of Pharmaceuticals for Human Use. Dose-response information to support drug registration.
84. Temple, R. (1989). Government viewpoint of clinical trials of cardiovascular drugs. *Med. Clin. N. Am.*, **73**, 495-509.
85. Sheiner, L.B. et al. (1991). A simulation study comparing designs for dose ranging. *Stat. Med.*, **10**, 303-321.
86. Paterson, J.W. et al. (1970). The pharmacodynamics and metabolism of propranolol in man. *Pharm. Clin.*, **2**, 127-133.
87. Ménard, J. (1993). Critical assessment of international clinical development programs for new antihypertensive drugs. *J. Hypertens.*, **11**, S39-S46.
88. Bengtsson, C. et al. (1975). Effect of different doses of chlorthalidone on blood pressure, serum potassium, and serum urate. *Br. Med. J.*, **i**, 197-199.
89. Berglund, G. and Andersson, O. (1976). Low doses of hydrochlorothiazide in hypertension: antihypertensive and metabolic effects. *Eur. J. Clin. Pharmacol.*, **10**, 177-182.
90. Carlsen, J.E. et al. (1990). Relation between doses of bendrofluazide, antihypertensive effect and adverse biochemical effects. *Br. Med. J.*, **300**, 975-978.
91. FDA. (1988). Division of Cardio-Renal Products. *Proposed Guidelines for the Clinical Evaluation of Antihypertensive Drugs*. Washington D.C., Government Printing Office.
92. George, C.F. et al. (1972). Pharmacokinetics of dextro, laevo and racemic propranolol in man. *Eur. J. Clin. Pharmacol.*, **4**, 74-80.
93. Editorial. (1995). ACE inhibitors reviewed. *Drug Ther. Bull.*, **33**, 1-3.
94. Meredith, P.A. et al. (1992). An individualised approach to optimising long-term antihypertensive therapy using concentration-effect analysis. In van Boxtel, C.J., Holford, N.H.G., and Danhof, M. (Eds.), *The In Vivo Study of Drug Action*, Elsevier Science Publishers B.V., Amsterdam.
95. Brunner, H.R. et al. (1983). Does pharmacological profiling of a new drug in normal volunteers provide a useful guideline to antihypertensive therapy? *Hypertension*, **5**, 101-7.
96. Campbell, D.J. (1987). Circulating and tissue angiotensin systems. *J. Clin. Invest.*, **79**, 1-6.
97. Cohen, L. and Kurtz, M.D. (1982). Angiotensin converting enzyme inhibition in tissues from spontaneously hypertensive rats after treatment with captopril or MK421. *J. Pharmacol. Exp. Ther.*, **220**, 63-9.
98. Williams, R.R. et al. (1991). Are there interactions and relations between genetic and environmental factors predisposing to high blood pressure? *Hypertension*, **18**, 129-137.
99. Lever, A.F. and Harrap, S.B. (1992). Essential hypertension: a disorder of growth with origins in childhood? *J. Hypertens.*, **10**, 101-120.
100. Perry, H.M. et al. (1966). Studies on the control of hypertension. 8. Mortality, morbidity, and remission during twelve years of intensive therapy. *Circulation*, **33**, 958-972.
101. Cameron, H.A. and Ramsay, L.E. (1984). The lupus syndrome induced by hydralazine: a common complication with low dose treatment. *Br. Med. J.*, **289**, 410-412.
102. Rose, M. and McMahon, F.G. (1990). Some problems of antihypertensive drug studies in the context of the new guidelines. *Am. J. Hypertens.*, **3**, 151-155.
103. Raftery, E.B. (1983). Understanding hypertension: the contribution of direct ambulatory blood pressure monitoring. In Weber, M.A. and Pickering, G.W. (Eds.), *Ambulatory Blood Pressure Monitoring*, Springer-Verlag, New York, pp. 105-116.

104. Stewart, M.J. and Padfield, P.L. (1992). Blood pressure measurement: an epitaph for the mercury sphygmomanometer? *Clin. Sci.*, **83**, 1-12.
105. Di Rienzo, M. et al. (1983). Continuous versus intermittent blood pressure measurements in estimating 24-hour average blood pressure. *Hypertension*, **5**, 264-269.
106. James, G.D. et al. (1988). The reproducibility of ambulatory, home and clinical pressures. *Hypertension*, **11**, 545-549.
107. Conway, J. et al. (1988). The use of ambulatory blood pressure monitoring to improve the accuracy and reduce the numbers of subjects in clinical trials of antihypertensive agents. *J. Hypertens.*, **6**, 111-116.
108. Mutti, E. et al. (1991). Effect of placebo on 24-h noninvasive ambulatory blood pressure. *J. Hypertens.*, **9**, 361-364.
109. O'Brien, E. et al. (1989). Ambulatory blood pressure measurement in the evaluation of blood pressure lowering drugs. *J. Hypertens.*, **7**, 243-248.
110. Casadei, B. (1991). Use of ambulatory blood pressure monitoring in pharmacological trials. *J. Hum. Hypertens.*, **5**, 1-4.
111. O'Brien, E. et al. (1991). Ambulatory blood pressure monitoring in the evaluation of drug efficacy. *Am. Heart J.*, **121**, 999-1006.
112. Staessen, J.A. et al. (1994). Clinical trials with ambulatory blood pressure monitoring: fewer patients? *Lancet*, **344**, 1552-1556.
113. Ihlen, H. et al. (1985). Changes in left ventricular stroke volume measured by Doppler echocardiography. *Br. Heart. J.*, **54**, 378-380.
114. Metcalf, M.J. and Rawlers, J.M. (1989). Stroke distance in acute myocardial infarction: a simple measurement of left ventricular function. *Lancet*, **i**, 1372-1373.
115. Webb, D.J. (1995). The pharmacology of human blood vessels. *J. Vasc Res.*, **757**, 1-26.
116. Thomas, S.H.L. (1992). Impedance cardiography using the Sramek-Bernstein method: accuracy and variability at rest and during exercise. *Br. J. Clin. Pharmacol.*, **34**, 467-476.
117. O'Rourke, M.F. (1994). Arterial mechanics and wave reflection with antihypertensive therapy. *J. Hypertens.*, **10**, S43-S49.
118. Laurent, S. et al. (1993). Isobaric compliance of the radial artery is increased in patients with essential hypertension. *J. Hypertens.*, **11**, 89-98.
119. Benjamin, N. et al. (1989). Local inhibition of converting enzyme and vascular responses to angiotensin and bradykinin in the human forearm. *J. Physiol.*, **412**, 543-555.
120. O'Kane, K.P.J. et al. (1994). Local L-N^{G}-monomethyl arginine attenuates the vasodilator action of bradykinin in the human forearm. *Br. J. Clin. Pharmacol.*, **38**, 311-315.
121. Aellig, W.H. (1994). Clinical pharmacology, physiology and pathophysiology of superficial veins. *Br. J. Clin. Pharmacol.*, **38**, 181-196 (Part 1) & 189-305 (Part 2).
122. Hand, M.F. and Webb, D.J. (1995). Assessment of the effects of drugs on the peripheral vasculature. In Nimmo, W.S and Tucker, C.T. (Eds.), *Clinical Measurement in Drug Evaluation*, John Wiley & Sons, Edinburgh, pp. 135-150.
123. Roberts, D.H. et al. (1986). The reproducibility of limb blood flow measurements in human volunteers at rest and after exercise by using mercury-in-Silastic strain gauge plethysmography under standardized conditions. *Clin. Sci.*, **70**, 635-638.
124. Webb, D.J. and Collier, J.G. (1987). Influence of ramipril diacid on the peripheral vascular effects of angiotensin I. *Am. J. Cardiol.*, **59**, 45D-49D.
125. Webb, D.J. et al. (1989). The potassium channel opening drug cromakalim produces arterioselective vasodilatation in the upper limbs of normal volunteers. *Br. J. Clin. Pharmacol.*, **27**, 757-761.
126. Haynes, W.G. and Webb, D.J. (1993). Venoconstriction to endothelin-1 in humans: the role of calcium and potassium channels. *Am. J. Physiol. (Heart Circ. Physiol.)*, **265**, H1676-H1681.
127. Vallance, P. et al. (1989). Effects of endothelium-derived nitric oxide on peripheral arteriolar tone in man. *Lancet*, **ii**, 997-1000.
128. Haynes, W.G. and Webb, D.J. (1994). Contribution of endogenous generation of endothelin-1 to basal vascular tone. *Lancet*, **344**, 852-854.
129. O'Connell, J.E. et al. (1992). Candoxatril, an orally active neutral endopeptidase inhibitor, raises plasma atrial natriuretic factor and is natriuretic in essential hypertension. *J. Hyperten.*, **10**, 271-277.
130. Vallance, P. et al. (1989). Nitric oxide synthesised from L-arginine mediates endothelium-dependent dilatation in human veins *in vivo*. *Cardiovasc. Res.*, **23**, 1053-1057.
131. Haynes, W.G. et al. (1994). Direct and sympathetically mediated venoconstriction in essential hypertension: enhanced response to endothelin-1. *J. Clin. Invest.*, **94**, 1359-1364.
132. Robinson, B.F. (1987). Assessment of the effects of drugs on the venous system in man. *Br. J. Clin. Pharmacol.*, **6**, 381-386.
133. Collier, J.G. et al. (1978). Comparison of effects of tolmesoxide (RX71108), diazoxide, hydrallazine, prazosin, glyceryl trinitrate and sodium nitroprusside on forearm arteries and dorsal hand veins of man. *Br. J. Clin. Pharmacol.*, **5**, 35-44.
134. Cockcroft, J.R. et al. (1993). Comparison of angiotensin-converting enzyme inhibition with angiotensin II receptor antagonism in the human forearm. *J. Cardiovasc. Pharmacol.*, **22**, 579-584.
135. Gifford, R.W. et al. (1989) Office evaluation of hypertension: a statement for health professionals by a Writing Group of the Council for High Blood Pressure Research, American Heart Association. *Circulation*, **79**, 721-731.

136. Garbe, E. et al. (1993). Clinical and statistical issues in therapeutic equivalence research. *Eur. J. Clin. Pharmacol.*, **45**, 1-7.

137. Lacourcière, Y. et al. (1994). Effects of modulators of the renin-angiotensin-aldosterone system on cough. *J. Hypertens.*, **12**, 1387-1393.

138. Friedman, L. et al. (1984). *Fundamentals of Clinical Trials*, (2nd ed). PSG Publishing, Littleton.

139. Moleur, P. and Boissel, J.-P. (1987). Definition of a surrogate endoint. *Controlled Clin. Trials*, **8**, 304.

140. Rawlins, M.D. (1995). Pharmacovigilance: paradise lost, regained or postponed? *J. R. Coll. Phys.*, **29**, 41-49.

Chapter 18

Drugs for Heart Failure

G. G. Belz and P. H. Joubert

CONTENTS

1 Introduction 237
1.1 Drugs for Heart Failure 238
1.1.1 Positive Inotropic Drugs 238
1.1.2 Vasodilators 239
1.1.3 Diuretics 240
1.1.4 ß-Adrenoceptor Antagonists 240
1.1.5 Major Safety Issues 240
1.1.6 Most Important Endpoints Relevant to Drug Trials 240
2 Studies in Healthy Volunteers 240
2.1 Selection Criteria 241
2.2 Safety Considerations 241
2.3 Methods 241
2.3.1 General Trial Design 241
2.3.2 Pharmacokinetic Issues 241
2.3.3 Pharmacodynamic Issues 241
2.3.3.1 Methods to Assess Cardiac Systolic Function 242
2.3.3.2 Assessment of Arterial Vasodilatory Drug Effects 243
2.3.3.3 Assessment of Vasodilatory Effects on the Venous Side 243
2.3.4 Assessment of Potency and of the Duration of Action of Competitive Antagonists 243
2.3.5 Relationship Between Pharmacodynamic Parameters and Efficacy 243
2.4 Controls 243
3 Patient Studies 244
3.1 Suitability 244
3.2 Selection Criteria 244
3.3 Safety Considerations 244
3.4 Methods 244
3.4.1 Pharmacokinetics 244
3.4.2 Surrogate Markers 245
3.4.2.1 Functional Assessment of Exercise Performance 245
3.4.2.2 Hemodynamics 246
3.4.2.3 Neurohumoral Regulation 246
3.5 Size and Duration of Trials 246
4 Decision Making 247
References 247

1 INTRODUCTION

Heart failure is a clinical syndrome characterized by the heart's inability to provide the tissues with an adequate blood supply in spite of the fact that there is sufficient venous return to the heart. Heart failure can involve the left ventricle (main features: fatigue and dyspnea), the right ventricle (main features: congestion of peripheral veins and edema), or both. Heart failure may develop acutely within minutes or hours (e.g., during a myocardial infarction) but is more frequently chronic. A rough classification of the severity can be obtained using the criteria of the New York Heart Association (Table 1). The prognosis of heart failure is poor and 20-50% of patients with severe heart failure (NYHA stages III+IV) die within

0-8493-9230-6/97/$0.00+$.50
© 1997 by CRC Press, Inc.

one year of diagnosis. Early and effective treatment is therefore extremely important. Heart failure has many causes (e.g., hypertension, coronary heart disease, and myocardial infarction, valvular disease, diseases of the myocardial cells) causing primary and secondary cardiomyopathies. All of these have as a common feature a disturbance of the function of the heart as a pump. This can readily be seen in an echocardiogram as a reduction of the ejection fraction (EF) of the left ventricle and enlargement of ventricular size.

Table 1 Criteria for NYHA Functional Classification

Functional Capacity (four classes)	
I	No limitation of physical activity *Ordinary physical activity does not cause undue fatigue, palpitation or dyspnea*
II	Slight limitation of physical activity *Comfortable at rest, but ordinary physical activity results in fatigue, palpitation, or dyspnea*
III	Marked limitation of physical activity *Comfortable at rest, but less than ordinary activity causes fatigue, palpitation or dyspnea*
IV	Unable to carry on any physical activity without discomfort *Symptoms of cardiac insufficiency may be present even at rest. If any physical activity is undertaken, discomfort is increased.*

The reduction of the performance of the heart in maintaining the circulation activates several compensatory neuroendocrine mechanisms which may initially maintain cardiac output but, however, soon induce further deterioration of circulatory function (Figure 1). An initial activation of the sympathoadrenergic system (indicated by increased plasma noradrenaline levels) and leading secondarily to an increased activity of the renin-angiotensin-aldosterone system (RAAS) give rise to many of the symptoms of heart failure such as tachycardia, arrhythmias, sodium and water retention, venous congestion, and edema. It has recently also been shown that circulating concentrations of endothelin are increased in patients with moderate to severe congestive cardiac failure[1] and that endothelin concentrations correlate with functional impairment. In chronic heart failure increased catecholamines induce a downregulation of cardiac ß-receptors, leading to further reduction in contractility and thus to further hemodynamic deterioration. Because the activated hormone systems induce vasoconstriction by several mechanisms (noradrenaline, angiotensin II, endothelin, sodium retention) the afterload of the left ventricle will also be increased. The failing heart is very sensitive to afterload changes and therefore will react with further reduction in its performance as a pump. Following this, the activation of the neuroendocrine mechanisms will further increase, resulting in a vicious cycle. An inhibition of the activated neuroendocrine mechanisms will, generally speaking, lead to clinical and prognostic improvement.

1.1 Drugs for Heart Failure

Several different principles are employed to treat heart failure (Figure 2). Each of these principles can be influenced by a variety of different drugs which differ with respect to their pharmacodynamic and kinetic properties.

1.1.1 Positive Inotropic Drugs

The oldest therapeutic approach is the use of cardiac glycosides of natural origin. Only a few of the many known cardiac glycosides have persisted as therapeutic agents: digoxin, digitoxin, and ouabain. Whereas these substances clearly differ with respect to their kinetics, it is a matter of debate whether they also differ in dynamic properties.[2] As recent studies clearly show the therapeutic effect of digoxin even in the presence of sinus rhythm,[3,4] the interest in compounds with a different dynamic profile and a broader therapeutic index may increase in the future. Other drugs with positive inotropic effects are: catecholamines and derivatives (e.g., dopamine, dobutamine); phosphodiesterase III (PDE III) inhibitors; and calcium sensitizers.

These substances, in addition to being positive inotropic, also have vasodilatory properties (so-called "inodilators"). Whereas for short-term administration (e.g., bridging) these substances may be useful, their long-term therapeutic benefit is questionable.

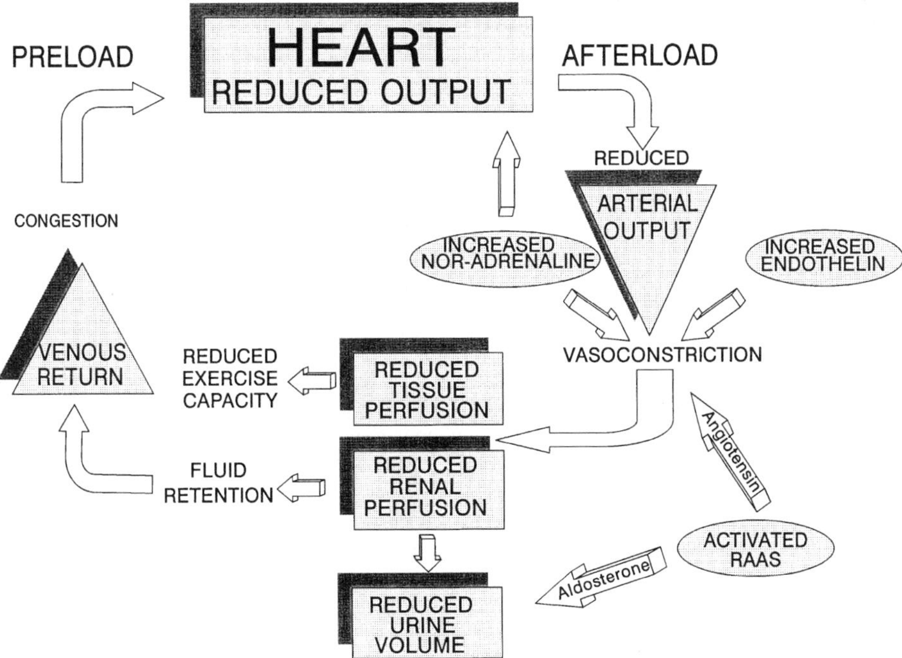

Figure 1 Simplified representation of the major pathophysiological features of congestive heart failure. Note that the neurohumoral counterregulatory mechanisms are shown in the ellipses.

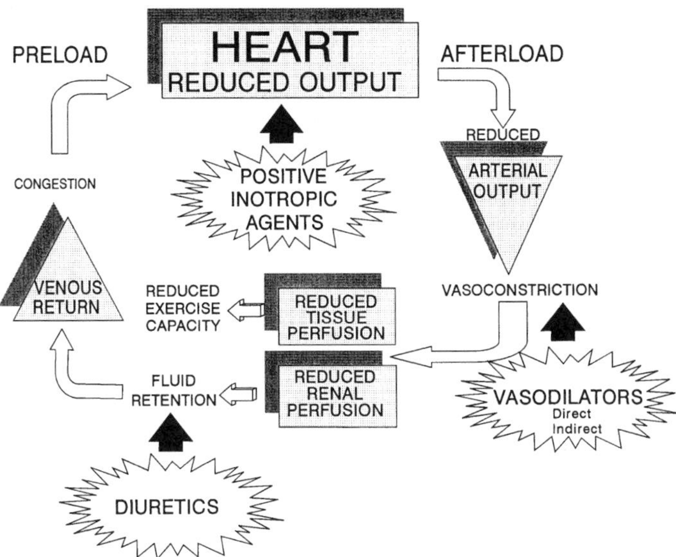

Figure 2 Major classes of drugs used for the treatment of congestive heart failure in the context of the main pathophysiologic features.

1.1.2 Vasodilators

Direct vasodilators acting on the arterial side (e.g., hydralazine) or on the venous side of the circulation (e.g., nitrates) produce acute effects, but their efficacy in chronic studies is unclear.[5] Indirect vasodilators, like ACE inhibitors, antagonize the effect of endogenous vasoconstrictors (AT II) and produce clear effects during both short- and long-term administration.[6,7]

1.1.3 Diuretics

Diuretics counteract the effects of an activated RAAS mainly by reversing the increased sodium and water retention. Due to the fact that diuretics themselves stimulate the RAAS, their effects are limited. A combination of diuretics with ACE inhibitors or with other inhibitors of the RAAS therefore has a very good pathophysiologic rationale.

1.1.4 ß-Adrenoceptor Antagonists

This principle, which at a first glance seems paradoxical, has been gaining importance during the last years. The underlying pathophysiological concept is based upon the occurrence of downregulation of adrenergic receptors during chronic sympathetic activation in heart failure. This results in the loss of the positive inotropic effects of the endogenous catecholamines. With very low doses of $ß_1$-selective antagonists, the receptors can be re-expressed and thereby the heart can redevelop a contractile response to noradrenaline.[8]

1.1.5 Major Safety Issues

Due to the poor prognosis of the disease and the high risk of naturally occurring acute and severe complications, e.g., ventricular fibrillation, it is necessary to perform studies under controlled conditions. If this principle is ignored, the causal relation between adverse events and treatment could either be overseen or overemphasized. Careful attention must, for instance, be paid to the potential for proarrhythmia which has been seen with many of the compounds considered useful in the treatment of heart failure.

1.1.6 Most Important Endpoints Relevant to Drug Trials

The most obvious hard endpoint for a study of the effect of interventions (medical or otherwise) is survival. There have been several studies with ACE inhibitors with a positive outcome for the treated group,[6,7] for PDE III inhibitors with a negative outcome,[9] and for calcium sensitizers with an equivocal outcome.[11] For digitalis glycosides such studies are ongoing. A useful endpoint is the worsening of heart failure after drug withdrawal, as seen with digoxin.[3] All these endpoints, however, have large time and budget requirements and are therefore a matter for studies in the later phases of drug development (phases III and IV).

In the early phases, studies should rely on surrogate parameters which:

1. Indicate and assess the effects of the compound (e.g., positive inotropism, vasodilatation, etc.). This type of research can most easily be done in healthy volunteers.
2. Can indicate an influence of the drug on the major independent prognostic factors such as EF, maximal oxygen uptake under physical exercise (VO_{2max}), VO_2, and plasma noradrenaline. Great care should also be taken to evaluate the safety profile of these substances in an early phase, to be able to stop development in the case of unacceptable clinical toxicity.

2 STUDIES IN HEALTHY VOLUNTEERS

Whereas the therapeutic efficacy of drugs for treatment of heart failure can only be tested in patients, studies in healthy volunteers in an early phase of the development can help:

1. To shorten the time of drug development.
2. To prevent patients from being treated with compounds which in man have unfavorable effects and/or a poor kinetic profile.
3. To establish the pharmacokinetic profile of a compound in man (e.g., suitability for chronic administration).
4. To establish the profile of pharmacologic effects, its dose effect or concentration/effect relationship and the time profile of action in man; since almost all substances used in treatment of heart failure have clear hemodynamic activities (e.g., positive inotropism, vasodilation) and/or can be characterized by an agonist/antagonist interaction (e.g., AT II antagonists) studies in healthy volunteers can provide essential data.
5. To evaluate in a clinical setting the pharmacokinetic and -dynamic interactions with other drugs which are frequently used in heart failure. Due to ethical considerations monotherapy with a new drug will only rarely be possible. Therefore co-administration with digitalis, diuretics, and/or ACE inhibitors will be unavoidable in most of the patients and these important drug-drug interactions need to be investigated at an early stage of development in healthy volunteers.

2.1 Selection Criteria

Although the target population, patients with heart failure, predominantly belongs to the advanced age groups, experience with many compounds has shown that data derived in healthy male volunteers between 18 and 35 years of age can be extrapolated to patients. Potential risks, e.g., arrhythmogenity are minimal in young volunteers.

2.2 Safety Considerations

Because the drugs used in heart failure, especially vasodilators and inodilators, may exert powerful actions (depending on the dose), all phase I studies must be performed in an in-house setting by investigators experienced in acute intervention in the case of an emergency.

Most of the untoward drug effects we have observed in such studies have been due to marked vasodilation, e.g., headache, palpitations, vomiting, general malaise, hypotension, collapse, and orthostatic hypotension. Though not considered as "serious," these effects can be very troublesome to the volunteers and may induce concern. Symptomatic treatment is frequently unavoidable.

2.3 Methods

2.3.1 General Trial Design

As in any other area of drug research, all studies to assess effects and/or efficacy must follow certain guidelines to avoid major mistakes.

Valid information can only be obtained from controlled studies. Studies of drug effects in healthy volunteers need at least a negative control (placebo) group. Positive control groups with substances of known mechanisms of action can be helpful to fit a new compound into an effect-spectrum of well-known substances. Due to the sensitivity of cardiovascular parameters such as heart rate, blood pressure, and cardiac output to environmental stimuli (e.g., noise, temperature, food, posture, pain, apprehension, etc.) experimental conditions need to be tightly controlled.

Efficacy studies in patients are more difficult to control. For ethical reasons monotherapy of test drug vs. placebo can only be done in studies of short duration where lack of therapy will have little effect on disease outcome. (One would, for instance, not do a placebo-controlled study for a new antiarrhythmic agent for ventricular tachycardia.) Studies of longer duration can be done vs. placebo only on the basis of an "add-on" treatment with drugs of proven efficacy (e.g., digitalis and/or diuretics, ACE inhibitors).

Nota bene: Before such "add-on" studies can be performed relevant drug interactions must be excluded. Small single dose studies usually have to precede multiple dose studies, but as heart failure is a chronic disease, the information that can be obtained from single doses is limited.

2.3.2 Pharmacokinetic Issues

Because heart failure, generally speaking, requires chronic therapy, the main route of administration will be oral (or maybe in the future also transdermal).

The key studies therefore have to use oral formulations. Intravenous formulations may be useful in emergency situations and for studying the acute hemodynamic effects of new drugs in the drug development program.

Because patients with heart failure will frequently have multiorgan disease, the influence of disease states on kinetics needs to be assessed, e.g., renal impairment, hepatic impairment, abnormalities in thyroid function, the heart failure itself (and especially peripheral venous congestion). Many of these issues, however, can be addressed by population methods during phase III of drug development, i.e., when the decision has been made to continue with trial drug development.

2.3.3 Pharmacodynamic Issues

In general, methods to assess pharmacodynamic drug effects in healthy volunteers should be noninvasive to allow safe and repetitive application. The methods must have a high sensitivity for detecting specific drug effects. They must also have a proven validity, and the value of such studies can be further increased by including positive controls. Drugs may affect cardiac performance by their ability to change contractility, pre- and afterload, or more frequently by a combination of effects on these variables. Methods exist for assessing cardiac systolic performance, venous dilatation and arterial dilatation in healthy subjects (Figure 3).

Many noninvasive methods for cardiovascular evaluation have been developed during recent years primarily for diagnostic purposes and for the evaluation of the course of cardiovascular dysfunction. Several of these techniques are used in clinical pharmacology. Four methods appear to be particularly

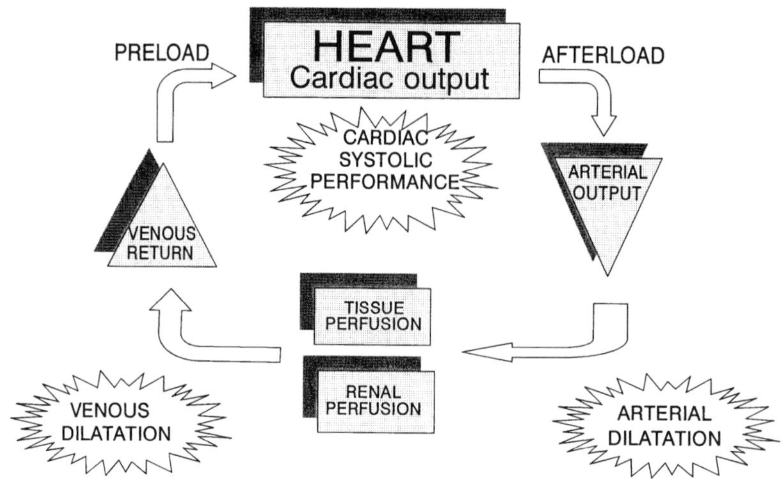

Figure 3 Major groups of parameters used for assessing the potential value of drugs for congestive heart failure in healthy volunteers.

suited for the noninvasive evaluation of cardiac systolic function: mechanocardiography (systolic time intervals), two-dimensional echocardiography, dual beam Doppler echoaortography, and transthoracic impedance cardiography.

2.3.3.1 Methods to Assess Cardiac Systolic Function

The measurement of systolic time intervals (STIs) is one of the oldest methods in noninvasive cardiology. This method depends on the simultaneous high speed registration of an ECG, phonocardiogram, and carotid pulse.[12]

There are three relevant intervals: PEP (pre-ejection period), LVET (left ventricular ejection time), and QS_2 (electromechanical systole). As these intervals (except for PEP) are strongly influenced by heart rate, a rate correction must usually be performed, designated by a c subscript (e.g., QS_{2C}).[13,14] In addition, PEP and LVET are strongly influenced by pre- and afterload, whereas QS_2 is almost independent of afterload and blood pressure. This interval, can be considered as one of the most valid reflections of cardiac contractility.[15-17]

STIs provide the highest sensitivity among many other noninvasive methods, including two-dimensional echocardiography, Doppler echocardiography, and electrical impedance cardiography.[18,19] As mentioned before STI measurements can be influenced by environmental factors such as food intake.[21] The rate correction is only valid for resting conditions and should not be used under stress which changes the slope and relation between HR and STIs.

Provided that conditions are standardized, STIs are highly reliable. In various studies dose- and concentration-effect relationships have been documented using this method for different drug groups, like digitalis glycosides, PDE III inhibitors, and others.[21-25]

Electrical impedance cardiography relies on the assessment of a differentiated electrical impedance signal (dz/dt). This method allows one to obtain a "stroke volume" equivalent and some other parameters like the Heather index: (dz/dt)/RZ.[26] In a study of the sensitivity of various methods, impedance cardiographic variables ranked second behind the STI.[18,19] The validity of the stroke volume obtained was high.[27] The changes in end-systolic volume, end-diastolic volume, and EF detected by two-dimensional echocardiography are far less sensitive with regard to the overall effects of isoproterenol. Doses four times higher than doses used with STIs were required to detect statistically significant changes.[18,19]

In spite of this relative lack of sensitivity, two-dimensional echocardiography remains of special value because it provides a more accurate (but not more sensitive) evaluation of the central cardiac loading conditions. Important advantages of both systolic time interval and impedance cardiography in contrast to the other two methods are: (1) their registrations require little observer intervention and (2) they can be repeated often without undue constraints or discomfort to the subjects; however, their signal analysis is tedious and subject to observer bias. In contrast to this the signal registration for Doppler echoaortograhy and two-dimensional echocardiography are highly observer-dependent, whereas their signal analyses are automated or semi-automated and thus are less subject to subjective bias.

These observer effects need to be taken into account; personnel require intensive training and continuous monitoring in terms of performance, consistency, and reproducibility.

2.3.3.2 Assessment of Arterial Vasodilatory Drug Effects

Many of the drugs used for the treatment of heart failure act via a reduction of afterload. This mechanism depends largely but not exclusively on arteriolar vasodilatation.

Arteriolar vasodilatation in general can be estimated using the total peripheral resistance (TPR), which represents the relation between blood pressure and cardiac output. Several noninvasive methods are available for assessment of cardiac output, e.g., electrical impedance cardiography, echoaortography, two-dimensional echocardiography.

To get insight into drug-induced regional vasodilation in specific arterial beds other methods have been developed such as strain gauge venous occlusion plethysmography for peripheral muscular blood flow.[28]

2.3.3.3 Assessment of Vasodilatory Effects on the Venous Side

Venous capacity and venous tone are determinants of the venous return to the heart and consequently determine cardiac preload. Venous tone in the extremities can be assessed by venous occlusion plethysmography.

It is possible using this method to assess drug effects (e.g., of nitrates) on the venous capacity.[29] A more direct method is the dorsal hand vein technique, which allows assessment of the effect of systemic and local drugs on the tone of human veins *in vivo*.[30-33] This method represents an *in vivo* technique in man similar to basic organ pharmacology. The local doses of drugs like vasoconstrictors are mostly below the threshold of systemic activity, thus allowing construction of complete dose effect curves *in vivo* in man.

2.3.4 Assessment of Potency and of the Duration of Action of Competitive Antagonists

Competitive antagonists may be assessed by their ability to antagonize the effects of agonists. The ACE inhibitors may be seen as competitive antagonists at the site of the ACE, as they compete for the binding site with angiotensin I[34] and ACE activity can be assessed by recording the blood pressure response to angiotensin I infusions.[35]

The situation is less complex when assessing ß-adrenoceptor antagonists or with angiotensin II antagonists.

Using this technique a half-life of the antagonist effect can be derived, which corresponds well to the duration of action.[34] Using various doses of the antagonist an apparent k_i dose can be derived which resembles the potency of an antagonist.[34] The therapeutic dose for a variety of antagonists had been found to be about 4 times k_i dose.

2.3.5 Relationship Between Pharmacodynamic Parameters and Efficacy

In general it is quite clear that the therapeutic efficacy of drugs for heart failure depend on certain pharmacodynamic effects, like positive inotropism, vasodilatation, Na excretion, and inhibition of neurohumoral reflexes. All these effects can be assessed and measured in healthy subjects and therefore the results obtained allow one to formulate a hypothesis about the therapeutic dose and the dosage interval with greater accuracy than the rather arbitrary approach used in the past. On the other hand, it has to be kept in mind that even when these effects are proven in man it only allows a prediction of the general therapeutic effects (and also some assessment of safety).

A definite decision about clinical efficacy can only be reached by clinical studies utilizing hard endpoints. One should keep in mind, for example, that PDE III inhibitors clearly showed positive inotropic and vasodilating effects in both healthy and heart failure subjects and were effective in acute clinical situations, but the effects in chronic studies were disappointing with decreased survival.

2.4 Controls

In testing dose-effect and time-effect relationships of new cardiovascular compounds in healthy volunteers the use of placebo controls is mandatory. Many of the variables used to assess drug effects show diurnal and other forms of variability, which may hide effects or produce false-positive results. The use and selection of positive controls are much more difficult to judge. Drugs like digitalis glycosides may be used as indicators of more or less pure positive inotropic effects. Vasodilators at the arterial side of the circulation like hydralazine may be useful for comparison in terms of pure vasodilation. All such studies must take into account the realities of dose-effect relationships. Frequently the observation of pharmacodynamic differences between a new drug and an old one are only due to different effects with noncomparable dose levels. To obtain data for the valid comparison of effect spectra of related substances, establishing dose-effect curves (ideally also concentration effect) is mandatory — but difficult and expensive.

3 PATIENT STUDIES

Early patient studies should not start until a sound database of pharmacokinetics and -dynamics in healthy volunteers is available. This information is vital in the selection of an appropriate initial dose and the dose interval for repetitive administration. From this it also is clear that a first entry-into-man study in this field cannot justifiably be done in patients if the necessary initial information can be obtained from healthy individuals. Patient studies become ethically justified when the patient has the possibility of some therapeutic benefit. Alternatively it is often possible to study the acute hemodynamic effects of new drugs invasively in patients undergoing routine diagnostic cardiac catheterization.

3.1 Suitability

In the field of heart failure early studies will most frequently be of single dose design or for a short period (e.g., one week) and will include dose ranging and also examine the safety and tolerability in the target population.

Heart failure is a chronic disease and treatment has to be given for long periods (mostly life long). Whether patients can obtain relevant therapeutic benefit in a short study is questionable. Furthermore, if there is an improvement in the patients condition and symptoms, it can be a rather difficult problem to withdraw the drug after completion of the study period.

3.2 Selection Criteria

For early patient studies one should restrict participants to NYHA II and III patients, since NYHA I does per definition not require treatment and NYHA IV are severely ill patients which are mostly unstable and require multitreatment. With NYHA II patients monotherapy with the new compound can usually be justified.

In NYHA III a basic treatment with conventional drugs (e.g., diuretics, digitalis, ACE inhibitors) cannot be stopped and the new drug has to be used "on top" of this treatment. Because heart failure is predominantly a disease of older age groups, the question of teratogenity usually does not play a role and the study population can include both males and females.

3.3 Safety Considerations

Heart failure is a severe disease with a poor prognosis. Acute decompensation, pulmonary edema, infarcts, cerebrovascular accidents, and sudden death may occur in the course of this disease and therefore also in the course of a study. There will always be the danger that in such a case, even though there may be no casual relationship between the experimental drug and the adverse event, such a relationship will be assumed by the patients, their relatives, and lawyers. To be on the safe side therefore early phase II studies with new compounds in patients with heart failure should be performed under in-house conditions with intensive observation of the patients before, during, and for an adequate period after the first administrations. Special attention has to be paid to the occurrence of arrhythmias which are frequent in patients with heart failure and which may be worsened by the treatment. As congestive heart failure is a disease with a poor prognosis, prolonged, uncontrolled open continuation of a completed trial should be avoided because of the potential negative influence on the safety database. If open continuation is foreseen it should be controlled.

Studies of the acute effects on hemodynamics and electrophysiology after i.v. administration in a catheter laboratory[36,37] are only justifiable when the new compound has a good safety and dynamic/kinetic profile in preclinical and normal volunteer pharmacology.

3.4 Methods

3.4.1 Pharmacokinetics

The pharmacokinetics of drugs may be influenced by heart failure itself, e.g., absorption could be reduced because of impaired hepatic and intestinal perfusion. This can only be evaluated in patients and should be known in an early stage of development. Determination of plasma kinetics will usually suffice. Only rarely will kinetics in other body fluids (e.g., urine or effusions) be necessary and useful. It should also be anticipated that pharmacokinetic changes may occur as heart failure improves.

3.4.2 Surrogate Markers

Hard endpoints for patients suffering from heart failure are death and/or clinical deterioration leading to hospitalization. These have, for example, been tested in phase III and IV studies with ACE inhibitors, PDE III inhibitors, nitrates, and hydralazine with varying results, a long duration, and prohibitive budgets.

In selecting appropriate surrogate endpoints which serve to help make early decisions about therapeutic efficacy in patients one has to take into account the high mortality rate in patients with heart failure. The impact of various indexes of disease severity on mortality has helped to establish the relative importance of the many parameters used to evaluate the severity of the disease. This has successfully been done in the Veterans Affairs Cooperative Vasodilator-Heart Failure Trials (V-HeFT I and II).[38,40] There are several determinants of prognosis in heart failure and EF, VO_2 peak, c/t ratio, and plasma noradrenaline that seem to be important independent prognostic factors. One usually assumes that influencing these variables in the "good" direction is also beneficial for the patient's prognosis, although this hypothesis does not hold true in all cases.

An improvement in these prognostic markers can be used to predict potential therapeutic benefit for a new drug.

For phase II studies one usually has to rely on the following surrogate endpoints (Figure 4): (1) functional assessment of exercise performance; (2) hemodynamics; and neurohumoral regulation.

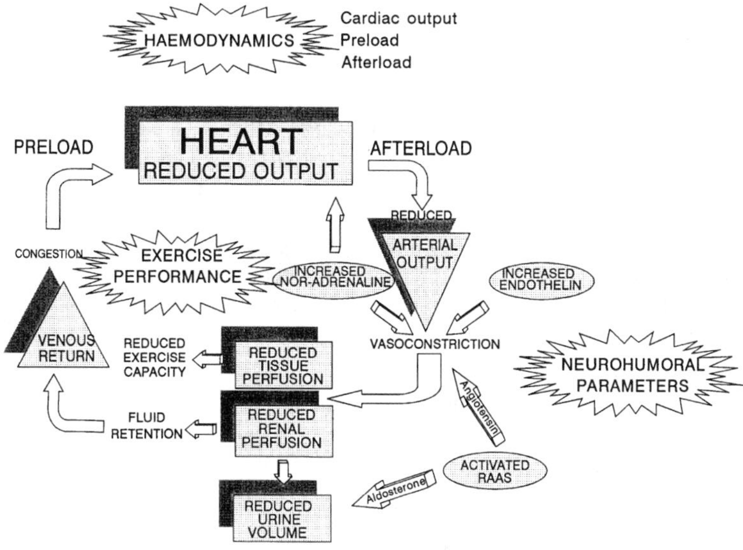

Figure 4 Major groups of parameters used as markers for assessing potential efficacy of drugs in early studies with congestive heart failure patients.

3.4.2.1 *Functional Assessment of Exercise Performance*

During aerobic (oxidative) metabolism the body tissues consume oxygen (O_2), while producing carbon dioxide (CO_2). Oxygen is taken up and CO_2 is eliminated via the lungs. The ratio between the volumes of CO_2 (VCO_2) to O_2 (VO_2), i.e., VCO_2/VO_2 is defined as the respiratory gas exchange ratio, R. Under normal resting conditions R equals from 0.75-0.85.[41]

Muscular work and the peripheral consumption of oxygen may rise to a degree where the cardiovascular system is no longer able to provide the muscles with sufficient oxygen. The muscles will then utilize the less efficient anaerobic metabolic pathway to increase its energy supply. Anaerobic metabolism produces lactate. The increasing intracellular lactate is buffered by bicarbonate and results in production of nonmetabolic CO_2, which increased the value of R in excess of normal. The onset of anaerobic metabolism during an exercise test can be defined as the point where an abrupt disproportionate increase in R occurs (R ± 1,0).

Simultaneous measurements of arterial lactate concentrations at that point show a concentration of ~4 mMol/l.

The anaerobic threshold is defined as the amount of O_2 uptake at the point where this abrupt change occurs. The ventilatory anaerobic threshold is a submaximal measure of aerobic capacity independent of individual motivation of patient and examiner and the ability of the patient in terms of physical performance (e.g., limited mobility due to arthrosis). The anaerobic threshold is reduced in heart failure.

An additional parameter derived from gas exchange measurements is the peak VO_2 under exercise from the final 0.5 min of exercise. When VO_2 rises to the level that exceeds the maximum pumping capacity of the cardiovascular system, i.e., cardiac output cannot be further increased, then the maximal oxygen uptake VO_{2max} is reached. The absolute values exceed those of the anaerobic threshold. In heart failure this VO_{2max} is clearly reduced.[41] Though VO_{2max} is not independent of individual motivation, i.e., it may be further increased by external stimuli (think of the galley slaves of old), it is a good predictor of prognosis. In the V-HeFT II study both, anaerobic threshold and VO_{2max} were assessed.[40] In spite of good arguments in favor of the anaerobic threshold, it was in comparison to VO_{2max}, not a more sensitive indicator of improvement in exercise performance.[40] A further technique for assessing gas exchange is noninvasive cardiopulmonary exercise testing (CPX test). A variety of equipment and protocols have been suggested. They all have in common:

1. Incremental physical stress testing; e.g., on a bicycle ergometer or on a treadmill
2. Assessment of VCO_2 and VO_2 either using mixed or breath-by-breath expired gas
3. Optimally a simultaneous measurement of the arterial lactate concentration, e.g., from the arterialized earlobe blood pressure, heart rate and ECG monitoring are, for safety reasons, mandatory during a CPX test

It is important to exclude a reduced pulmonary function in such patients, since it also will reduce VO_{2max} and anaerobic threshold. Usually a resting spirography will suffice.

3.4.2.2 Hemodynamics

The EF is that fraction of end-diastolic left ventricular volume which is ejected during systole. It depends on the measurement of end-systolic (ESV) and end-diastolic (EDV) volumes and is assessed by the ratio between (EDV-ESV)/EDV. These volumes can in clinical studies be obtained noninvasively by two-dimensional echocardiography or by radionuclide ventriculography. EF was shown to be a highly significant predictor of survival in the V-HeFT I and II studies.[39]

One rather simple and long established parameter quantification of the heart size is the cardiothoracic ratio (c/t) using a simple chest X-ray. The c/t ratio showed a highly significant prognostic power in the V-HeFT I and II studies.[40]

3.4.2.3 Neurohumoral Regulation

The neuroendocrine activation in heart failure leads to an increase in plasma noradrenaline levels. This sympathetic activation results in increased activity of the RAAS (with its consequences) and contributes to increased peripheral vascular resistance and increased left ventricular afterload and is responsible for further worsening of the pump function of the heart. The results from the V-HeFT II study clearly demonstrated that plasma noradrenaline is an independent predictor of prognosis in heart failure.[38] Drugs like hydralazine plus isosorbide dinitrate but not enalapril, cause increased plasma noradrenaline concentrations.[3,38] In the group treated with the ACE inhibitor the mortality was significantly lower. Differences in the survival were most significant when considering those patients showing the most intense change in plasma norepinephrine under treatment. These results indicate that the influence of new drug therapies on plasma noradrenaline should be considered as very important information in early patient studies.

3.5 Size and Duration of Trials

The big studies on the effects of ACE inhibitors vasodilators, inodilators, etc. comprised a large number of patients (e.g., V-HeFT I and II >600, >800 respectively) and were conducted over study periods of ~5 years. This type of study is not feasible for phase II of drug development. On the other hand, after only a 6-month study duration in the consensus trial a clear benefit was obvious. This shows that even in short time periods a positive result can sometimes be expected from hard endpoints.

Realistically one should plan for small, but realistic dose-finding trials in phase II (groups of $n \approx 10$), treating them with different doses of the new compound to establish the dose which produces an adequate therapeutic effect as assessed by markers and which is well tolerated. One should treat patients in this phase over a time span long enough to yield hemodynamic effects (>1 week) but not for too long to minimize risks.

Because pivotal studies have to follow such dose-finding studies, we think it appropriate to perform such phase II studies in an open (though controlled) fashion, allowing for quick adjustments and interim analysis where needed.

4 DECISION MAKING

To decide whether a new drug has therapeutic potential in congestive heart failure and warrants large phase III trials it is essential to have:

1. A full pharmacokinetic and pharmacodynamic profile including time-course of drug action (onset of activity) and dose-effect relationship of effects in humans.
2. Hemodynamic actions after single and after repetitive administration in patients with heart failure.
3. Limited potential for drug interactions with drugs that are commonly co-administered.
4. Evidence for efficacy during chronic treatment (>1 week) in terms of surrogate parameters of proven prognostic value (e.g., VO_{2max}, EF, plasma-noradrenaline).
5. Adequate data to support the dose and dose interval chosen.

Apart from these issues it should be clearly recognized that to convince regulatory authorities and to be able to make a major market impact a new drug should provide clear additional benefits (safety and/or benefit) to current standard therapy (digitalis, diuretics and ACE inhibitors).

REFERENCES

1. Wei CH, Lerman A, Rodenheffer RJ, McGregor CGA, Brandt RR, Wright S, Heublein DM, Kao PC, Edwards WD, Burnett Jr. JC: Endothelin in human congestive heart failure. *Circulation* 1994; 89:1580-1586.
2. Joubert PH: Are all cardiac glycosides pharmacodynamically similar? *Eur. J. Clin. Pharmacol.* 1990; 39:317-320.
3. Packer M, Gheorgiade M, Young JB et al.: Withdrawal of digoxin from patients with chronic heart failure treated with angiotensin-converting-enzyme inhibitors: RADIANCE study. *N. Engl. J. Med.* 1993; 329:1-7.
4. Uretsky BF, Young JB, Shahidi FD, Yellen LG, Harrison MC, Jolly MK: Randomized study assessing the effect of digoxin withdrawal in patients with mild to moderate chronic congestive heart failure: Results of the PROVED trial. *J. Am. Coll. Cardiol.* 1993; 22:955-962.
5. Ziesche S, Cobb FR, Cohn JN, Johnson G, Tristani F: Hydralazine and Isosorbide dinitrate combination improves exercise tolerance in heart failure. Results from V.HeFT I and V-Heft II. *Circulation* 1993; 87 Suppl VI:VI-56-VI-64.
6. The CONSENSUS Trial Study Group: Effects of enalapril on mortality in severe congestive heart failure: Results of the Cooperative North Scandinavian Enalapril survival study CONSENSUS. *N. Engl. J. Med.* 1987; 316:1429-1435.
7. The SOLVD Investigators: Effect of enalapril on survival in patients with reduced left ventricular ejection fraction and congestive heart failure. *N. Engl. J. Med.* 1991; 325:293-302.
8. Gottlieb S.S.: ß-blockers for heart failure: where are we now? *Curr. Opin. Cardiol.* 1994; 9:295-300.
9. Cohn JN: Inotropic therapy for heart failure: paradise postponed. *N. Engl. J. Med.* 1992; 320:729-731.
10. Curfman GD: Inotropic therapy for heart failure: An unfulfilled promise. *N. Engl. J. Med.* 1991; 325:1509-1510.
11. Feldman AM, Bristow MR, Parmley WW et al.: Effects of vesnarinone on morbidity and mortality in patients with heart failure. *N. Engl. J. Med.* 1993; 329:149-155.
12. Li Q and Belz GG: Systolic time intervals in clinical pharmacology. *Eur. J. Clin. Pharmacol.* 1993; 44:415-421.
13. Wolf GK, Belz GG: Methods of frequency-correction for systolic time intervals. *Basic Res. Cardiol.* 1981; 76:182-188.
14. Mäntysaari M, Länsimes E: Heart rate correction based on "universal" regression equation — erroneous conclusions when studying cardiac mechanical function during stress. *Eur. Heart J.* 1992; 13:1088-1091.
15. Stern HC, Matthews JH, Belz GG: Influence of dihydralazine induced afterload reduction on systolic time intervals and echocardiography in healthy subjects. *Br. Heart J.* 1984; 52:435-439.
16. Lewis RP, Rittgers SE, Forester WF, Boudoulas H: A critical review of the systolic time intervals. *Circulation* 1977; 56:146-158.
17. Joubert PH, Belz GG: Are pre-ejection period changes specific for inotropic effects? *Eur. J. Clin. Pharmacol.* 1987; 33:335-336.
18. Belz GG, Butzer, Erbel R, de Mey C, Nixdorf U, Schroeter V: Relative sensitivity of various noninvasive estimates of the effects of isoprenaline in man. *Clin. Pharmacol. Ther.* 1992; 51:172.
19. De Mey C, Belz GG, Nixdorf U, Butzer R, et al. Relative sensitivity of four noninvasive methods in assessing systolic cardiovascular effects of isoprenaline in healthy volunteers. *Clin. Pharmacol. Ther.* 1992; 52:609-619.

20. Belz GG: Systolic time intervals. A method to assess cardiovascular drug effects in man. In Kirch, E. Ed.: *Cardiovascular Effects of Histamine and H_2 Receptor Antagonists.* Zuckschwerdt, München 1994; p. 25-34.
21. Belz GG, Erbel R, Schumann K, Gilfrich HJ: Dose-response relationship and plasma concentrations of digitalis glycosides in man. *Eur. J. Clin. Pharmacol.* 1978; 13:103-111.
22. Schäfer-Korting M, Belz GG, Brauer J, Alken RG, Mutschler E: Digitoxin concentrations in serum and cantharides blister fluid: correlations with cardiac response. *Clin. Pharmacol. Ther.* 1987; 42:613-620.
23. Belz GG, Bliesath H, Essig J, Neumann N, Zech K, Wurst W: Differential effects of two dihydrophyridine calcium antagonists in humans. *Clin. Pharmacol. Ther.* 1992; 52:68-79.
24. Belz GG, Meinicke T, Schäfer-Korting M: The relationship between pharmacokinetics and pharmacodynamics of enoximone in healthy man. *Eur. J. Clin. Pharmacol.* 1988; 35:631-635.
25. Belz GG, Stern HC, Butzer R: Dose response following single administrations of a new cardiac performance enhancer Ro 13-6438 in normal volunteers. *J. Cardiovasc. Pharmacol.* 1985; 7:86-90.
26. Heather LW: A comparison of cardiac output values by the impedance-cardiograph and dye dilution in cardiac patients. In: National Aeronautics and Space Administration, Progress Report contract No. NAS9-4500, Houston, Texas, 1969.
27. Breithaupt K, Erb K, Neumann B, Wolf GK, Blez GG: Comparison of four non-invasive techniques to measure stroke volume: Dual-beam doppler echoaortography, electrical impedance cardiography, mechanosphygmography and M-mode echocardiography of the left ventricle. *Am. J. Noninvas. Cardiol.* 1990; 225:203-209.
28. Breithaupt K, Belz GG, Kempinski S, Schicketanz KH and Dieterich HA: The effect of oral enoximone on cardiac performance, calf arterial blood flow, and constrictor effects of norepinephrine infused into hand veins in humans. *J. Cardiovasc. Pharmacol.* 1990; 16:349-353.
29. Belz GG: Placebokontrollierte Studie zur Pharmakodynamik and Bioäquivalenz dreier Nitratpräparationen in: Hochrein H and Bussmann WD Eds.: *Nitrattherapie Perimed,* Erlangen Germany 1985; 55-61.
30. Aellig W: Clinical Pharmacology, physiology and pathophysiology of superficial veins I and II. *B. J. Clin. Pharmacol.* 1994; 38:181-196 and 289-305.
31. Belz GG, Beermann C, Schloss J, Neugebauer G: Influence of carvedilol on the responsiveness of human hand veins to noradrenaline and dinoprost. *Drugs* 1988; 36 Suppl. 6; 69-74.
32. Belz GG and Beermann C: Venodilatory effects of nicorandil in healthy volunteers. *J. Cardiovasc. Pharmacol.* 1992; 20 Suppl. 3.; S57-S58.
33. De Mey C, Breithaupt K, Seibert-Grafe M, Belz GG: Differential effects of the novel NO-donating drug pirsidomine and isosorbide dinitrate on the venous vascular bed. *Eur. J. Clin. Pharmacol.* 1994; 46:295-299.
34. Essig J, Belz GG, Wellstein A: The assessment of ACE activity in man following angiotensin I challenges: a comparison of cilazapril, captopril and enalapril. *Br. J. Clin. Pharmacol.* 1989; 27:217S-223S.
35. Joubert, PH, Brandt HD: Apparent racial difference in response to angiotensin I infusion. *Eur. J. Clin. Pharmacol.* 1990; 39:183-185.
36. Mitrovic V, Stöhring R, Schlepper M: The use of intravenous milrinone in chronic symptomatic ischemic heart disease. *Am. Heart J.* 1991; 121:1983-1994.
37. Mitrovic V, Petrovic O, Bahavar H, Neuzner J, Dietrich HA, Schlepper M: Anti-ischemic and hemodynamic effects of an oral single dose of 150 mg of the phosphodiesterase inhibitor enoximone in patients with coronary artery disease — Relation to plasma concentraton. *Cardiovasc. Drugs Ther.* 1991; 5:689-696.
38. Francis GS, Cohn JN, Johnson G, Rector TS, Goldman S, Simon A: Plasma norepinephrine, plasma renin activity and congestive heart failure. Relations to survival and the effects of therapy in V-HeFT I & II. *Circulation* 1993; 87 (Suppl. VI): VI-65-VI-70.
40. Cohn JN, Johnson G, Shabetai R, et al. Ejection fraction, peak exercise oxygen consumption, cardiothoracic ratio, ventricular arrhythmias, and plasma norepinephrine as determinants of prognosis in heart failure. *Circulation* 1993; 87 (Suppl. VI): VI-5-VI16.
41. Weber KT, Janicki IS: *Cardiopulmonary Exercise Testing.* WB Saunders, Philadelphia, 1986.

Chapter 19

Peripheral Arterial Disease

Jill J. F. Belch and Wolfgang Söhngen

CONTENTS

1 Introduction 250
2 Healthy Volunteers 252
  2.1 Selection Criteria 252
  2.2 Safety Considerations 252
  2.3 Methods 253
    2.3.1 General Trial Design 253
    2.3.2 Pharmacokinetic Issues 253
    2.3.3 Pharmacodynamics 253
      2.3.3.1 Vasodilatation 254
      2.3.3.2 Coagulation and Hemorrheology 255
      2.3.3.3 Blood Vessel Tone 256
        2.3.3.3.1 Iontophoresis 256
      2.3.3.4 Coagulation System 257
      2.3.3.5 Platelets, RBCs, and WBCs 258
        2.3.3.5.1 Platelets 258
        2.3.3.5.2 RBCs 258
        2.3.3.5.3 WBCs 259
      2.3.3.6 Fibrinolysis 259
  2.4 Controls 261
3 Patient Studies: Intermittent Claudication 261
  3.1 Suitability 261
  3.2 Selection Criteria 261
  3.3 Safety Considerations 264
  3.4 Methods 265
    3.4.1 Pharmacokinetics 265
    3.4.2 Surrogate Markers 265
      3.4.2.1 Clinical 265
      3.4.2.2 Laboratory 266
  3.5 Controls 266
  3.6 Size and Duration of Trials 266
4 Patient Studies: CLI 267
  4.1 Suitability 268
  4.2 Selection Criteria 269
  4.3 Safety 270
  4.4 Methods 270
    4.4.1 Pharmacokinetic Studies 271
    4.4.2 Surrogate Markers 271
      4.4.2.1 Laboratory 273
  4.5 Controls 273
  4.6 Size and Duration of Trials 273
5 Good Clinical Practice 273
  5.1 Steering Committee Meetings 274
Key Literature 274
References 274

0-8493-9230-6/97/$0.00+$.50
© 1997 by CRC Press, Inc.

1 INTRODUCTION

Atherosclerosis is the leading cause of obstructive arterial disease of the extremities. The prevalence of symptomatic disease increases with age. Its most common manifestation, intermittent claudication, affects between 1.5 and 7% of men aged between 40 and 60 years[1,2] and approximately 6% of men and 2% of women in the population aged 60 years and over[3,4] (Figure 1). Asymptomatic peripheral arterial occlusive disease (PAOD) occurs almost three times more frequently.[13] The disorder is more common in those who smoke cigarettes[14] and in those who have elevated blood lipids,[3] glucose,[7] and blood pressure.[10] Usually the first symptom is intermittent claudication which remains stable over time in the great majority of patients, particularly in those who reduce risks factors. In one Mayo clinic study approximately 90% had improved or showed no progression of their disease over time.[15] Others reported that 80% of patients remained stable over a period of 2-3 years.[16] However, the natural history of the disease is different for patients who continue to smoke or who have other risk factors such as diabetes mellitus. In one study of PAOD patients who smoked, 11% of patients who continued to smoke underwent amputation within 5 years. No limb loss was recorded for those who stopped smoking.[17] Furthermore, the amputation rate for diabetic patients is four times higher than that for their nondiabetic counterparts, again, over a 5-year period.[15]

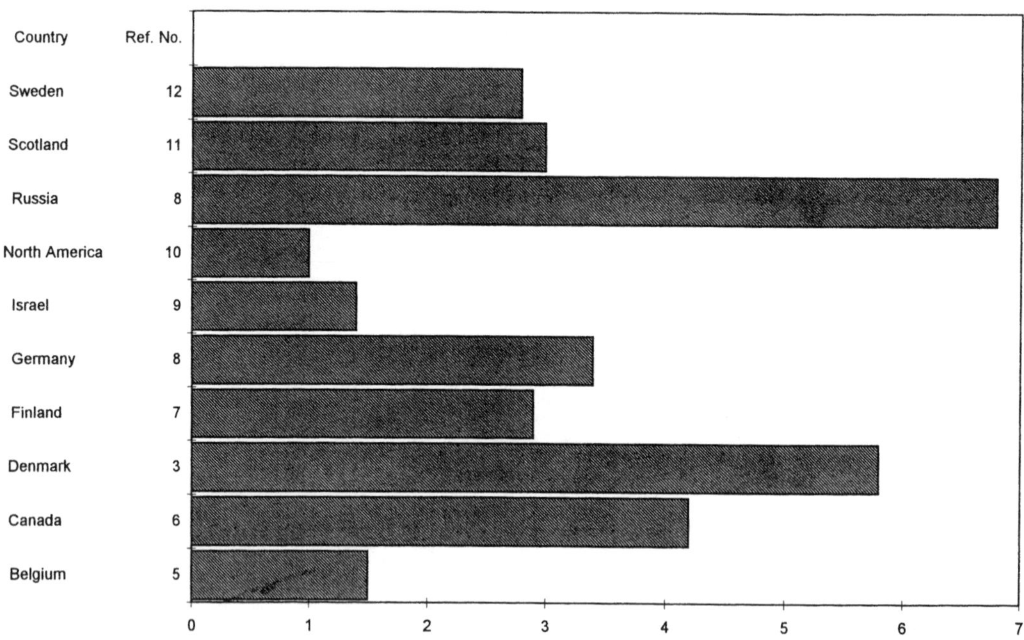

Figure 1 The prevalence of intermittent claudication.

It should be noted, however, that although intermittent claudication in most patients tends to remain stable, this disorder is associated with a high frequency of cerebraovascular events with a significant increase in mortality. In the Framingham Study[18] over a period of 14 years the average annual mortality for men with intermittent claudication was 3.9% compared to 1% in men without claudication. Survival rates were approximately 70-80% after 5 years, 40% at 10 years and only 26% at 15 years. Despite the data provided from the above studies the natural history of PAOD patients is relatively unknown compared to that of patients with coronary artery disease (CAD), and one of the inherent difficulties in planning studies in this area relates to the paucity of data on patient morbidity and mortality.

The symptoms of intermittent claudication are most commonly described by the patient as a pain or ache in one or both extremities, usually the legs, brought on by exertion and relieved by rest. The location of the pain depends upon the location of the arterial lesions. In patients with disease predominantly below the popliteal arteries discomfort may only be felt in the soles of the feet. If the disease is principally located in the superficial femoral arteries then the pain will appear in the calves. With aortoiliac disease the symptoms will also be felt in the thighs and buttocks. The amount of exercise required to precipitate the symptoms remains fairly constant over the shorter term and the patient's estimate of walking distance is usually fairly accurate, although standard walking tests must be carried out in therapy assessment studies. Walking speed is an important variable in the onset of symptoms and, if the pace is increased, the symptoms will occur sooner. Additional important factors are gradient of walk, symptoms being increased by a steep slope or stairs, and whether the patient is carrying a heavy weight. Use is made of these variables when designing the standard treadmill exercise test.

Occasionally the symptoms worsen abruptly due to rupture of an atherosclerotic plaque, thrombosis above a stenosis, or embolization from the vascular tree proximal to the limbs or heart. More usually progression of the disease, when it occurs, proceeds in a gradual fashion over months or years with minor deteriorations due to the above followed by gradual though not complete resolution due to the opening up of a collateral circulation. As can be seen from Figure 2 symptoms proceed through mild to moderate and finally to severe. Severe limb ischemia is estimated to affect between 500 and 1000 patients per million adults[19] depending on the definition used. Symptoms include pain on rest, relieved temporarily by dependency, trophic tissue changes such as ulceration, and finally tissue death/gangrene. The socioeconomic consequences of this severe form of PAOD are vast. In terms of quality of life the impact is great producing much suffering and inconvenience due to rest pain and loss of mobility. Furthermore, patients requiring amputation have a high postoperative mortality rate.[20] The survivors may suffer problems of physical handicap, severe financial consequences, and dependency upon others. The financial costs to the government are also high. A careful extrapolation from incidence data suggest that PAOD might account for approximately 5% of the total annual costs of all diseases.[21] Thus, risk factor modification, preventative medicine, and development and assessment of new forms of treatment should be actively encouraged.

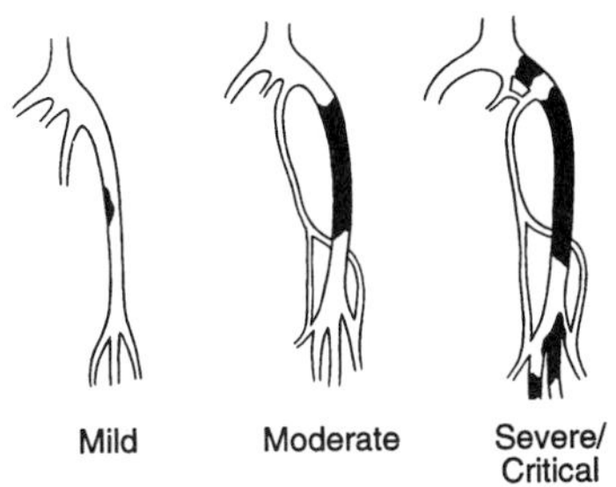

Figure 2 Progression of arterial disease.

Many drugs are promoted for the symptomatic treatment of intermittent claudication and severe limb ischemia and some have, in the past, obtained licenses when evidence of efficacy was insufficient or indeed lacking. Most of these compounds are primarily vasodilators. However, ischemic vascular beds are usually maximally dilated so vasodilator drugs can aggravate ischemia by diverting flow to nonischemic regions; the so-called "steal phenomenon."[22] Thus they are often promoted for their various additional properties such as beneficial effects on blood hemorrheology.[23] The usual endpoints for such therapeutic studies are walking distance to pain and maximum walking distance in intermittent claudication, and ulcer healing and relief of rest pain in severe limb ischemia.[24] Currently, however, more stringent criteria for drug registration are being prepared by both the European Commission (already in final form) and the Food and Drug Agency in North America. These are not yet published and are awaited with interest. For claudication these include a fixed percent improvement in walking distance, and for severe limb ischemia complete ulcer healing and/or a decrease in the amputation rate. These are discussed more fully later. Two major problems, however, hindering the development and assessment of drug therapy for PAOD are the distorted perceptions of patient need in intermittent claudication and quantification of drug benefits in severe limb ischemia. In the first of these there appears to be a double standard for claudication and angina pectoris (symptoms of the same process with approximately equal associated mortality risks) whose placebo response is also well documented.[25] Patients are equally disabled if they cannot walk because of pain in the legs as because of pain in the chest. Drugs are frequently withheld in the former but rarely in the latter. It has been suggested that severe lower limb ischemia is somewhat akin to cancer (Dr. G. Belcher, personal communication), any medical treatment we give is palliative relieving the symptoms for a limited period of time. With the symptomatic treatment for severe limb ischemia we are treating ulcers and pain, we do not attempt to cure the disease. Licensing body expectation should not therefore be too high. A 10% increase in survival produced by an anticancer drug allows a license as does a 5% reduction in mortality from myocardial infarction (MI). Perhaps the pendulum has swung too far in the critical appraisal of PAOD drug licensing when a 15% decrease in amputation and death rate fails to produce a license for the compound in some countries. One of the reasons for these problems is an apparent confusion as to whether therapies are aimed at symptomatic relief or prevention of progression of the underlying disease. The investigator should first decide which of these endpoints are being selected as they have many implications on study design, especially with regard to the sample size, i.e., several hundreds vs. several thousands of patients. The one does not, however, exclude the other and it is reasonable that drugs which prove to be successful in symptom relief should be evaluated in a second state of development for their efficacy in secondary disease prevention. Guidelines for these two approaches should be quite different and it should be noted that this chapter deals with the former, that is the relief of symptoms in the PAOD patient.

2 HEALTHY VOLUNTEERS

As with any drug development project the main task of phase I studies of drugs designed for PAOD treatment is to show safety, evaluate hemodynamics, pharmacokinetics, bioavailability in formulations other than intravenous preparations, and, if possible, decide on a rational dose for phase II studies. Pharmacodynamic assessments are also an important feature of phase I studies.

2.1 Selection Criteria

The types of volunteers suitable for studying a drug in this treatment area are similar to those used in most phase I studies. These include good health in the volunteer and, usually, male sex to prevent drug exposure to the developing fetus. Phase I studies in female volunteers are also necessary if the drug is going to be used in female patients, since it is important to find out whether dosing should be different. The first single and multiple dosing studies should be performed in healthy volunteers.

As PAOD is a disease of middle aged and elderly[2] the question should be posed as to whether phase I studies should be carried out in subjects ≥50 years of age or in young healthy volunteers. If the study is purely to answer questions of bioavailability and pharmacokinetics a young population can be studied, but if pharmacodynamics or safety is the primary issue then an older population should be selected. A study in elderly subjects does seem to be justified for a drug targeted toward PAOD in order to evaluate variation in pharmacokinetic parameters and suggest dose alterations, if required.

Although not accepted by all phase I units, we consider it to be important to include a placebo control in all phase I studies in order to minimize investigator bias.

2.2 Safety Considerations

The usual safety considerations for all phase I studies should be observed here. These include blood tests (RBC, WBC count, liver enzymes).

In addition to the above specific attention must be paid to the following areas: (1) effects of the drug on heart function and behavior; (2) potential alterations in blood pressure; and (3) renal handling of the compound.

Atherosclerosis is a multisystem disorder that affects several blood vessels in different organs simultaneously. Thus, the patient with PAOD may have concomitant CAD. Studies have demonstrated that the incidence of CAD in patients with claudication varies from between 25 to 90%.[25] Thus these patients may experience significant side effects from drugs which only minimally affect cardiac contractility, output, and conduction. In the same way the patients have a high incidence of cerebrovascular disease.[26] Men with chronic leg ischemia have a 5-year mortality two to three times higher than men of a similar age without PAOD; 50% die from ischemic heart disease, 15% of stroke, 10% abdominal vascular deaths, and only 25% die from noncardiovascular causes.[27] The presence of carotid vascular disease produces an enhanced risk of stroke with hypotensive agents. The morbidity and mortality following bypass surgery has both a coronary and carotid etiology,[28] and drugs which cause even modest alterations in blood pressure must be rigorously assessed. Another effect of blood pressure fall is attenuation of limb perfusion in a seriously ischemic limb. In such a limb elevated blood pressure may be providing the minimum required pressure for perfusion. Any hypotensive effect of a drug may thus contribute to increasing limb ischemia.[29]

In the patient with widespread atherosclerosis, it is to be expected that renal function might also be impaired. Drugs metabolized and/or excreted predominantly via a renal pathway may need a downward dose adjustment when introduced into patients and care should be taken to elucidate these pathways in the healthy volunteer.

Thus, a variety of assessments must be incorporated into the phase I studies of drugs destined for the PAOD market. Electrocardiograms and cardiac output should be routinely assessed during drug dosing. Twelve-lead ECG monitoring is easily applied as are noninvasive measures of cardiac output such as echocardiography. Routine blood pressure monitoring intermittently using a random zero sphygmomanometer or continuously through ambulant blood pressure monitoring can provide details regarding any hypotensive effect.[30] Pharmacokinetic studies will determine the renal metabolism/excretion profile. These studies will provide information to complement the work already obtained from animal and *in vitro* studies.

2.3 Methods

2.3.1 General Trial Design

Both single and multiple dose studies can be carried out although some simple precautions are required if certain pharmacodynamics aspects are to be evaluated. For example, if blood cell surrogate markers for vascular disease such as platelet aggregation are being measured a period of ten days must elapse between each single dose to exclude the antiplatelet effect persisting into the second dosing/placebo stage. In the same way freedom from drug therapy known to affect these markers must be for at least ten days prior to the study. Additionally, a number of drugs used in the treatment of PAOD have effects which persist after cessation of drug therapy for periods of weeks and months.[32-34] A cross-over design may be used for normal volunteer studies but they are, therefore, susceptible to treatment effects persisting into the placebo phase when active treatment is given first.[34]

2.3.2 Pharmacokinetic Issues

In general, pharmacokinetic procedures adapt well to the study of PAOD drug measurements. All the studies suggested above should be accompanied by pharmacokinetic measurements so that any drug effect can be correlated to plasma levels. The time of peak plasma levels should ideally correlate to the drug dosage (e.g., platelet inhibition) and changes in drug dosage/route of delivery should be considered if, for example, peak plasma levels correlate with adverse events that would limit the use of the drug. In the field of PAOD, however, plasma levels of agents currently used in this disease do not necessarily correlate with drug effect such as is seen in other areas, e.g., antibacterial activities with antibiotics. Thus it should be realized that pharmacokinetic as well as pharmacodydnamic measurements (see below) are more exploratory than predictive.

Plasma drug concentration measurement will provide dose-response curves, but it should be remembered that certain groups of compounds which may be of use in PAOD may require incorporation into cell membranes to exert an affect and evaluation of the drug levels within the cell membrane, usually red blood cells or platelets, may also be required.[32] While oral or transdermal formulations are preferred for claudication, severe limb ischemia may be well managed through the intravenous route.[33] Compounds useful in this area will probably include those with antiplatelet effects. As is often the case, therefore, the recommendation to take with food may be necessary. Furthermore, compliance of patients in taking their drug medication is not always guaranteed and thus the ideal drug should have the same pharmacokinetic profile regardless of whether the compound is taken before, during, or after a meal. Pharmacokinetic studies should be carried out both in the fasting and nonfasting state.

2.3.3 Pharmacodynamics

When designing normal volunteer studies the most difficult task is to decide on the scope and methods for pharmacodynamic measurements. Thus far there has been no unique pharmacodynamic quality that unambiguously predicts the effectiveness of a drug in later clinical studies in patients. Despite the fact that vasodilators proved that they truly vasodilated and that antiplatelet drugs had antiplatelet effects in phase I studies, this did not predict with any surety whether they were able to produce clinical benefit beyond doubt in later phase II/III trials. In PAOD there is no "gold standard" test which predicts efficacy and the range of surrogate markers delineated below have been selected on the basis of known mechanisms of blood flow and various epidemiological studies. Thus, vasodilatation might be expected to be beneficial if a "steal" effect can be avoided, and many studies have emphasized the importance of platelet aggregation,[34] white blood cell activity,[35] increased fibrinogen, and impaired fibrinolysis in predicting future cardiovascular events. At the present time, the best studied mechanisms of drugs used for the treatment of PAOD relate to vasodilatation and the alteration in blood hemorrheology. In the future drugs benefiting cell metabolism under ischemic conditions may also be available as may other drugs targeted to the atherosclerotic plaque. Obviously, the pharmacodynamic studies required depend upon the putative mode of action and will vary from compound to compound. This following section will relate mainly to vasodilatation and hemorrheological studies as most products currently under development are reported to possess these properties.

2.3.3.1 Vasodilatation

Intense vasodilatation will manifest by an increased heart rate and then a fall in blood pressure. In PAOD it is preferred that the compound have peripheral vasodilatory effects rather than central effects. This attenuates the fall in blood pressure and promotes flow to the extremities. Symptomatic side effects are likely to include facial flushing and headache accompanied by a sensation of warmth. Subjective quantification of flush has been used in the past in studies but is now replaced by objective measures. It should be noted that the techniques described below cannot be used with accuracy outside a temperature-controlled environment. The temperature of 24 ±1°C with a relative humidity of 50% ± 15% is a suitable example. Prior equilibration in this environment for between 20-30 min is required before the start of the tests.

1. Laser Doppler flowmetry (LDF): The principle underlying LDF is the same as is used in ultrasound to measure flow in vessels (see later). In this technique a narrow beam of monochromatic light is generated by a low power laser and carried by an optical fiber to the skin. Light hitting moving blood cells will undergo a slight Doppler shift but light hitting static structures will be unchanged (Figure 3). The magnitude and frequency distribution of the Doppler shift are directly related to the numbers and velocity of blood cells. Thus, a cell motion correlated single, the RBC flux, is obtained (number of RBCs × their average velocity). An output signal in volts linearly related to the RBC flux is generated. A number of manufacturers produce high quality equipment usually measuring the total microvascular flow to approximately 1 mm radius hemisphere of the dermis immediately below the probe head. The LDF signal is derived mainly from the movement of RBCs in the superficial plexus and capillary loops in the dermal pilae as well as arteriolar and shunt flow in the deeper dermis. While the majority of LDF machines measure flow over a small area, the newly developed scanning laser Doppler allows wider areas to be evaluated (Figure 4). During the past decade this method has become very popular as a means to evaluate skin microcirculation in humans,[36,37] nevertheless, certain considerations must be given to the interpretation of the output signals. The penetration depth given above is approximate and this and the measuring volume are essentially unknown and vary with physiological characteristics such as the amount of blood and the composition of the skin in the region investigated. Consequently a quantification of flow in ml/min^{1}/100 g^{-1} can only be obtained if certain specific conditions are fulfilled,[38] which is not the case for human skin.[39]

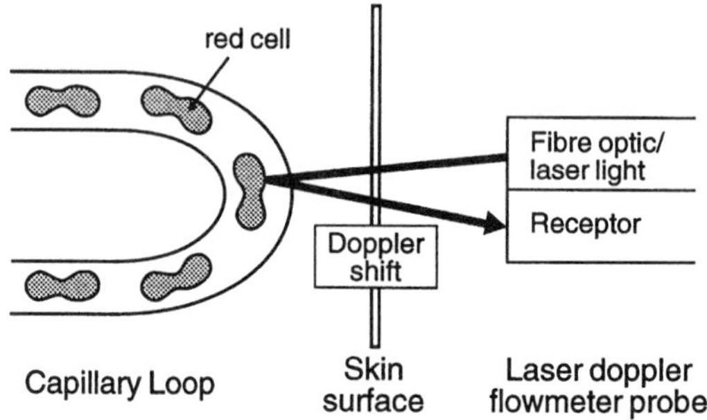

Figure 3 Laser Doppler flowmetry. (Reproduced from *Atlas of Peripheral Vascular Diseases,* 2nd edition, Times Mirror International Publishers, London. With permission.)

Furthermore, the zero value for the instrument cannot be used as a zero for living tissue. If the LDF probe is positioned over tissue in which blood flow has ceased the apparatus will still register a flow

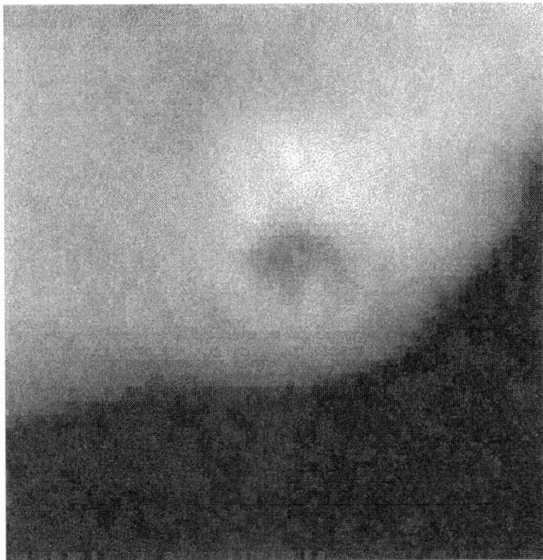
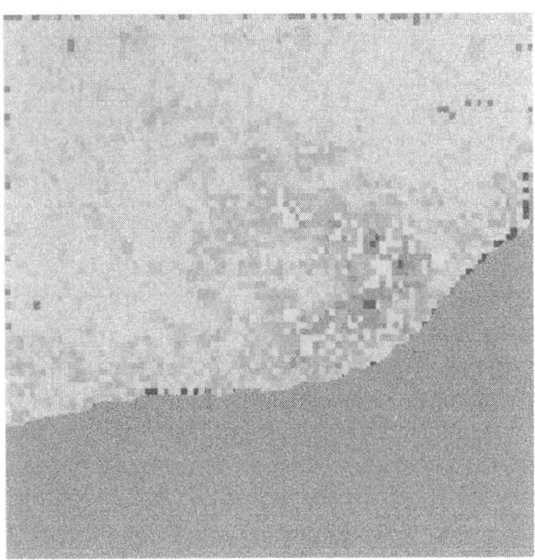

Figure 4 Scanning laser Doppler flowmetry showing an ischemic ulcer at the hallux, medial aspect. The capacity to heal was predicted by hyperemia surrounding the central portion. (Reproduced by kind permission of Moor Instruments Ltd.)

signal.[40] Marked variation in this biological zero can be seen over different tissues and in different areas of the same tissue.[41] Biological zero values should always be subtracted from the values recorded. Despite the above LDF is noninvasive and requires a minimum of patient preparation. Furthermore, the measurements occur directly and continuously with a very short response time (approximately 0.2 s) which makes it ideally suited for measuring mediated reflex changes in microcirculatory flow. LDF has also been compared with other flow measurement techniques and, in general, shows a good correlation. For example, LDF was shown to correlate well with venous occlusion plethysmography[42] and xenon-clearance.[43] Not all workers have found this concurrence, however,[44] and this highlights the complexicity of the microcirculation and that the use of a single measurement technique may not necessarily be optimum.

2. Dynamic nailfold capillary microscopy: This technique of *in vivo* observation of flow in skin capillaries has been adopted from the procedures used to assess the morphological appearance of skin capillaries at the nailfold. It has been developed by utilizing TV-microscopy and a video-photometric technique for analyzing the TV picture.[39,45] Analysis of blood cell velocity can be performed on an ordinary personal computer using a special software program.[46] As with LDF a number of variables can affect the results. There is again a need for equilibration prior to the study which must take place in a temperature-controlled room. Positioning of the patient is also of importance. When sitting, the transmural pressure is high and the blood filling of the capillaries is increased compared to that observed when the subject is in the supine position.
3. Thermography: This technique relies on the camera detection of skin temperature and is often used as an indication of blood flow by researchers.[47] Sophisticated quantification of skin temperature over defined areas allows estimates of warning and cooling times to be made with great accuracy. Nevertheless, the relationship between skin temperature and blood is complex. Skin temperature is not only dependent on blood flow but is also a function of arterial and venous blood temperature, the coefficient of heat transfer of the tissues, and environmental temperature. Thus a warm skin area may look "cool" using thermography if the skin is moistened with sweat, the latent heat of evaporation being subtracted from the warmth of the tissue by the camera. In inexperienced hands this is not a reliable method for assessing skin blood flow. In contrast, its usage by an expert aware of the drawbacks of this technique can produce useful results.

2.3.3.2 Coagulation and Hemorrheology

Although atherosclerosis is usually the basic underlying pathology in PAOD deterioration/progression in the symptoms of the disease can be mediated by changes in coagulation and thrombosis. Arterial occlusion is often due to obstructive thrombus, composed predominantly of platelets and fibrin, forming near to a vascular stenosis. There is no doubt that the occurrence of thrombosis in relation to pre-existing atherosclerotic plaque is the most important complicating event in the natural history of atherosclerosis and is responsible for the majority of clinical manifestations. Furthermore, where the vasculature is partially occluded or stenosed cell rheological properties become important. Platelet aggregates, hard RBCs, and adherent WBCs will all contribute to a decrease in flow in an already compromised vessel. It is for these reasons that PAOD therapies have been targeted toward the hemostatic/hemorrheological process. This can be schematically subdivided into four somewhat overlapping components all of which can be measured with reasonable accuracy to allow detection of drug effects. They are as follows. (1) the blood vessel; (2) the coagulation system; (3) platelet, RBCs, and WBCs; and (4) fibrinolysis.

2.3.3.3 Blood Vessel Tone

Vasoconstriction may be responsible for some of the clinical complications of thrombosis.[48] Among the mechanisms thought to be responsible for vessel contraction are neurogenic factors and blood chemistry such as adrenalin and endothelium-derived vasodilatation/vasoconstriction. Most vasodilatory responses can be measured as indicated above, but evaluation of the endothelial mechanisms need a more sophisticated approach. Table 1 documents endogenous vasoconstrictors and vasodilators. Those derived from the endothelium can either be measured in plasma/serum or indirectly assessed.

Table 1 Endogenous Vasodilators and Vasoconstrictors

Vasodilators	Vasoconstrictors
Prostacyclin (E)	Endothelin (E)
Other prostaglandins, e.g., PGE_1	Serotonin
NO/Endothelium derived relaxing factor (E)	Some prostaglandins, e.g., $PGF_2\alpha$
	Thromboxane A_2
	Adrenalin
	Sympathetic nerves

Note: (E) - endothelium derived.

Endothelin, first described in 1988,[49] is a potent vasoconstrictor peptide which does not belong to any previously known family but shows regional homologies to peptide neurotoxins that act on voltage-dependent ion channels. The physiological role of endothelin is not yet fully defined but recent accumulating evidence suggests that it may participate in the long-term regulation of vascular tone and may play a role in vascular diseases such as hypertension and arterial thrombosis.[50] Endothelins 1 and 2 can be measured in plasma after extraction using a radioimmunoassay. Work evaluating proendothelin and endothelin receptors site expression may also be relevant to this area in the future.

Radioimmunoassays are available to measure eicosanoid metabolites in plasma. 6-keto-$PGF_1\alpha$ is a stable metabolite of prostacyclin (PGI_2) and thromboxane B_2 (TXB_2) of TXA_2. Unfortunately these assays are subject to artifact when used to measure levels in blood although they may produce reliable results in *in vitro* experiments. One exception to this may be the 15-hydroxy-thromboxane B_2 assay which appears not to suffer these artifactual interferences when used to measure serum TXB_2.[51,52] Note, however, that serum TXB_2 reflects plasma and blood cell production of TXB_2 as it is measured after blood coagulation. Thus, a compound designed to stabilize platelet membranes and thus allow less TXA_2 release into plasma could not be adequately assessed using this assay.

Nitric oxide (NO) is an important mediator of blood vessel tone, nerve conduction, and immune function, but we are really only beginning to unravel its role in these processes. The majority of measurements of NO in man have involved the assay of high levels seen in inflammation and in sepsis, and this can be done with a variety of techniques such as the Greiss reaction or HPLC. However, the current challenge is to measure the low levels of NO which are likely to be found, and to be of pathogenic significance, in cardiovascular disease. The state-of-the-art technology is the assay of nitrite and nitrate by capillary electrophoresis.[53] It should be noted, however, that this assay development is in the early stages and a number of precautions require observation such as the elimination of dietary nitrite for 12 h before taking blood. Because the assays for NO are in the early stage of development, and thus validation, many workers are selecting the technique of iontophoresis for assessment of endothelial-dependent and independent vasodilatation.

2.3.3.3.1 Iontophoresis

The technique of iontophoresis uses an electrical charge to transfer small quantities of pharmacological agents directly across the skin surface. This technique is particularly suited to studying microcirculatory control mechanisms because it avoids the effects of local trauma and any potential hazards of systemic drug administration. The quantity of drug delivered depends on the charge of the ion, it's molecular weight, the strength of the electrical current, and duration of current flow.[54] Briefly, the system consists of an active platinum loop electrode contained within an iontophoretic chamber and an indifferent electrode both of which are linked to a current generator. An LDF is used to measure the response with a hole through the center of the iontophoresis chamber acting as the fiberoptic probe holder. The solution for iontophoresis is injected into a well inside the chamber. Direct iontophoresis of acetycholine can be used to measure endothelium-dependent microvascular vasodilatation[54,55] and sodium nitroprusside to measure myogenic vasodilatation,[56] while indirect iontophoresis of acetylcholine through stimulation of nociceptive C fibers and resultant local axon reflex allows assessment of neurogenic vasodilatation.[54,57] Figure 5 shows the trace obtained after iontophoretic application of acetylcholine. This vasodilatory response can be modified by disease and drugs. This technique is reasonably simple to utilize although there can be marked inter- and intrasubject variations in the time-course of the response curves. This necessitates a certain number of subjcts be enrolled for study purposes.

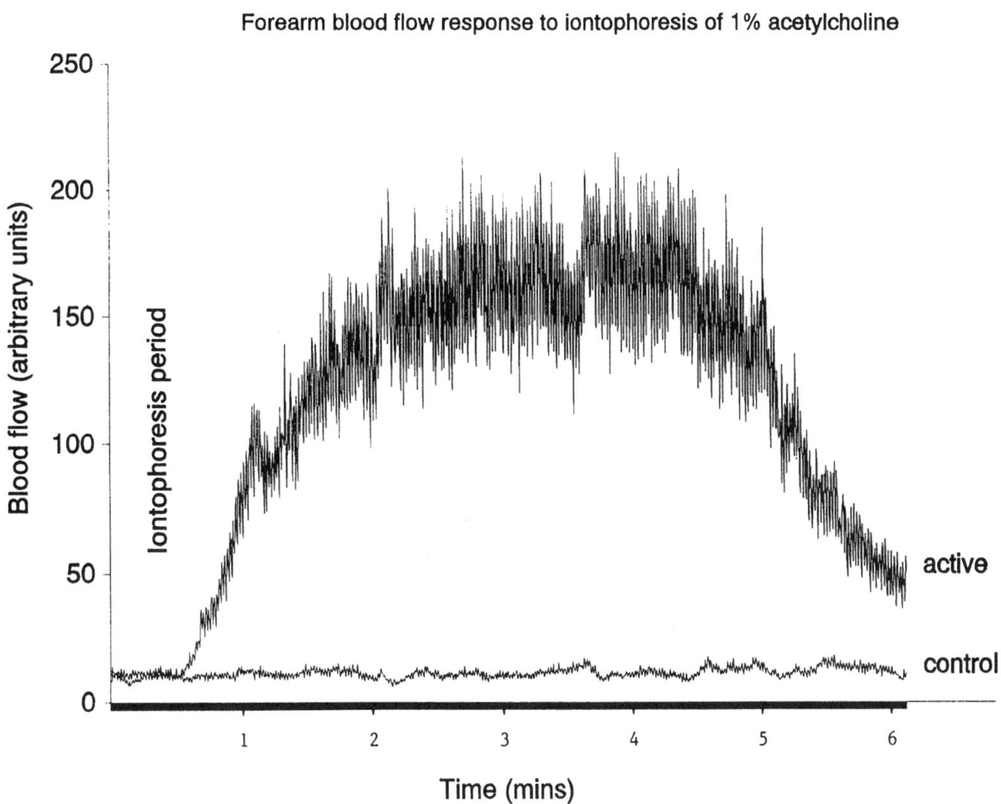

Figure 5 Vasodilatation after iontophoretic application of acetycholine measured by laser Doppler flowmetry.

2.3.3.4 Coagulation System

The role of the coagulation system in hemostasis is to provide stability to the platelet plug by the formation of a network of insoluble fibrin. The system comprises of a stepwise series of proenzyme conversions, each enzyme sequentially activating the proenzyme next in line. Interacting with this procoagulant mechanism are a series of physiological anticoagulant mechanisms that exert a dampening effect. Specific assays of individual factors both activated and not are available as are "global" tests of function such as the prothrombin time (PT), activated partial thromboplastin time (APTT), and international normalized ratio (INR). Also in regular routine use are specific tests for the physiological anticoagulants such as antithrombin III, heparin co-factor 2, alpha-2 macroglobulin, alpha-2 antiplasmin, and proteins C and S. Drug affects on these measures can be fairly easily evaluated as the above tests are available in the majority of hematology laboratories. It is not within the scope of this chapter to fully document these assay techniques, but the reader can refer to detailed methodology textbooks as listed under key publications at the end of the chapter.

2.3.3.5 Platelets, RBCs, and WBCs

2.3.3.5.1 Platelets

Some commonly used tests of platelet behavior are listed in Table 2. Some of these tests involve relatively little trauma to the platelet and therefore the information they give is likely to be relevant to platelet behavior *in vivo*. Other tests, although providing greater insight into underlying mechanisms, involve more drastic interference with the platelet such as anticoagulation, cell separation, and exposure to foreign surfaces. They allow selected phenomena to be studied at the cost of removal of other influences. As with tests of coagulation the reader is directed to the key references from methodology textbooks. Nevertheless, as the platelet aggregation assays are currently so integral in the testing of new compounds for PAOD these are outlined below.

Table 2 Tests of Platelet Behavior

Survival	Release
Count	• β Thromboglobulin
Volume	• Platelet factor 4
Adhesion	• Thromboxane B_2
• P-selectin	• Serotonin
• IIb/IIIa	Bleeding time
Aggregation	
• Platelet rich plasma	
• Whole blood	

Platelet aggregation in platelet rich plasma (PRP) is based on the following principle. When an aggregating agent is added to vigorously stirred PRP previously prepared by centrifugation, the formation of platelet clumps produces a decrease in optical density which can be measured making serial readings with a photoelectric absorptiometer.[58] Platelet aggregation in PRP is a simple and usually reliable technique for the testing of a drug's antiplatelet effect. It is, however, subject to artifactual influences when used by the inexperienced. For example, large gauge needles must be used for venepuncture, which must take place following minimum tourniquet pressure. Tests must be completed well within 2 h of sampling which includes the time taken to transfer the sample to the laboratory, the 15 min of centrifugation to prepare the PRP, and later 10 min of centrifugation for the preparation of platelet-poor plasma. Platelet aggregation in PRP is time consuming and may be liable to artifact due to the blood centrifugation procedure required. Additionally, the platelets are studied in isolation, in the absence of other cells. Platelet aggregation in whole blood is a sensitive reproductive method of measuring platelet aggregation originally measured using specific whole blood platelet aggregometers[59] but now using a standard Coulter counter.[60] A count of the number of single platelets is made before and after the addition of a platelet aggregant. The initial platelet count is expressed as 100% and the numbers of single platelets remaining after aggregation are expressed as a percent of this initial count. This omits the centrifugation procedure of PRP aggregation, allows interaction of all blood cell types, and a series of experiments can be completed within 15 min of venepuncture. As with all tests of platelet behavior it should be remembered that there is a diurnal variation in platelet aggregation and that platelet aggregation is affected by a high fat meal.[61] These factors must be considered when study design is being discussed.

2.3.3.5.2 RBCs

The most commonly used tests to evaluate the effect of RBCs on blood flow are red cell deformability and whole blood viscosity (at both high and low shear rates). RBC deformability can be measured by a variety of techniques often using a filtration method.[62] In this assay RBCs are forced to filter through micropores which have a diameter smaller than that of a normal RBC. RBCs which are capable of shape change (deforming) require less force to cross the pores than those which are rigid, and some drugs used in the treatment of PAOD have been found to decrease red cell diameter (RCD).[63] In recent times, however, the realization that WBC contamination of the suspension has contributed to the abnormal results has lessened the popularity of the test as a potential surrogate marker for vascular disease.

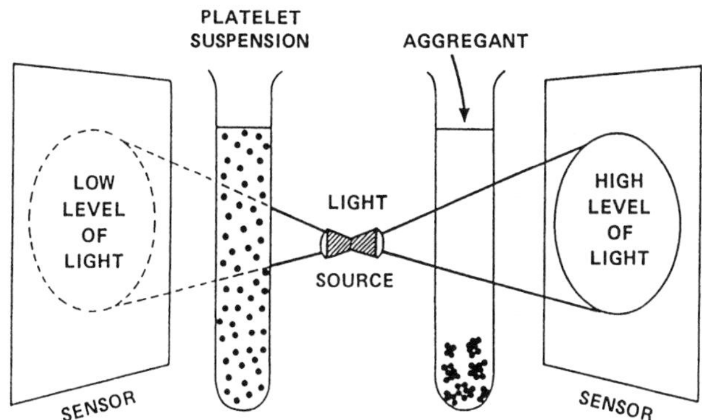

Figure 6 Principle of platelet aggregation using the photometric technique of Born.

2.3.3.5.3 WBCs

In contrast, the importance of the WBC in relation to vascular disease has increased over recent years,[64] and suggestions that beneficial effects can be expected from drugs which also alter WBC behavior are being investigated. Epidemiological studies suggest that the WBC count is a powerful and persistent predictor of cardiovascular events.[65] A high WBC count in the "normal range" is a predictor of future amputation in critical limb ischemia.[35] There are several possible explanations as to why the WBC may contribute to PAOD and these include: (1) the physical obstruction of the blood vessel by the WBC, (2) release of noxious chemicals such as free radicals (FRs), and (3) interaction of the WBC with other blood constituents.

WBC deformability can be measured using techniques similar to those used in evaluating RBC deformability. WBC aggregation can also be performed, and as with the platelet, this can be either in a separated cell population[66] or in whole blood.[67] The advantages of the whole blood WBC aggregation technique are the same as those for whole blood platelet aggregation, i.e., speed, absence of artifact from cell separation procedures, and interactions of all blood cell types. The basis for these tests are also identical except that the aggregant affects WBC behavior, e.g., FMLP vs. ADP.

If a WBC becomes trapped in the microcirculation it can deliver a variety of insults to the blood vessel lining (Table 3). The chemical substances released from the WBC would normally be used in the protection of the organism against microbial invaders, but such defense mechanisms can promote vascular injury and disease. These substances include elastase, leukotrienes,[64] and FRs.[68] Of these, the most frequently investigated in PAOD are the FRs, their products, and scavengers. Direct measurement of FRs is difficult without sophisticated electron spin resonance/magnetic resonance imaging techniques. Thus, it is usual to measure products of FR reactions such as lipid peroxides and conjugated dienes.[69,70] Earlier spectrophotometric assay methods for lipid peroxides are now being replaced by HPLC techniques allowing more sensitive results in drug studies.[71] The antioxidant status of the blood can be assessed individually again by HPLC assay of various antioxidants such as vitamin C[72] and vitamin E.[73] A technique which gives a global assessment of antioxidant potential is also available.[74] Direct scavenging of radicals can be assessed though this is best carried out *in vitro*,[75] as normal volunteers have a very low baseline level of FR production and to show changes within the normal population requires very large numbers.

While some of the above assays are reasonably straightforward others require either sophisticated techniques or knowledge of methodological pitfalls. For example, as with other blood constituents important in vascular disease, there are diurnal variations in FR markers[76] and WBC behavior is affected by exercise and posture.[77] The reader is directed for further guidance to the methodology handbooks in the references.

2.3.3.6 Fibrinolysis

Plasma fibrinolysis has been shown to be defective in patients with PAOD[78] and certain fibrinolytic markers predict vascular events within a population. Fibrinolysis can be assessed when measuring the overall fibrinolytic activity of the plasma or more usually by assaying individual factors involved in the fibrinolytic pathway (Figure 7). When evaluating PAOD therapies the two most commonly measured

Table 3 Chemicals Released From WBCs Which May Affect Vascular Damage

Toxic oxygen species	Lysosomal enzymes
Hydroxyl radical	Elastase
Superoxide anion	Plasminogen activator
Singlet oxygen	Collagenase
Hydrogen peroxide	
Lipids	
Leukotrienes	
13 HODE	
Eicosanoids	
Platelet activating factor	

components of fibrinolysis are tissue plasminogen activator (tPA) and plasminogen activator inhibitor (PAI). Plasma tPA and PAI activity can be detected using chromogenic assays. As with all these assay systems certain precautions must be included in the study design. The fibrinolytic process varies throughout the day[51] and is affected by exercise and eating.[79] Simple precautions such as standardizing the time of day, presampling rest time, and ensuring a fasting state can greatly minimize artifacts. It is also possible to measure stimulated fibrinolysis by applying the technique of venous occlusion.[78] This diminishes the importance of the potentially variable baseline by allowing maximum production of tPA and maximum inhibition of PAI to be estimated. If a fibrinolytic effect of the drug itself is to be assessed then the breakdown products of fibrin (ogen), fibrin degradation products, and D-dimer can be evaluated. It is, however, important to stress once again that normal volunteer studies have a limited role in the pharmacodynamic evaluation of PAOD drugs and nowhere is this more obvious than in the process of fibrinolysis. If only small amounts of fibrin are being formed such as occurs normally, then to evaluate a drug for a minor fibrinolytic effect can be very difficult. Only minute changes will be seen in a normal population and very large numbers are thus required.

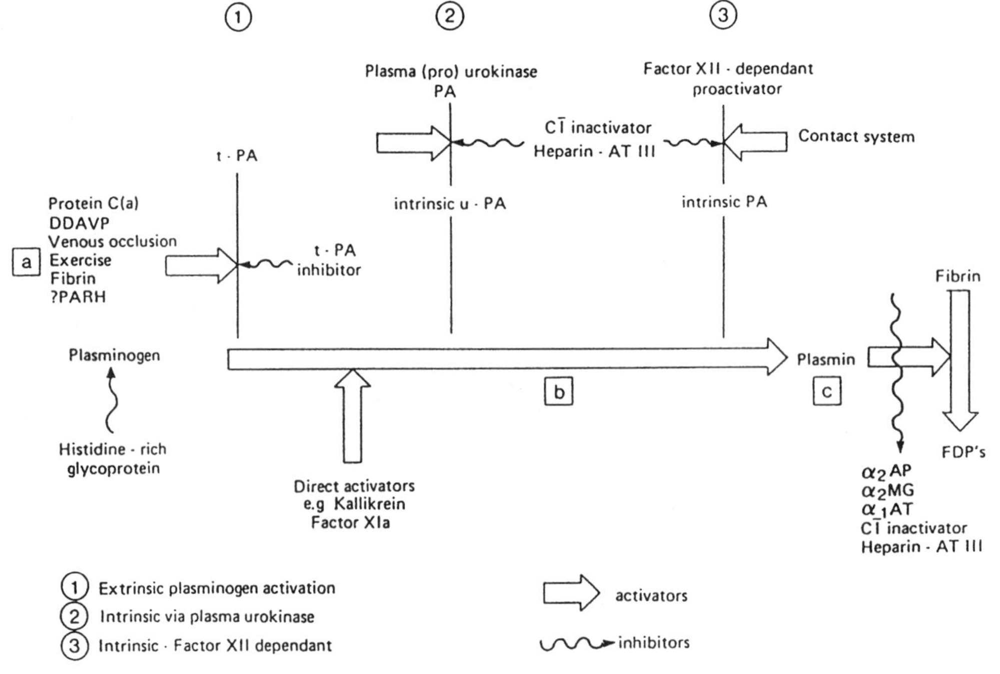

Figure 7 The fibrinolytic pathway.

2.4 Controls

Due to the variability in the baseline of the above tests combined with their significant diurnal variation, control studies are considered essential in this area. As no absolute gold standard drug exists, this is ethically acceptable. Furthermore, as the compounds already licensed for PAOD have many different modes of action, a comparator can be difficult to find. We recommend that phase I studies should be placebo controlled. Certainly drugs with vasodilator potential can be compared to conventional vasodilators and antiplatelet drugs with established chemicals such as aspirin. It must be remembered, however, that action against these surrogate markers for vascular disease does not predict effectiveness in later clinical studies. While these tests may shed light on various mechanisms of action no surrogate hemodynamic or hemorrheological measurement can be used as a primary endpoint in efficacy studies.

Table 4 Classification of Fontaine

Stage I	Asymptomatic disease
Stage IIa	Ischemia induced by exercise producing the symptoms of intermittent claudication after walking 200 m, relieved by rest
Stage IIb	Ischemia induced by exercise producing the symptoms of intermittent claudication before a distance of 200 m has been reached, relieved by rest
Stage III	Ischemic symptoms/pain at rest, i.e., rest pain
Stage IV	Trophic ulcers and gangrene

3 PATIENT STUDIES: INTERMITTENT CLAUDICATION

There are extensive varieties of disease manifestation and endpoints occurring in PAOD. Two of the major symptoms are intermittent claudication and rest pain in critical limb ischemia (CLI), both stages of the same process but with very different therapeutic aspirations, endpoints, and surrogate markers. Classification of the various stages of PAOD has been made by Fontaine[80] and this is illustrated in Table 4. It should be noted that Fontaine himself did not separate between IIa and IIb and this was introduced later by German angiologists. A number of publications give various claudication distances separating these two groups though none is definitive. A claudication distance of ≤200 m is regarded as severe claudication and is often used as the cutoff in clinical studies. In claudication, improving walking distance to pain is a useful aid but so too is decreasing the restenosis rate following angioplasty and/or improving quality of life issues. In CLI after considering whether the compound is aimed at acute or chronic disease presentation, the selection of an endpoint may relate to decreased rest pain, ulcer healing, vascular graft survival, or fall in the amputation rate. Thus, it can be seen that intermittent claudication and CLI are best considered separately.

3.1 Suitability

Early entry of the drug into a patient population is recommended for compounds targeted to the PAOD population. The surrogate markers for vascular disease such as platelet aggregation and vasodilatory responses will be "normal" in a healthy volunteer population. It can be difficult, therefore, to show alteration of these measures within a normal range using drug therapy. It is thus preferred that such surrogate markers be evaluated as soon as possible in the patient population. In some situations, the "success" of conventionally utilized interventions may not be very great and it may be judged therefore that comparison to surgery and percutaneous transluminal angioplasty (PTA) should be a feature of phase II rather than phase III studies. Safety aspects, however, must be fully explored prior to patient exposure for the reasons documented earlier.

3.2 Selection Criteria

One of the first considerations which should be addressed is whether the patient does truly have occlusive vascular disease. The diagnosis of claudication is based on the clinical symptoms outlined earlier combined with objective measures suggestive of peripheral blood flow obstruction. These include inability to palpate peripheral pulses, ankle brachial Doppler pressure indices (ABPI), and arteriography.

The clinical measures are very subjective and are not adequate for use as selection criteria. For example the symptoms of pain on walking can result from venous claudication and orthopedic problems such as sciatica, spinal stenosis, and arthritis. Similarly, the palpation of peripheral pulses is very subjective suffering from inter- and intrapersonal variation and can be affected by anatomical features such as obesity and edema. For this reason, patients being enrolled into claudication studies must have objective evidence of lower limb vascular occlusion. Arteriography remains the best method of providing structural information about the arterial tree upon which decisions regarding the technical aspects of proposed treatment can be made, for example, PTA. However, angiography is an invasive technique with a small but definite risk of complications such as anaphylaxis, thrombosis, embolization, and hematoma.[81] Therefore, unless the clinician in charge of the patient has decided that an operation or PTA will be carried out if a suitable lesion is detected, the patient may not have had an angiogram. It would be difficult to justify angiography on ethical grounds for study purposes alone. An acceptable compromise is to ask for an angiogram to have been carried out within the past one year prior to the study. This angiogram should show evidence of occlusive disease. This allows the investigator to ensure a correct diagnosis of PAOD but does not, of course, provide acceptable baseline data for study of disease progression.

More recently, Duplex ultrasound scanning has been used to detect and mark the presence of PAOD. This technique combines B-mode imaging and a pulsed Doppler into one instrument.[82] The former uses the reflection of ultrasound from tissue interfaces rather than from blood movement as in the Doppler technique. A high-resolution image of the vessel can be obtained together with spectral analysis of the blood flowing within the vessel. This combination of the simultaneous structural and flow information obtained noninvasively has resulted in duplex scanning replacing angiography in some cases of arterial disease, for example, in carotid disease.[83] In some centers duplex scanning is also replacing lower limb arteriography, but it should be remembered that visualization may be difficult in obese patients and that a significant amount of technical expertise is required for meaningful data to be collected.[84]

The most commonly applied screening test for PAOD of the lower limb is the ABPI.[85] In this technique Doppler ultrasound enables blood flow to be monitored in the lower limb arteries and in conjunction with a sphygmomanometer allows measurement of the ankle systolic blood pressure. To measure this pressure a sphygmomanometer cuff is wrapped around the lower limb and the cuff inflated to a supra-systolic level. The cuff is then slowly deflated and the onset of return of blood flow as detected by the Doppler probe equals the ankle systolic blood pressure. Doppler ankle pressures are often expressed as a ratio of the brachial systolic pressure, the ABPI. This index allows comparisons to be made over time in the same patient (a change of 0.15 is considered significant) and from patient to patient. Healthy subjects have an ABPI of ≥1.0 while in claudicants it is usually <0.9. Arterial calcification, common in diabetic patients, may give falsely elevated ratios due to incompressible vessels. Toe blood pressures are less likely to be affected by calcification and are recommended when studying diabetic populations. They do require specialized cuffs, however, and are more difficult to measure routinely. Drug treatment targeted to symptomatic relief is unlikely to affect the ABPI as this is a coarse measure of macrocirculatory flow. The ABPI can, however, be combined with exercise which increases the sensitivity of the test.[86] Enhanced muscle blood flow required by the precise process will result in a fall in ABPI which returns to normal over a measurable time.

Once the diagnosis of PAOD has been established demographic considerations should be taken into account. An age of ≥40 or 45 years should be an enrollment criteria to exclude patients with the inflammatory vascular disease, thromboangiitis obliterans (Buerger's disease). Patients of either sex can be enrolled but the majority will of course be male.

The nature of concomitant drug therapy must be established and exclusion made of patients receiving vasoactive drugs as a treatment for their PAOD. The high incidence of CAD in these patients[25] will mean that a significant proportion will be taking vasoactive drugs for angina and for ethical reasons these should not be stopped unless significant interactions/side effects are to be expected. A four-week washout period following such drug withdrawal is usually considered appropriate. In contrast, because of the widespread and justified use of aspirin in these patients, exclusion of patients on aspirin therapy would be difficult for two reasons. First, while it may be possible to stop aspirin in the short-term, longer term studies would be considered unethical because of the well-recognized beneficial effects of antiplatelet drug therapy in diminishing vascular events[87] and the need for vascular surgery.[88] Secondly, if such an exclusion were made the very small numbers of patients not receiving aspirin for clinical reasons would prejudice the enrollment rate. It is therefore recommended that any drug being considered as a symptomatic treatment for PAOD should be evaluated in patients receiving aspirin. The usual exclusion of unsuitable subjects should also be made. These include relevant laboratory abnormalities, concurrent diseases making survival to the end of the study unlikely, and participation in clinical trials of any other drug within the last three months. As an exercise test is likely to be a primary endpoint, patients whose walking performance is decreased for reasons other than arterial disease should be excluded. The high incidence of vascular disease elsewhere might produce exercise-limiting angina and poor mobility through stroke. Cigarette smoking will induce lung disease as well as arterial problems and dyspnea may also limit exercise tolerance.

Exclusion should also be made of patients who have just had or about to have interventions which may alter their ability to exercise. This includes vascular surgery and/or PTA within six months of the study or patients in whom such procedures are being planned and which will occur during the course of the study.

Risk factor modification must also be addressed as it is recognized that disease in patients with unmodified risk factors progresses much more quickly than in those in whom risk factors have been addressed.[17] The majority of patients with PAOD are smokers or ex-smokers.[14] Significant numbers and sound randomization procedures should ensure they are equally distributed between active and placebo groups. More difficult to ensure or indeed desire is that smoking remains a constant phenomenon throughout the study period. Active encouragement toward smoking cessation should be continued for ethical reasons. Sadly experience suggests that few heed this advice and thus smoking cessation does not become a confounding factor during clinical trials. Hyperlipidemia is becoming better recognized as a risk factor for PAOD[3] and most units will test for this and modify the lipid profiles with diet and drugs. Thus, patients enrolled in claudication studies using vasoactive drugs will be normolipemic either naturally or through medication. Studies of lipid-lowering agents will target newly presented patients about to enter the risk modification protocol.

Diabetes mellitus affects 25% of people in the Western world. The incidence of PAOD in diabetic patients is 14% over two years[89] and 45% by 20 years.[90] In one study 37% of lower limb amputations were carried out in diabetic patients compared to 4% age-matched, nondiabetic controls.[91] In therapeutic studies a decision must be made whether to exclude diabetic patients or to ensure appropriate randomization within groups. This is particularly important in view of a generally held though poorly substantiated opinion that diabetic patients respond less well to drug therapy for cardiovascular disease. The current recommendation is for these patients to be included in all studies.

The inclusion/exclusion criteria for a study in PAOD are the action and risks of a drug which are already known. There are many factors which will influence the treatment effect in PAOD. Those which probably have the most profound effect have not yet been fully explored. It is for this reason that minimization techniques should be used in order to ensure that an imbalance within patient groups of various factors will not influence the outcome of any study. Minimization means that all groups of treatment should have represented within them the same proportions of sex, cigarette smokers, diabetes, history of interventions, time of onset of disease, etc. This minimization approach increases study duration time but does produce a scientifically valid study. The method of minimization has been described by Taves[92] but has not been utilized to the extent that might have been anticipated. The complicated logistics involved may be one reason for its poor utilization. On the other hand, it is the widespread assumption that randomization will ensure an even spread of patient attributes that underpins our current enrollment procedures. It is not well established that the absence of statistically significant differences within patient groups does not infer absence of an important clinical effect.

Table 5 Randomization by Minimization

Factor	Level	No. on Treatment	No. on Treatment	Next Patient
		A	B	
Sex	Male	30	31	x
	Female	10	9	
Diabetes	Diabetic	18	17	
	Nondiabetic	22	23	x
Cardiac output	MI in history	31	32	x
	No MI in history	9	8	
Ankle blood pressure	Doppler pressure > 50 mmHg	19	21	x
	Doppler pressure < 50 mmHg	18	22	x
Marginal totals		157	163	

Minimizing should be used when minimizing bias in each treatment group is important. Treatments are equalized within levels prior to entering a patient into a trial. "Levels" are the above-mentioned influencing factors such as diabetes vs. no diabetes, male vs. female, acute MI history vs. none, etc. Assume that we have the following factors, and their distribution, in a given study population of a study where 80 patients are recruited. Because Group A has the lowest number of subjects the next patient will be assigned to Group A if he has the described criteria X. For practical reasons it is the best approach to let the first 40 patients of a given 400-patient study be randomly assigned to Group A or B as is the usual procedure in any study. The patient characteristics should be reported to the statistical center and the following patients will then be assigned according to the marginal totals of the whole study population at any time during the study. It is quite obvious that this approach needs detailed planning and the inclusion of a central statistics center. Nevertheless, with telephone registration and/or telefax this is not a valid argument against such an approach. An example of how this can be achieved is given in Table 5.

3.3 Safety Considerations

Adverse drug events occurring during the course of the treatment should be carefully recorded throughout all study phases including data about their nature, frequency, intensity, and relevance. Although adverse reactions occur reasonably frequently within this group of patients, particularly so in the group to be described later (CLI), many adverse reactions will be rare and large sample sizes will be necessary to detect them. Thus the combination results from all studies preferably those which address efficacy is recommended for final safety analysis. It is usual practice to ensure that the randomized double-blind comparative trials with efficacy endpoints are followed by a longer drug exposure in open conditions. The draft European Community Guidelines[93] on clinical testing requirements for drugs for long-term use suggest that at least 100 and, if possible, 300 patients should be treated with a new drug for one year to establish the incidence and importance of adverse effects. The casual relationship and outcome must be reported for all adverse events.

Healthy volunteer studies should have already provided data in respect to cardiovascular and renal effects of a particular compound. Depending on the pharmacological and toxicological activity of a drug, specific attention should be paid to any adverse event which may be expected on the basis of these activities. Particular attention must be paid to the assessment of drug effects on myocardial function and blood pressure. For reasons outlined earlier PAOD patients are very susceptible to subtle drug effects due to the presence of vascular disease in arteries other than those in the limb.[25] Renal function should have been addressed by the enrollment criteria of normal laboratory values, but a simple measure of plasma urea and creatinine levels may mask a subclinical but relevant renal impairment if a drug is excreted through this organ. Initial single-dose studies are recommended in PAOD patients to assess these safety issues.

As the primary clinical endpoint in these claudication studies is often pain-free walking distance a further problem relating to the co-existence of CAD may arise. In our own experience 30% of 62 claudicants being considered for enrollment to a clinical study were excluded because of abnormalities on their ECGs recorded while walking to claudication pain. No consensus exists on how well documented the co-existing CAD should be prior to enrollment into clinical studies or on whether patients with abnormal coronary arteries should be excluded from drug studies. The American Heart Association recommends that all PAOD patients undergoing treadmill testing for claudication should have ECG monitoring. Resuscitation facilities should also be available. Difficulty occurs in obtaining adequate patient recruitment if these subjects are totally excluded from clinical studies. Furthermore, and most importantly, as the majority of the target population will have CAD the first introduction of a drug into such patients should be under the strictly controlled and monitored auspices of a Good Practice study.

Intermittent claudication is a chronic disease and these patients frequently receive concomitant treatments for other disorders such as angina and chronic obstructive airways disease. It is therefore mandatory to perform drug interaction studies including both pharmacokinetic and pharmacodynamic measurements. Such studies should be performed taking into account the drugs most frequently used for the management of these patients.

The techniques used for measuring adverse events should be similar over the whole development period of the drug since, by doing so, an overall safety analysis can be carried out. A good exercise for this approach is to write a hypothetical summary of product characteristics at each stage of development, incorporating data from previous trials and phase I studies comparing the drug with other drugs currently being used for the treatment of PAOD and/or adverse experienced during surgical or PTA intervention.

3.4 Methods

As with normal volunteer studies, studies in patients can evaluate either single or multiple drug doses. The dose and therapeutic schedule should be selected according to the results of previous studies and usually three dose levels (low, medium, and high) are assessed. These studies should be carried out in selected patients with strict inclusion and exclusion criteria. The same precautions apply as for healthy volunteer studies, for example, wash-out periods for drugs known to affect surrogate markers and caution regarding persistence of effects in a cross-over design.[34] For major therapeutic studies aimed at drug registration, a cross-over design is not recommended due to interference from factors such as progression of the disease.

Certain design features should be incorporated into studies whose endpoints are clinical efficacy. If possible, the trials should last a minimum of six months and primary and secondary efficacy criteria should be assessed every one or two months during the treatment period. The development of tolerance (tachphylaxis) should be investigated as should "rebound phenomenon" seen after the withdrawal of some drugs.

3.4.1 Pharmacokinetics

Plasma concentrations of drugs will provide information on pharmacokinetic issues, although specific cellular assays may be required depending on intracellular drug penetration.[32] Pharmacokinetic studies will also assess patient compliance when carried out in larger patient populations. Oral formulations are preferred for the long-term symptomatic management of claudication and the effect of food on absorption should be considered. Transdermal application is also an attractive though underdeveloped drug delivery route for this group. However, it may be that the local vasodilatation induced by a number of compounds used for this indication might be disturbing for the patients. Studies would also be required to determine whether satisfactory plasma levels of the compound could be achieved.

3.4.2 Surrogate Markers

3.4.2.1 Clinical

In claudication Fontaine Stage II the main efficacy criteria are pain-free and absolute walking distances. Pain-free walking distance is a reasonable measure as it is the onset of pain that limits functional activity. It is, however, influenced by subjective factors such as pain threshold, patient motivation, etc. The absolute walking distance can also be measured, but it can be affected by factors other than claudication such as fatigue, dyspnea and angina. Most exercise testing in claudicants is now performed on a treadmill. The speed and gradient of most treadmills varies and it is important that these are standardized for each trial. A slower rate allows enrollment of frail patients but needs a longer time for exercise to induce pain. The same is true for a lower gradient. A fast rate and steeper slope precipitates symptoms more quickly but may not be well tolerated by the elderly. A reasonable rate would be 4 km/h with a gradient of 10 degrees.[87] Appropriate numbers of such tests should be carried out at intervals until sufficiently reproducible results are obtained before randomization. Unfamiliarity with the treadmill and other factors can produce a significant "learning" curve. The maximum change between the two tests in the run-in phase immediately prior to enrollment should be ≤25%.

Consideration should also be given to the pain-free walking distance itself. Patients with claudication after 200-300 m have a different and better progression rate than those with distances shorter than 100 m. Furthermore, they are more likely to experience so-called "walk through" phenomenon. While claudicants with all ranges of walking distance can be studied it is recommended that separate studies be planned for those with a walking distance of ≤100 m and >100 m. Treadmill tests should be performed under standardized enrollment conditions, time of day, and preferably carried out by the same investigator during the trial.

Walking distance has been used as the primary efficacy criteria in most claudication studies. Nevertheless, it should be remembered that it is in fact a surrogate endpoint as far as effect on progression of disease and patient well-being is concerned. Thus future studies in claudication will have to show an additional effect on quality of life (QoL). There is no internationally accepted QoL;[94] nevertheless, such questionnaires are available but must be validated prior to being used in pivotal studies. One suggested approach in the meantime is to begin with a standard QoL questionnaire such as the SF36[95] and modify it for the specific needs of the PAOD patient. It should be remembered that PAOD patients are often elderly and may have accompanying cerebrovascular disease. It is therefore important to keep the questionnaire simple. The questionnaire that we currently employ was considered straightforward by those of us involved in the study design; nevertheless, many patients were unable to fill in the questionnaire without help. It should be remembered that the FDA is not in favor of complicated QoL assessments and prefers a global assessment with few questions answered by both the physician and patient. In our experience the improvement of walking distance on the treadmill best correlates with the patient's feeling of whether or not he has achieved his stated personal aim at the commencement of the study.

3.4.2.2 Laboratory

It is unrealistic to expect symptomatic drug treatment to alter the baseline ABPI. However, some workers suggest that measuring the time taken for the pressures to return to this baseline following a standard exercise test may be of use.[86] Vasodilatation and microcirculatory effects can be evaluated as described for healthy volunteers. While LDF, thermography, and capillaroscopy are perhaps considered more relevant in the study of CLI, these tests can also be evaluated in claudicants. Some precautions need to be observed, however. With LDF most of the signal in healthy volunteers is generated by the movement of RBCs. In some pathological conditions, for example, leukemia and thrombocythemia, a large proportion of the signal is produced by the movement of WBCs and platelets.[36] Furthermore, the highest biological zero values are found in the PAOD patient and may be as much as 80% of the resting flow value. Thus, this random part of the signal becomes more significant in areas with diminished blood flow.[41] It is imperative that biological zero is recorded and subtracted when this technique is used in clinical practice.

In contrast, the blood tests of coagulation, hemorrheology, and fibrinolysis may produce more rewarding results when evaluated in patients as compared to healthy volunteers. Abnormalities of platelet behavior, white cell aggregation and release, and fibrinolysis are well documented and normalization of these abnormal results can illustrate potential mechanisms of actions of the compound. As acute exercise appears to enhance some of these abnormalities sampling pre- and post a treadmill test standardized for duration may be a useful way of observing drug effects. It should be remembered, however, that most patients will be on aspirin therapy[88] and this limits the value of platelet aggregation and release tests in these groups of subjects.

3.5 Controls

Any approach to drug therapy for limb ischemia must take into account the natural history of the disease, making controlled trials essential. It is hardly surprising that in such a common disease with a wide variety of pathophysiological variables many drugs have been used to try to alter or improve these factors. In the U.K. the drugs currently registered for use in claudication are treated with some skepticism.[96] This is broadly true in North America although in other parts of Europe outside the U.K. drug treatment is widely used. Contrary to the statement in the recent British National Formula that "no controlled studies have shown any improvement in walking distance,"[97] large controlled studies have shown positive results for naftidrofuryl,[98] oxpentifylline,[99] and ticlopidine.[100] Although the average increase in pain-free walking distance may be small, though statistically significant, some individual patients can do very well. For this reason in some countries placebo-controlled studies are acceptable whereas in others comparisons with one of the above is required. There is no doubt that placebo-controlled studies may be considered scientifically more rigorous and these studies are currently required for registration in North America and some parts of Europe. In North America it is additionally required to have at least one study with pentoxyphylline as a comparator. Nevertheless, choice of control is of less importance than the controlled aspect of the study itself.

A more difficult concept to control for is exercise training. Exercise standardized by treadmill[101] has been shown to improve exercise tolerance in claudicants in a number of controlled studies.[102] Unfortunately, only 25% of patients with claudication are able to undertake exercise training programs for the same reasons as some patients cannot carry out standard treadmill testing in drug studies, e.g., the presence of chronic obstructive airways disease, angina, arthritis, poor motivation, etc. Thus, it is not feasible to ensure patients are exercise trained before inclusion and difficult to include an exercise arm into the study design due to the poor compliance. If, however, this is considered to be an essential comparator it could be dealt with in phase III. It is more important to ensure that the claudication itself has been present for at least six months and that the patient has been given advice regarding the advisability of exercise during this time.

3.6 Size and Duration of Trials

Choice of patient numbers and the duration of each study depends upon endpoint selection. In claudication these can include various pharmacokinetic measures, dose ranging and tolerance studies, and evaluation of clinical surrogate markers. These include objective measures of blood flow, tests of coagulation and hemorrheology, and walking distances. Depending upon the purported action of the drug other specific endpoints might be selected, e.g., restenosis following PTA. For each of these, various details are required to allow power calculation estimates to be made. These include proposed change from baseline which reflects a significant improvement and inter- and intrapersonal variation of the tests (standard deviations). Other factors may need to be considered such as whether the proposed study is between subjects or within subjects, the number of centers participating in a multicenter study, and the number of primary endpoints selected. Guidelines for European readers regarding these points can be obtained from the European Commission.[103]

Each laboratory should be able to provide the above details on particular tests to allow calculations to be made. For example, in our laboratory LDF studies require 42 patients per study group when predicting a 30% improvement in flow in actively treated patients compared to placebo controls. The coagulation and hemorrheological tests have inter- and intra-assay variations of between 3 and 7.5% and depending on whether the study is between or within subjects number requirements to show a 20% benefit range approximately from 10 individuals to 37 in each of two groups. Well-established software packages are available for such estimations and no study should proceed without power calculation of population numbers. The clinical endpoints of pain-free walking distance and absolute walking distance have wide standard deviations within the claudicant population and larger study numbers are required. Nevertheless, it should be remembered that no surrogate hemodynamic or hemorrheological measurement may be used as a primary efficacy endpoint for registration purposes. There should be at least 50-60 patients per group enrolled into the study in order to generate a database that is large enough to make power calculations for later phase III studies. The following examples of power calculations may provide useful illustrations.

For these power calculations, the question that is being asked is whether or not the treatment effect is statistically significant. This question may be only weakly related to the issue of clinical benefit. We should be asking whether or not a treatment effect is *clinically* significant,[104] but this is not possible at the present time as clinically significant benefit has not yet been defined in this group of patients. Recommendations have been made that the sample size should be set to ensure that the estimate of effect size will be reported not only with adequate power but also with appropriate precision through the use of confidence intervals.[105]

Duration of study will depend upon preliminary registration details. Remember, however, that some compounds take up to three months to show clinical efficacy in this indication. A minimum follow-up period of six months should be selected.

Interim analysis might be useful to evaluate treatment effects after a certain period of the treatment, but it will inevitably weaken the statistical power of the study and thus greater patient numbers must be included into the original patient number calculations.[106] It should be noted that the regulatory agencies discourage interim analysis and this fact also has to be carefully noted during the planning of a successful drug development strategy. If an interim analysis is required it should be treated in the same way as having an additional primary endpoint, e.g., α adjusted from 0.05 to 0.025 for 2 and further to 0.0125 if 3 endpoints or additional analyses.

4 PATIENT STUDIES: CLI

CLI may be acute, acute on chronic, or chronic. The two former groups present with a painful white leg as clinical emergencies and at present are treated either by surgery or thrombolysis.[107] These approaches are not covered in this chapter and it should be remembered that specialized and occasionally different safety considerations, pharmacodynamics, and endpoints will need to be considered if studies in these areas are required.

Intermittent claudication may progress to critical lower limb ischemia, although CLI can arise de novo in some situations. Chronic lower limb ischemia (CLI) may have a number of different causes. The prognosis for each of these forms varies and may range from spontaneous resolution to limb loss/amputation. A severe form, chronic critical limb ischemia where threat to limb viability occurs is of major importance as the vast majority of lower limb amputations are performed because of it.[106] While CLI may merely be a progression from claudication attempts have been made to specifically define CLI to improve the comparability between clinical trials. In the Fontaine staging CLI covers grades III and IV, that is the presence of rest pain then trophic ulcers and/or gangrene. It is considered, however, that Fontaine staging[80] for CLI is too loose to allow meaningful comparisons between clinical practice in geographically different sites and between clinical studies. For this reason a European Consensus document on CLI was devised with input from eight specialist European societies.[29] The definition of CLI in this document is as follows:

> "Critical limb ischemia in both diabetics and nondiabetic patients is defined by either of the following two criteria: persistent recurrent rest pain requiring analgesics for more than two weeks, with an ankle systolic pressure of ≤50 mmHg and/or a toe systolic pressure of ≤30 mmHg; or ulceration or gangrene of the foot or toes with an ankle systolic pressure of≤50 mmHg and a toe systolic pressure of ≤30 mmHg."

There is no doubt that the consensus process has considerably strengthened approaches to scientific study of CLI and provided a first class management strategy for this disorder. It is an extremely valuable working document and is recommended reading for European workers. Nevertheless, it is accepted that this consensus process is still ongoing and needs to consider the following.

In North America current practices make some of the recommendations unacceptable. Additionally, the North Americans have made their own attempts at classification of lower limb ischemia.[108] It is recognized that any further revisions of the document must attempt to reconcile these differences.[109] A further problem with the Consensus Document is that the majority of large studies in severe limb ischemia have not used the consensus definition and it remains questionable as to whether the same results in terms of therapeutic benefit would have been obtained if they had. The European PARTNER concept studies[33] consist of five placebo and one PGE_1-controlled trial designed to evaluate efficacy of a prostacyclin analog. A side issue arose from these studies because the entry criteria were designed in parallel with the consensus process. Concern was expressed that the Consensus Document definition of CLI was too limiting and patients with pressures above the Consensus Document cutoff, i.e., ankle pressures between 50 and 60 mmHg were compared to those at or below the Consensus Document cut-off point (<50 mmHg). In the placebo-treated groups approximately 50% fulfilled the criteria for Consensus Document CLI and 50% did not. When the percentage of major amputations ± death was evaluated 40% of patients who fulfilled the consensus definition had a major amputation compared to 31% of those who were above it, i.e., these 31% did have CLI and defining CLI as an ankle pressure of <50 mmHg excludes these patients.

Thus, if one adheres to the Consensus Document criteria for inclusion, true cases of CLI may be excluded and studies may exclude a CLI patient population who might significantly benefit from treatment. Thus while the Consensus Document is admirable in its aims and in many of its recommendations, Fontaine grades III and IV are still used as a method for selecting patients for CLI studies. The Consensus Document has shown us, however, that entry ABPIs ± toe pressures must be strictly defined for each study.

The gold standard limb salvage treatment for CLI is the application of interventional techniques such as bypass grafting and angioplasty. In almost all cases of chronic CLI due to arterial occlusion the atheromatous lesions are mainly situated below the inguinal ligament. The majority of these patients will be offered some sort of revascularization procedure. However, a number of patients with CLI cannot for various reasons be offered such a procedure. Data in the 1970s[110] suggested that up to 30% of patients were not suitable for intervention, but more recent work suggests that these numbers have fallen and that <10% have inoperable disease.[111] This number, however, may be increased by considering patients who are inoperable by virtue of concurrent health problems such as CAD and chronic obstructive airways disease. For those in whom revascularization is not possible progression to amputation may occur. Using the available figures for progression of claudication to amputation the total amputation figures in the U.K. may be in excess of ten thousand per annum.[112,113] The need for pharmacological treatments for CLI in order to avoid amputation is reflected in these figures and also in the in-hospitality mortality rate following major leg amputation. Between 3 and 10% of patients undergoing below knee amputation die postoperatively and the figure is estimated to be approximately 20% when the amputation level is above the knee.[112] Nevertheless, such studies are difficult and specific points of guidance are given below.

4.1 Suitability

Due to the large numbers required for meaningful therapeutic studies in CLI as much supportive work as possible should be completed before embarking on such a major study. This includes studies in healthy volunteers, those with risk factors for vascular disease and claudication (for laboratory evaluation of surrogate markers). Safety aspects must be actively considered before the introduction of the drug into patients with CLI. Only patients who are not suitable for revascularization procedures should be considered for the study. The decision to treat by surgery, PTA, or medical management is not an easy one. It depends not only on objective patient and disease-related factors but also on the local situation in the hospital, its equipment, and the expertise of the various physicians and surgeons. To make decision making even more difficult the best treatment option is sometimes a combination of various modalities. Examples are the combination of surgery and angioplasty, surgery and thrombolysis, and thrombolysis followed by PTCA or surgery. Patients suitable for a drug trial could be those in whom surgery, PTCA, or combined therapy is not being considered.

4.2 Selection Criteria

As with claudication studies, age should be >40-45 years to exclude inclusion of patients with thromboangiitis obliterans (Buerger's disease). Patients with CLI tend to be on average about ten years older than their claudicant counterparts and care should be taken not to limit the upper age limit too severely. While drugs for use in the elderly may need certain extra registration requirements, patient recruitment for CLI studies can be difficult and should not be additionally hampered by unnecessary age restrictions. Any sex can be enrolled into these studies, the vast majority of female patients will be past childbearing age. The diagnosis of CLI secondary to PAOD should also be established. Arteriography within one year is acceptable but most patients will have had a recent investigation during consideration for revascularization procedure. In patients with ulceration an ischemic origin must be determined as far as possible thus excluding subjects with predominantly venous or neuropathic ulcers. Both of these two latter tend to produce ulceration in classical positions, but this is not always the case and exclusion should be made of patients with a significant past history of deep vein thrombosis or major peripheral neuropathy.

An ABPI is also helpful in suggesting an obstructive etiology with the lowest pressure reading being taken for inclusion. The selection of a particular ABPI/ankle pressure should be made after discussion with the investigating clinician. Using Fontaine grades III and IV[80] as selection criteria provides no guidance for ABPI measures, but the Consensus Document recommendation of <50 mmHg ankle pressure may prevent sufficient numbers being recruited[109] and also allow a majority of "endstage" disease to be enrolled, as discussed earlier.[33] Conversely patients with near normal ABPIs are unlikely to have significant vascular disease unless vessel stiffening is present. Thus, ulceration with ABPI ≥0.8 suggests a nonischemic cause for the ulceration. Suggested maximum ankle systolic pressure measures to be used for patient exclusion/inclusion range from between 50-80 mmHg. Because of the previously discussed vessel stiffening secondary to diabetes mellitus a toe pressure should also be selected. This allows diabetic patients with ABPIs greater than the cutoff to be included on the basis of toe pressures alone. As low toe pressures may be secondary to vasospasm in the microcirculation a temperature-controlled environment is optimum when these measures are being carried out. Where this is not possible gentle warmth can be applied after the detection of a low toe pressure to determine whether the pressure can be increased by vasodilatation secondary to warmth. Extreme care must be taken when applying any degree of heat to the ischemic limb as it cannot be rapidly removed as blood flow is minimal. Temperatures >37°C should be avoided. A toe pressure between 30-50 mmHg could be acceptable.[33]

Because of the debate in this area it might be considered that ischemia should be further confirmed by measuring transcutaneous oxygen pressure ($tcpO_2$), a value of ≤20 mmHg indicating critically ischemic tissues. The $tcpO_2$ measurements are made using commercially available microcathode systems. The electrode is attached to the skin by a self-adhesive ring. Oxygen is reduced at the platinum cathode to produce a current proportional to the partial pressure of oxygen at the electrode surface.[114] The probe temperature is thermostatically controlled to produce maximal arterialization of the skin circulation and diffusion across it. Theoretically attractive, there are some difficulties relating to reproducibility of sequential results using this technique. Nevertheless, it can be usefully employed by those with experience in its use. As with LDF there are changes after exercise and with posture,[115] and precautions regarding these aspects and a temperature-controlled environment are required.

Patients in CLI studies who fulfill the above ankle/toe pressures ± $tcpO_2$ estimations may be considered for enrollment into studies. Additionally, however, the clinical symptoms of rest pain ± ischemic ulceration ± minor gangrene must also be present. The pain must be present at rest, usually temporarily alleviated by dependency and should have been present for a minimum period of two weeks. Patients should be described as having chronic stable rest pain. Those whose pain is of short duration may rapidly deteriorate or sponaneously improve. As with ulceration a neuropathic origin for the pain should be excluded as far as possible. Exclusion should also be made of patients who are progressing rapidly or whose symptoms warrant urgent amputation, e.g., rapidly spreading infection, septicemia, or overt osteomyelitis. It is preferred that any significant infection within the ulceration should be treated before enrollment into the study as removal of infection can produce rapid resolution of symptoms and failure to treat can lead to a rapid worsening of the condition.

While a past history of reconstructive surgery or PTA should not exclude patients from these studies, patients with a very recent history of these interventions are not considered to be fully stable and a period of time should be allowed to elapse before enrollment. The optimum time is not yet known but should certainly not be less than two weeks. Lumbar sympathectomy or epidural stimulation within this time period should also lead to exclusion of this patient from the study.

Again, as with studies in claudication good randomization procedures and sufficient numbers will ensure that risk factors such as smoking, hyperlipidemia, and diabetes mellitus are distributed equally within the study groups. The clinical suspicion that patients with diabetes mellitus and CLI do not respond as well to drug treatment as those without diabetes has not been substantiated in clinical trials of CLI.[116,117]

General exclusion criteria also apply here such as significantly abnormal laboratory values, other clinical trial participation within three months, inability to give informed consent, concurrent therapy with similar mechanisms of action as the study drug and patients who, for reasons other than having reached an endpoint, are unlikely to complete the full study. The ability of these patients to continue in any study is severely limited by their extraordinary high mortality (Figure 8). This is illustrated in one study where there was a 30% increase in mortality rate over time when compared to a normal population.[118]

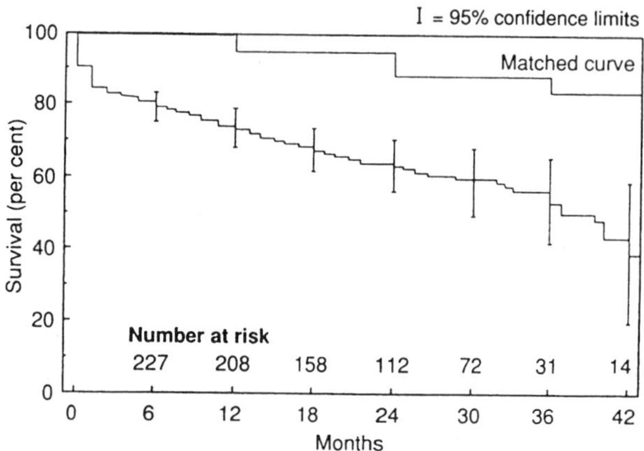

Figure 8 Mortality rates in critical CLI. (Reproduced from *Critical Limb Ischaemia,* Cambridge Medical Publications, Worthing, U.K., 1991. With permission.)

4.3 Safety

It is the very high mortality from cardiovascular events which alerts the investigator to the stringent caution and early evaluation of cardiovascular effects required for this very sick population. Patients with CLI invariably have CAD, carotid, and renal artery disease.[119] A further safety issue which should be considered here is that any delay in a necessary amputation can cause significant problems to the patient. CLI threatens both life and limb if toxic symptoms secondary to the tissue death are ignored or prolonged unnecessarily.

4.4 Methods

A parallel study design is preferred due to the nature and likely progression of the disease. Often the action of the compound is such that vasoactive side effects are to be expected and a cross-over study may allow unblinding by an alert patient. A wash-out period for prohibited drugs is also required. The nature of CLI is such that the four-week wash-out period required for claudication studies is not feasible here; 48 h is often selected and may be reasonable.

Standard therapy for all patients irrespective of treatment allocation should be provided. This includes optimum control of pain, infection, cardiac failure with arrythmias or edema, and local wound care. Studies with clinical endpoints will, by necessity, be multicenter and it will not be possible to agree to a standard protocol for the above considerations acceptable to all parties. It is usual to agree that standard therapy as applied by each center should continue throughout the duration of the study.

As with claudication studies, duration should be for a minimum of six months. If amputation rate is used as an endpoint a one-year study duration is more likely to show treatment effects.[120] As these patients may have trophic lesions and be generally unwell they are often inpatients, nevertheless, there is no necessity for this in terms of study design and, if applicable, outpatients can be enrolled. It is known, however, that bedrest can produce clinical benefit in CLI as can the more frequent wound care received as an inpatient and randomization procedures must ensure equal numbers of both in- and outpatients in each arm of the study.

The study schedule must include regular assessments, initially weekly and thereafter at four-week intervals even when the patients have completed the active drug treatment phase of the study. A potential study schedule is shown in Figure 9.

	VISIT																		
ASSESSMENT	Pre Study	Days 1–7	Wk 2	Wk 3	Wk 4	Wk 8	Wk 12	Wk 16	Wk 20	Wk 24	Wk 28	Wk 32	Wk 36	Wk 40	Wk 44	Wk 48	Wk 52	End of Treatment	4 Wks Post treatment
Inclusion/Exclusion	X																		
Demographic Data	X																		
Medical History	X																		
Clinical Status	X																		
Aorto–Angiography	X																		
Chest X–Ray	X																	X	
Doppler Pressures	X																	X	
Haemodynamics	X	X	X	X	X	X	X	X	X	X	X	X	X	X	X	X	X		
Trophic lesions	X				X	X	X	X	X	X	X	X	X	X	X	X	X	X	
Rest pain/Analgesics	X				X	X	X	X	X	X	X	X	X	X	X	X	X		
ECG	X																	X	
Clinical Chem./Haem. (safety)	X				X		X			X							X	X	X
Concom. Disease	X				X	X	X	X	X	X	X	X	X	X	X	X	X		
Concom. Medication	X				X	X	X	X	X	X	X	X	X	X	X	X	X		
Adverse Events		X	X	X	X	X	X	X	X	X	X	X	X	X	X	X	X	X	
Study Medic. Details		X	X	X	X	X	X	X	X	X	X	X	X	X	X	X	X	X	

Figure 9 Example of a study schedule for a CLI study.

4.4.1 Pharmacokinetic Studies

Only absolutely essential pharmacokinetic studies should be carried out on this patient group due to the severe nature of the consequences of disease progression, i.e., amputation. Additionally in the majority of Western countries pharmacotherapy is already available and licensed for this indication and ethical considerations might suggest studies without therapeutic endpoints should be avoided. The majority of pharmacokinetics can be carried out in the less severely affected claudicant population or, indeed, in elderly healthy controls.

4.4.2 Surrogate Markers

As a general rule the primary endpoints should be "hard," i.e., clinically relevant, and as easy as possible to measure so that the centers with large patient numbers but less sophisticated laboratories can participate. Examples of this in CLI are need for surgery or amputation ± death. Death may be measured as death from all causes or vascular death. Death as an endpoint in intervention studies in CLI implies that the primary aim of the study is secondary prevention. This is not justified since there is no casual or time relationship between amputation and death. Of 859 CLI patients in controlled clinical studies, 296 patients required amputation and only 38 patients of the 90 patients who died had required an amputation. Additionally, only 18 of these patients underwent an amputation procedure within 30 days prior to death (Table 6). Death as an outcome measure has implications toward sample size. The requirement for huge patient numbers are probably not justified at the early stage of drug development.

Rest pain should be quantified using standard procedures such as visual analog scales or point scores. Such quantification should be undertaken by both patient and clinician. Accurate recording of analgesic

Table 6 Outcome in 859 CLI Patients (Fontaine Stages III-IV)

Mortality	n = 90/859	Sample size for a 20% (10.5% = >8.5%) event reduction (n = 3473/group)
All amputations	n = 295/859	Sample size for a 20% (34.3% = >27.4%) event reduction (n = 731/group)
Disabling amputations	n = 222/859	Sample size for a 20% (25.8% = >20.1%) event reduction (n = 888/group)
Patients died and amputated before death (any time)	n = 38	4.4% of all patients 42.2% of those who died 12.8% of those with (any) amputation 17.1% of those with disabling amputation
Patients died and amputated before death (≤30 days)	n = 18	2.1% of all patients 20.0% of those who died 6.1% of those with (any) amputation 8.1% of those with disabling amputation
Patients died and amputated before death (≤7 days)	n = 8	0.9% of all patients 8.8% of those who died 2.7% of those with (any) amputation 3.6% of those with disabling amputation

type and consumption is essential if the patient record of pain experienced is to be meaningful. It should be noted that the enrollment of the patient into the study often leads to a change in analgesic consumption as the pain severity becomes better recognized. The enhanced analgesic dose provided may decrease rest pain without true clinical benefit from the study drug. While a measure of rest pain is recommended it is recognized that this is a "soft" endpoint open to the effects of many variables such as patient mood, motivation, presence of neuropathy, and time of day.[121]

Ulcer size measurement is also considered a soft endpoint, although attempts have been made to "harden" this measure. In addition to documenting whether the patient and blinded clinician believe the ulcer to be improving, worsening, or undergoing no change, the ulcer is usually photographed in a standard fashion using a technique which includes a measuring rule within the picture frame. It should be noted, however, that photo documentation is very difficult indeed to interpret at the end of the study. Planimetry, where a transparent cover is placed over the ulcer and traced is the most commonly used measure of ulceration. One technique allows the transparent cover to be placed over the ulcer but a second cover is then placed upon the first and the circumference of the ulcer drawn onto the second cover which can then be inserted into the case record form for later analysis. The first cover which will have been contaminated by ulcer constituents can be discarded. Measurement of ulcer circumference, diameter, or area have all been evaluated in CLI studies and computer software packages are now available allowing more accurate quantification of these measures. Planimetry does not, however, address ulcer depth. Volume can be measured by filling the ulcer crater with a nonirritant gel using a measuring syringe filled with a set amount of gel. The volume will be measured in milliliters of gel required to fill the ulcer crater. Graded ulcer scores are also available.[33] Uncertainty remains, however. If multiple ulcers are present which should be measured, should only the largest ones be assessed? How does one address the common situation of an ulcer between the toes which is not measurable by the above techniques? Also to be considered is the endpoint of ulcer healing to be selected. Should this be total healing or partial healing? Most recent studies of CLI have selected between 30-50% healing as their endpoint,[116,117] and while this may be statistically significant the endpoint should also be clinically significant to the patient. It is possible that partial ulcer healing could be used as a surrogate marker for efficacy when screening products but that studies with amputation and death as their primary endpoints should be required for registration. A balance must be sought between an unprofitably high cost of drug development and certainty of drug clinical benefit. Amputation rate should always be assessed in these studies even if not selected as a primary endpoint. As with ulcer healing, amputation scores are available which combine amputation numbers with a scoring system for the level.[33]

QoL questionnaires can also be useful but the same problems are attached to QoL questionnaires for CLI as for intermittent claudication. It is recommended that an additional global assessment score such as better/same/worse should be measured in response to standard questions. These questions should be addressed to both physician and patient.

4.4.2.1 *Laboratory*

Laser Doppler flowmetry,[36] thermography,[47] and $tcpO_2$ measures[114] can all be used as surrogate markers for drug efficacy as outlined in the two earlier segments. These cannot, however, be used as primary endpoints in major efficacy studies or for registration purposes. This is also true for tests of coagulation and hemorrheology. As with claudicants, patients with CLI should be taking aspirin if tolerated[88] and this limits the value of platelet aggregation and release tests.

4.5 Controls

Controlled studies are essential in CLI as the number of variables applicable to ulceration, for example, localization, spontaneous healing rates, and presence of infection all vary from lesion to lesion. Thus, studies must either contain large patient numbers which lead to long recruitment periods and/or tight inclusion/exclusion criteria which lead to poor recruitment.[122] No matter which approach is selected controls must be included as part of the design. The proposed registration documents for North America and Europe request placebo-controlled studies. There is some difficulty experienced because of this ruling, however. In certain countries where other compounds are registered for use in CLI, ethical committees are requiring the use of active controls such as naftidrofuryl forte and dextran. Dialogue is needed between these two groups as at present industry and the medical profession have two equal but opposite pressures exerted upon them when designing studies. Studies against surgery or PTA could be considered if phase II studies suggest an efficacy level comparable to these already accepted interventions.

4.6 Size and Duration of Trials

As with the studies in claudication size and duration of the trial depend on endpoints selected, although inoperable CLI has been dealt with here. Other endpoints, such as graft stenosis reduction following bypass surgery, will require different population sizes to those evaluating amputation rate. Again, the number of centers participating in the study and the number of primary endpoints will also influence population requirements. The following examples may be useful.

In a study comparing low dose, high dose, and placebo effects, the following may apply. Assuming a drop-out rate of no greater than 30% and a placebo response rate of 50%, recruitment of 120 patients per group provides a power of 0.90 to detect a difference between ulcer healing rates of 25% (drug rate 25%, $\alpha = 0.05$ two-tailed). One hundred and twenty patients per group for a three-arm trial relates to ulcer healing and will be too small even for phase II to show any trend of effect on amputation. Since this is the ultimate endpoint in CLI, one would need at least 600 patients per treatment arm to provide information on potential amputation effects.

5 GOOD CLINICAL PRACTICE

It must be clear to all those interested in planning intervention studies in PAOD that such studies will be lengthy, costly, and with a high inherent risk of failure. Although there are (draft) guidelines for the completion of such studies being prepared by various regulatory bodies there are no existing guidelines that are based on large pools of data taken from placebo-controlled studies. It is thus imperative that any study design should be discussed with the appropriate regulatory body. These agencies, however, are dependent upon published opinion such as the consensus paper on CLI.[29] Such opinions are often being modified by workers in the field and may not be appropriate even a few years after their publication. If a company has already treated hundreds of patients with the same condition with another compound than the data obtained from these studies should be used in support of future study designs, although this would mean that approval for registration would only be for this well-defined target population.

All studies should be performed according to the European/FDA Good Clinical Practice Guidelines. These include such items as written or witnessed oral informed consent from the patient and has implications for both the clinician and the study monitors. Monitoring should be performed at least every 4–6 weeks in each center. Source data verification must be documented, the percentage of errors calculated, and audits performed by an independent quality assurance unit in selected centers such as the involved departments of the sponsor, the involved clinical research organizations, or any other third party. Direct source data verification necessitates the viewing of case record forms and as such requires permission from the patient. Source data verification can also be carried out using a cross-check method where the monitor has no direct access to the patient's data. This can be completed without patient consent.

5.1 Steering Committee Meetings

Steering Committee Meetings must be arranged on a regular basis before and during the study in order to discuss problems arising from the study and to improve data quality. Because studies in CLI in particular are so complicated, an average of three Steering Committee Meetings per year seems to be a minimum requirement. The agenda of the meetings could contain the following:

- Review of the study protocol (and necessity for changing inclusion and exclusion criteria)
- Practical problems with the study
- Good Clinical Practice and its consequences
- Discussion of adverse events
- Scientific update
- Defining publication strategies

The numbers required for meaningful studies in this area are such that good and meaningful work can rarely be carried out in a single center. Multicenter, often multinational, studies are now the norm for evaluation of treatments for peripheral vascular disease and such designs can cause problems of their own. As career advancement can depend on research publications or M.D. theses, those of us in research units have a duty to provide the facilities for these to our junior staff. In a multicenter study not all workers can be co-authors of the finished piece of work. If no publication is on the horizon a less motivated junior can enroll infrequently and/or inappropriately. One method of ensuring that sufficient numbers and quality of patients be enrolled is to allow adjunctive studies of an area of particular interest to that unit, e.g., effect of the drug on WBC behavior. Furthermore, although cumbersome we believe that a footnote documenting both the center's leader and juniors should be included in the major publication. Publication/presentation strategy should be discussed in a round table fashion with each group, if possible, being allocated a role. Working Party meetings should rotate throughout the centers if geographically possible. The chairman should be elected and his/her role carefully defined. If such guidelines are not observed the risk is run of the study being carried out by busy, poorly motivated, and poorly supervised juniors.

KEY LITERATURE

1. Galland, R. B., Clyne, C. A. C. (Eds.), *Clinical Problems in Vascular Surgery,* Edward Arnold, London, 1993.
2. Bloom, A. L., Forbes, C. D., Thomas, D. P., Tuddenham, E. G. D. (Eds.), *Haemostasis and Thombosis 3rd Edition.* Churchill Livingstone, Edinburgh, 1994.
3. Vane, J., O'Grady, J. (Eds.), *Therapeutic Application of Prostaglandins.* Edward Arnold, London, 1993.
4. Second European Consensus Document on Chronic Critical Leg Ischaemia. *Circulation,* 84(4): 1-22, 1991.
5. Belcaro, G., Hoffmann, U., Bolhinger, A., Nicolaides, A. (Eds.), *Laser Doppler,* Medorion Publishing Company, London, 1994.

REFERENCES

1. Kannel, W. B., Shurtleff, D. The Framington study. Cigarettes and the development of intermittent claudification. *Geriatrics,* 28, 61, 1973.
2. Widmer, L. K., Greensher, A., Kannel, W. B. Occlusion of peripheral arteries: a study of 6,4000 working subjects. *Circulation,* 30, 836, 1964.
3. Schroll, M., Munock, O. Estimation of peripheral arteriosclerotic disease by ankle blood pressure measurements in a population study of 60 year old men and women. *J. Chron. Dis.,* 34, 261, 1981.
4. Crigui, M. H., Fronek, A., Barrett-Connor, E. et al. The prevalence of peripheral arterial disease in a defined population. *Circulation,* 71, 510, 1985.
5. De Backer, I. C., Kornitizer, M., Sobolski, J., Denolin, H. Intermittant claudication — epidemiology and natural history. *Acta Cardiol.,* 34, 115, 1979.
6. Dagenais, G. R., Maurice, S., Robitaille, N. M., Gingras, S., Lupein, P. J. Intermittant claudication in Quebec men from 1974-1986: the Quebec Cardiovascular Study. *Clin Invest. Med.,* 14, 93, 1991.
7. Reunanèn, A., Takkunen, H., Aromaa, A. Prevalence of intermittant claudication and its effect on mortality. *Acta Med. Scand.,* 211, 249, 1982.
8. Bothig, S., Metelisa, V. I., Barth, W. et al. Prevalence of ischaemic heart disease, arterial hypertension and intermittant claudication, and distribution of risk factors among middle-aged men in Moscow and Berlin. *Cor. Vasa.,* 18, 104, 1976.
9. Gofin, R., Karic, J. D., Friedlander, T. et al. Peripheral vascular disease in a middle-aged population sample. The Jerusalem Lipid Research Clinic Prevalence Study. *Int. J. Med.,* 23, 157, 1987.

10. Pomrehn, P., Duncan, B., Weissfeld, L. et al. The association of dyslipoproteinaemia with symptoms and signs of peripheral arterial disease. The Lipid Research Council Prevalence Study. *Circulation,* 73 (Suppl. 1), 100, 1986.
11. Fowkes, F. G. R., Housley, E., Riemersma, R. A. et al. Smoking, lipids, glucose intolerance and blood pressure as risk factors for peripheral atherosclerosis compared with ischaemic heart disease in the Edinburgh Artery Study. *Am. J. Epidermiol.,* 135, 331, 1992.
12. Isacsson, S. Venous occlusion plethysymography in 55-year-old men: a population study in Malmo, Sweden. *Acta Med. Scand.,* 537 (Suppl.), 1, 1972.
13. daSilva, A., Widmer, L. K. (Eds): *Occlusive Peripheral Arterial Disease Diagnosis. Incidence, Course and Significance.* Hans Huber, 1981.
14. Levy, L. A. Smoking and peripheral vascular disease. Epidemiology and podiatric perspective. *Podiatr. Med. Assoc.,* 79, 398-402, 1989.
15. Schadt, D. C., Hines, E. A. Jr., Juergens, J. L. et al. Chronic atherosclerotic occlusion of the femoral artery, *JAMA,* 175, 937, 1961.
16. Imparato, A. M., Kim, G., Davidson, T. et al. Intermittant claudication: its natural course. *Surgery,* 78, 795, 1975.
17. Juergens, J. L., Barker, M. W., Hines, E. A. Jr. Arteriosclerosis obliterans: review of 520 cases with special reference to pathogenic and prognostic factors. *Circulation,* 21, 188, 1960.
18. Kannel, W. B., Skinner, J. J., Schwartz, M. J., Shurtleff, D. Intermittent claudication: incidence in the Framington Study. *Circulation,* 41, 875, 1970.
19. Lasila, R., Lepantalo, M., Lindfors, O. Peripheral arterial disease — natural outcome. *Acta Med. Scand.,* 220, 295, 1986.
20. Pell, J. P., Fowkes, F. G. R. et al. Quality of life following lower limb amputation for peripheral arterial disease. *Eur. J. Vasc. Surg.,* 7, 448, 1993.
21. Widmer, L. K. (Ed). *Critical Ischaemia: The Disease.* Worthing: Professional Postgraduate Services Europe Ltd., 1991.
22. Galland, R. B., Kline, C. A. C., Edward, A. *Clinical Problems in Vascular Surgery.* London, 1994.
22a. Coffman, J. D. Vasodilated drugs in peripheral vascular disease. *N. Engl. J. Med.,* 300, 713, 1979.
23. Perhoniemi, V., Salmenkivi, K., Sundberg, S., Johnson, R., Gordin, A. Effects of flunarizine and pentoxifylline on walking distance and blood rheology in claudication. *Angiology,* 3, 366, 1984.
23a. Bloom, A. L., Forbes, C. D., Thomas, D. P., Tuddebham, E. G. D. *Haemostasis and Thrombosis,* 3rd edition. Churchill Livingstone, Edinburgh, 1994.
24. Vane, J., O'Grady, J. *Therapeutic Application of Prostaglandins.* Edward Arnold, London, 1993.
25. Hertzer, N. R., Bevan, E. G., Young, J. R. et al. Coronary artery disease in peripheral vascular patients. A classification of 1000 coronary angiograms and results of surgical management. *Ann. Surg.,* 199, 223, 1984.
26. Diehl, J. T., Cali, R. F., Hertzer, N. R. et al. Complications of abdominal aortic reconstruction. An analysis of perioperative risk factors in 557 patients. *Ann. Surg.,* 197, 49, 1983.
27. Dormandy, J., Mahir, M., Ascady, G., Balsano, F., De Leeuw, P., Blombery, P. et al. Fate of the patient with chronic leg ischaemia: a review article. *J. Cardiovasc. Surg.,* 30, 50, 1989.
28. Goldman, L., Caldera, D. L., Southwick, F. S. et al. Cardiac risk factors and complications in one-cardiac surgery. *Medicine,* 57, 357, 1978.
29. Second European Consensus Document on Chronic Critical Leg Ischaemia. *Circulation,* 84(4), 1, 1991.
30. Sonecha, T. N., Nicolaides, A. N. The relationship between intermittant claudication and coronary artery disease — is it more than we think? *Vasc. Med. Rev.,* 2, 137, 1991.
31. Verhaeghe, R. Antiplatelet Drugs in Crit. Leg Ischaemia. *Crit. Ischaem.,* 2 No. 3, 26, 1992.
32. Belch, J. J. F. The role of the white blood cell in thrombosis. (Editorial). Current Medical Literature. *Thrombosis,* 3(3), 63-67, 1993.
33. Belch, J. J. F., Diehm, C., Henry, M., Rieger, H., Rudofsky, G., Frings, M., Hornig, F., Sohngen, W. Evaluating treatment of critical limb ischaemia: for the European PARTNER concept study groups. *Crit. Ischaem.,* 2(4), 4, 1993.
34. Diehm, C., Abri, O., Baitsch, G. et al. Illoprost, ein stabiles. Prostacyclin Derivat bei arterieller Verschlußkrankheit im Stadium IV. *Dtsch. Med. Wochenschr.,* 114, 783, 1989.
35. Belch, J. J. F., Frings, M., Voleske, P., Söhngen, W. Neutrophil count in amputation in critical limb ischaemia. *Int. J. Angiol.,* 7, 48, 1994.
36. Tooke, J. E., Ostergren, J., Fagrell, B. Synchronous assessment of human skin microcirculation by laser Doppler flowmetry and dynamic capillaroscopy. *Int. J. Microcirc. Clin. Exp.,* 2, 277, 1983.
37. Wilkin, J. K. Periodic cutaneous blood flow during postocclusive reactive hyperaemia. *Am. J. Physiol.,* 250:(*Heart Circ. Physiol.,* 19): H 765, 1986.
38. von Ahn, H. C. Measurement of gastrointestinal blood flow with laser Doppler flowmetry — an experimental and clinical study. *Linkoping Uni Med Dissertat,* No. 226, Vimmerby, Sweden: VTT-Frafiska, 1986.
39. Fagrell, B., Microcirculation of the skin. In: Mortillaro, N. Ed., *The Physiology and Pharmacology of the Microcirculation,* Volume 2, 133, 1984.
40. Caspary, L., Creutzig, A., Alexander, K. Biological zero in laser Doppler fluxmetry. *Int. J. Microcirc. Exp.,* 7, 367, 1988.

41. Fagrell, B., Intaglietta, M., Tsai, A. G., Ostergren, J. Combination of laser Doppler flowmetry and capillary microscopy for evaluating the dynamics of skin microcirculation. In: Mahler F., Messmer, K., Hammersen, F. Eds. Techniques in clinical copular microscopy. *Prog. Appl. Microcirc.*, Basel: Karger, 11, 30, 1986.
42. Johnson, J. M., Taylor, W. F., Shepherd, A. P. et al. Laser Doppler measurement of skin blood flow: comparison with plethysmography. *J. Acta Physiol.*, 56(3), 798, 1984.
43. Holloway, G. A., Watkins, D. W. Laser Doppler measurement of cutaneous blood flow. *J. Invest. Dermatol.*, 69, 306, 1977.
44. Engelhart, M., Petersen, L. J., Kristensen, J. K. The local regulation blood flow evaluated simultaneously by ^{133}Xenon washout and laser Doppler flowmetry. *J. Invest. Dermatol.*, 91, 451, 1988.
45. Fagrell, B., Intaglietta, M., Fronek, A. A microscopic television system for studying flow velocity in human skin capillaries. *Am. J. Physiol. Heart Circ. Physiol.*, 2(3), H318-21, 1977.
46. Fragrell, B., Eriksson, S. E., Malmstrom, S., Sjolund, A. Computerized data analysis of capillary blood cell velocity. *Int. J. Microcirc. Clin. Exp.*, 7, 276, 1989.
47. Barnes, R. B. Thermography of the human body, *Science*, 140, 870, 1963.
48. Oliva, P. B., Breckenridge, J. C. Arteriographic evidence of coronary arterial spasm in acute myocardial infarction. *Circulation*, 56, 366, 1977.
49. Yanagisawa, M., Kurihara, H., Kimura, S. et al. A novel potent vasoconstrictor peptide produced by vascular endothelial cells. *Nature*, 332, 411, 1988.
50. Kanno, K., Hirata, Y., Emori, T. et al. Endothelin and Raynaud's phenomenon. *Am. J. Med.*, 90, 130, 1991.
51. Bridges, A. B., McLaren, M., Saniabadi, A. R., Fisher, T. C., Belch, J. J. F., Circadian rhythm of endothelial cell function, red blood cell deformability and dehydrothromboxane B_2 in healthy volunteers, *Blood Coag. Fibrinol.*, 2, 447, 1991.
52. Hanss, J. G., Taylor, G. W. Metabolism and toxicology of the prostaglandins. In: *Therapeutic Applications of Prostaglandins.* Vane, J., O'Grady, J. Eds. Edward Arnold, London, 1993, p. 37-48.
53. Leone, A. M., Francis, P. L., Rhodes, P., Moncada, S. A rapid and simple method for the measurement of nitrite and nitrate in plasma by high performance capillary electrophoresis. *Biochem. Biophys. Res. Commun.*, 200, 951, 1994.
54. Westerman, R. A., Widdop, R. E., Hannaford, J. et al. Laser Doppler velocimetry in the measurement of neurovascular function. *Aust. Phys. Eng. Sci. Med.*, 11, 53, 1988.
55. Furchgott, R. F., Zawadzki, J. V. The obligatory role of endothelial cells in the relaxation of arterial smooth muscle by acetylcholine. *Nature*, 288, 373, 1980.
56. Westerman, R. A., Widdop, R. E., Low, A., Hannaford, J., Kozak, W., Zimmet, P. Noninvasive tests of neurovascular function: reduced axon reflex responses in diabetes mellitus of man and streptozotocin-induced diabetes of the rat. *Diab. Res. Clin. Prac.*, 5, 49, 1988.
57. Walmsley, D., Wiles, P. G. Assessment of the neurogenic flair response as a measure of nociceptor C fibre function. *J. Med. Eng. Technol.*, 14, 194, 1990.
58. Born, G. V. R., Aggregation of platelets by ADP and its reversal. *Nature*, 194, 927, 1962.
59. Saniabadi, A. R., Lowe, G., Belch, J. J. F., Barbenel, J. C., Forbes, C. D. A platelet counting technique to study platelet aggregation in whole blood: application to pathologically low platelet counts. *Platelets*, 1, 151, 1990.
60. McLaren, M., Bancroft, A., Alexander, W., Belch, J. J. F. Platelet aggregation in whole blood: Comparison between Clay Adam ultraflow-100 and Coulter haematology analyser T-540. *Platelets*, 1, 95, 1990.
61. Belch, J. J. F., Saniabadi, A., McLaren, M., McLaughlin, K., Forbes, C. D. Acute platelet changes after a saturated fat meal and their prevention by UK38,485, a potent thromboxane synthetase inhibitor. *Lipids*, 22(3), 159, 1987.
62. Saniabadi, A. R., Fisher, T. C., Belch, J. J. F., Forbes, C. D. A study of the effect of dipyridamole on erythrocyte deformability using an improved filtration technique. *Clin. Haemorheol.*, 10, 263, 1990.
63. Saniabadi, A. R., Fisher, T. C., McLaren, M., Belch, J. J. F., Forbes, C. D. Effect of dipyridamole along and in combination with aspirin on whole blood platelet aggregation, PGI_2 generation and red cell deformability *ex vivo* in man. *Cardiovas. Res.*, 25(3), 177, 1991.
64. Belch, J. J. F. Vasculitis (Editorial). *Vasc. Med. Rev.*, 3, 1-2, 1992.
65. Grim, R. H., Cohen, J. D., Smith, W. M., Falvo-Gerard, L., Neaton, J. D. Hypertension management in the multiple risk factor intervention trial (MRFIT) 6 year intervention results from men in special intervention and normal care groups. *Arch. Intern. Med.*, 145, 1191, 1985.
66. Territo, M. C., Monocyste-macrophage function in leucocyte function methods. In: *Haematology*, Cline, M. J., Ed., Churchhill Livingstone, London, 1981, p. 53-83.
67. Fisher, T. C., Belch, J. J. F., Barbenel, J. C., Fisher, A. C. *In vitro* human whole blood granulocyte aggregation. *Clin. Sci.*, 76, 183, 1989.
68. Lau, C. S., Scott, N., Brown, J. E., Shaw, W., Belch, J. J. F. Increased activity of oxygen free radicals during reperfusion in patients undergoing percutaneous peripheral artery balloon angioplasty. *Int. Angiol.*, 10(4), 244, 1991.
69. Jennings, P. E., McLaren, M., Scott, N., Saniabadi, A., Belch, J. J. F. The relationship of oxidative stress to thrombotic tendency in type 1 diabetic patients with retinopathy. *Diab. Med.*, 8, 860, 1991.
70. Belch, J. J. F., Chopra, M., Hutchinson, S., Lorimer, R., Sturrock, R. D., Forbes, C. D., Smith, E. Free radical pathology in chronic arterial disease. *Free Rad. Biol. Med.*, 6(4), 375, 1989.
71. Halliwell, B., Gutteridge, J. M. C. *Free Radicals in Biology and Medicine.* Oxford: Oxford University Press, 1985.

72. Hernanz, A. High-performance liquid chromatographic determination of ascorbic acid in serum using paired-ion chromatography and UV spectrophotometric Detection. *J. Clin. Chem. Clin. Biochem.*, 26, 459, 1988.
73. Lehmann, J., Martin, H. L., Improved direct determination of alpha- and gamma-tocopherols in plasma and platelets by liquid chromatogrphy, with fluorescence detection. *Clin. Chem.*, 28/8, 1784, 1982.
74. Belch, J. J. F., Bennett, I., Speirs, T. O., Cree, I. A., McLaren, M., Thrope, G. H. Clinical validation of a chemiluminescence assay for the measurement of global antioxidant capacity of biological fluids, submitted for publication.
75. Bridges, A. B., Scott, N. A., Belch, J. J. F. Probucol, a superoxide free radical scavenger *in vitro*. *Atherosclerosis*, 89, 263, 1991.
76. Bridges, A. B., Fisher, T. C., Scott, N., McLaren, M., Belch, J. J. F. Circadian rhythm of white blood cell aggregation and free radical status in healthy volunteers. *Free Rad. Res. Commun.*, 16(2), 89, 1992.
77. Bridges, A. B., McLaren, M., Scott, N. A., Pringle, T. H., McNeill, G. P., Belch, J. J. F. Circadian variation in white blood cell aggregation and free radical indices in men with stable ischaemic heart disease. *Eur. Heart J.*, 13, 1632, 1992.
78. McLaren, M., Jennings, P. E., Forbes, C. D., Belch, J. J. F. Fibrinolytic response to venous occlusion in diabetics with and without micro-angiopathy compared to normal age and sex matched controls. *Fibrinolysis*, 4(2): 116, 1990.
79. Fearnley, G. R., Balmforth, G., Fearnley, E. Evidence of a diurnal fibrinolytic rhythm: with a simple method of measuring natural fibrinolysis. *Glynn Si*, 16, 645, 1957.
80. Fontaine, R., Kim, M., Kieny, D. Die chirurgische Behandlung der peripheren Durchblutungsstörungen. *Helv. Chir. Acta*, 5/6, 499, 1954.
81. Hessel, S. J., Adams, D. F., Abrams, H. L. Complications of angiography. *Radiology*, 138, 273, 1981.
82. Evans, D. H., McDicken, W. N., Skidmore, R., Woodcock, J. P. *Doppler Ultrasound: Physics Instrumentation and Clinical Application*. John Wiley, Chichester, 47, 1989.
83. Flanigan, M., Schuler, J. J., Vogel, M., Borozan, P. G., Gray, B., Sobinsky, K. R. The role of carotid Duplex scanning in surgical decision making. *J. Vasc. Surg.*, 2, 15, 1985.
84. Legemate, D. A., Teeuwen, C., Hoeneveld, H., Eikelboom, B. C. The value of Duplex scanning compared with angiography and pressure measurement in the assessment of aorto iliac arterial lesions. *Br. J. Surg.*, 78, 1003, 1991.
85. Yao, J. S. T., Hobbs, J. T., Irvine, W. T. Ankle systolic pressure measurements in arterial disease affecting the lower extremisties. *Br. J. Surg.*, 56, 676-679, 1969.
86. Berglund, B., Eklund, B. Reproducibility of treadmill exercise in patients with intermittent claudication. *Clin. Physiol.*, 1, 253-256, 1981.
87. Goldhaber, S. Z., Manton, J. E., Stampfer, M. J. et al. Low-dose aspirin and subsequent peripheral arterial surgery in the Physicians' Health Study. *Lancet*, 340, 143, 1992.
88. Antiplatelet Trialists Collaboration. Secondary Prevention of Vascular Disease by prolonged antiplatelet treatment. *Br. Med. J.*, 296, 320, 1988.
89. Beach, K. W., Bedford, G. R., Bergelin, R. O. et al. Progression of lower extremeity arterial occlusive disease in type II diabetes mellitus. *Diab. Care*, 11, 464, 1988.
90. Melton, I. J., Macken, K. M., Palumbo, J. et al. Incidence and prevalence of clinical peripheral vascular disease in a population based cohort of diabetic patients. *Diab. Care*, 3, 650, 1980.
91. Lieberg, E., Persson, B. M. Age, diabetes and smoking in lower limb amputation for arterial occlusive disease. *Acta. Orthop. Scand.*, 54, 383, 1983.
92. Taves, D. R., Minimization: a new method of assigning patients to treatment and control groups. *Clin. Pharmacol. Ther.*, 15, 443-453, 1974.
93. Guideline on Clinical Testing Requirements for Drugs for longterm use. The Rules governing medicinal products in the European Community, 3, 163, 1989.
94. Pocock, S. J. A prospective on the role of Quality of Life Assessment in clinical trials. *Contr. Clin. Trials*, 12, 257, 1991.
95. Garrat, A. M., Ruta, D. A., Abdalla, M. I., Buckingham, J. K., Russel, I. T. The SF 36 Health Survey Questionnaire: an outcome measure suitable for routine use within the NHS? *Br. Med. J.*, 306, 1440-1444, 1993.
96. Housley, E. Management of claudication in five words. Smoking and keep walking. *Br. Med. J.*, 296, 1483, 1988.
97. British National Formulary, 22, 85, 1991.
98. LeHert, P., Riphagen, F. E., Ganand, S. The effect of naftidrofuryl on intermittent claudication: a meta analysis. *J. Cardiovasc. Pharmacol.*, 16, 81, 1990.
99. Lindgarde, F., Gelnes, R., Bjorkman, H., Adielsson, G., Kjellstrom, T., Palmquist, I., Stavenow, L. Conservative drug treatment in patients with moderately severe chronic occlusive peripheral arterial disease. *Circulation*, 80, 1549, 1989.
100. Arcan, J. C., Panak, E., Ticlopidine in the treatment of peripheral occlusive arterial disease. *Semin. Thromb. Haemostas.*, 15, 167, 1989.
101. Hiatt, W. R., Regensteiner, J. G., Hargarten, M. E., Wolfel, E. E., Brass, E. P. Benefit of exercise conditioniong for patients with peripheral arterial disease. *Circulation*, 81, 602, 1990.
102. Hiatt, W. R., Wolfel, E. E., Regensteiner, J. G. Exercise in the treatment of intermittant claudication due to peripheral arterial disease. *Vasc. Med. Rev.*, 2, 61, 1991.
103. Note for guidance on biostatistical methodology in clinical trials in application for marketing authorization for medical products. European Commission Directorate General 3 Industry, Industrial Affairs, Consumer Goods Industries Pharmaceuticals.

104. Zweig, H. M., Campbell, G. Receiver-operating characteristics (ROC) plots: A fundamental tool in clinical medicine. *Clin. Chem.*, 39, 4, 561-577, 1993.
105. Borenstein, M., The case for confidence intervals in controlled clinical trials. In: *Controlled Clinical Trials,* Elsevier Science, New York, 15, 411, 1994.
106. PMA biostatistics and medical ad hoc committee on interim analysis, interim analysis in the pharmaceutical industry. *Contr. Clin. Trials.*, 14, 160-173, 1993.
107. Belch, J. J. F., Mackay, I. R., Hillis, S. Thrombolysis in peripheral vascular disease. *Vasc. Med. Rev.*, 4(2): 111, 1993.
108. Ad hoc committee on reporting standards Society for Vascular Surgery, North American Chapter, International Society for Cardiovascular Surgery: Suggested standards for reports dealing with lower extremity ischaemia. *J. Vasc. Surg.*, 4, 80, 1986.
109. Edmonds, M. The next stage for the consensus document. An international debate at 16th WCIUA, Paris, September 1992. *Crit. Ischaem.*, 3, 1, 1992.
110. Vollmar, J. Moglichkeiten und Grenzen der chirurgischen Behandlung arterieller Verschlußkrankheiten. *Therapiewoche,* 6, 394, 1972.
111. Sorensen, S., Schsroeder, T. When revascularization is not possible, arterial reconstruction still remains the treatment of choice. *Crit. Ischaem.*, 3, 1, 1994.
112. Dormandy, J. A., Ray, S. A. The fate of amputees. *Vasc. Med. Rev.*, 5, 331, 1994.
113. Amputation statistics for England, Wales and Northern Ireland. Statistics and Research Division of the DHSS, London: HMSO, 1987.
114. Franzeck, U. K., Talke, P., Bernstein, E. F. et al. Transcutaneous PO_2 measurements in Health and Arterial Occlusive Disease. *Surgery,* 91, 156, 1982.
115. Holdich, T. A. H., Reddy, P. J., Walker, R. T., Dormandy, J. A. Transcutaneous oxygen tension during exercise in patients with claudication. *Br. Med. J.*, 292, 1625, 1986.
116. Guilmot, J. L., Diot, E. Treatment of lower limb ischaemia due to atherosclerosis in diabetic and non-diabetic patients with Iloprost, a stable analogue of prostacyclin: results of the French multicentre trial. *Drug Invest.*, 3(5), 351-359, 1991.
117. Diehm, C., Hübsch-Müller, C., Stammler, F., Intravenöse Prostaglandin E_1-Therapie bei Patienten mit peripherer arterieller Verschlußkrankheit (AVK) im Stadium III — eine doppelblinde, plazebokontrollierte Studie. In: Heindrich, H., Böhme, H., Rogatti, W., (Eds) *Prostaglandin E_1 Wirkung and Therapeutische Wirksamkeit.* Heidelberg: Springer, 133, 1988.
118. Hoofwijk, A. The fate of the patient with critical limb ischaemia. The literature lacks an overall picture of the fate of the patient with critical limb ischaemia. *Crit. Ischaem.*, 1, 3, 15, 1991.
119. Sonecha, T. N., Nicolaides, A. N. The relationship between intermittant claudication and coronary artery disease — is it more than we think? *Vasc. Med. Rev.*, 2, 137, 1991.
120. Loosemore, T. Meta-analysis of the major Iloprost studies. *Int. Angiol.*, in press.
121. Kadambari, R. Critical leg ischaemia and the mind. *Crit. Ischaem.*, 2, 4, 23, 1993.
122. The Ciprostene Study Group. The effect of Ciprostene in patients with peripheral vascular disease (PVD) characterized by ischaemic ulcers. *J. Clin. Pharmacol.*, 31, 81, 1991.

Part VI. Assessment of Drug Effects on the Respiratory System

Chapter 20

Anti-Asthmatic Drugs

A. M. Edwards

CONTENTS

1 Definition of Asthma 281
2 Measurements of Airflow Limitation 282
3 Evaluation of Anti-Asthmatic Drugs in Man 282
3.1 Bronchial Challenge Experiments 283
3.1.1 Principles 283
3.1.2 Conclusion 284
4 Therapeutic Trials 284
4.1 Objectives 284
4.2 Trial Design 284
4.3 Selection of Patients 284
4.3.1 Age 285
4.3.2 Asthma Type 285
4.3.3 Current Therapy 285
4.3.4 Pulmonary Function Tests 286
4.3.5 Severity of Symptoms 286
4.3.6 Bronchial Reactivity and Reversibility 287
4.4 Methodology 287
4.4.1 Patient Selection 287
4.4.1.1 New Member of an Existing Class of Drug 287
4.4.1.2 Novel Compounds 287
4.4.2 Previous Therapy 287
4.4.3 Criteria for Entry into Test Treatment Period 288
4.4.4 Baseline Period 288
5 Measurements of Efficacy 289
5.1 Primary Variables 289
5.1.1 Patients' Global Opinion of Efficacy 289
5.1.2 Patients' Assessment of Asthma Symptoms 289
5.1.3 Daily Peak Flow Readings 289
5.1.4 Pulmonary Function Tests 289
5.1.5 Daily Use of Rescue Inhaled Bronchodilators 289
5.2 Secondary Variables 289
5.2.1 Clinician's Global Opinion of Efficacy 289
5.2.2 Clinician's Assessment of Severity of Asthma 289
6 Number of Patients 289
7 Statistical Methods 290
8 Setting 291
9 Data Analysis 291
10 Conclusion 291
References 291

1 DEFINITION OF ASTHMA

Asthma is a chronic inflammatory disorder of the airways in which many cells play a role. The inflammation results in airflow obstruction which varies both with time and as a result of treatment. The obstruction results partly from constriction of the bronchial smooth muscle and partly from swelling of

0-8493-9230-6/97/$0.00+$.50
© 1997 by CRC Press, Inc.

the bronchial mucosa and the presence of bronchial mucus. The swelling of the bronchial mucosa is due both to edema and to cellular infiltration, characteristically with eosinophils but also with mast cells, polymorphonuclear leukocytes, macrophages, and lymphocytes. The condition is also characterized by an increase in airway responsiveness to a variety of stimuli.

Specific trigger factors cause short- and long-term changes in airways' caliber. They are airborne and ingested allergens such as house dust, house dust mite, animal danders, pollens, fungal spores, and a variety of foodstuffs. Nonspecific triggers which cause short-term changes are exercise, cold air, and atmospheric pollutants such as car fumes, cigarette smoke, and aerosols. Longer term alterations can be induced by infections both viral and bacterial.

It is not known what the exact relationship is between these trigger factors and the functional alterations of mucosal inflammation and bronchial muscle constriction, but it would seem likely that allergens and infections will produce predominantly inflammation, whereas the nonspecific triggers will result in bronchoconstriction. However, as it has been shown that even in mild asthmatic patients requiring little or no treatment a chronic inflammatory state of the bronchial mucosa exists, it is possible that both play a part in most circumstances.

One of the consequences of the inflammatory changes in the bronchial mucosa and characteristic of asthma is that patients show an abnormal bronchoconstrictive response to bronchial challenges with histamine and methacholine. This abnormal response, known as bronchial hyperreactivity or bronchial hyperresponsiveness, is used both to identify potential asthmatic subjects in epidemiological studies and to measure the effects of treatment. In recent years attention has focused on substituting 4.5% saline as a bronchoconstrictive agent as it may be more specific for asthma.[1]

The clinical consequences of these pathological changes and functional disturbances are the characteristic symptoms of asthma, wheeze, shortness of breath, cough, morning tightness and, in the chronic state, the symptoms limit the ability to carry out normal day-to-day activities and cause disturbances in sleep. These subjective symptoms are associated with measurable changes in airflow, which not only varies seasonally, according to the predominance of allergenic factors, but also shows a characteristic diurnal variation.

2 MEASUREMENTS OF AIRFLOW LIMITATION

Variable airways obstruction, being a characteristic of asthma, means that measurement of airway function forms an important part of the evaluation of drugs for the treatment of asthma. It is beyond the scope of this chapter to give a detailed evaluation of the various measurements that can be made. In short-term experiments in man, measurements of both large airway function: peak expiratory flow rate, PEFR; forced expiratory volume in 1 s, FEV_1; and forced vital capacity, FVC and also those of small airway function — forced expiratory volume between 25% and 75% of vital capacity, $FEF_{25\text{-}75}$; and partial expiratory flow rate, pEFR are commonly used. Whereas in longer term experiments, those measurements that can be repeated frequently (FEV_1, PEFR) are most often used. In some cases more sophisticated measures of airway function are needed.[2,3]

Measurements of airway function exhibit an exaggerated diurnal variation in asthmatic patients, the amplitude of which varies according to disease severity. In short-term experiments examining possible treatment effects, this factor also has to be taken into account.

The purpose of this introduction is to emphasize three important factors when considering evaluating the effects of anti-asthmatic drugs.

1. Asthma is a disease of mixed functional pathology in which the key defect — airflow limitation — stems from both inflammatory edema and muscle bronchoconstriction.
2. Asthma is a disease in which the pathology, the functional consequences of the pathology, and the clinical symptoms are subject to inherent intra- and interpatient variability.
3. All asthmatic patients will be taking some type of medication which will have some effect on the pathology, functional measurements, and clinical measurements of their disease. These effects have to be taken into account and allowed for in any study.

3 EVALUATION OF ANTI-ASTHMATIC DRUGS IN MAN

The initial studies of any anti-asthmatic compound in man will be to characterize the absorption, distribution, metabolism, and excretion of the compound, and its single- and repeated-dose tolerance in healthy volunteers. The next series of studies will be bronchial challenge studies, which will investigate the ability of the compound to block or attenuate the bronchoconstricting effects of a number of agents, including inhaled antigen, exercise, sulfur dioxide, sodium metabisulfite, adenosine monophosphate, bradykinin, histamine, and methacholine. The relationship between these challenges and asthma is not known, and, as such, they are not necessarily predictive of the ability of a drug to be useful in asthma. However, they are useful to explore the pharmacological profile of the compound and to investigate the protective effect of different dose sizes and how long that protective effect lasts.

3.1 Bronchial Challenge Experiments

Full details of the standards to which these studies should be given are provided in more detailed texts.[4-7] The principles that must be followed in any experiment of this type are listed below.

3.1.1 Principles

1. The subjects used in the experiment must be cooperative, be stable, and have given written informed consent to participate in the study.
2. They should be adult asthmatic patients with baseline pulmonary function as measured by FEV_1 within ±20% of their predicted normal.
3. Their pulmonary function should not fluctuate over the period of the experiment by more than ±10%. This will exclude patients with severe asthma and those on large doses of medication or medications.
4. They should not have any other disease and should not have a history (within 6 weeks) of a recent viral or other infection that affects the respiratory tract.
5. Patients whose asthma is exacerbated by a seasonal allergen (pollens and fungal spores) should not be used in experiments during or near to the time of year when these pollens or fungal spores are prevalent. Similarly, patients allergic to avoidable allergens (cats, dogs, horses) should avoid such contact during the period of the experiment.
6. Measurements of bronchial hyperreactivity should not vary by more than ±10% during the period of the experiment. (Bronchial hyperreactivity is usually determined using bronchial challenges with increasing doses or concentrations of solutions of histamine or methacholine.) The level of hyperreactivity is expressed as either the concentration of histamine or methacholine, or the dose of either substance that on inhalation produces a 20% fall in pulmonary function. These are shown, respectively, as the PC_{20} (histamine:methacholine) or the PD_{20} (histamine:methacholine).
7. Where possible, anti-asthmatic treatments that are likely to influence the effects of the challenge should be discontinued before each challenge. Because of the dangers of withdrawing prophylactic treatments such as corticosteroids (oral or inhaled), chromones and sustained-release theophyllines, either patients who are taking these routinely should be excluded or, if this is not possible, the dose of their treatments and the timing of each dose should be fixed each day and maintained throughout the period of the experiment. (Inhaled β_2-agonists should be discontinued 12 h before each challenge, oral β_2-agonists 24 h before, and antihistamines 72 h before.)
8. Each challenge should be conducted under the same conditions, in the same environment, and at the same time each day. The whole experiment, which will usually involve at least four challenges (two controls, active treatment preceding challenge, placebo treatment preceding challenge), should be conducted over as short a time-scale as possible, with at least 3 days but not more than 7 days between each challenge.
9. The challenges should only be carried out in specialist units or laboratories staffed by personnel who are skilled and experienced in the techniques involved and who are capable of dealing with any medical emergency should it arise. Patients should be kept under observation throughout the period of the experiment and resuscitation equipment should be available to deal with any respiratory or cardiovascular emergency. Patients should not be permitted to leave the laboratory until their pulmonary function has returned to normal predicted values and these values have been sustained for at least 60 min. Patients should be sent home with an inhaled bronchodilator with instructions on its use in case an unexpected delayed reaction should occur. Patients should also be issued with a peak flow meter and instructed to take readings regularly (four times daily) throughout the experiment. Any fluctuation from normal would require contact with the doctor conducting the experiment.
10. The measurements to be used can be any appropriate measurement of pulmonary function that will change as a result of the challenge (FEV_1, PEFR, pEFR, $FEF_{25\text{-}75}$). The severity of the challenge should be chosen so that it produces a reduction of FEV at its maximum of between 20 and 30%. The two control challenges should be within ±5% of each other.

11. The evaluation of the results will determine the protective effect of the compound as compared with a matching placebo. The treatments should be randomized in a double-blind fashion and given at the same fixed time before the challenge. The protective effect may be expressed as

$$\frac{100\text{x max. \% fall in } FEV_{1.placebo} - \text{max. \% fall in } FEV_{1.active}}{\text{max. \% fall in } FEV_{1\text{-}placebo}}$$

A drug that provides at least 50% protection in at least 80% of patients is worthy of further trials. For a drug that is going to be administered at 6-h intervals, at least 50% protection should still be present at 6 h and for a drug to be administered 12 h, 50% protection should still be present at 12 h.

3.1.2 Conclusion

Bronchial challenge experiments are not predictive of efficacy of a drug in asthma. It is unlikely that the mechanism whereby inhaled antigen induces bronchoconstriction is the same mechanism whereby inhaled sulfur dioxide induces bronchoconstriction. However, such experiments are useful in establishing the pharmacological profile of any compound and also in determining the minimum effective protective dose of a compound and the length of time that protection lasts.

Bronchial challenge experiments are not without their dangers and should only be carried out under specialist units with properly trained staff. Patients should be kept under continual supervision and only allowed home when normal. Patients should be aware of who to contact and how, should any unexpected delayed reaction occur.

4 THERAPEUTIC TRIALS

The short-term therapeutic trial (4–6 weeks) is the definitive experiment that will determine the therapeutic potential of an anti-asthmatic drug. These trials have to be conducted under precisely defined circumstances in carefully selected patients and the remainder of this chapter will define these conditions. Trials to establish the position of a new drug in the therapy of asthma and trials to compare a new drug with existing treatments will need to be of longer duration (3–12 months).

4.1 Objectives

The objectives of the study must be clearly stated. In most cases they should be to compare the safety and efficacy of drug X with drug Y in the management of patients with bronchial asthma. Drug X will be the test drug and drug Y will be either a matching placebo or another active treatment.

4.2 Trial Design

The trial should be a randomized double-blind parallel group design in which the group treated with the new drug X is compared with the group treated with the control drug Y (placebo or another active treatment).

The test treatment period should be a minimum of 28 days and should be preceded by a baseline period of at least 14 days. During the baseline period, patients will continue to take their existing therapy unchanged.

Before the baseline period there may be a run-in period during which existing therapy may be altered in order to induce a defined level of symptomatology.

For these early trials, it is not considered appropriate to use trial designs of the cross-over type, even with a wash-out period, because of the difficulty in interpreting any changes in a disease with so much in-built inter- and intrapatient variability.

4.3 Selection of Patients

The selection of patients for these early trials is of paramount importance. It is likely that in these early studies women of childbearing age will be excluded and the trials will be carried out in men. It is essential that considerable trouble be taken to select patients who are homogeneous with respect to the variables listed in Table 1.

Each of these variables will be used in the evaluation of the test treatment and each of them may have some bearing on the response to the test treatment. Unless considerable attention is paid to the selection of patients, ambiguous or equivocal results may be obtained, giving rise to both type I and type II errors.

Table 1 Invariables for Which Trial Subjects Must be Homogenous

Age
Type of asthma
Allergic
Nonallergic
Length of asthma
Starting in childhood
Starting in adult life
Type of treatment currently being taken
Patients on inhaled and/or β_2 agonists alone
Patients on theophyllines
Patients on corticosteroids
Patients on sodium cromoglycate/nedocromil sodium
Patients on ketotifen or other oral anti-asthmatic drugs
Severity of asthma as judged by pulmonary function
Performed at the clinic
Performed daily during the baseline period
Severity of asthma as judged by symptoms recorded daily by the patient
Asthma at night
Asthma during the day
Severity of asthma as judged by bronchial reactivity
Reversibility of asthma

4.3.1 Age

Asthma appears to change with age, with nonallergic mechanisms playing a more important role with increasing age. Asthma which starts in adult life (e.g., over the age of 25) may be different from asthma which starts in childhood. Patients should therefore be selected within a fairly narrow age band (not more than 20 years), and for those whose asthma started in childhood, the age range 20-40 years is suitable. If patients with late-onset asthma are selected, the age range 35-55 years is probably more suitable.

4.3.2 Asthma Type

The presence or absence of evidence of an allergic cause is important and it is preferable to select either all allergic patients or all nonallergic patients. The presence of allergy should be confirmed by either skin tests or tests for specific IgE, and there should be historical evidence of the asthma worsening when the patient is exposed to the antigen. Patients with perennial asthma symptoms are preferable to those with seasonal asthma only.

4.3.3 Current Therapy

The treatment a patient is currently receiving will have a major effect on that patient's asthma and their response to any new treatment.

Inhaled β_2-agonists are usually used to treat acute symptoms on an "as required" basis, and the number of times they have to be used during the day and during the night is an important measure of the severity of their asthma. Patients who do not need to use their rescue inhaled bronchodilator daily and use it less than three times a week have mild asthma; those who use it daily have moderate asthma; and those who use it more than 3–4 times a day have severe asthma. Some patients use inhaled bronchodilators as their only treatment and may use a regular dose, irrespective of need, with additional doses taken for acute symptoms. In some countries patients use short-acting theophyllines as rescue therapy and the used daily dose of these may be handled in the same way as inhaled β_2-agonists.

The use or not of oral β_2-agonists and short-acting theophyllines appears to be of less importance and patients may continue to take them. The daily dose should remain fixed throughout the trial.

Patients maintained on sustained-release theophyllines with the dose adjusted to achieve and maintain serum theophylline levels within a defined range and who use either inhaled bronchodilators or short-acting theophyllines for rescue therapy should be selected on the basis that this is their sole treatment.

Patients using inhaled corticosteroids and/or oral corticosteroids should be selected because they all take either inhaled or oral, or both, and the dose should have remained constant for the previous 3 months. Patients requiring large doses of oral corticosteroids (greater than 10 mg prednisone or equivalent per day) are best avoided in early trials, as are patients who need repeated courses of oral corticosteroids. Patients taking inhaled corticosteroids should take them within the same dose range; for example, ≤400 μg of beclomethasone dipropionate (BDP) or equivalent per day (mild asthma), 400-1000 μg of BDP per day (moderate asthma), and 1000 -2000 μg of BDP per day (severe asthma). Patients requiring larger doses than this are best avoided.

With regard to sodium cromoglycate, ketotifen, and nedocromil sodium either all patients may be taking them or none.

All of these treatments may or may not be adjusted as part of the trial design. If they are not to be changed, then the dose and dose frequency must remain fixed throughout the baseline and test treatment periods.

4.3.4 Pulmonary Function Tests

Pulmonary function tests should be carried out each time the patient visits the clinic and 2–3 times daily. The baseline pulmonary function tests can be used to categorize the severity of asthma and will also be used to measure the effectiveness of treatment.

Full spirometry should be carried out during each clinic visit. During the baseline period, the pulmonary function tests carried out at the clinic should not vary by more than 10% and all patients should be within a 20% band of predicted normal values, i.e., within 80–100% predicted normal or 60–80% predicted normal. Current international guidelines define patients as follows: mild asthma — FEV_1 or PEFR >80% predicted normal values with a diurnal variability of <20%; moderate asthma — FEV_1 or PEFR 60–80% predicted normal values with a diurnal variability of 20–30%; and severe asthma — FEV_1 or PEFR <60% predicted normal values with a diurnal variability of >30%. All pulmonary function tests should be standardized according to recognized international standards.[9,10]

During the baseline period and throughout the trial, patients will be asked to measure and record their peak expiratory flow rate on three occasions each day: immediately after rising in the morning; between 1600 and 1800 h; and on going to bed.

The mean daily peak expiratory flow rate should not vary by more than ±10% during the baseline period and all patients should fall within a 20% band of predicted normal values.

4.3.5 Severity of Symptoms

Although maintenance of pulmonary function within the range of predicted normal values is the ultimate aim of anti-asthma treatment, patients can still have symptoms of cough and wheeze despite normal lung function. Daily assessment by the patient of asthma-related symptoms has proved to be a valuable tool in the evaluation of anti-asthma drugs. Many scales have been devised and used but that given in Table 2 has proved to be both representative of asthma symptoms, recognized by patients of varying ability and to be sensitive enough to recognize change in asthma severity both spontaneously and as a result of treatment.

Table 2 Scale of Severity of Asthma Symptoms

Score	Description
Daytime Asthma	
0	No symptoms during the day
1	Occasional wheeze or breathlessness quickly relieved by bronchodilator aerosol
2	Wheezing or short of breath most of the day but did not interfere with usual activities
3	Wheezing or short of breath most of the day; interfered to some extent with usual activities
4	Asthma very bad; could not go to work or school or engage in usual activities at all
Night-Time Asthma	
0	No symptoms
1	Awoke once in the night because of wheezing or cough; awake for less than an hour; did not need to use a bronchodilator aerosol
2	Awoke once in the night because of wheezing or cough; awake for less than an hour but needed to use a bronchodilator aerosol to get back to sleep
3	Awoke once for more than an hour or awoke more than once because of wheezing or cough
4	Awake for most of the night because of wheezing or cough

Other scales can be found in the literature. Visual analog scales are not considered to be reliable. Once a scale has been fixed, it should be used in all trials.

4.3.6 Bronchial Reactivity and Reversibility

All asthmatic patients have reactive airways which can be measured by either a histamine or methacholine dose response. This reactivity is also reflected in a response to a single dose of an inhaled bronchodilator. Patients should be within the same broad range of bronchial reactivity and should all have evidence of reversibility to an inhaled bronchodilator ≤15%.

4.4 Methodology

4.4.1 Patient Selection

The type of patient to be selected for trials will depend upon the stage of development of the compound and the type of drug under development.

4.4.1.1 New Member of an Existing Class of Drug

If the test drug to be evaluated is a new member of an existing class of compound (corticosteroid, chromone, oral anti-asthma) then it may be possible to establish efficacy and safety on the basis of substitution of an established member of that class. Patients will need to be selected who are all currently maintained on the same existing drug and the new compound is substituted on a double-blind, randomized basis. In these circumstances it is very important that all patients fit within a defined band of entry criteria with respect to symptom severity, pulmonary function, existing therapy, and use of rescue medication. Their asthma should also have been stable without severe exacerbation or change of therapy for at least 3 months.

Symptom severity may be on the basis of mean severity scores during the baseline period or that scores are recorded of >1 on at least 4 days of the last week of the baseline. Pulmonary function can be defined on the basis of reference to predicted normal and diurnal variation recorded during the baseline and rescue bronchodilators on the basis of daily usage during the final week of the baseline. It may also be necessary to include some criteria of reversibility of pulmonary function in order to ensure that patients are asthmatic.

Consideration will have to be given to the number of patients that need to be included and the length of the trial in order to ensure that a true comparison of the new drug and the existing one can be made. It has been shown in previous trials that up to 20% of asthmatic patients can be maintained well on a placebo treatment for up to a year.

4.4.1.2 Novel Compounds

If the compound to be evaluated is a new class of compound of unproved efficacy then it will probably be necessary to establish absolute efficacy using a placebo control. In these circumstances it will be necessary to select a group of patients who have a sufficient level of symptom severity and below-normal pulmonary function for an effect to be demonstrated as compared to placebo.

In most hospital clinics where such trials are likely to be conducted, the majority of patients who will be suitable for clinical trials are likely to be well controlled on their existing treatment with little room for improvement. In these circumstances a run-in period can be used during which a proportion of existing medication will be removed, in order to produce a slight but controlled worsening of asthma symptoms. Deterioration in asthma can be severe, life-threatening, and unpredictable particularly if changes in medication are made. To reduce medication in a stable asthmatic can be hazardous but in some trial situations there is no alternative. This is a difficult ethical decision, but provided that stable, cooperative, well-controlled patients who are fully informed have immediate access to emergency services at any time of the day and night, are within easy reach of the hospital, and give written consent are selected then such a design is considered justified and the risks small. Full discussion with both patients and close relatives and with a properly constituted ethical committee will be required.

The run-in period should not need to be any longer than 4 weeks with patients being seen weekly and a defined deterioration in either symptoms or pulmonary function or both during the previous week being the entry criteria. Patients will then enter a baseline period at that level of treatment.

4.4.2 Previous Therapy

1. Patients on β_2-agonists alone. Oral β_2-agonists should be stopped and inhaled bronchodilators used on an as required basis.

2. Patients on sustained-release theophyllines. These should be stopped and patients be given either immediate-release theophyllines or inhaled ß$_2$-agonists, to be used on an as required basis.
3. Patients on inhaled corticosteroids. The withdrawal of any corticosteroid treatment has to be undertaken cautiously. Any dose reduction should not be greater than 25% of the starting dose and not more frequently than every 2 weeks. Patients needing daily doses of inhaled corticosteroids in excess of 1200 μg of BDP or equivalent should not be included. Suggested dose reductions are given in Table 3. Patients should be seen weekly during this phase and if there is any evidence of worsening asthma in excess of that required by the protocol, the patient should be withdrawn from the trial and returned to their previous dose of inhaled corticosteroids. A short course of oral corticosteroids may be required to stabilize the patient again. All patients to be given inhaled ß$_2$-agonists to be used on an as needed basis.
4. Patients on chromones (sodium cromoglycate, nedocromil sodium). Like the corticosteroids these drugs should also be reduced step-wise during the run-in period. The current dose should be reduced initially to 50% then to 25% and then to 0.

Table 3 Suggested Dose Reductions for Inhaled Corticosteroids

Starting Dose (g)	Reduced Dose (g)
1200	1000
1000	800
800	600
600	500
500	400
400	300
300	200
200	150
150	100
100	50
50	0

4.4.3 Criteria for Entry into Test Treatment Period

Criteria need to be defined for when a patient's asthma has sufficiently worsened for entry into the test treatment period. As soon as these criteria have been satisfied, the patient may be entered into the test treatment phase.

Suggested criteria are as follows:

1. Mean daily score for either day or night asthma of 1.5 or greater over 7 days.
2. Mean morning PEFR over 7 days 10–20% lower than that over the last 7 days of the baseline period.
3. 10–20% increase in the total daily use of inhaled ß$_2$-agonist.

These are relatively small changes, but they are quantifiable and are produced as a result of treatment withdrawal and can be reversed within a 28-day period by an effective anti-asthma treatment. Induced changes any greater than these are likely to be associated with unstable asthma, and patients should be withdrawn from the trial.

It is very important that once the definitions of the entry criteria are agreed that they become absolute and any patient that does not comply is withdrawn.

4.4.4 Baseline Period

The baseline period is used to establish that the patients comply with the entry criteria, get used to the measurements they have to make, and to provide the baseline values which will be altered by the test treatment or treatments. During the baseline period existing treatment will be maintained constant apart from the rescue bronchodilator usage. At least two clinic visits should be made for baseline pulmonary function, reversibility, and bronchial hyperreactivity readings. In addition, blood and urine samples will be taken for baseline readings.

5 MEASUREMENTS OF EFFICACY

Data will be collected throughout the trial — run-in, baseline, test treatment phases — and will be used to determine whether the test treatment is efficacious.

5.1 Primary Variables

5.1.1 Patient's Global Opinion of Efficacy

At the end of the trial, each patient will be asked to score on a 1-5 scale the efficacy of the test treatment they received:

1 Very effective
2 Moderately effective
3 Slightly effective
4 No effect
5 Made condition worse/withdrawn because of worsening asthma

5.1.2 Patients' Assessment of Asthma Symptoms

Patients will keep a daily diary card, recording the severity of their symptoms. It is usual to include 2-3 symptoms each on a 0-4 scale, as in Table 4.

5.1.3 Daily Peak Flow Readings

Using a suitable portable peak expiratory flow meter, patients should record their peak expiratory flow rate at least twice and preferably three times a day (on waking; between 1600 and 1800 h; on retiring to bed). The morning reading should be taken before the first dose of the inhaled bronchodilator or of the test treatment. All patients should use the same peak flow meter.

5.1.4 Pulmonary Function Tests

Carried out at each clinic visit: FEV_1; FVC; PEFR.

5.1.5 Daily Use of Rescue Inhaled Bronchodilators

The patients should record their use (doses or puffs) of inhaled bronchodilator used each day: the 24-h total and the number of doses used between rising in the morning, retiring at night, and during the night.

5.2 Secondary Variables

5.2.1 Clinicians' Global Opinion of Efficacy

On same scale as patient.

5.2.2 Clinicians' Assessment of Severity of Asthma

At each clinic visit, after examining the patient, examining the diary cards, and conducting the pulmonary function tests, the clinician should make an evaluation of the severity of the asthma on that day using the following scale:

1 Very severe
2 Severe
3 Moderately severe
4 Mild
5 No symptoms

6 NUMBER OF PATIENTS

The number of patients will need to be fully discussed with the statistician associated with the trial and will depend upon the circumstances. The following considerations are relevant.

In trials which involve the worsening of symptoms during the run-in period, the null hypothesis approach will state that neither treatment will produce an improvement in the asthma. It is unlikely that any improvement that does take place will be to a position better than baseline values. For the variables used, the maximum improvement from run-in is likely to be:

For diary card symptoms	20–30%
For daily PEFR	10–15%
For inhaled bronchodilator use	10–15%
For clinic asthma severity	15–20%
For global efficacy	20% difference

If the comparative treatment is placebo, there will need to be sufficient patients included to detect differences of this magnitude if the active treatment is efficacious. Placebo-controlled trials of longer than 3 months' duration are probably not justified or necessary.

If the trial design is a comparison between two active treatments, one of which is of proven efficacy and comparative treatment is another active treatment, then sufficient patients will be needed to provide 90% power of showing the two treatments to be equivalent. A minimum of 6–8 weeks treatment is necessary for such trials and trials of up to 12 months of this design will probably be necessary.

7 STATISTICAL METHODS

The data collected in this type of study consist of daily recordings of symptom severity, PEFR readings, use of inhaled bronchodilators, and global opinion of efficacy.

Table 4 Patients' Daily Diary Cards for Recording the Severity of Symptoms

Daytime Asthma	
0	No symptoms during day
1	Occasional wheeze or breathlessness quickly relieved by bronchodilator aerosol
2	Wheezing or short of breath most of the day but did not interfere with usual activities
3	Wheezing or short of breath most of the day; interfered to some extent with usual activities
4	Asthma very bad; could not go to work or school or engage in usual activities at all
Night-Time Asthma	
0	No symptoms
1	Awoke once in the night because of wheezing or cough; awake for less than an hour; did not need to use a bronchodilator aerosol
2	Awoke once in the night because of wheezing or cough; awake for less than an hour but needed to use a bronchodilator aerosol to get back to sleep
3	Awoke once for more than an hour or awoke more than once because of wheezing or cough
4	Awake for most of the night because of wheezing or cough
Morning Tightness	
0	None
1	Slight; awoke at usual time; chest tight but did not need to use bronchodilator aerosol
2	Awoke at usual time; chest tight and needed to use bronchodilator aerosol
3	Awoke earlier than usual because of asthma and needed to use bronchodilator aerosol once between waking and measuring morning PEFR (one dose = two inhalations)
4	Awoke earlier than usual because of asthma and needed to use bronchodilator aerosol more than once between waking and measuring morning PEFR
Cough (Day)	
0	None
1	Occasional coughing but not troublesome
2	Frequent coughing but it did not interfere with usual activities
3	Frequent coughing, interfering to some extent with usual activities
4	Distressing cough most of the day
Cough (Night)	
0	None
1	Occasional coughing but not troublesome
2	Frequent coughing but it did not interfere with sleep
3	Frequent coughing, interfering to some extent with sleep
4	Distressing cough most of the night

For all diary card data, changes from the last week of baseline or the last week of run-in, as compared with the last 2 weeks of the treatment period, are compared. Two-tailed tests should be used throughout at the 5% level of significance. For full details, readers are referred to a standard reference on statistical evaluation of clinical trials.[11,12]

Patients who have to be withdrawn from the trial during the test treatment phase owing to worsening of asthma should be included in all analyses, provided that they take at least 7 days of the test treatment. Endpoint analysis is then undertaken, using the mean of the last 3 days prior to withdrawal.

8 SETTING

These preliminary trials should be conducted in hospital outpatient clinics staffed by clinicians experienced in the management of asthma and with adequate staff to provide 24-h coverage. Special trial clinics should be arranged and there should be close attention to ensuring that all patients know who to contact and how to contact them, should their asthma deteriorate. Arrangements for immediate inpatient care should be available, with the availability of full resuscitation if needed.

9 DATA ANALYSIS

The basis of the analysis is that the drug under evaluation either produces an improvement in the primary efficacy variables as compared to a placebo or another active drug or maintains the existing level of primary efficacy variables. Against a background of need and cost effectiveness other means of handling the data are being used. These include the percentage of symptom-free days and/or nights, the number of days on which a rescue bronchodilator was needed, percentage reduction in dose of rescue bronchodilator, and in longer term studies the number of acute exacerbations and hospital and doctor visits.

10 CONCLUSION

The early evaluation of anti-asthmatic drugs in man presents a challenge of attention to detail and organization. The inherent variability of asthma does not lend itself to routine pharmacological examination and the lack of complete understanding as to the mechanisms involved does not allow any short-term or single-dose studies to be predictive. Considerable preclinical knowledge on any new compound has to be obtained to allow up to 4 weeks' administration in man before any assessment of clinical efficacy can be undertaken. The conduct of the first 28-day trials must be meticulous, so that a true assessment can be made before large numbers of patients with what is a potentially dangerous condition are exposed to an untried and unproved treatment.

REFERENCES

1. Smith, C.D. and Anderson, S.D. (1989). Inhalation provocation tests using non-isotonic aerosols. *J. Allergy Clin. Immunol.*; 84: 781-790.
2. Tattersfield, A.E. and Keeping, I.M. (1979). Assessing change in airway caliber-measurement of airway resistance. *Br. J. Clin. Pharmacol.* 8: 307-319.
3. Pride, N.B. (1979). Assessment of changes in airway caliber. Test of forced expiration 8: 193-203.
4. Chai, H., Farr, R.S., Froehlich, L.A., Mathison, D.A., McLean, J.A., Rosenthal, R.R., Sheffer, A.L., Spector, S.L. and Townley, R.G. (1975). Standardisation of bronchial inhalation challenge procedures. *J. Allergy Clin. Immunol.*, 56, 323-7.
5. Eggleston, P.A., Rosenthal, R.R., Anderson, S.A., Anderton, R., Bierman, C.W., Bleecker, E.R., Chai, H., Cropp, C.J.A., Johnson, J.S., Konig, P., Morse, J., Smith, L.J., Summers, R.J. and Trantlein, J.J. (1979). Guidelines for the methodology of exercise challenge testing of asthmatics. *J. Allergy Clin. Immunol.*, 64, 642-5.
6. Cropp, G.J.A., Bernstein, I.L., Bouchsey, H.A., Hyde, R.W., Rosenthal, R.R., Spector, S.L. and Townley, R.G. (1980). Guidelines for bronchial inhalation challenges with pharmacologic and antigenic agents. *ATS News*, Spring 11-19.
7. Eiser, N.M., Kerrabijn, K.F. and Quanjer, P.J. (1983). Guidelines for standardisation of bronchial challenges with (non-specific) bronchoconstricting agents. *Bull. Eur. Physiopathol. Res.*, 19, 495-514.
8. International Consensus Report on Diagnosis and Treatment of Asthma. National Heart, Lung and Blood Institute, National Institutes of Health, Bethseda, MD: 1990; Publication No. 92-3091.
9. Lung function testing: selection of reference values and interpretional strategies. A statement of the American Thoracic Society (1991). *Am. Rev. Resp. Dis.* 144: 1202-1218.
10. Standardised lung function testing. (1991). *Eur. Resp. J.*; 6 (Suppl.) 16: 1-100.
11. Altman, D.G. *Practical Statistics for Medical Research.* London, Chapman and Hall 1991.
12. Pocock S.J. *Clinical Trials: A Practical Approach.* Chichester, Wiley 1983.

Part VII. Assessment of Drug Effects on the CNS

Chapter 21

Measurement of CNS Effects

Finian Kelly and J. Raymond Bratty

CONTENTS

1 Introduction ... 295
2 Neurophysiological Measurements ... 296
  2.1 Q-EEG Classification of Psychotropic Drugs ... 296
  2.2 Central Bioavailability and Pharmacodynamic Relationships ... 296
  2.3 Methodological Considerations ... 297
3 Psychometric Testing ... 297
  3.1 Healthy Volunteers or Patients? ... 298
  3.2 Methodological Considerations ... 298
  3.3 Critical Flicker Fusion ... 299
  3.4 Vigilance Tasks ... 299
  3.5 Reaction Time Tests ... 300
  3.6 Digit Symbol Substitution ... 300
  3.7 Memory Tests ... 300
  3.8 Driving Tests ... 300
4 Saccadic Eye Movements/Body Sway ... 301
  4.1 Saccadic Eye Movement Analysis ... 301
  4.2 Body Sway ... 301
5 Rating of Subjective Feelings ... 301
6 Conclusions ... 302
References ... 302

1 INTRODUCTION

The principal aims of measurement of the central nervous system (CNS) effects of an investigational drug are prediction of therapeutic effects and prediction of unwanted effects. Preclinical investigation of a drug, both in general testing and in specific models predictive of clinical activity, will have provided a basis on which to anticipate the effects of a drug when it is used in healthy volunteers and in patients with the target illness. Early phase studies, usually in healthy volunteers, will provide the first evidence of whether a drug's properties are carried through into man. It is important to remember that it is not only psychotropic drugs which exert effects on the CNS; many drugs whose primary actions are on other organ systems may have secondary effects on the CNS, for example, certain antihistamines and antihypertensives. Therefore assessment of all new drugs should include at least a primary evaluation of possible CNS effects in phase I and early phase II studies.

Phase I studies in healthy volunteers will provide evidence of CNS adverse events such as sedation, drowsiness, dizziness, insomnia, or excitation. However, these effects may be apparent only at doses at the upper extremes of the putative therapeutic level. Specific objective psychopharmacological assessment techniques are required to measure the CNS effects of investigational drugs over a range of dose levels which should correspond with the expected therapeutic range in patients, thus providing data which may assist in determining the appropriate dose range for phase II studies.

The effects of a drug on the overall neurophysiological activity of the brain can be measured by electroencephalographic (EEG) techniques. The effects on CNS functions such as vigilance, cognition, memory, and behavior can be measured by psychometric testing. Saccadic eye movement analysis and body sway measurement, which are essentially psychomotor tests, and are both very sensitive to CNS drug effects, are discussed separately. Subjective rating scales can provide additional data on sedation, arousal, and mood changes which will complement the findings of the objective measures. This chapter

0-8493-9230-6/97/$0.00+$.50
© 1997 by CRC Press, Inc.

will therefore review measurement of CNS effects under the headings: neurophysiological measurements; psychometric testing; saccadic eye movement/body sway; and subjective assessments.

Disease-specific measurement instruments will not be discussed as these are appropriately dealt with in specific chapters elsewhere in this text.

2 NEUROPHYSIOLOGICAL MEASUREMENTS

Electroencephalography has been used extensively for over 40 years in the evaluation of the effects of drugs on brain function. Its use is based on the assumption that if an investigational drug has effects on brain function, it will influence the waking EEG of healthy volunteers who take the drug. The EEG is attractive as a research tool because it is a safe, repeatable, noninvasive, and objective measure of brain function. Electroencephalographic signals are recorded on tape, generally for periods up to 24 h. Subsequent quantitative analysis by computerized techniques using power density spectral analysis provides the record of the quantitative pharmaco-EEG (Q-EEG).

The most widely used application of pharmaco-EEG has probably been in the classification of psychotropic drugs, which is based on the different alteration of EEG patterns seen with different classes of drugs. Q-EEG has also been used to measure the central bioavailability of a drug and to determine the relationship with the drug's pharmacodynamic actions. EEG can provide data which allows a topographical representation of brain activity. Other practical applications of the EEG which have been described include comparison of the effects of two enantiomers, comparisons between different formulations of the same drug, and determination of the efficacy of benzodiazepines in alcohol withdrawal.

2.1 Q-EEG Classification of Psychotropic Drugs

The observation that drugs with clinically different actions altered the EEG to a measurably different extent lead to an evaluation of the use of the EEG in classification of drugs. Specific EEG profiles for antipsychotic, anxiolytic, antidepressant, psychostimulant, and nootropic drugs have been described,[1,2] allowing comparison between the profile of an investigational drug and that of psychotropic drugs whose effects have been well characterized. Data generated will have implications for prediction of both the behavioral effects of new chemical entities and their potential therapeutic applications. Good examples of the use of EEG in classification of psychotropic drugs have been reported by Herrmann and colleagues.[3,4] The investigational drugs savoxepine, a putative antipsychotic, and levoprotiline, a putative antidepressant, were shown to be similar to that of established antipsychotic and antidepressant drugs, respectively. However, as an example of the limitations of the pharmaco-EEG in predicting therapeutic effects of investigational compounds, the same authors have reported the profile of the investigational drug, maroxepine.[5] Features of both antidepressants and antipsychotics were seen on pharmaco-EEG recordings, and there were also features indicative of a strong sedative potential. However, efficacy was not proven in either depression or psychosis, and the drug was stimulating rather than sedative, thereby demonstrating that pharmaco-EEG is not infallible in predicting the therapeutic potential of drugs.

Classification of psychotropic drugs by pharmaco-EEG is further limited by the fact that it is possible to classify drugs only into those categories which were retrospectively used in establishing the original classification. New drugs, such as selective dopamine or serotonin receptor antagonists, will not necessarily fit into the established categories, thus limiting the application of EEG classification.

An unresolved question in measurement of the effects of drugs on pharmaco-EEG is whether the EEG reflects diffuse changes secondary to drug administration, or reveals specific drug activity indicative of therapeutic potential.[5] The relevance of the EEG changes of specific drug categories to their therapeutic effects on their respective clinical syndromes have not been adequately explained. The pharmaco-EEG profiles of drugs in patients might well be different from those seen in healthy volunteers, who are the usual subjects for such studies, as might the profiles on chronic dosing, and these remain areas for further research.

2.2 Central Bioavailability and Pharmacodynamic Relationships

Pharmaco-EEG allows an objective assessment of CNS bioavailability of a drug. The EEG is very sensitive to drug-induced changes in vigilance, and at the most basic level it can provide the simple, but essential, information that a drug is affecting the human CNS, when there is minimal evidence of CNS drug activity on objective and subjective clinical measures. The time-course of the pharmacodynamic actions of an investigational drug on the CNS can be measured and this can be correlated with its behavioral and cognitive effects. The data provided can be used as a solid basis for deciding on the dose schedule of the drug, or to allow comparison of the pharmacodynamics of different formulations of the same drug. The behavioral toxicity of a drug can also be correlated with the pharmaco-EEG activity, allowing definition of the CNS toxicity of compounds under investigation.

2.3 Methodological Considerations

Pharmaco-EEG studies are usually conducted in healthy volunteers in order to avoid the possibly confounding effects of illness in patients; the limitations of this constraint have been referred to above. A double-blind, placebo-controlled, cross-over experimental design should be used, with subjects randomized to the test drug, usually at a range of doses. The wash-out period between drug administration sessions should be long enough to allow elimination of the drug and any active metabolites. The effects on Q-EEG are compared with placebo; if there is a standard drug from the therapeutic category of the investigational drug which has a well-characterized Q-EEG profile, this should also be included as an active comparator. Subjects must be free of effects of other drugs, including caffeine, alcohol, and recreational drugs. EEG recordings will be made before drug intake and at appropriate time intervals thereafter for up to 24 h. Blood samples should be taken at the same time intervals for estimation of plasma levels of the drug in order to establish the pharmacokinetic-pharmacodynamic relationship. A battery of psychometric tests should also be performed, and safety data, including vital sign measurements and adverse events, should be recorded at regular intervals.

3 PSYCHOMETRIC TESTING

Of the vast array of psychometric tests which have been described in the literature,[6] some of the more frequently used will be described in this section, with a focus on practical aspects of their use. All psychometric tests must have a sound theoretical, methodological, and psychological basis, but a detailed review of the theoretical and methodological basis for psychometric tests is beyond the scope of this text.

Psychometric tests are used to assess the effects of drugs on behavior and cognition. An individual test will usually assess more than one aspect of behavior and thus may provide information on a drug's effects on information processing, sensorimotor coordination, reaction time, reasoning, skilled behaviors, or aspects of memory. However, no single test will adequately simulate complex performance tasks and a selection of tests must be used in order to evaluate the full range of CNS activity which might be affected by a drug. It is therefore usual to use a performance test battery to assess both the overt and more subtle behavioral effects of drugs. There is no single standardized human performance assessment battery and individual researchers use their preferred range of tests. The use of different tests and different methodologies in measuring behavioral effects of drugs has rightly been criticized because it makes valid comparisons between studies very difficult.[6,7]

The development of psychopharmacological methods of assessing the behavioral effects of drugs has given rise to the concept of "behavioral toxicity," a term used to describe the adverse effects of a drug which are either new behavioral deficits or exacerbations of pre-existing ones. Behavioral toxicity may have serious consequences for patients, particularly in performing complex tasks such as driving or operating machinery. It must therefore be identified by appropriate experimental performance studies which reflect the way the drug will be used by patients.

All psychometric tests included in a performance battery should have been rigorously validated and must be reliable, in order to allow the benefit and risk of drugs to be established. Some tests which are widely used lack adequate information on their validation and must not be accepted as valid simply because of long and frequent use. The increasing use of microcomputers in performance testing has led to electronic adaptation of pencil and paper tests. It is necessary that such microcomputer adaptations are validated in their own right, even if the original pencil and paper test was fully validated.[8]

Simple psychometric tests have frequently been developed as pencil and paper tests.[9] The ease of administration and replication, coupled with the lack of complex equipment, make such tests attractive, though many are now being adapted for use as part of a microcomputer battery of tests. Computerized test batteries can be designed for use by healthy volunteers or by patients with a specific diagnosis. For example, a computerized assessment system for use in assessing cognitive function in patients with dementia has been described by Simpson and colleagues.[10] This comprises cognitive tasks measuring choice reaction time, vigilance, and the sensitivity and speed of digit, word, and picture recognition.

3.1 Healthy Volunteers or Patients?

Psychometric testing in the early stages of drug development will be carried out in healthy volunteers because of the greater experimental control which is possible. A patient's illness is likely to have confounding effects on performance. For example, CNS arousal level has been shown to be decreased in depressed patients,[11] and it may be impossible to distinguish the effects of drug from the effects of illness on decrements of performance.

However, since most users of drugs are patients, it is essential to evaluate the effects in this population.[12] Differences between healthy elderly volunteers and patients with dementia in the dose range of experimental antidementia drugs which were well tolerated have been reported,[13,14] and it is likely that such differences would also manifest on psychometric testing. Therefore, generalization to patients of results from studies in healthy volunteers is not always valid, particularly if the dosing schedule, or duration of treatment, in volunteers differs from that which will be used in patients. Studies in patients will allow improvements in performance, resulting from alleviation of disease processes which themselves might have hindered performance, to be measured.

Nonpatient volunteers who have personality features relevant to the investigational drug are another option for testing of psychotropic drugs.[15] For example, subjects who have high anxiety traits, which can easily be assessed by such instruments as the State-Trait Anxiety Inventory (STAI),[16] might be suitable for assessment of a drug which is intended for anxiolytic use. Use of such subjects theoretically might allow an evaluation of aspects of the illness without the confounding effects of the disease itself.

It is also possible to induce disease symptoms in healthy volunteers in an attempt to mimic illness or provide a surrogate measure. Thus memory impairment induced by scopolamine and its reversal by an anticholinergic drug, has been reported.[17]

3.2 Methodological Considerations

Several methodological factors must be taken into account when designing studies to assess behavior and cognition. The tests will be performed in human beings whose behavior is neither consistent nor stable and there will have to be adequate experimental control for the effects of sex, age, circadian rhythm, and personality on behavior. Additionally, in studies in patients, disease effects must also be taken into account.

A double-blind, placebo-controlled experimental design is usual. In studies of acute drug effects a cross-over design is often used and it is essential that an adequate period of time intervenes between test sessions to allow for the elimination of drug. In calculating this time period, the possibility of longer CNS activity than would be expected by plasma levels should be taken into account. EEG data may be of value in determining the duration of central activity of the test drug. Use of a positive control is desirable as it will be of value in determining the sensitivity of the study measures; for example, a study finding that an investigational drug lacks sedative effects would be strengthened by the finding in the same study that a comparator benzodiazepine was definitely sedating. Similarly, a drug with cardiovascular activity and no known CNS effects was shown to be devoid of effects on CNS function despite such prominent associated CNS adverse events as headache; in the study impairments of both objective and subjective CNS activity was shown with the comparator drug, diazepam.[18]

In studies in healthy volunteers it is essential that there are controls for the effects of psychoactive substances other than the test drug. Thus, subjects should be free of the effects of alcohol, nicotine, and caffeine at the time of testing and should not have a history of use of psychoactive drugs, whether legal or illegal. Initial screening for drug and alcohol use, and at random intervals during the study, is advisable. Subjects should be screened for disease states which might affect CNS function. Screening for human immunodeficiency virus (HIV) infection may be advisable, as subtle cognitive changes may be present before other manifestations of the disease, but exclusion of subjects with HIV risk factors, such as a history of drug abuse or high risk sexual activity, may be unnecessary.[19]

Age may be of significance in evaluating drug effects. Some studies show that middle aged subjects have greater performance decrements than younger subjects,[20,21] though this is not always a consistent finding.[22,23] Therefore generalization from one age group to another is not always possible and the effects on performance should be tested in as wide an age group as will potentially use the drug.

In studies in healthy volunteers, whether young or elderly, it is unlikely that there will be an inability to perform the test battery. Studies in patients, however, should take into account the physical ability to perform tests which may involve button pressing or other motor activities. This is particularly true for elderly patients with cognitive impairments, although patients with dementia were not limited in their ability to use a computerized assessment system.[10] Certain cognitive and psychomotor deficiencies are likely to be present in patients suffering from other illnesses, including depression and psychotic disorders, and these should also be taken into account in assessing the results of psychometric tests in these populations.

Gender differences are not always considered when assessing the effects of drugs on performance and many studies are conducted in healthy male volunteers only. This is a serious criticism, since many psychotropic drugs will be used widely in a female patient population and generalization of effects from one gender to the other is not always possible. The gender difference in itself is important, but also scant regard has been paid to the influence of the hormonal changes of the menstrual cycle on the effects of drugs on behavior and cognition. Regulatory agencies increasingly require fuller information on gender differences in the effects of drugs and this should be taken into account in planning study programs.

Personality traits can influence performance on psychometric tests, as has been demonstrated for critical flicker fusion threshold testing.[24,25] A recent study suggests that the personality profile of healthy volunteers may not mirror that of the general population.[26] In healthy volunteers, the influence of personality can be minimized by using personality inventories, such as the MMPI, as part of the screening process. Specific mood traits can be excluded by using an appropriate instrument which has been validated for this purpose; for example, the trait questionnaire of the Spielberger State-Trait Anxiety Inventory,[16] a 20-item, self-rated instrument, can be used to detect subjects with high levels of anxiety as part of their usual personality.

Psychometric tests may be subject to practice and learning effects, especially those tests which involve the coordination of sensory and motor systems. Prior to entering a study subjects should be trained until they reach a level beyond which there is no further improvement in their performance, thereby eliminating learning effects. Pencil and paper tests also are subject to practice and learning effects and parallel examples should be used to prevent subjects remembering the test from one session to the next.

The duration of treatment with a drug is critical for assessing possible tolerance to wanted or unwanted drug effects, and for evaluating changes in psychometric test results in patients which may be due to improvement in cognitive function as the drug induces symptom remission.[12] Many studies of CNS effects of drugs are rightly criticized for extrapolating conclusions, based on acute treatment in healthy volunteers, to patients who may have pre-existing cognitive deficits as part of their disease process, and who will take dugs for a much longer period than that tested in the study.

3.3 Critical Flicker Fusion

Critical flicker fusion threshold (CFF), which measures CNS arousal or activation, is one of the most widely used tests of psychomotor function.[6,27] It is a sensitive, valid, and reliable measure of the capacity of an individual to process information and has been shown to have a marked sensitivity to drug effects. It is lowered by a range of drugs which affect performance and in several studies has been shown to be closely related to the subjective decrease in alertness caused by those drugs. Impairment of CFF can be due to an effect on the cortical mechanisms involved in flicker detection or due to a failure in concentration.

In measuring CFF, subjects look at a flashing light and are required to discriminate flicker. The point at which the light appears to be continuous is termed the threshold and provides a measure of overall CNS arousal and activity. CFF measures are dependent on age, sex, and personality of subjects, and differ with circadian variation in CNS activity. Therefore these factors must be carefully controlled. A criticism of the use of CFF is that subjects or patients often appear to have performed the test while viewing the flickering light source with unrestricted vision. Changes in pupillary diameter will change the measurement of CFF.[28] Similarly, drugs which cause either pupillary miosis[29] or mydriasis[30] can lower or raise CFF. It is therefore essential to take into account the possible effects of drugs on pupillary size and the testing environment, and to use an artificial pupil when testing CFF.

Unfortunately there has been little standardization of CFF assessment procedures and this makes valid comparisons between the data reported in different studies difficult. However, in a review of studies which did use similar assessment procedures, consistency was demonstrated across several classes of drugs.[27]

3.4 Vigilance Tasks

In many psychometric tests, an assessment of vigilance of the individual subject or patient is an integral component. These tests include simple pencil and paper tests such as letter cancellation tests, which involve primary simple reflexes that measure both the processing of sensory information and the speed of psychomotor reaction.[31] Other simple tests of vigilance include symbol copying tests, letter cancellation, and the number matching test.[32]

3.5 Reaction Time Tests

Reaction time tests evaluate the speed of motor responses, usually by requiring the subject to press a button in response to a stimulus. The number of correct responses and the latency in time to respond are measured. Both simple and choice reaction time tests have been described.[7]

In simple reaction time tests, motor response is evaluated. In choice reaction time tests, both accuracy and speed of reaction time are tested. Choice reaction time tests assess sensorimotor performance by adding a recognition time component.[33]

3.6 Digit Symbol Substitution

The digit symbol substitution test (DSST), originally described as part of the Wechsler adult intelligence test,[34,35] is one of the most widely used objective measures of sedation. The original test is a pencil and paper test and its popularity in clinical studies is probably linked to the simplicity of the test. Subjects are presented with a form in which the numbers 0 to 9 are presented in random order surmounting empty boxes into which the subject places the symbol corresponding to the respective number indicated by a code at the top of the form. The test requires sustained attention and concentration and evaluates psychomotor speed of response and recognition of sensory information. The test is unaffected by memory.[36] Although the results of DSST testing are highly variable between studies and drugs, in general it is a sensitive measure of psychomotor impairment due to sedative drug effects. However, it may be less sensitive than other tests when peak levels of drug have not been achieved or when concentrations are falling.[9] The symbol copying test can be used to assess the motor component of the DSST, using the same symbols but requiring the subject to just copy them.

3.7 Memory Tests

Memory is not a unitary function and different forms of learning and memory are subserved by different brain functions. Memory systems are not independent, but operate in close interaction with one another. Drug-induced memory impairment may be due to an effect on either memory mechanisms or an earlier stage of information processing. Effects on the earlier stages of information processing may be due to either sedation or impairment of attention. The latter can be detected by visual tasks, including DSST, which will provide evidence of a defect in visual information processing. A high correlation between sedation and memory impairment has been shown.[37,38] It is possible that the cognitive affects of drugs are due to sedation rather than memory impairment,[39,40] but in several studies it has not been possible to disassociate these effects. However, a full test battery should be able to provide some evidence of those defects which are due to sedation, impaired attention, and impaired memory.

Simple tests which measure memory functions include free recall, for example, of word lists which are presented visually at a set rate, followed by a short period during which the subject can write down as many words as can be remembered. Memory scanning tasks test short-term memory. Backwards digit span is a very simple test of short-term memory. The Sternberg memory scanning task[41] is a test in which a series of different digits are presented, followed by a single digit which the subject has to indicate if recognized from the preceding series. The paired-associated learning task is a test of verbal reasoning and intermediate term memory, and the Buschke selective reminding task[18,42] is a test of long-term memory.

3.8 Driving Tests

Driving is a complex psychomotor task which involves both motor and higher CNS components, and which has been shown to be impaired by many drugs. Simulated driving tests can be considered as complex tests of reaction time. They measure hand to eye coordination and involve higher CNS functions in decision making. Operating a motor vehicle in traffic is possibly the most demanding and potentially dangerous psychomotor task which will be performed by patients. Methodological guidelines for assessing the effects of drugs on driving performance have been proposed by a body of internationally recognized experts.[43] There was agreement that studies designed to predict a psychoactive drug's effects on driving performance should always measure the effects after multiple doses administered according to the proposed therapeutic regimen. In order to validly predict a drug's effects on driving, a screening battery should include separate tests which measure divided attention, sustained attention, continuous perceptual motor coordination, and discreet choice reaction time. Rigorous and comprehensive laboratory performance testing should be followed by the application of the most realistic test that can safely be applied in a driving simulator, on a course closed to traffic, or on real roads in normal traffic.

4 SACCADIC EYE MOVEMENTS/BODY SWAY

4.1 Saccadic Eye Movement Analysis

Saccadic eye movements occur when a person follows a target moving abruptly from one point to another. They are the fastest and best controlled movements of which the human body musculature is capable,[44] and they are under the control of several CNS structures.[45,46] Saccadic eye movement analysis provides a sensitive measurement of the CNS effects of drugs.[47] They can be frequently and quickly measured, and once initiated, they are independent of the attempts of the subject to control or alter his saccades.[48,49] Effects on saccadic eye movements have been observed in normal volunteers with a wide range of drugs, including barbiturates, benzodiazepines, opiates and related compounds, carbamazepine, amphetamine, and ethanol.[47] Saccadic eye movement analysis can be used in conjunction with other psychometric tests to provide a comprehensive profile of a drug's CNS effects, and they can also be used to provide an estimation of a drug's duration of action.

4.2 Body Sway

Body sway is a fundamental homeostatic mechanism arising from the regulatory activity of control loops involved in the maintenance of balance, drawing on the main sensory systems which are involved in the maintenance of balance (proprioception, enteroception, the vestibular system and vision).[50] Sway is increased in the elderly and in children and several factors have been shown to have an influence on body sway, including height and weight, anxiety and neuroticism, pain and muscle weakness, and disease states. Various drug treatments have been shown consistently to affect body sway, as has ethanol.[50]

Several methods are available to objectively quantify the effects of psychoactive drugs on body sway. These include mechanical devices, balance platforms, and noncontact techniques. The most useful measures are the mean amplitude, sway path, and sway area.[51] Fourier analysis is used to quantify body sway.

Body sway is a particularly sensitive objective measure of the effects of ethanol, which has been shown to have consistent effects. It has also been shown to be a sensitive measure of the effects of benzodiazepines, particularly in the elderly where it may manifest as increased ataxia.[52,53] Although it has been proposed that body sway might be a useful measure of sedative drug activity,[52] a review of relevant studies did not support this,[50] with only higher doses of sedative tricyclic antidepressants affecting body sway and chlorpromazine not at all. Drugs with anticonvulsant activity tend to increase body sway but not all are markedly sedative.

Body sway increases with age and it has been used to provide an objective index of the potential benefits of cerebral activators. It is increased in dementia and has been proposed as a marker of progression of the disease and of the therapeutic effects of drugs. It may have further potential as an objective measure of performance in studies in elderly subjects.

Body sway should be regarded as an objective measure of CNS function and a useful test for inclusion in a battery of tests for studies in human psychopharmacology, though the value of its use alone is limited.

5 RATING OF SUBJECTIVE FEELINGS

Many scales are used in clinical trials to rate the subjective effects of drugs. Both self-rated scales, which are simpler for the investigator to administer, and structured questionnaires, have been used to measure mood changes. However, not many scales have been validated fully in the healthy volunteer population in which they are frequently used. Visual analog scales are simple to use and have been widely used in measurement of subjective feelings, to assess the subjective sedative and mood effects of investigational drugs. One of the best of these sets of scales which is very commonly used includes 16 items, for each of which two dimensions of feelings (e.g., alert-drowsy) are separated by a 100-mm line.[54] Subjects mark the line at a point which corresponds with the magnitude of the effect on that particular item. Analysis should be by the method described by Bond and Lader,[54] in which a principal component analysis of this scale has identified three factors: alertness, contentment, and calmness.

Other self-rating scales which have been described include the Aggression Rating Scale which consists of 13 bipolar visual analog scales measuring feelings of hostility.[55] The STAI[16] measures both trait anxiety and current levels of state anxiety. It consists of a 20-item, self-rating scale which assesses current levels of tension and apprehension, and is appropriate for use in both healthy volunteers and patients. Adverse events should be recorded in response to a general, nondirective question. However, a specific rating scale may also be of value, particularly in healthy volunteers. An example is the Bodily Symptoms Scale[56] consisting of 14 visual analog scales requiring subjective ratings of such symptoms as dryness of the mouth, concentration, and irritability.

6 CONCLUSIONS

The measurement of CNS effects should be regarded as an essential component of a comprehensive assessment of the safety and toxicity of all new drugs. In the case of putative psychotropic agents, such assessment will be more detailed and may provide important data on the therapeutic potential of the investigational compound. An assessment battery should include valid and reliable tests, with both objective and subjective measures included. There should be adequate controls for variables such as gender, age, and personality, which can affect test results, and there must be a sound testing environment. Measurement of CNS effects should, as far as possible, reflect the way in which drugs will be used and should therefore include assessments in patients over adequate durations of treatment. Greater standardization of testing procedures would be of benefit to research in this field, allowing more valid interstudy and interdrug comparisons.

REFERENCES

1. Fink M. EEG and human psychopharmacology. *Electroenceph. Clin. Neurophysiol.* 1963; 15: 133-137.
2. Itil T (ed). *Psychotropic Drugs and the Human EEG.* Karger, Basel 1974: 377.
3. Hermann WM, Schärer E, Delini-Stula A. Predictive value of pharmaco-electroencephalography in early human-pharmacological evaluations of psychoactive drugs. *Pharmacopsychiatry* 1991; 24: 196-205.
4. Hermann WM, Schärer E, Wendt G, Delini-Stula A. Pharmaco-EEG profile of levoprotiline. *Pharmacopsychiatry* 1991; 24: 206-213.
5. Hermann WM, Schärer E, Wendt G, Delini-Stula A. Pharmaco-EEG profile of maroxepine. *Pharmacopsychiatry* 1991; 24: 214-224.
6. Hindmarch I. Psychomotor function and psychoactive drugs. *Br. J. Clin. Pharmacol.* 1980; 10: 1189-209.
7. Kunsman GW, Manno JE, Manno BR, Kunsman CM, Przekop MA. The use of microcomputer-based psychomotor tests for the evaluation of benzodiazepine effects on human performance: a review with emphasis on temazepam. *Br. J. Clin. Pharmacol.* 1992; 34: 289.301.
8. Hindmarch I. Instrumental assessment of psychomotor functions and the effects of psychotropic drugs. *Acta Psychiatr. Scand.* 1994; 89 (Suppl. 380): 49-52.
9. Stone BA. Pencil and paper tests — sensitivity to psychotropic drugs. *Br. J. Clin. Pharmacol.* 1984; 18: 15S-20S.
10. Simpson PM, Surmon DJ, Wesnes KA, Wilcock GK. The cognitive drug research computerised assessment system for demented patients: a validation study. *Int. J. Geriat. Psychiatr.* 1991; 6: 91-102.
11. Siegfried K, Jansen W, Pahnke K. Cognitive dysfunction in depression. *Drug Dev. Res.* 1984; 4: 533-553.
12. Freeman H, O'Hanlon JF. Acute and subacute effects of antidepressants on performance. *J. Drug. Dev. Clin. Pract.* 1995; 7: 7-20.
13. Cutler NR, Sramek JJ, Murphy MF, Nash RJ. Implications of the study population in the early evaluation of anticholinesterase inhibitors for Alzheimer's disease. *Ann. Pharmacother.* 1992; 26:1118-1122.
14. Cutler NR, Sramek JJ, Murphy MF, Nash RJ. Alzheimer's patients should be included in Phase I clinical trials to evaluate compounds for Alzheimer's disease. *J. Geriat. Psychiatr. Neurol.* 1992; 5:192-4.
15. Kleinknecht RA. Psychomotor skills. *Br. J. Clin. Pharmacol.* 1984; 18: 39S-41S.
16. Spielberger CD, Coruch RL, Lushene RE. Manual for State-Trait Anxiety Inventory. Florida State University, Tallahassee, 1968.
17. Wesnes K, Anand R, Simpson P, Christmas L. The use of a scopolamine model to study the potential nootropic effects of aniracetam and piracetam in healthy volunteers. *J. Psychopharmacol.* 1990; 4(4): 219-232.
18. King DJ, Bell PM, Bratty JR, McEntegert DJ. Preliminary study of the effects of flosequinan on psychomotor function in healthy volunteers. *Int. Clin. Psychopharmacol.* 1991; 6:155-168.
19. Jagathesan R, Lewis LD, Mant TGK. A retrospective analysis of the prevalence of HIV seropositivity and its demographics in the normal healthy volunteer population of a phase I clinical drug study unit. *Br. J. Clin. Pharmacol.* 1995; 39: 463-464.
20. Raskin A, Friedman AS, Dimascio A. Effects of chlorpromazine, imipramine, diazepam and phenelzine on psychomotor and cognitive skills of depressed patients. *Psychopharmacol. Bull.* 1983; 19: 149-152.
21. Mattila MJ. Interactions of benzodiazepines on psychomotor skills. *Br. J. Clin. Pharmacol.* 1984; 18: 21S-26S.
22. Nicholson AN, Stone BM. Zopiclone: sleep and performance studies in healthy man. *Pharmacology* 1983; 27 (Suppl. 2): 92-97.

23. Nicholson AN, Stone BM. Efficacy of zopiclone in middle age. *Sleep* 1987; 10 (Suppl. 1): 35-39.
24. Krugman H. Flicker fusion frequency as a function of anxiety reaction: an exploratory study. *Psychosomat. Med.* 1947; 4: 269-72.
25. Goldstone S. Critical flicker fusion measurements an anxiety levels. *J. Exp. Psychol.* 1955; 49: 200-2.
26. Farre M, Lamas X, Cami J. Sensation seeking amongst healthy volunteers participating in phase I clinical trials. *Br. J. Clin. Pharmacol.* 1995; 39: 405-409.
27. Hindmarch I. Critical flicker fusion frequency (CFF): the effects of psychotropic compounds. *Pharmacopsychiatry* 1982; 15 (Suppl. 1); 44-48.
28. Smith JM, Misiak H. Critical flicker frequency (CFF) and psychotropic drugs in normal human subjects — a review. *Psychopharmacology* 1976; 47: 175-182.
29. Danjou P, Warot D, Hergueta T, Lacomblez L, Bouh P, Puech AJ. Comparative study of the psychomotor and antistress effects of ritanserin, alprazolam and diazepam in healthy subjects: some trait anxiety-independent responses. *Int. Clin. Psychopharmacol.* 1992; 7(2): 73-79.
30. Deijen JB, Loriaux SM, Orlebeke JF, DeVries J. The effects of paroxetine and maprotiline on mood, perceptual-motor skills, and eye movements in healthy volunteers. *Acta Psychiatr. Scand.* Suppl; 1989; 350:41.
31. Bond AJ, Lader MH. Residual effects of hypnotics. *Psychopharmacology* 1972; 25: 117-132.
32. Wesnes K, Simpson P, Kidd A. An investigation of the range of cognitive impairments induced by scopolamine 0.6 mg s.c. *Hum. Psychopharmacol.* 1988; 3: 27-41.
33. Wesnes K, Simpson P, Christmas L. The Assessment of Human Information — Processing Abilities in Psychopharmacology. In: *Human Psychopharmacology Measures and Methods* (Eds. Hindmarch I, Stonier PD) John Wiley & Sons, Chichester 1987.
34. Wechsler D. Manual for the Wechsler adult intelligence scale. Psychological Corporation, New York; 1955.
35. Wechsler D. A manual for the Wechsler adult intelligence scale (revised). Psychological Corporation, New York; 1981.
36. Lezak M. *Neuropsychological Assessment.* 2nd edition, Oxford University Press, New York 1971.
37. Hommer D, Matsou V, Wolkwitz O. Benzodiazepine sensitivity in normal human subjects. *Arch. Gen. Psychiatr.* 1986; 43: 542-551.
38. Hommer D, Weingartner H, Breier A. Dissociation of benzodiazepine-induced amnesia from sedation by flumazenil pretreatment. *Psychopharmacol. Bull.* 1993; 112(4): 455-460.
39. Curran HV. Benzodiazepines, memory and mood: a review. *Psychopharmacology* 1991; 105: 1-8.
40. Curran HV, Birch B. Differentiating the sedative, psychomotor and amnesic effects of benzodiazepines: a study with midazolam and the benzodiazepine antagonist, flumazenil. *Psychopharmacology* 1991; 103: 519-523.
41. Subhan Z, Hindmarch I. Effects of zopiclone and benzodiazepine hypnotics on search in short-term memory. *Neuropsychobiology* 1983; 12: 244-48.
42. Buschke H, Fuld A. Evaluating storage and retrieval in disordered memory and learning. *Neurology* 1974; 24: 1019-1024.
43. Vermeeren A, deGier JJ, O'Hanlon JF. Methodological guidelines for experimental research on medicinal drugs affecting driving performance: an international expert survey. Maastricht: Institute for Human Psychopharmacology, University of Limburg, Technical Report 93-27, 1994.
44. Fuchs AF, Kaneko CRS. A brain stem generator for saccadic eye movements. *Trends Neurosc.* 1981; 283-286.
45. Luschei ES, Fuchs AF. Activity of brain stem neurones during eye movements of alert monkeys. *J. Neurophysiol.* 1972; 35: 445-461.
46. Keller EL. Participation of medial pontine reticular formation in eye movement generation in monkeys. *J. Neurophysiol.* 1974; 37: 316-332.
47. Griffiths AN, Marshall RW, Richens A. Saccadic eye movement analysis as a measure of drug effects on human psychomotor performance. *Br. J. Clin. Pharmacol.* 1984; 18: 735-825.
48. Becker W, Fuchs AF. Further properties of the human saccadic system: eye movements and correction saccades with and without visual fixation points. *Vision Res.* 1970; 9: 1247-1258.
49. Baloh RW, Konran HR, Sills AW, Honrubia V. The saccade velocity test. *Neurology* 1975; 25: 1071-1076.
50. McClelland GR. Body sway and the effects of psychoactive drugs. *Hum. Psychopharmacol.* 1989; 4: 3-14.
51. Hufschmidt A, Dichgans J, Mauritz KH, Hufschmidt M. Some methods and parameters of body sway quantification and their neurological applications. *Arch. Psychiat. Nervenkr.* 1980; 228: 135-150.
52. Swift CG. Postural instability as a measure of sedative drug response. *Br. J. Clin. Pharmacol.* 1984; 18: 875-905.
53. Swift CG, Ankier Mr, Pidgen SI, Robinson A, Robinson J. Single dose pharmacokinetics and pharmacodynamics or oral loprazolam in the elderly. *Br. J. Clin. Pharmacol.* 1985; 20: 119-128.
54. Bond A, Lader M. The use of analog scales in rating subjective feelings. *Br. J. Med. Psychol.* 1974; 47: 211-218.
55. Bond AJ, Lader MH. A method to elicit aggressive feelings and behavior via provocation. *Biol. Psychol.* 1986; 22: 69-79.
56. Bond AJ, Feizollah S, Lader MH. The effects of D-fenfluramine on mood and performance, and on neuroendocrine indicators of 5-HT function. *J. Psychopharmacol.* 1995; 9(1): 1-8.

Chapter 22

Antiepileptic Drugs

Joe Mercer and Gwilym Hosking

CONTENTS

1 Introduction 305
2 Healthy Volunteers 306
2.1 Inclusion Criteria for Healthy Volunteer Studies 306
2.2 Safety Considerations 307
2.3 Methods 307
2.3.1 General Trial Design 307
2.3.2 Pharmacokinetics 307
2.3.2.1 First Single Dose Administration 307
2.3.2.2 First Multiple Dose Administration 308
2.3.2.3 Radiolabel Study 308
2.3.2.4 Food 308
2.3.2.5 Drug Interactions 308
2.3.3 Pharmacodynamics Issues 309
2.4 Controls 309
3 Phase I and II Studies 310
3.1 Early Evidence of Clinical Efficacy 310
3.2 Early Open Label Studies 310
3.3 Controlled Clinical Trials 311
3.3.1 Cross-Over Design 311
3.3.2 Alternative Add-On Trial Design 311
3.3.3 Enriched Parallel Design 312
3.3.4 Outcome Measures 312
3.3.5 General Study Issues 312
4 Monotherapy 312
4.1 Previously Treated 313
4.2 Previously Untreated 313
4.3 Alternative Monotherapy Designs 313
4.4 Concentration-Controlled Design 313
4.5 "Low Dose Active Control" ("Attenuated" Active Control Design) 313
4.6 Presurgical Evaluation 313
5 "Newer" Outcome Measures 314
References 314

1 INTRODUCTION

Epilepsy is a symptom complex reflecting paroxysmal cerebral dysrhythmia of either identifiable etiology (symptomatic), unidentifiable etiology (cryptogenic), or no apparent etiology (primary or idiopathic). As such it is not the name of a specific pathological state. Symptoms will vary according to the site(s) of the dysrhythmia (focal or generalized) and the general state of the brain, e.g., in terms of maturity or metabolic state.

Pathophysiological processes that give rise to the symptom complex of epilepsy vary and are in most instances still unidentified. In recent years, however, transmitter systems have been identified and knowledge of these systems has given a basis for rational antiepileptic drug (AED) design based on the relationship between symptoms and functional mechanisms.

0-8493-9230-6/97/$0.00+$.50
© 1997 by CRC Press, Inc.

The final clinical evaluation of new potential AEDs still relies heavily upon an empirical approach using clinical endpoints. For the most part these will be the response of seizures to the administration of the drug. There are virtually no surrogate markers of efficacy.

The chronic administration of drugs acting on the central nervous system (CNS) demands rigorous attention to adverse events (AE) involving the CNS and other systems. In general, AEDs should act at a presynaptic site; receptor antagonism often induces unacceptable AEs.

Apart from determining the risk/benefit ratio for new AEDs, reasonable attempts should be made to demonstrate its effects on the quality of life of patients.

2 HEALTHY VOLUNTEERS

Epilepsy is a chronic disorder usually requiring an extended duration of drug therapy and for which there are currently no recognized surrogate markers for drug efficacy in healthy volunteers.

A number of issues must be addressed in the early phases of clinical development of AEDs so that the decision to proceed to full clinical development is made with the right data. It is necessary to show that the compound is tolerated by man at therapeutically relevant plasma concentrations and that the pharmacokinetics of the drug are clinically acceptable. It is essential to gain information on the tolerability and pharmacokinetics of multiple doses of the compound in order to be able to predict reasonably the dosing regimen required in the clinical efficacy studies. Many AEDs induce their own elimination and that of other AEDs after multiple doses and this possibility must be addressed by *in vitro* studies and if necessary in specific interaction studies.

As AEDs are intended for chronic administration and plasma concentrations kept within a therapeutic window, the effect of food on the bioavailability, as well as the effects of age and organ function on the kinetics of the drug should be determined. These studies can usually wait until the final development decision is made.

Special studies should be scheduled at this early stage to assess the penetration of the compound into the brain and to try to determine the probable clinically effective dose prior to the start of the efficacy studies. The impact of any unwanted CNS effects of the compound should also be addressed as many AEDs have significant sedative potential which may limit their commercial success.

As patients with epilepsy are usually on long-term therapy with drugs such as phenytoin (PHT) or carbamazepine (CBZ), studies in healthy volunteers allow information about the drug to be collected in a setting without interference from underlying pathology or concomitant medication. As placebo-controlled studies are not possible in epileptic patients, a further advantage of studying healthy volunteers is that the new drug can be compared to placebo. Furthermore, clinical pharmacology studies are often intensive with a tight schedule requiring a high degree of cooperation and commitment and, in some studies, extensive training, which is easier to attain with healthy volunteers.

The collection of well-controlled data on an AED is important during the initial studies which should establish the dose and concentration at which adverse drug effects become unacceptable, and to help to determine whether the compound under investigation warrants further development.

As it is ethically and practically difficult to assess the effect of multiple drugs given over extended periods to volunteers, it is prudent to include a population pharmacokinetic analysis strategy in the design of the phase II and III studies. This allows major drug-drug interactions to be identified, and if indicated, specific studies to be designed to quantify these effects.

A number of techniques are available to assess the effects of AEDs in the CNS. Data obtained from these techniques reflect the character of the side effects of the drugs more closely than the therapeutic effect. These are valuable in making predictions about the effects of these drugs on measures associated with activities involved in every day living.

2.1 Inclusion Criteria for Healthy Volunteer Studies

Appropriate inclusion criteria for volunteer studies employed to support the regulatory submission of the compound under development should be dependent on the target patient population. As patient populations with epilepsy are heterogeneous, both young and elderly volunteer populations should be studied. Ideally, early studies should, if possible, include both males and females and adequate representation from all racial groups.

In early studies, the results of reproductive toxicology studies may not be available, precluding the early inclusion of women. Male volunteers are also favored at this stage because of the difficulty in detecting early pregnancy and the absence of confounding factors such as hormonal fluctuations and use of oral contraceptives that might alter drug metabolism. Other inclusion/exclusion criteria are similar to those usually employed for phase I studies.

2.2 Safety Considerations

Dosing with certain AEDs, including PHT, CBZ, and lamotrigine (LTG), have been associated with a small but significant incidence of rash. Allergic drug reactions are of concern in healthy volunteers given the philosophy that the volunteers' health should not be affected by the administration of the novel compound. The mechanism by which rash is produced is unclear and probably not consistent between drugs so it is prudent to maintain a particularly close monitoring of the volunteers' white cell counts. However, the number of volunteers involved in early phase studies and the short nature of the duration of administration of the drugs means that rash will necessarily be a rare event and may not be detected even if the compound is immunogenic. However, consideration should be given to excluding volunteers who have a history of allergic drug reactions.

Subjective adverse experiences related to the CNS effects of AED drugs are common and effects on mood should also be assessed. Adverse experience probes of the form: "Do you feel different from usual or unwell in any way" should be used. These will elicit details of the adverse experiences without leading or prompting the volunteer. AE probes should be scheduled to include all phases of the pharmacokinetic (PK) profile of the drug with particular attention to the absorption and distribution phases. Volunteers should also be encouraged to report spontaneously any drug effects they feel as these may be related to the presence of active metabolites with a very different PK profile than that of the parent drug.

Specific visual analog scales for the assessment of mood changes in volunteers are available, often in computerized form. The scales of Bond and Lader (1974)[1] are able to detect changes related to mental and physical sedation and tranquilization with good sensitivity. More objective tests of performance can be administered in early phase studies (see Section 2.3.3), but study designs required to optimize the sensitivity of these tasks are not appropriate at this stage of development (see below) and so only preliminary information can be derived.

2.3 Methods

2.3.1 General Trial Design

The dose escalation usually employed during the first administration of the compound to man should include a placebo group when assessing CNS active compounds such as AEDs. The CNS activity of these compounds should be determined as early as possible and the nature of the investigation guided by preclinical pharmacology and toxicology.

2.3.2 Pharmacokinetics

An appropriate standardized blood sampling schedule should be developed as soon as possible in the development cycle to aid comparisons to be made between studies. This should include rapid blood sampling during the absorption phase, the characterization of C_{max}, and of any distribution phase. AEDs are designed to penetrate the brain and may be preferentially concentrated there, so a marked but rapid drug distribution phase is likely. The sampling schedule should extend up to about 10 half-lives of the longest lived drug-related compound.

Adequate pharmacokinetic data from phase I studies are important because an elimination half-life which allows one or, at most, twice a day dosing is an advantage and a short half-life might preclude further development or require development of a suitable formulation.

The first administration of LTG to man, for example, suggested that the compound was well absorbed orally and had linear PK over the range studied with an elimination half-life of around 24 h.[2]

An early study with vigabatrin,[3] by contrast, showed rapid absorption with linear PK in the dose range 1-3 g and with a predominantly renal route of elimination as unchanged drug. However, both enantiomers of vigabatrin have relatively short half-lives (≈7 h) suggesting multiple daily doses might be required or that a sustained release formulation of the drug would need to be developed.

2.3.2.1 First Single Dose Administration

The primary issues to be resolved in an initial study are whether the drug is well tolerated at doses likely to be in the therapeutic range and whether the pharmacokinetics of the drug are satisfactory. Effects on the cardiovascular system and clinical pathology should be assessed and adverse experiences documented.

Preliminary data should be obtained on the effects of the AED in the CNS (e.g., mood changes, sedation and performance impairment or enhancement). Although these data will not be definitive due to the study design, the data obtained are invaluable in the calculation of statistical power of further studies.

A double-blind, placebo-controlled, dose-escalation study design allows a clear profile of the subjective and objective tolerability and pharmacokinetics of the compound to be established and the nature of the linearity and dose proportionality of the PK of the drug as well as the basic PK parameters such as half-life and clearance to be characterized.

The first administration of lamotrigine to man suggested that the compound was well absorbed orally and had linear PK over the range studied with an elimination half-life of around 24 h.[2] The adverse experience profile included nausea, somnolence, dizziness and diplopia but suggested that, at therapeutic doses, few adverse experiences related to CNS effects of the drug could be expected.

2.3.2.2 First Multiple Dose Administration

The first multiple dose administration study allows the definition of the steady-state pharmacokinetics, which is essential in terms of drugs such as AEDs which are taken chronically.

If the AED induces its own metabolism then the actual steady-state PK parameters will differ from those predicted from single doses and may necessitate higher doses than predicted to achieve therapeutic plasma concentrations. It is a definite advantage in drug development terms if autoinduction does not occur, and the presence or absence of this property might influence the full development decision.

On the other hand, a long half-life with multiple dosing will lead to accumulation of the compound and may result in a high incidence of adverse events if too high a dose is selected.

If CNS-related adverse experiences were detected in the initial study it may be possible to assess whether tolerance to these effects develops over the dosing period. If there are CNS-related AEs, to be able to demonstrate the rapid development of tolerance is an advantage.

2.3.2.3 Radiolabel Study

Studies using radiolabeled AEDs are used to quantify the rates and routes of elimination of a compound and to identify the complete spectrum of metabolites. Knowledge of all metabolites in man is invaluable in assessing the robustness of the toxicological profile of the AED built up by screening in animal species, and the data may prompt further pharmacology and toxicology studies.

A study using ^{14}C-lamotrigine indicated that 95% of an administered LTG dose was eliminated in the urine as a glucuronide[4] while it was shown that gabapentin is not metabolized by man and is excreted exclusively in the urine.[5]

2.3.2.4 Food

The effect of food on drug AED absorption can influence the decision to proceed with development as highly variable absorption can lead to difficulty in controlling plasma levels and therapeutic effect.

The oral bioavailability of LTG in volunteers is around 97%,[6] suggesting that factors known to increase bioavailability will have no detectable effect. In contrast, the oral bioavailability of gabapentin is approximately 60%,[7] which suggests that food might significantly improve the absorption of gabapentin.

Frisk-Holmberg et al.[8] have shown that vigabatrin PKs are unaffected by food in young volunteers suggesting that vigabatrin may be administered at times convenient to the patient and no effect on food on absorption has been seen in volunteers after the administration of felbamate.[9] The bioavailability of valproate after the administration of the prodrug valpromide has been found to be increased after food,[10] although it is unclear whether this is due to an increase in valpromide absorption or to an increase in the extent of the typical 70-80% conversion of valpromide to valproate.

2.3.2.5 Drug Interactions

Interactions related to enzyme induction require extended multiple dosing for meaningful assessment. The risk to volunteers must be carefully assessed and the feasibility of conducting such a study in patients should be examined. However, the nature of the patient population and confounding factors such as concomitant medication, compliance, and the risk of affecting the control of seizures may require that a volunteer study be carried out.

Many AEDs induce their own metabolism and may alter the PK of concomitantly administered AEDs. A multiple dose kinetics study (see above) addresses the first issue while an interaction study assessing the influence of multiple dosing with the AED on the clearance of antipyrine is a standard method of defining hepatic enzyme induction.

A specific early assessment of the impact of simultaneous use of the compound under development and standard AEDS such as CBZ and PHN is important. Studies using single doses of these compounds can be conducted rapidly in healthy volunteers but do not reflect the clinical use of these agents and a more appropriate study design employs multiple drug doses. The use of full therapeutic doses of CBZ and PHT is associated with a number of adverse experiences which may be unacceptable in healthy volunteers and so the use of subtherapeutic doses should be considered.

The effects of therapy with the standard AED on the kinetics of the novel compound can be best assessed in patients using population pharmacokinetic analysis during the phase II studies.

Any interaction between the AED and the oral contraceptive pill should be assessed as early as possible. A significant impact of concomitant administration will require dosage recommendations to be altered and may even lead to a contraindication, unacceptably limiting the market for the compound.

2.3.3 Pharmacodynamics Issues

As there are no surrogate markers for clinical efficacy of AEDs in healthy volunteers, studies in this area are limited to assessing the CNS-related adverse experiences associated with the compounds and to investigating how administration of these drugs may affect the quality of life of the patients. Ideally, these studies require the use of placebo-controlled, randomized cross-over study designs employing positive controls. These parameters often show marked interindividual variability and it is preferable to do cross-over studies with each volunteer acting as their own control. Studies of this type require close control of experimental conditions and careful attention to the psychological state of the volunteers. Specialized laboratories and equipment are required to obtain reproducible results and these studies are difficult to conduct. A wide variety of performance tasks are available. These tasks are usually derived from psychological tests and assess drug effects on a number of cognitive levels from reaction times to complex syntactic skills. Hamilton et al.[11] examined the effects of LTG and CBZ on a battery of psychometric tests and were able to make recommendations on LTG dosing to reduce the incidence of unwanted effects. Curran et al.[12] used psychometric testing to identify an improvement of psychometric performance and concentration but not memory after the administration of 150 or 300 mg oxycarbazepine b.i.d. for 15 days to healthy volunteers.

Sequential EEG measurements can be used to produce a time-course of drug effect which can be used to derive a concentration-effect relationship with the measured plasma drug concentration. Similarly, evoked potentials produced by light, sound, or electrical stimulation can be used to determine objective drug effects. Evoked potentials have also been used to identify slowing of nerve conduction by AEDs,[13,14] which has been suggested to be related to the development of peripheral neuropathies after long-term therapy with PHT.

Appreciation of the value of positron-emission tomography (PET) and nuclear magnetic resonance (NMR) is growing as these methods become sensitive enough to directly measure the concentrations of the drug or drug targets in the brain. This allows the derivation of relationships linking the anticonvulsant effect and the effect site and plasma concentrations. This can lead to improved predictions of the dose required for therapeutic benefit with consequent savings in time in the design and conduct of the drug efficacy studies. Rothman et al.[15] used 1H NMR to compare the concentrations of GABA in the occipital lobe of volunteers and patients receiving vigabatrin (an inhibitor of GABA transaminase) and found significantly elevated GABA levels in the brains of the patients.

2.4 Controls

It is important to include placebo controls in studies of AEDs in volunteers. The nature of AEDs means that subjective adverse experiences will be encountered and it is vital to be able to interpret these by comparing with data from volunteers under the same experimental conditions.

The inclusion of a positive control in a study is also important. These are normally used in well-controlled studies examining specific drug effects, such as psychometric performance, rather than in the earlier phase studies. The positive control demonstrates that the experimental setup is sensitive to drug effects and allows comparison with the effects of a reference standard therapy. Those most often used in AED development are PHT and CBZ.

3 PHASE I AND II STUDIES

The object of early phase drug studies using healthy volunteers is to provide appropriate information upon which the clinical development of the compound can be based and upon which the commercial attractiveness of the novel compound can be assessed. The design of the pivotal efficacy studies can be significantly improved by data from these studies leading to enormous savings in time and money. However, it is important that the design of these studies is firmly based on the particular characteristics of the compound and the requirements of the project and not on the design of a "shopping list" of studies which have been conducted previously with other drugs.

3.1 Early Evidence of Clinical Efficacy

Preliminary evidence of efficacy in man may be obtained using electrophysiological models with single-dose studies. As electroencephalogram (EEG) discharge rates, even if high, vary greatly from moment to moment, they need to be assessed for no less than 24 h, and will therefore usually require telemetric monitoring.

Binnie[16] investigated the effects of single doses of LTG. In an open study of 5 patients he counted EEG spikes every 30 min with telemetry over an initial 24-h period. Following this a single dose of LTG was administered. All patients demonstrated a reduction of interictal spike frequency of between 78 and 98% after LTG administration. The effect lasted for the full 24 h.

Jawad et al.[17] had similarly suggested an efficacy for LTG when a reduction in interictal spikes was seen in a controlled single-dose comparison between LTG, placebo, and diazepam.

The range of flicker frequencies which produce epileptic discharges in photosensitive patients is relatively stable or fixed and is referred to as the "photosensitivity range" of the individual. Binnie[18] studied six patients with a single dose of LTG and demonstrated a reduction in the photosensitivity range in all six, and its abolition in two. Later he confirmed that this was not a nonspecific effect of a sedative drug.[19]

3.2 Early Open Label Studies

Before embarking on a series of controlled randomized studies (see below) smaller studies of the test drug in patients with poorly controlled seizures should be considered. This may be in an open label or in a controlled fashion. These studies should:

1. Be a preliminary evaluation of the drug's safety profile and potential efficacy in the epileptic patient
2. Further define the dose range for the clinical development program
3. Determine pharmacokinetics in chronically medicated patients

The test drug is added to concomitant AED therapy initially as a single dose (see above) followed by a step-wise increase to a maximum tolerated dose (MTD). If the test drug exhibits pronounced drug interactions then the add-on phase can be followed by a response-related gradual withdraw of previous therapy. Evaluation parameters may include:

1. Change in seizure frequency
2. Adverse reactions
3. Serum levels of test drug and concomitant AEDs
4. Monitoring of laboratory tests
5. Evaluation of drug interactions

Patients chosen must be compliant and should be thoroughly investigated to identify cardiac, renal, hepatic, or active psychiatric disorders. Patients with progressive neurological conditions and women of childbearing age are excluded.

It is vital to be able to classify the patient's seizures, preferably according to the International Classification of Seizures,[20] and if possible the International Classification of Epilepsy and Epileptic Syndromes.[21] Patients may be included irrespective of the number of different seizure types. It is preferable that they should take only one concomitant therapy, although two or three may be acceptable.

The number of patients should be small and they should be carefully monitored. The MTD should be defined first from single-dose studies before repeated dosing. PK analyses should be undertaken with recording of serum levels of drugs. Frequency of dosing and size should be determined not only from these studies but also from the earlier volunteer studies. Evaluation of the test drug should be as much as possible against specific seizure types, hence some preference for patients with single seizure types.

Generally these studies should last no longer than one or two months. The exact length will be dependent on seizure frequency and the PK characteristics of the test drug.

3.3 Controlled Clinical Trials

Although controlled clinical trials of a new antiepileptic drug are now accepted as both standard and essential practice, up until the last decade few AEDs had been tested in this way. In 1982, Gram[22] identified 51 controlled trials, substantially more than the two identified by Coatsworth[23] a decade earlier. Since Gram's review the number of controlled clinical trials has increased markedly.

The concept of controlled clinical testing in the early stages of the clinical development program is now accepted practice and preferable to large numbers of nondefinitive studies with potentially overlapping results.[24]

Conventional early phase II antiepileptic drug trials are usually placebo controlled add-on studies using multiple periods within patients ("cross-over") design or single period parallel groups ("parallel") design.

3.3.1 Cross-Over Design

In practice these studies typically involve two 3-month treatment periods, one on placebo and the other on the test AED. Documentation of an initial baseline period of a stable co-medication dosing regime is required. Between the two study phases there has to be a wash-out period sufficiently long (typically four weeks) to ensure that there is no carry-over effect of the active test drug and not so short that there is a risk of withdrawal seizures. A second wash-out period will be required after the second phase. A typical cross-over study would last about 40 weeks.

Cross-over studies, although widely used, do have some disadvantages:

1. Dropout rates for whatever reason may be problematic, particularly if they occur late.
2. Even with all the precautions taken the effect of the test drug may be considerable and much more than anticipated so that a lasting change occurs thus distorting the seizure responsiveness in the two different placebo phases.
3. "Regression toward the mean" first described by Galton in 1885 is relevant in epilepsy when patients may often be recruited into trials when the seizures are particularly poorly controlled and that thereafter there may be a spontaneous tendency toward a decrease in seizure severity. Conversely though those with a low seizure frequency may experience an increase.[25] There are a number of ways to avoid the problems (to some degree) of regression toward the mean. Patients may be recruited to studies irrespective of current seizure frequency but then stratified according to initial seizure frequency before randomization. Baseline periods should be of sufficient duration, the duration of the study phases may be either very short or very long and the "response conditional cross-over design" may be introduced (see below) in which there is incomplete cross-over.
4. Ethical difficulties may occur if patients show a clinically significant reduction of seizures during the first phase. Crossing over may be refused by the patient. Again the "response conditional cross-over design" addresses itself to this real problem as only patients with an "insufficient" response actually cross-over.

Cross-over trials also have certain advantages:

1. They are able to overcome the difficulties of intersubject variation and factors known to affect prognosis.
2. Within subject cross-over trials give greater power. A parallel group study is likely to require 3-6 times the number of subjects to achieve the same statistical power as a cross-over study. This feature of cross-over studies alone is likely to assure its continued use even though many theoretical considerations favor the parallel group design.

3.3.2 Alternative Add-On Trial Design

Response conditional cross-over designs are those in which subjects are randomized initially to placebo or active test drug and remain on these if there is a specified reduction in seizure frequency with respect to baseline. Patients are only transferred to an alternative treatment if they have not responded. If the test drug is efficacious the number of subjects receiving placebo should be very small.

3.3.3 Enriched Parallel Design

Patients commence add-on therapy with the test drug under open label conditions. AEs may be closely monitored and the dosings increased until seizure control is achieved or tolerance or lack of tolerance encountered. The patients that respond will enter a double-blind controlled phase in which they are randomized to either placebo or active test drug. It will be important to ensure that withdrawal seizures are avoided. Only subjects that respond will be entered into the controlled phase.

3.3.4 Outcome Measures

In these early phase II studies the primary objectives will be evaluation of efficacy through controlled randomized trials with secondary objectives to find the active dose range and a further evaluation of the safety profile.

The evaluation parameters may include:

1. Change in seizure frequency
2. Change in seizure free intervals
3. Change in seizure duration
4. Change in seizure pattern
5. Change in functional capacity
6. Percentage of responders
7. Adverse reactions
8. Serum/plasma levels of test drug, important metabolites, and concomitant AEDs
9. Monitoring of laboratory tests

3.3.5 General Study Issues

Patients may be in- or outpatients with epilepsy refractory to existing AED therapy despite maximal doses given.

Drug compliance is essential, and epileptic histories must be well documented, including classification of seizures.

Cardiac, renal, or hepatic disorders should be identified and the patient excluded as well as those with expanding cerebral tumors or progressive neurological disorders. If there has not been any teratogenicity demonstrated in the animal data patients of both sexes may be entered, but women of child-bearing potential must use reliable methods of contraception.

Previous response to AEDs should be documented. Patients with a concomitant and non-AED therapy which may interfere with evaluation or cause toxicity of the test drug should be excluded.

The size of the sample should be determined on the basis of seizure frequency and expected reduction and this will be influenced by experience in the late phase I/exploratory studies (see above). The length of studies also depends on seizure frequency. This may range from one week with EEG monitoring for absence seizures to at least 3 months for partial or generalized seizures with a frequency with three to four a month. A prospective baseline should be initiated with seizure frequency evaluated with telemetry in the case of absences and with a seizure diary in other cases.

The use of EEG is not recommended either for the evaluation of the baseline stage or subsequently except in the case of absence epilepsy.

Serum levels of the test AED and concomitant AEDs should be monitored together with relevant laboratory tests. Particular care will be needed as drug-drug interactions may produce an efficacy or a toxicity picture that is very different from when the test drug was used in a monotherapy setting.

4 MONOTHERAPY

Monotherapy studies may be conducted in previously untreated, previously treated, or as part of a continuation study in patients from controlled add-on studies. In patients who have been previously treated the general principle has been to add the test AED or the comparator AED following randomization. After completion of the double-blind phase, the previous therapy can be gradually withdrawn in responders.

For previously untreated patients randomization may be to test drug, to placebo, or a comparator reference drug.

Evaluation parameters are as described in Section 3.3.4.

4.1 Previously Treated

Typically the patient will be one with incomplete seizure control despite maximum doses of one drug. Good compliance is crucial.

The test drug is administered in a randomized double-blind fashion and the pre-existing therapies in those that favorably respond may be withdrawn.

Sample size will be determined from seizure frequency and the response expected on the basis of the response in the early phase II studies. A prospective baseline is essential and treatment duration must be such as to allow adequate evaluation of a persistence of AED effect. These studies may be open.

4.2 Previously Untreated

For those who have not previously been treated the situation is a little more complex.

With clear proof of efficacy in a drug prone to marked drug interactions, patients may be evaluated in a monotherapy design with the variable evaluated being the interval to the next seizure. Typically the add-on design for previously untreated patients is a blinded parallel group design in which established AED is administered systematically in association with the test drug or a placebo according to a randomized sequence.

4.3 Alternative Monotherapy Designs

Monotherapy studies with new drugs have been much less common than controlled add-on studies. Such monotherapy studies have virtually always been against active controls and this has usually resulted in a no difference outcome, which could mean that both drugs are either effective or ineffective.

The U.S. Food and Drug Administration has expressed increasing unwillingness to accept this type of study.[26]

4.4 Concentration-Controlled Design

This type of study is difficult to perform, but valuable if there is a clear concentration/effect relationship and a variable relationship between dose and concentration. This design has been employed in studies of sodium valproate.[27]

4.5 "Low Dose Active Control"("Attenuated" Active Control Design)

This has to be recognized as a particularly controversial design recently exploited in studies of felbamate.[28] The test medication was introduced and escalated over one week with progressive reduction of co-medication over 4 weeks before assessing a possible response. Escape criteria were specified in advance, requiring standard medication to be resumed if seizures increased to an unacceptable level. Patients with a history of status epilepticus were excluded. The control in this study was a low and subtherapeutic dose of valproate used as an "active placebo."

In this study 40% of patients on the test drug had to receive "escape" therapy, in contrast to 78% on the low dose valproate.

Ethical concerns with this design are dealt with by the inclusion criteria that eliminate patients with severe epilepsy, and by escape criteria.

4.6 Presurgical Evaluation

A true monotherapy placebo-controlled study is possible by making use of patients admitted to hospital for presurgical evaluation and who will have their existing AEDs reduced or withdrawn. AED reduction enables seizures to occur that can be recorded and further evaluated by telemetry. Such a study design has been utilized in the evaluation of felbamate.[29]

Preset escape criteria are essential. The patients in such settings are in an unstable state and there may be only a brief interval between capturing sufficient seizures to meet the needs of preoperative assessment and the onset of serial seizures demanding immediate control. The test drug in such a trial should act quickly; if several days are needed to build up a therapeutic concentration the opportunity to prove an effect may be missed. In some it may prove impossible to assess monotherapy if seizure frequency increases rapidly before the existing medication is fully withdrawn. To avoid this problem test treatments could be introduced prior to withdrawal of the existing medication. However, for those who respond to the test drug the period of telemetry may have to be prolonged.

5 "NEWER" OUTCOME MEASURES

There is more to the management of epilepsy than simply a reduction in seizure frequency. The severity of seizures is for some patients as important or more so than their frequency. A reduction in severity may mean that a patient no longer falls, no longer loses consciousness, is incontinent, or has such complex confusional states.

The mental and emotional state of the patient may be enhanced (or not) by the test drug possibly as a consequence of some intrinsic properties of the drug through its effect on an epileptic process or some nonepileptic process.[30]

Together or separately these more qualitative changes may be grouped under the general heading of quality of life. The instruments for the measurement of quality of life are still at a very early stage of development but are being used more frequently in AED trials, as are measures of health economics or resource usage. It is anticipated that regulatory bodies, health authorities, and clinicians are going to expect to see these types of data more frequently.

REFERENCES

1. Bond, A., Lader M., The use of analogue scales in rating subjective feelings. *Br. J. Med. Psychol.*, 47, 211, 1974.
2. Cohen, A. F. et al., Lamotrigine, a new anticonvulsant; pharmacokinetics in normal humans, *Clin. Pharmacol. Ther.*, 42, 535, 1987.
3. Schechter, P. J., Clinical pharmacology of vigabatrin, *Br. J. Clin. Pharmacol.*, 27, 19S, 1989.
4. Peck, A. W., Clinical pharmacology of lamotrigine, *Epilepsia*, 32, S9, 1991.
5. Vollmer, K.-O. et al., Pharmacokinetics and metabolism of gabapentin in rat, dog and man, *Drug Res.*, 36, 830, 1986.
6. Yuen, W. C., Peck, A. W., Lamotrigine pharmacokinetics: oral and iv infusion in man, *Br. J. Clin. Pharmacol.*, 29, 242, 1988.
7. Vollmer, K.-O., et al., Pharmacokinetic profile and absolute bioavailability of the new anticonvulsant gabapentin, *Adv. Epileptol.*, 17, 209, 1989.
8. Frisk-Holmberg, M. et al., Effect of food on the absorption of vigabatrin, *Br. J. Clin. Pharmacol*, 27, 23S, 1989.
9. Gudipati, R. M. et al., Effect of food on the absorption of felbamate in healthy male volunteers, *Neurology*, 42, 332, 1992.
10. Pisani, F. et al., Increased dipropylacetic acid bioavailability from dipropylamide after food, *Epilepsia*, 23, 115, 1982.
11. Hamilton, M. J. et al., Carbamazepine and lamotrigine in healthy volunteers: relevance to early tolerance and clinical trial dosage, *Epilepsia*, 34, 166, 1993.
12. Curran, H. V. et al., Cognitive and psychomotor effects of oxcarbazepine, *Epilepsia*, 32, 56, 1991.
13. van Wieringen, A. et al., Comparison of the effects of lamotrigine and phenytoin on the EEG power spectrum and cortical and brainstem-evoked responses of normal human volunteers, *Neuropsychobiology*, 21, 157, 1989.
14. Lamb, R. J. et al., The acute effects of phenytoin and lamotrigine on nerve conduction velocity and latency of the somatosensory evoked potential in healthy volunteers, *Br. J. Clin. Pharmacol.*, 36(2), 170P, 1993.
15. Rothman, D. L. et al., Localised 1H NMR measurements of gamma-aminobutyric acid in human brain *in vitro*, *Proc. Natl. Acad. Sci. U.S.A.*, 90, 5662, 1993.
16. Binnie, C., Preliminary evaluation of potential antiepileptic drugs by single-dose electrophysiology and pharmacological studies in patients, *J. Neural Transm.*, 72, 259, 1988.
17. Jawad, S., Oxley, J., Yuen, W., and Richens, A., The effects of lamotrigine, a novel anticonvulsant on interictal spikes in patients with epilepsy, *Br. J. Clin. Pharmacol.*, 22, 191, 1986.
18. Binnie C., Acute effects of lamotrigine (BW430C) in persons with epilepsy, *Epilepsia*, 22, 248, 1986.
19. Binnie, C., Kasteleun-Nolste-Trenite, D., De Korte, R. Photosensitivity as a model for acute anti-epileptic drug studies. *Electroencephalogr. Clin. Neurophysiol.*, 63, 35, 1986.
20. Commission on Classification and Terminology of the International League Against Epilepsy, proposal for revised clinical and electrocochleographic classification of epileptic seizures, *Epilepsia*, 22, 289, 1981.
21. Commission on Classification and Terminology of the International League Against Epilepsy, proposal for revised classification of epilepsies and epileptic syndromes, *Epilepsia*, 30, 389, 1989.
22. Gram, L., Bentsen, K. D., Parnas, J. et al., Controlled clinical trials. A review, *Epilepsia*, 23, 491, 1982.
23. Coatsworth, J. J., Studies on the clinical effect of marketed antiepileptic drugs. *NINDS* Washington, U.S. Government Printing Office, Monograph No. 12, 1971.
24. Gram, L., Schmidt, D., Innovative designs of controlled clinical trials in epilepsy, *Epilepsia*, 34 (Suppl. 7), S1, 1993.
25. Spilker, B., Segreti, A., Validation of the phenomena of regression of seizure frequency in epilepsy, *Epilepsia*, 25, 443, 1984.
26. Leber, P., Hazards of inference: the active control investigation, *Epilepsia*, 30, S37, 1989.

27. Gram, L., Wulff, K., Rasmussen, K.E. et al., Valproate sodium: a controlled clinical trial including monitoring of serum levels, *Epilepsia,* 18, 141, 1977.
28. Faught, E., Sachdeo et al., Felbamate monotherapy for partial-onset seizures: an active controlled trial, *Neurology,* 43, 688, 1993.
29. Bourgeois, B., Leppik, I. E. et al., Felbamate: a double-blinded controlled trial in patients undergoing pre-surgical evaluation of partial seizures, *Neurology,* 44, 693, 1993.
30. Smith, D., Baker, G., Davies, G., Dewey, M., Chadwick, D. W., *Epilepsia,* 34, 252, 1993.

Chapter 23

Anxiolytics and Hypnotics

G. R. McClelland

CONTENTS

1 Introduction 317
2 Pharmacokinetics and Metabolism — Healthy Volunteers 318
3 Pharmacodynamics — Healthy Volunteers 319
  3.1 Psychomotor Function 319
  3.2 Electroencephalography 321
  3.3 Sleep Studies 321
  3.4 Mode of Action 322
  3.5 Normal Elderly 322
  3.6 Safety 322
  3.7 Tolerance, Rebound, and Withdrawal 322
  3.8 Interaction Studies 322
4 Patient Studies 323
  4.1 Study Design 323
  4.2 Tolerance 323
  4.3 Withdrawal Reactions and Rebound Insomnia/Anxiety 323
  4.4 Pharmacokinetics and Metabolism Assessments 324
  4.5 Pharmacodynamics 324
5 Decision Making 324
  5.1 Development of a Hypnotic 324
  5.2 Development of an Anxiolytic 325
References 326

1 INTRODUCTION

In recent years drugs used to treat anxiety disorders (anxiolytics) and sleep disorders (hypnotics) have received a great deal of attention from regulatory authorities, the legal profession, the media, and consequently the general public. This interest has been primarily directed at the benzodiazepine class of drugs and the physiological and psychological effects that may occur after stopping treatment. Anxiety and insomnia remain the two most common disorders of the central nervous system (CNS) encountered by primary care physicians. However, a consequence of the adverse publicity is a decrease in prescribing drug treatment and it has recently been predicted by Menlo Biomedical Associates that 23% of the CNS prescription market enjoyed by anxiolytics will shrink to 7% by the year 2005.

The anxiolytic and hypnotic market continues to be dominated by benzodiazepines. The advantages of benzodiazepines include useful and rapid efficacy, few somatic side effects, and safety in overdose.[1] Most of the benzodiazepines have been on the market for several years and are no longer protected by patent and are subject to generic competition, consequently, the cost of treatment is relatively low. Therefore, any new treatment faces the difficult task of having, in a declining market, to demonstrate a significant improvement in safety and/or efficacy, compared with the benzodiazepines, in order to achieve a price which would enable the recouping of research and development costs.

It is clear that in the 1990s there has been, and will continue to be, a decrease in the number of new compounds being developed for the treatment of anxiety and insomnia. Nevertheless, there continues to be significant advances in the understanding of these disorders and the mechanisms by which they can be treated. Several new molecular entities are being developed which could indeed be shown to possess superiority over the existing treatments. The mechanisms of action of these new potential drugs include $5HT_{1A}$ agonists, $5HT_2$, and $5HT_3$ antagonists, potentiation of adenosinergic transmission, cholecystokinin

0-8493-9230-6/97/$0.00+$.50
© 1997 by CRC Press, Inc.

B receptor antagonists, ACE inhibitors, and drugs acting on the neuropeptide Y system. In addition there remains significant research into drugs with partial agonist properties at benzodiazepine receptors, or agonists targeted at a particular subset of benzodiazepine or GABA receptors.

Sedation, sleep, and general anaesthesia are generally regarded as being part of the same continuum of CNS depression, and as hypnotics are capable of producing such a CNS depression they are often indicated for the treatment of anxiety. Similarly, there is a significant overlap of drugs used in the treatment of depression and anxiety (particularly phobias). This chapter will concentrate on the development of drugs whose initial target indication is that of anxiety or sleep disorders.

There are many ways in which sleep disorders (dyssomnias) have been classified. The four general headings used by the Diagnostic and Statistical Manual (DSMIIIR) produced by the American Psychiatric Association and by the World Health Organization in the International Classification of Diseases (ICD-9CM) and Guidelines for the Clinical Investigation of Psychotropic Drugs[2] are as follows:

1. Disorders of initiation and maintaining sleep (insomnia)
2. Disorders of excessive somnolence (hypersomnia)
3. Disorders of the sleep-wake cycle
4. Dysfunctions associated with sleep, sleep stages, or partial arousals (parasomnia)

Hypnotics are suitable for study in the treatment of insomnia only.

The DSMIIIR lists many disorders under the general heading of anxiety disorders — generalized anxiety disorders, panic disorder, agrophobia, social phobia, simple phobia, post-traumatic stress disorder, and obsessive-compulsive disorder. The treatment of phobias and post-traumatic stress disorder primarily involves nondrug, psychological treatments; anxiolytics may, however, provide useful supportive treatment.

This chapter will describe the investigations that need to be performed in the early clinical evaluation of new anxiolytics (particularly for the treatment of generalized anxiety disorders) and hypnotics, both in healthy, nonpatient, volunteers and in patients.

2 PHARMACOKINETICS AND METABOLISM — HEALTHY VOLUNTEERS

The ideal hypnotic for the treatment of most insomnias would be a drug which produces a rapid onset of sleep, promotes the maintenance of sleep for a short period, and then allows an immediate return to the normal awake state; at present no such compound is available. Generalized anxiety disorder and some insomnias, such as insomnia related to psychiatric disorders, may require a different pharmacodynamic profile, involving a prolonged anxiolytic action but with minimal daytime sedation. Panic disorders can be treated by drugs with the latter profile, however, they could also be treated at the beginning of a panic attack by a drug with a very rapid onset and short duration of action.

Pharmacokinetic data are therefore particularly valuable in the early clinical evaluation of these drugs, with the desired pharmacokinetic profile dependent upon the particular disorder, and in the case of panic, the intended treatment regimen (chronic or as required). Most new regimens for the treatment of anxiety or insomnia should have a rapid onset of action and consequently will have to possess a rapid rate of absorption.

Measurement of plasma concentrations will reveal distribution to the highly vascular tissues. The brain is a highly vascular organ and so hypnotics and anxiolytics should be able to cross the blood-brain barrier with ease. Thus plasma concentration should parallel brain concentration.

After absorption, the drug is distributed to the poorly vascular tissues, such as voluntary muscle, and then eliminated by metabolism and excretion. The duration of pharmacodynamic activity is generally determined by the drug concentration in the brain, with the therapeutic effect ceasing when the concentration falls below a threshold. If this threshold is passed during the distribution phase, then the pharmacodynamic effect of a single dose will be short. If the threshold is passed during the elimination phase, then the pharmacodynamic effect should parallel the elimination half-life.

Another pharmacokinetic variable, important in the early volunteer studies, is the possibility of accumulation. Hypnotics and anxiolytics are often taken for periods of days, if not weeks, and therefore drugs with a long residence time/half-life will accumulate.

Plasma drug concentrations are not always predictive of the incidence or severity of residual daytime impairment.[3] For instance, temazepam has an elimination half-life of approximately 10 h, yet a 20-mg oral dose has been reported to cause no residual sequelae after an overnight ingestion.[4] In their recent review Kunsman et al.[5] stated that to date, a strong correlation between the impairment or trend toward impairment indicated in these studies and the level of drug or metabolites in body fluids has not been established for temazepam or other benzodiazepines. Thus pharmacokinetic data on the parent compound can provide valuable supporting information in early volunteer studies. However, they cannot replace the use of sensitive, objective, pharmacodynamic assessments.

The formation of active metabolites may be particularly important to both the duration of drug effect and the possibility of accumulation. Flurazepam, for instance, has a plasma half-life of 2-3 h, however, its active metabolite *N*-desalkyl flurazepam has a half-life of approximately 100 h.[6] In his *Handbook of Clinical Pharmacokinetic Data*, Jack,[7] shows that half of the anxiolytics and hypnotics currently in use have active metabolites. It is therefore important to identify both potential active metabolites by performing a ^{14}C (mass balance) study and have developed assays to quantify plasma concentrations of active metabolites very early in development.

3 PHARMACODYNAMICS — HEALTHY VOLUNTEERS

It is difficult to extrapolate from healthy volunteers to patients with most psychotropic drugs, as the intended therapeutic effect is often hard to identify by an action in an unimpaired subject. Hypnotics are probably the easiest of psychotropic drugs to study in normal subjects, as the intended therapeutic action (sedation) can be observed and quantified.

Assessment of anxiolytic properties are more difficult. It is possible to subject healthy volunteers to an anxiety-provoking stimulus but the repeated administration of such a stimulus, as is required in most well-controlled volunteer studies, leads to desensitization (e.g., a changing baseline). Such stimuli that have been utilized include riding a ferris wheel,[8] anticipation of pain,[9] and watching anxiety-provoking films.[10] Pharmacological stimuli should be more reproducible, with lactic acid, cholecystokinin, and pentagastrin having been used recently as models of anxiety in healthy volunteers, with the anxiety thus generated being prevented by treatment with potential anxiolytics.[11]

Assessment of CNS function in healthy volunteers, in the very first study in man, can provide very useful early information. In addition, the later use of pharmacological models of anxiety may also provide vital data on the dose response curve, and enable the prediction of doses to be investigated in the first patient, efficacy, studies.

3.1 Psychomotor Function

It is important that the objective and subjective measurements of CNS function are sensitive and reproducible. There are many tests that have been used to assess sedation in man. Fifteen years ago Hindmarch,[12] in a relatively limited review, listed over 50 such tests. It is inappropriate to use only one or two tests which measure a restricted range of CNS functions. A full battery of tests should be employed to cover the range of functions and ought to include assessment of alertness, cognitive function, reaction times, and memory.[2,5,13]

Different tasks are more sensitive than others to different psychotropic drugs. McClelland and Jackson[14] studied a range of psychotropic drugs using a broad battery of tests, and found that the three drugs studied with hypnotic/anxiolytic properties, amylobarbitone, ethanol, and oxazepam, correlated well with one another but could be differentiated clearly from other classes of psychotropics. The objective tests most sensitive to these hypnotics were, choice reaction time, a rapid information processing task (Figure 1), and a manipulative motor task; least sensitive were digit span and elapsing time estimation.

One particularly valuable method to study the time-course of anxiolytic/hypnotic drug activity in healthy volunteers is saccadic eye movement. This technique is particularly useful for studying the time of onset of drug effect, as continuous testing for an hour or more is possible, as demonstrated with intravenous diazepam and lorazepam.[15]

Subjective assessments, particularly visual analog scales (e.g., a 10-cm horizontal line with opposite adjectives at either end, and the subject having to mark the line at a point which represents their current feeling), are often as sensitive to sedative drug effects as objective measures.[17] It is therefore important that subjective measures are included in any test battery.[12] The time-course of the subjective effects usually parallel the objective effects,[18] as illustrated in Figures 1 and 2.

These objective and subjective measures of CNS function are clearly useful in providing information on the onset and duration of effect. They can also be used to produce dose-response curves such that the minimum effective dose is established. Another advantage with the use of a test battery is that any new potential psychotropic drug can be compared with previously studied standard drugs.

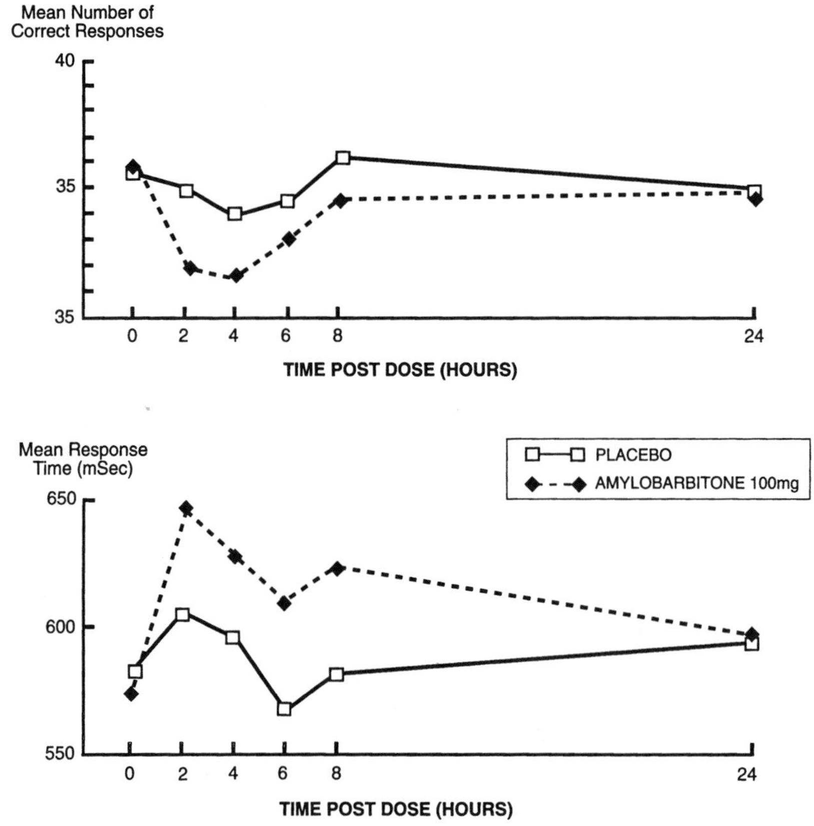

Figure 1 The effect of amylobarbitone on a rapid information processing task, after oral administration to 12 normal volunteers. (From McClelland, G.R., Raptopoulos, P., (1986). *Br. J. Clin. Pharmacol.* 22, 227-228P. With permission.)

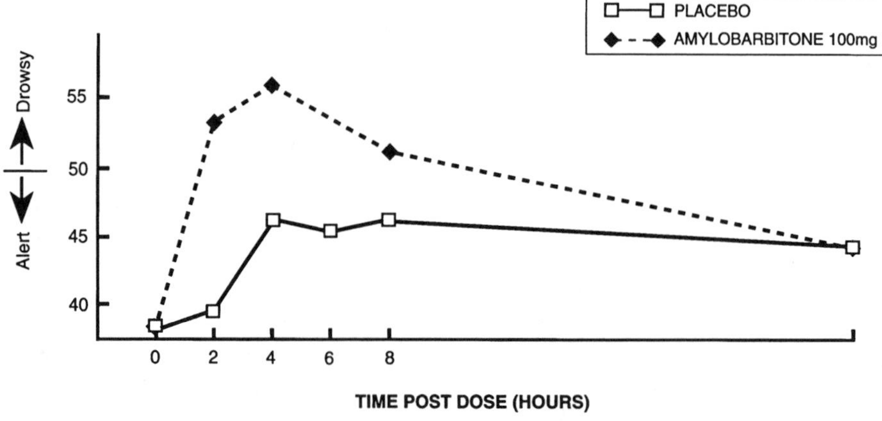

Figure 2 The effect of amylobarbitone on a bipolar visual analog scale for alert/drowsy after oral administration to 12 normal volunteers. (From McClelland, G.R., Raptopoulos, P., (1986). *Br. J. Clin. Pharmacol.* 22, 227-228P. With permission.)

3.2 Electroencephalography

The computer analyzed (or quantitative) electroencephalogram (EEG) has been used to study psychotropic drugs following the pioneering work of Fink and Itil.[19,20] Several workers have now confirmed that the EEG can be useful when classifying psychoactive drugs by their action on the different EEG frequencies,[21] and to study the time-course of CNS effects.[22] The EEG profile of anxiolytic/hypnotics being a decrease in alpha waves (8-12 Hz) and an increase in delta (0-4 Hz) and slow beta activity, as exemplified by the benzodiazepine anxiolytic ketazolam,[23] shown in Figure 3.

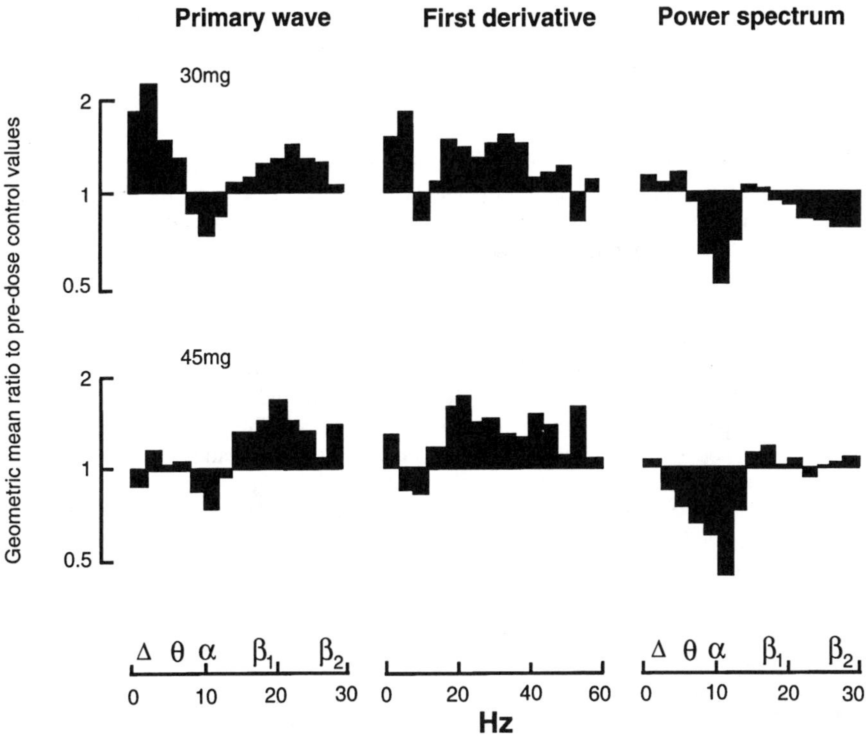

Figure 3 Mean ratio to predose control values of the EEG 24 h after oral ketrazolam (30 and 45 mg) to 9 normal volunteers. (From McClelland, G.R., Sutton, J.A., (1985) *Psychopharmacologia* 85, 306-308. Copyright Springer-Verlag GmbH & CaKG. With permission.)

There are examples of psychotropic drugs, such as nomifensine, where the EEG changes do not correlate with pharmacokinetics.[24] However, this work by Saletu and co-workers[24] on nomifensine and benzodiazepines, showed that psychometric measures correlated with the EEG rather than the pharmacokinetics. This emphasizes the relative importance of the pharmacodynamic assessment of psychotropic drugs.

The P300 component of the auditory evoked potential is known to be a useful indicator of cognitive function[25,26] and has been shown to be a more sensitive index of the effects of midazolam than standard psychomotor tests.[27]

3.3 Sleep Studies

Sleep studies in healthy volunteers with both new potential hypnotics and anxiolytics can provide useful data, prior to patient studies. The relative homogeneity of the normal volunteer population, and possibly reduced trial-related anxiety levels, does mean that studies of hypnotics on sleep can be performed with fewer subject numbers than in an insomniac patient population. Situational insomnia can be reliably induced in such studies by artificial means, for instance, by playing records of traffic noise. Such reproducibility is a potentially valuable method of studying the dose-response curve of a hypnotic in one form of insomnia.

Sleep studies should include basic measures such as onset of sleep, speed of awakening, number of night time awakenings, and the volunteers' subjective assessment of sleep quality. Subjective measures particularly useful are visual analog scales, as in the Leeds Sleep Evaluation Questionnaire.[28] EEG recordings can provide objective measures of the onset and offset of sleep, time spent in each of the four sleep stages, and the amount of rapid eye movement (REM) sleep.

3.4 Mode of Action

Information on the possible mode of action of new hypnotics can be gained during the early clinical studies, by using specific pharmacological tools. Flumazenil is a specific benzodiazepine receptor antagonist, with little, if any, intrinsic activity in normal subjects.[29] Flumazenil can be used to prevent/reverse the effects of a new hypnotic/anxiolytic, and thus reveal any central benzodiazepine receptor agonistic activity.

3.5 Normal Elderly

Insomnia is more commonly reported in the elderly than the young[30] and they are twice as likely to be receiving a hypnotic.[31] In addition aging is associated with an increased sensitivity to, and prolongation of, activity of most psychotropic drugs.[31] It is therefore important to compare the pharmacokinetics and pharmacodynamics of new hypnotics and anxiolytics in normal elderly and young subjects.

3.6 Safety

The standard monitoring of hematology, blood chemistry, the cardiovascular system, adverse events, and routine physical examinations should be included in all studies with new hypnotics/anxiolytics.

Other areas that require specific investigation for new drugs include the existence of any "hangover" effect (i.e., impaired performance the morning after night-time administration) and even the existence of any impairment of performance when wakened during the night. Such studies should employ a battery of tests of performance similar to those used in the acute measurement of volunteers.

Ataxia is a common side effect of many hypnotics and anxiolytics and may be related to an increase in potentially hazardous, falls, particularly in the elderly.[32,33]

Body sway can be measured objectively by various methods including a balance platform, and is very sensitive to the effects of alcohol and benzodiazepines.[34] The inclusion of an objective measurement of body sway in early volunteer studies may therefore determine the extent of this undesirable side effect.

Respiration is affected by hypnotics and anxiolytics. Mechanisms include a direct depressant effect via the CNS, and a reduction of resting tone of the airway muscles. The most vulnerable time for an adverse effect to occur is during sleep when arterial oxygen concentrations are lowest. It is therefore advisable to include the noninvasive measurement of respiration and oxygenation during early sleep studies in the laboratory.

Specific studies of a possible induction of hepatic drug-metabolizing enzymes and of plasma protein binding may be necessary where there are chemical, pharmacological, or clinical reasons for believing an interaction could occur (see Section 3.8).

3.7 Tolerance, Rebound, and Withdrawal

Most hypnotics and anxiolytics seem to produce pharmacological tolerance with repeated administration and rebound actions upon withdrawal. This has led to regulatory authorities requiring that these drugs are restricted to use for no more than 2-4 weeks. Studies to investigate such potential problems can be performed in normal subjects. However, even the positive effects of hypnotics are not always clearly shown in normal subjects[35] let alone any possible tolerance or rebound.[36] An explanation, provided by Lee and Lader[36] for their inability to demonstrate rebound with the benzodiazepines quazepam and triazolam, was that such effects are difficult to demonstrate in normal subjects in contrast to insomniacs. The use of standardized, validated, sensitive rating scales such as that developed by Merz and Ballmer[37] might provide valuable information on withdrawal potential in volunteers.

3.8 Interaction Studies

Hypnotics and anxiolytics are commonly taken with other drugs, particularly in the elderly. It is likely that they will have an additive effect with other drugs having a sedative action and with alcohol. However, interactions between hypnotics/anxiolytics and drugs other than alcohol and psychotropics are uncommon and of little clinical significance.[31]

The main interaction study that must be performed is with alcohol, so that the extent of any interaction can be determined.

4 PATIENT STUDIES

4.1 Study Design

The initial studies in patients will usually be performed in the relatively young (under 65 years old) who are in all other respects healthy. Such studies start with the intensive monitoring of the effects of single doses before progressing to repeated administration. The main purpose of these initial studies is to define the therapeutic range for investigation in later phase II and phase III studies.

Hypnotics, in particular, are often prescribed to the elderly and therefore at the time of registration the database should contain a high percentage of elderly patients. The inclusion of healthy elderly subjects in early studies will facilitate their inclusion in late phase II studies. As the elderly often receive several other medications, it is also important to assess any possible drug interactions before commencing large multicenter trials. While most interaction studies can be performed in animals and any potential interaction assessed in normal subjects, some interaction studies have to be performed in patients (e.g., potential interaction with digoxin).

Perhaps more than any other treated conditions there is a significant placebo response in the treatment of insomnia and anxiety.[38] It is therefore vital that a matched placebo is included in most, if not all, patient studies. A positive control, in the form of an established hypnotic/anxiolytic will assist in the evaluation of relative efficacy and safety.

The two main designs used in clinical trials are parallel and cross-over. Each has advantages and disadvantages. In the treatment of both insomnia and anxiety there is often a significant carry-over effect between the two arms of cross-over studies, and this results in the efficacy data from the second period being excluded from statistical analysis, thus effectively reducing the study to a parallel design. It is therefore proposed that the optimal general trial design of hypnotics and anxiolytics is a parallel study of two (or more) doses of the new drug, against placebo and a standard.

Studies are often restricted to a short duration of dosing; however, in clinical practice hypnotics and anxiolytics are often prescribed for up to one month and some patients do receive long-term treatment for many months or years. The main clinical trials should be performed with treatment periods of up to 4 weeks. However, it has been recommended that studies of prolonged treatment, for up to a year, are performed.[2] The inclusion criteria and various study designs have recently been reviewed extensively.[39]

4.2 Tolerance

During periods of prolonged treatment, tolerance to the efficacy of a hypnotic or anxiolytic can develop, but the significance of this phenomenon has recently been questioned. The reduction in efficacy can appear after just two weeks' treatment,[41,42] and careful monitoring of efficacy during repeat dose studies is therefore important.

4.3 Withdrawal Reactions and Rebound Insomnia/Anxiety

Upon cessation of any drug treatment rebound effects are not uncommon, for benzodiazepines, rebound insomnia is related to rebound anxiety and withdrawal syndromes.[43] Others[44] have suggested that tolerance and dependence result from the same adaptive mechanisms. However, Reynolds et al.[45] have shown that administration of the benzodiazepine, clobazam, can result in a tolerance to its anticonvulsant property without producing dependence (e.g., withdrawal reactions). Tolerance and dependence, therefore, appear to be independent of each other.

Even the newer hypnotics such as quazepam, zolpidem, and zopiclone, seem to cause rebound insomnia, although probably to a lesser extent than the classic hypnotics.[46] It is therefore important that studies with new hypnotics and anxiolytics assess both tolerance and dependence. The most frequently reported effects upon withdrawal include: anxiety, depression, somatic symptoms such as muscle trembling and muscle pain, malaise, weight loss, sweating, perceptual disturbance, sensory intolerance, hallucinations, psychosis, and seizures.[47-48]

The occurrence of any withdrawal reactions must be carefully monitored for any new hypnotic/anxiolytic. The Food and Drug Administration in the U.S. recommends three nights' monitoring after cessation of treatment with hypnotics to assess any rebound insomnia.[49] However, longer periods of (at least two weeks) monitoring are required to study all aspects of potential withdrawal problems.

A spontaneous reporting of withdrawal symptoms may lead to great differences between investigators in frequency of occurrence, a standardized method of assessment is advisable, such as the Withdrawal Symptom Scale which has been developed by Merz and Ballmer[37] and used in both a normal population, and together with the Withdrawal Symptom Questionnaire,[50] in benzodiazepine-treated patients.[47]

4.4 Pharmacokinetics and Metabolism Assessments

Because hypnotics and anxiolytics are widely used in the elderly, it is likely that many patients will be suffering from some degree of impairment of renal and/or hepatic function. As a minimum it is necessary to study the pharmacokinetics in patients with well-characterized hepatic and renal impairment during phase II and/or phase III as part of a population pharmacokinetic approach. Alternatively, the pharmacokinetics may be studied in separate studies in hepatic and renally impaired patients. It will certainly be important that, at the time a product license is applied for, there is a sufficient number of elderly subjects within the database.

4.5 Pharmacodynamics

The pharmacodynamic measures used in patient studies, both objective and subjective, are essentially those discussed earlier for nonpatient volunteers.

Sleep studies in the laboratory are clearly an important part of the early patient studies of both hypnotics and anxiolytics, however, for longer term studies it is impractical to keep patients in a laboratory, and it may also be necessary to have a longer baseline period for patients than with volunteers. It will also be necessary to characterize the type and extent of any insomnia each patient suffers from. It can be argued that laboratory studies are done in an artificial environment, and although studies with the patient at home must rely on subjective assessments, this is a better reflection of the clinical situation. One way in which this difficulty in obtaining objective sleep measures in clinical trials can be solved is to use ambulatory EEG recorders with either a standardized visual inspection or with automated analyzers. An even simpler, and perhaps equally valid, method is to monitor movement with wrist-worn sensors.[51]

The most common methods of measuring anxiolytic efficacy are with rating scales, completed by both the medical staff and the patient. Numerous rating scales have been developed to measure anxiety, but the most widely accepted are the Clinical Global Impression,[52] the Hamilton Anxiety Scale,[53] and patient rating with the Hopkins Symptom Checklist.[54]

5 DECISION MAKING

It is evident from the above that there are many methods available to examine the pharmacodynamic effects of hypnotics and anxiolytics, in both healthy volunteers and patients. In a recent review Roth et al.[55] state that "no norms or therapeutic targets for these various measures of hypnotic efficacy are available" and that for methodologies to study sleep "no single method at this time is considered sufficient." This is a situation which provides both advantages, in terms of opportunities for scientific investigation, and disadvantages for decision making in drug development.

It is therefore especially important for these drugs that prior to starting a clinical trial the primary outcome measure must be established. Indeed it is important that a target profile be established for any new drug prior to entering clinical development. The target profile will need to consider the known pharmacological properties of the new hypnotic/anxiolytic and the intended marketing strategy.

5.1 Development of a Hypnotic

A potential clinical target profile for a new hypnotic could include the following:

1. Greater than 50% reduction in sleep onset
2. Plasma concentration half-life/mean residence time less than 2 h
3. No active metabolites
4. Psychomotor/cognitive performance equivalent to placebo if woken within 2 h of sleep onset
5. No rebound insomnia
6. No amnestic properties
7. Cardiopulmonary, ataxia, and other adverse effects less than with existing treatments
8. Lack of tolerance over 6 weeks

A simplified clinical development plan to evaluate a new drug with the above target profile could consist of the following:

1. Entry-into-man, single dose in healthy volunteers
   Establish pharmacokinetic profile
   Establish effects on a limited range of tests of psychomotor function/EEG
   Establish lack of major adverse events
   Assess amnesic properties

2(a). Repeat dose sleep laboratory study in patients (if a center is identified with the appropriate facilities and ability to rapidly conduct the study)
   Investigate efficacy dose range
   Investigate "hangover" effect
   Establish repeat dose pharmacokinetics
   Establish lack of major adverse events on repeat dosing

2(b). Perform mass balance study
   Establish metabolic profile

3(a). Study range of doses in outpatients for 2 weeks' treatment (plus 2 weeks follow-up) in a placebo-controlled study
   Establish efficacy dose range
   Establish lack of "hangover" effect
   Establish lack of rebound
   Investigate range of adverse events

3(b). Perform alcohol interaction study in healthy volunteers
   Establish lack of interaction

4. Perform two separate phase III trials of one dosage of the new drug against the leading competitor hypnotics and against placebo, being allowed to continue with extended treatment for up to one year
   Establish long-term safety profile
   Establish market position

Each of the proposed studies will provide information that could enable the making of Go/No Go development decisions. Such studies should also provide regulators with sufficient clinical information to consider a Produce License Application for a hypnotic, together with other studies generally required for any new drug.

5.2 Development of an Anxiolytic

A potential target profile for an anxiolytic could include the following:

1. A decrease by more than 4 points on the Hamilton Anxiety Scales[53] greater than that achieved by placebo
2. Lack of any daytime psychomotor impairment
3. Duration of action sufficient to permit once daily dosing
4. Absence of the development of tolerance or rebound anxiety
5. Cardiopulmonary, ataxia and other adverse effects less than with existing treatments

A simplified clinical development plan to evaluate a new drug with the above target profile could consist of the following:

1. Entry-into-man, single dose in healthy volunteers
   Establish pharmacokinetic profile
   Establish effects in a limited range of tests of psychomotor function/EEG
   Assess amnestic properties
   Establish lack of major adverse events

2. Repeat dose study with a range of doses in healthy volunteers, including the application of a model of anxiety at the beginning and end of treatment
   Estimate efficacious dose range
   Establish repeat dose pharmacokinetics

3(a). Study a range of doses in outpatients with 2-4 weeks' treatment (plus 2 weeks follow-up) against placebo
   Establish acute efficacy dose range
   Establish lack of psychomotor impairment
   Establish lack of tolerance

Establish lack of rebound

3(b). Perform alcohol interaction study in healthy volunteers
Establish lack of interaction

4. Perform two separate phase III trials of one dose of new drug against the leading anxiolytic and placebo treatment with treatment for 6 months with an optional extension for a further 6 months
Establish long term safety
Establish market position

Each of the proposed studies will provide information that could enable the making of Go/No Go development decisions. Such studies should also provide regulators with sufficient clinical information to consider a Product License Application for a new anxiolytic, together with other studies generally required for any new drug.

REFERENCES

1. Lader, M., (1994). Treatment of anxiety. *B.M.J.* 309, 321-324.
2. WHO-Guidelines (1986). Guidelines for the clinical investigation of psychotropic drugs (WHO). *Pharmacopsychiatry* 19, 395-399.
3. Harvey, S.C., (1985). Hypnotics and Sedatives. In: *The Pharmacological Basis of Therapeutics,* 7th edition. Eds. A. Goodman Gilman, L.S. Goodman, T.W. Rall, F. Murad. Macmillan, New York.
4. Nicholson, A.N., (1986). Hypnotics and transient insomnia. In: *Drugs and Driving.* Eds. J.F. O'Hanlon and J.J. de Gier. Taylor & Francis, London.
5. Kunsman, G.W., Manno, J.E., Manno, B.R., Kunsman, C.M., Przekop, M.A., (1992). The use of microcomputer-based psychomotor tests for the evaluation of benzodiazepine effects on human performance: a review with emphasis on temazepam. *Br. J. Clin. Pharmacol.* 34, 289-301.
6. Jochemsen, R., van Boxtel, C.T., Hermans, J., Breimer, D.D. (1983). Pharmacokinetics of 5-benzodiazepine hypnotics in the same panel of healthy subjects. In: *Clinical Pharmacokinetics of 5-Benzodiazepine Hypnotics.* R. Jochemsen Doc. Disc. J.H. Pasmans, The Hague.
7. Jack, D.B., (1992). *Handbook of Clinical Pharmacokinetic Data.* Macmillan, Basingstoke.
8. Laties, V.G., (1959). Effects of meprobamate on fear and palmar sweating. *J. Abnorm. Soc. Psychol.* 59, 155-161.
9. Uhr, L., Miller, J.G., (1959). Experimental determined effects of envylcamate on performance, autonomic response, and subjective reactions under stress, *Ann. J. Med. Sci.* 240, 204-211.
10. Pillard, R.C. and Fishers, (1967). Effects of chlordiazepoxide and secobarbitol on film induced anxiety. *Psychopharmacologia* 12, 18-23.
11. Traub, M., Lines, C., Ambrose, J., (1993). CCK and anxiety in normal volunteers. *Br. J. Clin. Pharmacol.* 36, 504P.
12. Hindmarch, I., (1980). Psychomotor function and psychoactive drugs. *Br. J. Clin. Pharmacol.* 10, 189-209.
13. Roehrs, T., Merlotti, L., Zorick, F., Roth, T., (1994). Sedative, memory and performance effects of hypnotics. *Psychopharmacolgia.* 116, 130-134.
14. McClelland, G.R., Jackson, D., (1987). Automated testing of the effects of drugs on cognitive function. Pres. XIth International Meeting of Pharmaceutical Physicians, Brighton.
15. Griffiths, A.N., Marshall, R.W., Richens, A., (1984). Saccadic eye movement analysis as a measure of drug effects on human pscychomotor performance. *Br. J. Clin. Pharmacol.* 18, 735-825.
16. Tedeshi, G., Smith, A.T., Dhillion, S., Richens, A., (1983). Rate of entrance of benzodiazepines into the brain determined by eye movement recording. *Br. J. Clin. Pharmacol.* 15, 130-107.
17. Bond, A.J., Lader, M.H., (1973). The residual effects of flurazepam. *Psychopharmacologia.* 32, 223-235.
18. McClelland, G.R., Raptopoulos, P., (1986). Paroxetine and amylobarbitone, effects on psychomotor performance. *Br. J. Clin Pharmacol.* 22, 227-228P.
19. Fink, M., (1969). EEG and human psychopharmacology. *Ann. Rev. Pharmacol.* 9, 241-258.
20. Itil, T.M., (1974). Quantitative pharmacoelectroencephalography. Use of computerised cerebral bipotentials in psychotropic drug research. In: *Modern Problems of Pharmacopsychiatry.* Vol. 8: Psychotropic drugs and the human EEG. Ed. T.M. Itil, Karger, Basel.
21. Herrmann, W.M., (1982). Development and critical evaluation of an objective procedure for the electroencephalographic classification of psychotropic drugs. In: *Electroencephalography in Drug Research.* Ed. W.M. Herrmann, Gustav Fischer, Stuttgart.
22. Fink, M., (1982). Quantitative pharmaco-EEG to establish dose-time relations in clinical pharmacology. In: *Electroencephalography in Drug Research.* Ed. W. M. Herrmann, Gustav Fischer, Stuttgart.
23. McClelland, G.R. and Sutton, J.A., (1985). Pilot investigation of the quantitative EEG and clinical effects of ketazolam and the novel antiemetic nonabine in normal subjects. *Psychopharmacologia.* 85, 306-308.
24. Saletu, B., Grunberger, J., Taeuber, K., Nitsche, V., (1982). Relation between pharmacodynamics and -kinetics: EEG and psychometric studies with cinolazepam and nomifensine. In: *Electroencephalography in Drug Research.* Ed. W.M. Herrmann, Gustav Fischer, Stuttgart.

25. McClelland, G.R., (1995). Reaction times and the evoked potential. Pres. 29th Annual Meeting European Society of Clinical Investigation, Cambridge.
26. Signorino, M., D'Acunto, S., Angeleri, F., Pietropaoli, P., (1995). Eliciting P300 in comatose patients. *Lancet* 345, 255-256.
27. Engelhardt, M., Friess, K., Hartung, E., Sold, M., Dierks, T., (1992). EEG and auditory evoked potential P300 compared with psychometric tests in assessing vigilance after benzodiazepines sedation and antagonism. *Br. J. Anaesth.* 69, 75-80.
28. Parrott, A.C., Hindmarch, I., (1978). Factor analysis of a sleep evaluation questionnaire. *Psych. Med.* 8, 325-329.
29. Brogden, R.N., Goa, K.L., (1988). Flumazenil. A preliminary review of its benzodiazepine antagonist properties, intrinsic activity and therapeutic use. *Drugs* 35, 448-467.
30. Bixler, E.O., Kales., Soldatos, C.R., Kales, J.D., Healey, S., (1979). Prevalence of sleep disorders in the Los Angeles metropolitan area. *Am. J. Psychiatr.* 136, 1257-1262.
31. Lader, M.H., (1986). The use of hypnotics and anxiolytics in the elderly. *Int. Clin. Psychopharmacol.* 1, 273-283.
32. Swift, C.G., (1984). Postural instability as a measure of sedative drug response. *Br. J. Clin Pharmacol.* 18, 875-905.
33. Ray W.A., Griffin, M.R., Schaffner, W., Baugh, D.K., Melton, L.J., (1987). Psychotropic drug use and the risk of hip fracture. *N. Engl. J. Med.* 316; 363-369.
34. McClelland, G.R., (1989). Body sway and psychoactive drugs: a review. *Hum. Psychopharmacol.* 4; 3-15.
35. Stanley, R.O., Tiller, J.W.G., Adrian, J., (1987). The psychomotor effects of single and repeated doses of hypnotic benzodiazepines. *Int. Clin. Psychopharmacol.* 2, 317-323.
36. Lee, A., Lader, M., (1988). Tolerance and rebound during and after short-term administration of quazepam, triazolam and placebo to healthy human volunteers. *Int. Clin. Psychopharmacol.* 3, 31-47.
37. Merz, W.A., Ballmer, W., (1983). Symptoms of barbiturate/benzodiazepine withdrawal syndrome in healthy volunteers: Standardised assessment by a newly developed self-rating scale. *J. Psychoactive Drugs* 15, 71-84.
38. Spinweber, C.L., Johnson, L.C., (1982). Effects of triazolam (0.5 mg) on sleep, performance, memory and arousal threshold. *Psychopharmacologia* 76, 5-12.
39. Rickels, K., Noyes Jr., R., Robinson, D.S., Schweizer, E., Uhlenthuth, E.H., (1994). Evaluating drug treatments of Generalized Anxiety Disorder and Adjustment Disorders with anxious mood. In: *Clinical Evaluation of Psychotropic Drugs: Principles and Guidelines.* Eds. R.F. Prien and D.S. Robinson, Raven Press, New York.
40. Logan, K.E. and Lawrie, S.M., (1994). Long term use of hypnotics and anxiolytics may not result in increased tolerance. *BMJ.* 309, 742-743.
41. Kales, A., Bixler, E.O., Kales J.D., Scharf M.B. (1977). Comparative effectiveness of nine hypnotic drugs: sleep laboratory studies. *J. Clin. Pharmacol.* 17, 207-213.
42. Kales, A., Soldatos, C.R., Bixler, E.O., and Kales, J.D., (1983). Rebound insomnia and rebound anxiety: A review. *Pharmacology.* 26, 121-137.
43. Lader, M.H., Lawson, C., (1987). Sleep studies and rebound insomnia: methodological problems, laboratory findings and clinical implications. *Clin. Neuropharmacol.* 10, 291-312.
44. Feely, M.P., Haigh, J.R.M., (1988). Differences between benzodiazepines. *Lancet* i, 1460.
45. Reynolds, E.H., Heller, A.J., Ring, H.A., (1988). Clobazam for epilepsy. *Lancet* ii, 565.
46. Lader, M., (1992). Rebound insomnia and newer hypnotics. *Psychopharmacologia* 108, 248-255.
47. Schmauss, C., Apelt, S., Emrich, H.M., (1987). Characterisation of benzodiazepine withdrawal in high and low dose dependent psychiatric in patients. *Brain Res. Bull.* 19, 393-400.
48. Duncan, J., (1988). Neuropsychiatric aspects of sedative drug withdrawal. *Hum. Psychopharmacol.* 3, 171-180.
49. F.D.A. Guidelines (1977). *Guidelines for the Clinical Evaluation of Hypnotic Drugs.* U.S. Government Printing Office, Washington D.C.
50. Tyrer, P., Rutherford, Huggett, T., (1984). Benzodiazepine withdrawal symptoms and propanolol. *Lancet* 1, 520-522.
51. Borbely, A.A., (1984). Ambulatory motor activity monitoring to study the time course of hypnotic action. *Br. J. Clin. Pharmacol.* 17, 835-865.
52. ECDEU Assessment Manual Published by the U.S. Department of Health and Welfare (1976).
53. Hamilton, M., (1959). The assessment of anxiety states by rating. *Br. J. Med. Psychol.* 32, 50-55.
54. Derogatis, L.R., Ronald, S., Rickles, K., Uhlenhuth, E.H., Covil, (1974). In: *Psychological Measurements in Psychopharmacology.* Eds. P. Picket and R. Olivier-Martin. Karger, London.
55. Roth, T., Roehrs, T.A., Vogel, G.W., Dement, W.C., (1994). Evaluation of hypnotic medications. In: *Clinical Evaluation of Psychotropic Drugs: Principles and Guidelines.* Ed. R.F. Prien and D.S. Robinson. Raven Press, New York.

Chapter 24

Antidepressants

Jasper Dingemanse

CONTENTS

1 Introduction 330
2 Phase I Studies 330
  2.1 Safety and Tolerability 331
  2.2 Pharmacokinetics 331
  2.3 Pharmacodynamics 331
    2.3.1 Amine Pressor Tests 331
    2.3.2 Tests of Autonomic Nervous System Function 332
    2.3.3 Psychomotor Performance 332
    2.3.4 Electroencephalography 332
    2.3.5 Imaging Techniques 333
  2.4. Pharmacokinetic-Pharmacodynamic Modeling 333
  2.5 Interactions 333
  2.6 Stereoisomerism 334
3 Phase II Studies 334
  3.1 Safety and Tolerability 334
  3.2 Methodology 334
    3.2.1 Population and Diagnosis 334
    3.2.2 Concomitant Drug Treatment 335
    3.2.3 Assessments 335
    3.2.4 Design of Studies 335
    3.2.5 Onset of Therapeutic Response 336
    3.2.6 Duration of Studies 336
    3.2.7 Sample Size 336
    3.2.8 Data Analysis 337
    3.2.9 Measurement of Plasma Levels 337
  3.3 Markers of Depression 337
    3.3.1 Neurotransmitters and Their Metabolites 337
    3.3.2 Trace Amines 337
    3.3.3 Amino Acid Profiles 337
    3.3.4 Platelet Markers 337
    3.3.5 Neuroendocrine Markers 338
    3.3.6 Sleep Markers 338
    3.3.7 Imaging Techniques 338
    3.3.8 Conclusion 338
  3.4 Concentration-Response Relationships 338
  3.5 Alternative Approaches in Dose Finding 338
  3.6 Drug Compliance 339
  3.7 Pharmacoeconomics 339
  3.8 Overdose 339
  3.9 Antidepressant Drug Trials in Special Populations 339
    3.9.1 Gender 339
    3.9.2 Pregnancy 339
    3.9.3 Age 340
4 Other Indications 340

0-8493-9230-6/97/$0.00+$.50
© 1997 by CRC Press, Inc.

5 Antidepressant Drugs of the Future 340
5.1 Ideal Antidepressant Drug Profile 340
5.2 New Mechanisms of Action 340
6 Conclusions 341
Acknowledgments 341
References 341

1 INTRODUCTION

Depression is a serious and common disorder. Its lifetime prevalence is approximately 10% and successful suicide occurs in about 15% of depressed patients.[1]

A consensus conference on antidepressant drug trials defined an antidepressant as a drug that has been shown, in comparison with placebo, to improve all symptoms characteristic of the depressive syndrome in at least a subgroup of patients with recognized depressive disorder of at least moderate severity.[2] From a regulatory point of view a drug is considered an antidepressant only when it is shown to be effective in the treatment of major depressive episodes.[3]

Two different classes of effective antidepressant drugs, viz. the tricyclic antidepressants (TCAs) and monoamine oxidase inhibitors (MAOIs), were discovered by serendipity in the 1950s. For both drug classes the increase of the availability of monoamines at synapses is the proposed mode of action. Most antidepressant drugs which followed are structurally and/or pharmacologically very similar to early drugs.[4] The most recent extensions to the therapeutic armamentarium in depression are selective serotonin reuptake inhibitors (SSRIs) and reversible inhibitors of MAO-A (RIMAs).[4,5] Both classes, however, represent only a narrowing of the spectrum of pharmacological actions of their classical congeners. In general, progress has been made predominantly with regard to the side effect profile rather than efficacy.[6] As 60-70% of depressed patients improve on antidepressant drugs compared to 20-40% on placebo,[7] there is still room for improvement in their efficacy profile.

The development of antidepressants with a novel mechanism of action is severely impaired by a lack of understanding of the biological basis of depression and the way existing antidepressant drugs elicit their therapeutic effects.[8] Evidence from animal and clinical studies suggests that all antidepressants produce similar qualitative adaptive changes in adrenergic and serotonergic transmission during chronic treatment in parallel with the development of the therapeutic response.[9] The role of dopamine in depression remains unclear.[10] The acute pharmacological profiles of the different drug classes can, however, differ widely.

2 PHASE I STUDIES

The primary objective of the phase I development of new antidepressant drugs is to determine their safety and tolerability profile. This type of information is usually collected from single and multiple ascending dose studies in healthy volunteers. Studies in elderly volunteers are particularly appropriate as the elderly form an important target group among depressed patients and such studies provide information on age which can be a variable which influences the response to antidepressant drugs. A viable approach is to conduct the single ascending dose study in young and the multiple ascending dose study in elderly volunteers. It is advisable to evaluate pharmacokinetics and pharmacodynamics after the first dose to identify potential differences in the elderly before the start of the multiple dosing regimen.

With the introduction of new well-tolerated antidepressant drugs, the issue of poor tolerability of antidepressants in healthy volunteers compared to depressed patients, as often reported for the TCAs, has lost its significance as a consideration in antidepressant drug development.

The incorporation of suitable pharmacodynamic response measures in early studies is useful provided they bear some relationship to the therapeutic response in depressed patients.[11] Obviously, real measures of efficacy can only be obtained in a depressed patient population. Phase I studies offer a unique, and perhaps the only, opportunity to obtain knowledge of pharmacokinetic and pharmacodynamic characteristics and their interrelationship over a wide dose range of the new drug.[12] Some of these doses, i.e., in the low range and close to the maximum tolerated dose, are unlikely to be administered again in subsequent studies. The information generated by integrated pharmacokinetic-pharmacodynamic studies in phase I should be of great value in narrowing the dose range to be employed in phase II and can contribute to the decision whether the drug is a viable candidate for further clinical development.

2.1 Safety and Tolerability

New antidepressant drugs intended for use in a broad population of depressed patients should in the first instance have an excellent safety and tolerability profile.

Safety and tolerability in healthy volunteers are to be assessed by standard methods like reporting of adverse events, measurement of vital signs, physical/neurological examination, and determination of clinical laboratory parameters. Particular attention should be given to those events expected on the basis of preclinical studies or which are known to be of clinical relevance for similar drugs, e.g., gastrointestinal events with the SSRIs or orthostatic hypotension with TCAs.

The adverse events recorded in the multiple dose study are of interest in judging the development of either tolerance or an increase in intensity, e.g., due to drug accumulation upon multiple dosing.

2.2 Pharmacokinetics

Many aspects of the pharmacokinetics of a new antidepressant in man can already be established before the start of the first clinical pharmacology study, such as protein binding and by *in vitro* techniques such as human hepatocytes.[13] Early elucidation of metabolic pathways in man will indicate the drugs or drug classes with which clinically relevant interactions are likely to occur.

Detailed reviews of the pharmacokinetics of classical antidepressants have appeared.[14] Due to the pronounced interindividual pharmacokinetic variability and some evidence for concentration-response relationships, therapeutic drug monitoring for these drugs is often advocated.

Polymorphic hydroxylation reactions contribute significantly to the pronounced variability in the pharmacokinetics (particularly the clearance) of TCAs.[15] In principle, patients of the poor metabolizer phenotype are more liable to experience adverse effects on standard doses, whereas extensive metabolizers are at risk of therapeutic failure. Simple phenotyping or genotyping tests are of value in interpreting the pharmacokinetics of a new antidepressant drug undergoing polymorphic drug oxidation.[16] However, a large retrospective study of patients taking imipramine did not show a correlation between the debrisoquine oxidation capacity and the frequency or intensity of side effects.[17] Although the pharmacogenetic differences in the metabolism of most SSRIs per se are probably of little clinical relevance in terms of adverse clinical effects, they may be extremely important with regard to serious interactions with drugs metabolized by the same isozymes.[18] This feature of even new-generation drugs illustrates the importance of elucidating in detail the metabolic pathways of new chemical entities and their interference with the metabolism of other drugs.[19]

With the exception of fluvoxamine, moclobemide, and paroxetine all the currently available antidepressant drugs form one or more active metabolites during *in vivo* biotransformation in humans.[20,21] Such metabolites may contribute to both therapeutic and toxic effects. The mechanism of action of the metabolites may be similar to or different from that of the parent compound. The metabolism of tertiary to secondary amine tricyclic antidepressants is, e.g., associated with a shift in the ratio of serotonin/noradrenaline reuptake inhibition. Differences between *in vitro* and *in vivo* potency can point to the presence of active metabolites formed *in vivo*. Studying active metabolites of existing and new antidepressants might even pave the way to improve pharmacotherapy.[22] The most common pharmacodynamic response measures are schematically presented in Figure 1.

2.3 Pharmacodynamics

Historically, pharmacodynamic testing of antidepressant drugs in phase I studies mainly focused on the biochemical characterization of the drug to confirm the mechanism of action previously elucidated in animals.[23] Because the brain is not accessible for direct measurement of neurotransmitters and/or their metabolites, indirect methods have to be employed. Such methods are of particular value for therapeutic studies since this offers the possibility of establishing correlations with changes in severity of depression. These measures used are described in Section 3.3.

2.3.1 Amine Pressor Tests

The noradrenaline uptake inhibiting properties of an antidepressant can be investigated in healthy volunteers by intravenous administration of sympathomimetic amines. The sensitivity to the directly acting noradrenaline is increased, and to indirectly acting tyramine is decreased.[24] These pressor tests are conducted by consecutive administration of ascending doses of amines until a predefined increase in systolic blood pressure (usually 30 mmHg) has been attained. Plasma concentrations of TCAs and their effect on tyramine pressor tests correlate quite well. It should be realized, however, that this is merely an assessment of the peripheral effects of antidepressants.

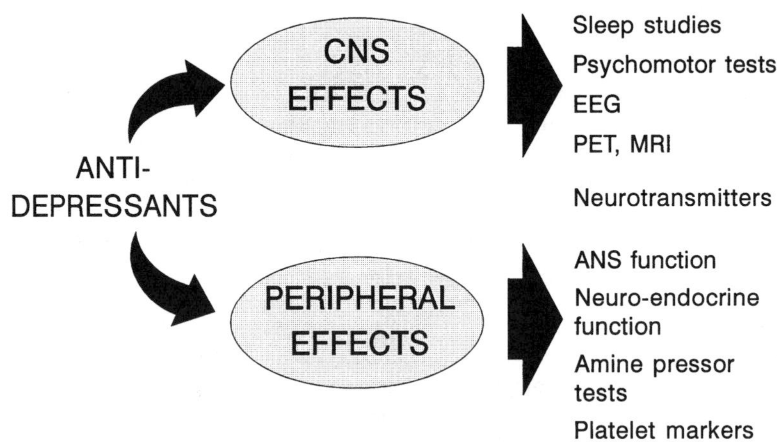

Figure 1

2.3.2 Tests of Autonomic Nervous System Function

Effects of drugs on the autonomic nervous system can, among others, be investigated by assessment of pupillary responses to adrenergic and cholinergic agents.[25] Autonomic effects of antidepressant drugs with a differentiation between muscarinic and adrenergic functions have also been assessed.[26] This type of study is more easily interpreted in healthy volunteers because depressive illness itself is often associated with disturbances of autonomic function.[27]

2.3.3 Psychomotor Performance

Since most of the classical antidepressant drugs have detrimental effects on cognitive and psychomotor performance, usually attributed to their anticholinergic action, the effects of new drugs on variables like vigilance, attention, and memory should be investigated.[28,29] Psychopharmacological studies should assess the "safety" of the antidepressant with reference to its clinical usage pattern, i.e., at therapeutic doses and under conditions which are close to real life. Healthy volunteers have frequently been tested following a relatively low single dose.[30] It is still a matter of debate whether a battery of laboratory tests measuring a spectrum of CNS functions[31] or actual highway driving mainly measuring the standard deviation of the lateral position[32] permits a better measure of real-life car handling ability. Figure 2 shows the mean standard deviation of the lateral position as a function of distance driven on treatment days 1 and 8 of a multiple dosing regimen with moclobemide 200 mg b.i.d., mianserin 10 mg t.i.d., and placebo. Mianserin affected driving, while moclobemide could not be distinguished from placebo.[33] A clear preference for a particular psychometric test cannot be expressed, since only few of them have been well validated.[34] Such studies are normally conducted in healthy volunteers because of the necessity for standardized conditions. However, the outcome of these studies cannot always be easily extrapolated to depressed patients.[35] Most studies fail to consider sufficiently that depression per se will have adverse effects on cognitive functions and memory.[30,36]

Because many ambulant patients in general practice might also consume small amounts of alcohol when treated with antidepressants, the possibility of an interaction with alcohol should also be investigated with respect to psychomotor and cognitive performance.[37] The same holds true for the concomitant intake of antidepressants and sedatives/hypnotics.

2.3.4 Electroencephalography

Quantitative pharmaco-electroencephalography (EEG) theoretically offers promising perspectives as a marker of antidepressant drug effects since it focuses directly on the target organ, the human brain.[38] Time- and dose-response relationships could also be constructed, thereby facilitating the establishment of relationships between pharmacokinetics and pharmacodynamics. One of the reasons that pharmaco-EEG methods are infrequently employed in studies with new antidepressants is that the EEG profile can only be judged by comparing it to that of existing antidepressants. The possibilities and limitations of the technique in postulating hypotheses about therapeutic efficacy of psychoactive drugs in man have been reported extensively.[39-41]

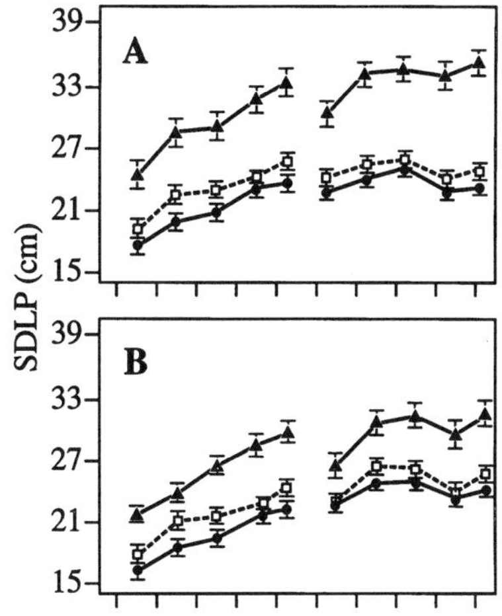

Figure 2 Mean SDLP ± SE as a function of distance traveled in each condition on the first (A) and eighth (B) treatment day. The functions are broken at mid-test where the subjects reversed their direction of travel. ------□------ placebo; --■-- moclobemide; —▲— mianserin. (From Ramackers, J. G., *Psychopharmacology,* 106, 562, 1992. With permission.)

2.3.5 Imaging Techniques

In vivo nuclear magnetic resonance spectroscopy and positron-emission tomography (PET) hold potential for research in psychiatry.[42-44] These sophisticated techniques are still in their childhood and as yet have limited predictive capability. They may be of value in obtaining knowledge of brain levels and brain receptor occupancy of psychotropic drugs, respectively.

2.4 Pharmacokinetic-Pharmacodynamic Modeling

Pharmacokinetic-pharmacodynamic modeling, i.e., the establishment of relationships between concentration and pharmacological response, can be of great value in improving the understanding of drug action in clinical psychopharmacology,[45,46] and providing information on appropriate dose selection and insight into the factors causing variability in drug response.[47]

2.5 Interactions

In the treatment of depression polypharmacy is quite common. In a recent prescription database study it was shown that about 20% of patients on antidepressant drugs were treated with other psychotropics.[48] The combination of two antidepressants from different classes is not unusual. Relevant drug interactions with antidepressants have been comprehensively described earlier.[49] Severe interactions have been reported between drugs of the MAOI and SSRI type.[50] When developing new drugs belonging to the same or similar class this should be taken into account and further investigated if needed.[51] Potential interactions with commonly used drugs, both on a prescription and over-the-counter basis, have also to be considered. Interaction studies are best performed in healthy volunteers since only then clean pharmacokinetic and pharmacodynamic data can be gathered. In depressed patients the use of other drugs and underlying symptomatology are often confounding factors. However, in the patient situation, population data and therapeutic drug monitoring may be valuable to discover and quantify drug interactions as was recently demonstrated with data collected on amitriptyline and nortriptyline in almost 3000 patients.[52]

When considering drug interactions, not only simultaneous but also serial administration of drugs has to be studied, since there may be a persistent or delayed pharmacokinetic and/or pharmacodynamic influence long after administration of a drug has been discontinued. In the case of fluoxetine and classical MAOIs the very long elimination half-life of (nor) fluoxetine and the irreversible inhibition of MAO, respectively, are responsible for these phenomena. Although the SSRIs are very similar pharmacodynamically, pharmacokinetic differences are pronounced. With respect to drug interactions sertraline has the lowest liability to interfere with the metabolism of other drugs.[53] Additive or synergistic therapeutic effects when antidepressants are combined can often be explained by a pharmacokinetic interaction.[54]

The effect of food should also be studied. The "cheese effect," due to interaction with tyramine-containing foodstuffs, was the reason for the rapid decline in popularity of the classical MAOIs. This potential problem had to be adequately investigated for drugs belonging to the new class of RIMAs.[55] Because gastrointestinal side effects may occur with antidepressants, the timing of drug and food intake may influence the side effect profile and may need to be studied.

When considering drug interactions it is crucial not to forget that alcohol and smoking can also interfere with the pharmacokinetics and pharmacodynamics of various psychotropic medications.[56] The effect of smoking on drugs has been less well studied than that of alcohol. The primary pharmacodynamic interaction of smoking with psychotropic agents seems to be the decreased drowsiness experienced by smokers compared to nonsmokers due to the central nervous system stimulating effects of tobacco smoking.

2.6 Stereoisomerism

Many antidepressant drugs, including the SSRIs citalopram and fluoxetine, are administered as racemates although practically nothing is known about their stereoselective activity and metabolism. Amine pressor tests in healthy subjects show a clear distinction between the optically active isomers of the tetracyclic antidepressant oxaprotiline.[57] Enantiomers can differ both in pharmacodynamic and pharmacokinetic properties.[58] Therefore, assay methods which do not differentiate between the different compounds in a racemic mixture may lead to meaningless results and conclusions.

3 PHASE II STUDIES

Phase II development of an antidepressant drug should obtain information on the safety and tolerability in the target population, explore dose-response relationships, and identify a therapeutic range to be employed in phase III studies.

3.1 Safety and Tolerability

From a regulatory point of view, safety and tolerability remain key issues during phase II.[59] Although extensive information on a broad dose range should have become available from phase I studies, special attention should be paid to adverse events to which depressive patients may be particularly prone. Because most patients will be treated in an ambulant setting, monitoring cannot be as intense as during phase I, but physical examination and determination of clinical laboratory parameters should be conducted at regular intervals. Direct questioning regarding specific types of adverse effects and particularly sexual function should be considered since these are often not reported spontaneously.

3.2 Methodology

The methodological problems in the therapeutic evaluation of antidepressant drugs have long been recognized.[60] Several standards, guidelines, and consensus reports on the methodology of assessing the efficacy of antidepressant drugs have appeared.[2,3,8,61-63]

3.2.1 Population and Diagnosis

Most depressed patients seek help from primary care physicians rather than psychiatrists.[64] Underrecognition and misdiagnosis of depression are quite common.[65] For the diagnosis of depression and its subtypes three major psychiatric systems are used.[63] The most widely applied diagnostic system is the Diagnostic and Statistical Manual (DSM) of Mental Disorders, now in its 4th edition.[66] The other widely applied systems are ICD-9/10 (International Classification of Diseases) and RDC (Research Diagnostic Criteria). Benefits and limitations of these systems have been discussed as well as approaches to improving current classification methods.[67]

Applying stricter criteria than those given by the DSM can have a positive influence on the outcome of clinical trials.[68] Comorbidity of anxiety and personality disorders frequently complicates a differential diagnosis.[69] The duration of the depressive episode and the psychiatric history should be recorded since these can influence the response rate. Phase II trials should preferably be conducted with hospitalized patients.[2] The report on the antidepressant drug trial should give a clear description and justification of the classification approaches in the case of diagnostic subgroups to allow assumptions on the generalization of results.[70] It should be stressed that the in- and exclusion criteria of study protocols should be realistic and really clinically relevant, otherwise patient recruitment may turn out to be difficult or even impossible.[71]

3.2.2 Concomitant Drug Treatment

A complete drug history including over-the-counter drug use is necessary when considering a patient to be included in an antidepressant drug trial. This is essential to rule out both drug and disease contributions to depression, and also to avoid drug-drug interactions. Sometimes it is better to continue long-term medication (e.g., benzodiazepines) than to induce withdrawal symptoms during an antidepressant drug trial. However, it is important that all concomitant treatments are considered in the evaluation of the trial.

3.2.3 Assessments

There is no consensus on the improvement needed in clinical status of depressed patients to conclude on the antidepressant efficacy of a drug. The Hamilton Rating Scale for Depression[72] and the Montgomery and Asberg Depression Rating Scale[73] are the scales most frequently employed in antidepressant drug trials. Others are the Beck Depression Inventory and the Zung Self-Rating Depression Scale.[74] However, their use and interpretation are not without pitfalls.[70] Most of the scales were primarily designed for patients with endogenous forms of depression and improvement in a total score does not necessarily indicate antidepressant action. Moreover, it should be realized that some adverse effects can influence the total score. Similar problems are inherent to other rating scales for depression, including the Clinical Global Impression Scale which generates ratings of both illness severity and clinical improvement. In exploratory studies, comprehensive scales are preferable whereas later in development short scales may be used for hypothesis testing.[2] Different outcome measures for the assessment of antidepressant drug response can be identified. The most commonly used measures are: (1) a relative reduction of baseline score on a rating scale, (2) a fixed endpoint cut-off score on a rating scale, and (3) a combination of these two criteria.[75,76] Particularly in short-term trials, a fixed, severity-independent, cut-off score can lead to unwanted biases if treatment groups are not controlled for severity.[76] The sensitivity of discrimination between active treatment and placebo is increased when aiming solely for a percentage reduction of baseline score, and it can therefore be employed with smaller sample sizes.

3.2.4 Design of Studies

Before embarking on a large phase II program it is useful to first conduct some exploratory studies in depressed patients unless the phase I studies have resulted in clear indications about the dose range to be tested in phase II.[77] Exploratory studies, which may be of open or single-blind design, are essential for hypothesis generation.

Placebo-controlled parallel group studies are considered to be the design of choice to test the efficacy of a new antidepressant since depressive episodes tend to spontaneously remit, partially or fully. It is the only guarantee against an ineffective drug being introduced into the market.[78] Patients with a significant suicide risk and those with marked functional impairment raise ethical problems. Several other ethically less controversial designs for controlled trials have been proposed, but they have methodological problems.[78] Strong placebo responders can usually be detected in an initial 1-2 week period of placebo treatment before allocation to trial medication. Since a single design cannot fulfill all the phase II objectives, fixed-dose and dose-titration designs are usually combined.[79]

It is important to explore the full potential therapeutic dose range, guided by the findings in phase I. A pivotal part of phase II development should be a well-conducted dose-finding study.[80] It is striking that even with the TCAs and irreversible MAOIs, which have been in clinical use for more than 30 years, relatively few dose-response studies have been performed.[77] Fixed-dose designs are well suited for attempts to establish concentration vs. clinical response/toxicity relationships, whereas titration designs within predefined dose ranges are more relevant to clinical settings.[81] Dose changes have to be implemented on the basis of operationalized criteria. For antidepressant drugs in phase II an efficacy dose escalation design is often chosen, in contrast to phase I titration studies where the decision to administer the next higher dose is based on tolerability considerations. The analysis of both efficacy and safety in titration studies require special evaluation techniques.[82] The pace of dose titration needs to be specified. There is a dearth of trials investigating the value of reaching the maximum antidepressant dose within one week of treatment to shorten the time necessary to observe the full drug effect.

Comparison of the new antidepressant against reference drugs is usually performed during later phases of clinical development. Special precautions have to be taken in trials in which a new drug is compared only with a reference drug.[83,84] Both the choice of reference drug and its dosage have to be carefully considered to avoid type I or type II errors.[70] Reference drugs are quite often administered at less than adequate dosage in comparative trials involving new antidepressants.[85] This fate often befalls TCAs when in a flexible dose study the patient or the treating physician is sensitive to side effects occurring at relatively low doses. At least 150 mg imipramine daily, or its equivalent, should be administered.[86]

3.2.5 Onset of Therapeutic Response

Clinical trials with new antidepressant drugs frequently report a quicker onset of clinical effect compared to TCAs, but these claims often do not hold. The time-course of antidepressant response is seldom well explored since it requires frequent assessments and a careful selection of doses. Particularly when dose titration is applied, it is extremely difficult to compare the onset of response for two antidepressants. It has been suggested that the early onset response can predict the outcome for the duration of the trial.[87]

3.2.6 Duration of Studies

For most antidepressant drug trials, four weeks is sufficient to determine if a drug is effective in initially controlling acute symptoms, but definitely not to determine its efficacy in treating the entire depressive episode.[88] A significant proportion of patients, irrespective of diagnostic subtype, who show no clear-cut response at four weeks show improvement compared to placebo at six weeks. During the first two weeks of a study the likelihood of responding to drug or placebo is roughly equal.[88] The chance of improving with drug therapy increases with time, whereas the chance of improving with placebo treatment does not increase (Figure 3). Two-phase drug trials in which the trial period in responding patients is extended from 6-12 weeks can further increase the statistical discrimination between active drug and placebo.[89] For high scorers on rating scales the observation period has to be adjusted to fully evaluate the potential of a new antidepressant.[76]

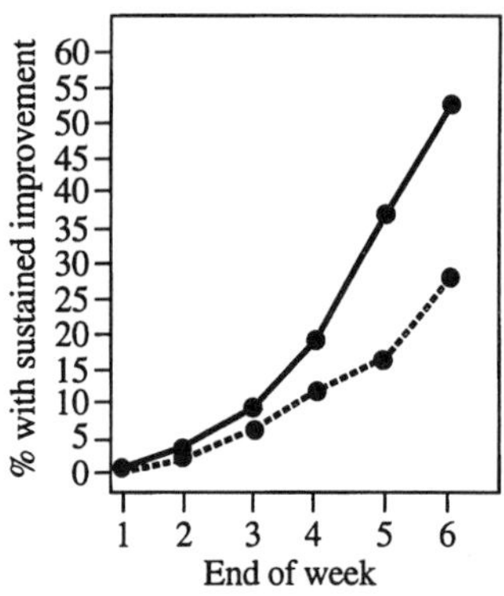

Figure 3 Life table showing percent of patients who showed improvement and sustained this improvement throughout a six-week study. Patients receiving drug are indicated by solid line (n = 113); patients receiving placebo by a broken line (n = 103). (From Quitkin, F. M., *Arch. Gen. Psychiatry,* 41, 238, 1984. With permission.)

Evidence has been accumulating that, in order to prevent relapse and recurrence, depressed patients after a first or second depressive episode should be treated with full-dose antidepressants for at least 6-12 months.[9] The prophylactic effects of antidepressants are usually studied in phase III or IV. Since DSM lists dysthymia as a separate entity, research interest in this area is growing.[90] Guidelines or design, assessment and evaluation of long-term trials in psychiatry have recently been reported on as a result of a consensus conference.[91]

3.2.7 Sample Size

A primary outcome criterion for antidepressant efficacy should be specified prior to study conduct for the statistical determination of sample size. This is based on the likelihood of type I or type II error, what is regarded as a clinically significant difference, and an estimate of the outcome variance for the control group. For placebo-controlled studies the number of patients needed to test the efficacy of new drugs is generally 10-20 times lower than when using reference drugs which puts the ethical issue into another perspective.[78]

Due to the variability of depression, many studies of antidepressant drugs are done with an insufficient number of patients. This is particularly true for studies focusing on efficacy, concentration-response relationships, and the value of biological markers.

Multicenter trials are often the only way to achieve adequate numbers of patients. These studies require intense training of all investigators involved to ensure that the common protocol is strictly followed and that the same criteria are used by all centers. The importance of interrating training cannot be overemphasized.[94]

3.2.8 Data Analysis

Different types of analysis have been used in trials evaluating antidepressants such as "completer analyses," "endpoint analyses" (or intent-to-treat analysis), and "survival analyses."[70,92] The latter approach is particularly useful for studies of longer duration. For studies of antidepressants that yield ambiguous results "pattern analysis" of the timing and duration of patients' responses can be useful.[93]

In pooling data from multicenter studies, detection of a center by treatment interaction should initiate a search for the specific factor(s) responsible for the interaction. In large multicenter trials the seasonal rhythmicity in the occurrence of acute depressive episodes should be considered. The increasing popularity of meta-analyses warrants caution, even if the studies used the same treatments and outcome measures (e.g., Reference 95) because the literature is biased toward positive studies.[96]

3.2.9 Measurement of Plasma Levels

Monitoring of drug concentration is helpful in compliance control and explaining nonresponse or side effects. It will facilitate attempts to establish concentration-response relationships.

3.3 Markers of Depression

The ultimate aim of a marker would be to predict accurately the response to antidepressant treatment. This should lead to a more rational selection of specific drugs for individual patients. Markers can be separated into clinical and biological predictors of treatment response. Among the clinical predictors chronicity of depression, high "neuroticism," psychotic features, and comorbidity are associated with a poor response.[97] Severity of illness seems the single most important predictor of an antidepressant drug's short-term efficacy relative to placebo.[98]

3.3.1 Neurotransmitters and Their Metabolites

Biochemical parameters focusing on metabolites of central monoamines (MHPG, 5-HIAA, HVA), their precursors, and the enzymatic processes have been disappointing as predictive markers.[99] As is common in the field of drug markers, earlier reports had been more positive.[100] There has been a shifting interest from noradrenaline to serotonin as the major neurotransmitter thought to be involved in the etiology of depression.

3.3.2 Trace Amines

Several trace amines (phenylethylamine, tryptamine, *m*- and *p*-tyramine) have been claimed to play a role in the etiology of depression and in the mode of action of antidepressant drugs. Some of these amines and/or their metabolites have been proposed as state and trait markers for depression.[101]

3.3.3 Amino Acid Profiles

Plasma amino acid profiles have been proposed as a predictor and marker of treatment response but results have been inconsistent,[102] and their applicability is controversial.

3.3.4 Platelet Markers

Platelets have been proposed as a model of CNS neurons[103] and appear to be suitable for studying neuronal α_2-adrenergic receptor regulation.[104]

Effective antidepressant therapy with MAOIs was originally thought to require 85% or more inhibition of platelet MAO.[105] The advent of the RIMAs which do not inhibit MAOB and therefore platelet MAO have, however, well-established antidepressant efficacy.

High affinity binding of tritiated imipramine or paroxetine to platelets has been suggested as a specific biological marker of depressive disorders and of the course of antidepressant therapy. These binding sites are associated with the serotonin transporter.[106] Many contradictory reports on the value of this marker have appeared, but there is now growing consensus that they cannot be considered as markers of clinical remission.[107] Recently, defective platelet L-tryptophan transport was proposed as a state-dependent marker of depression.[108]

3.3.5 Neuroendocrine Markers

Numerous endocrine abnormalities are found in depressive illness and several have been proposed as useful markers in depression therapy. The dexamethasone suppression test[109] and thyrotropin-releasing hormone stimulation test[110] have been most widely applied but their clinical utility is questionable.[111,112] Currently pineal function is an important focus of investigation.[113]

In an attempt to refine the neuroendocrine approach, nocturnal hormone secretion was measured under the influence of antidepressant drugs.[114,115] Elevated cortisol and blunted testosterone secretion were reported as state markers of acute depression. The influence of age and gender in employing neuroendocrine probes has not always been considered.[116]

3.3.6 Sleep Markers

Although most types of depression are associated with sleep disturbances, the large variability complicates their use as a disease marker. Most antidepressant drugs have an influence on the total sleep time and the latency to rapid eye movement (REM) sleep.[117] This effect, however, occurs before the antidepressant response is manifested.[115]

3.3.7 Imaging Techniques

Sophisticated brain imaging techniques like PET may prove to be of help in the search for biological markers in depression. Particular attention has thus far been given to the metabolic rate in different parts of the cortex.[118]

3.3.8 Conclusion

At present there are no useful markers of depression, and the choice of an antidepressant drug for an individual patient is largely empirical. In investigating the value of markers, more attention should be devoted to longitudinal studies in which the specific marker is followed over a long enough time period.[119] The availability of a robust biological marker would greatly improve the validity, reliability, and reproducibility of drug trials, but in the light of the manifold clinical manifestations of depression this remains a Utopian concept.

3.4 Concentration-Response Relationships

The APA Task Force report[120] concluded that there seems to exist a crude relationship between antidepressant effect and plasma level for only a few TCAs which have been extensively investigated (imipramine, desipramine, and nortriptyline). The vast majority of studies exploring concentration-antidepressant response relationships have been retrospective in design. Complicating factors concerning concentration-response relationships of antidepressants are design-, disease-, and drug-related.[45] To the latter belong the dose range studied, (inter)active metabolites, and plasma protein binding. Bioassays to quantify all pharmacologically active forms of a drug have been set up to improve the establishment of concentration-effect relationships, however, so far without much success.[121] It has been hypothesized that the componential approach which views the disorder in structural terms (emotional, behavioral, perceptual, cognitive, and somatic) is likely to be more useful in establishing concentration-response relationships than the common unitary model of depression.[8] A recent study on clomipramine reported on the monitoring of plasma concentrations of the parent compound and three active metabolites and their positive use for predicting clinical outcome.[122]

Although many attempts were made, there is no convincing evidence of a relationship between plasma concentrations of any of the SSRIs and clinical efficacy.[19]

Besides the classical concentration-antidepressant response studies, it is strongly recommended that integrated pharmacokinetic-pharmacodynamic studies are not limited to healthy volunteers only, since different baseline conditions may exist in the target population.[47] This type of study can augment the information obtained through standard dose-response methods.[12] Moreover, kinetic-dynamic investigations can be very useful in special patient subgroups such as the elderly and patients with liver or renal disease.

3.5 Alternative Approaches in Dose Finding

Population pharmacokinetic approaches may be helpful in the early individualization of antidepressant dosing when there is some knowledge of the concentration-response relationship.[123] Dose-response relationships can be investigated by population-based analyses in which the data of all individuals undergo a pooled analysis with the goal of assessing the influence of disease or demographic variables on the distribution of dose-response parameters.[124] The ultimate aim of this type of approach is to provide dosing information for special populations.[125] Randomized concentration controlled clinical trials have been proposed in which the patients are not randomized to fixed doses but to steady-state drug concentrations.[126]

3.6 Drug Compliance

A factor which has been grossly neglected in the evaluation of clinical trials is the fact that many patients do not take their medication as prescribed.[127] In patients with mental illness, noncompliance rates are likely to exceed 50%.[128] Also drug compliance in the elderly can be assumed to be relatively low.[129]

Therapeutic drug monitoring of antidepressants may assist in the assessment of compliance. It is often suggested that the fact that therapeutic drug monitoring is being performed per se already increases patient compliance. Sophisticated methods for measuring compliance may be particularly useful in outpatient studies and can provide more reliable information than drug level measurements since the latter do not describe the pattern of ingestion.[130] However, satisfactory solutions on how to handle partial compliance in the evaluation of clinical trials have as yet not been provided.

3.7 Pharmacoeconomics

Quality of life and pharmacoeconomic measures are playing an increasingly important role in the development of drugs.[131] A cost-benefit analysis should take into account all social and health factors, in addition to the cost of medication. A new antidepressant may, although more expensive, be associated with a better tolerability profile and therefore a better compliance which in turn leads to fewer visits to the physician and a reduced risk of overdose.[132]

3.8 Overdose

If possible, knowledge of the tolerability of the antidepressant at high doses should come from phase I studies in healthy volunteers. Classical antidepressants like the TCAs have received extensive attention with regard to their overdose toxicity, and cardiotoxic effects have been investigated in detail.[133] The fatal toxicity index (number of deaths per 1 million prescriptions) is much lower for the second generation antidepressants.[134,135] Recently it was calculated that a switch in first line treatment from TCAs to SSRIs could save the lives of at least 300 patients per year in the U.K.[136]

Attempts should be made to obtain as much information as possible on intentional or accidental overdoses during phase II. This includes close monitoring of the clinical status of the patient and drug level determinations in plasma. Mixed overdoses of antidepressants which are relatively safe per se can lead to a fatal outcome and should be considered as well.[137]

3.9 Antidepressant Drug Trials in Special Populations

The population of depressed patients in antidepressant drug trials is usually quite mixed and the evaluation of the study results should take into account subpopulations such as female and elderly patients.

3.9.1 Gender

Women seek treatment and receive psychotropic medication more frequently than men.[138] Therefore, it is remarkable that little research has been conducted on gender differences in therapeutic effects and side effects of psychotropic drugs. Reviews of the existing literature on differences in pharmacokinetics and pharmacodynamics suggested that young women have an enhanced response to nontricyclic antidepressants.[116,139] Generally, the administration of exogenous hormones and the menstrual cycle phase can interact with medications.[140] The dearth of investigations to look for pertinent gender differences is partially caused by the fact that much of the phase I work is conducted in young men. A recent FDA guideline draws attention to this phenomenon and encourages the early initiation of drug trials in females.[141]

3.9.2 Pregnancy

Pregnancy is usually an exclusion criterion for participation in clinical trials with antidepressant drugs. A large multinational epidemiological study on the use of psychotropic drugs in pregnancy indicated that antidepressants were prescribed to only 0.1% of the nearly 15,000 women interviewed.[142] Although avoiding psychotropic drugs is recommended, benefits may outweigh the risks. With the exception of lithium, no psychotropic drugs have a demonstrated teratogenic potential.[116] However, it is unknown whether drug treatment during pregnancy has subtle effects on the developing brain.

The reluctance with respect to the prescription of antidepressant drugs to pregnant women and the ethical implications will make it virtually impossible to investigate the effects of these drugs in this population.

3.9.3 Age

Depression is a relatively common condition in the elderly and is associated with considerable morbidity and mortality. Approximately 10% of persons aged 65 or older living in the community have important symptoms of depression.[143] The identification and treatment of depression may be more difficult in the elderly than in younger patients because of comorbidity and concurrent drug therapy.[144] A commonly advocated approach is to initiate therapy in elderly at lower doses than usually recommended for younger adults. Because antidepressants show a large degree of interindividual variability in drug clearance, it is difficult to attribute differences to age per se. However, for many drugs clearance is reduced in the elderly[145] and it is assumed that drug sensitivity is increased.[146] It is generally believed that the geriatric population is especially vulnerable to cardiovascular and anticholinergic side effects. With respect to the former, postural hypotension and the associated potential for falls and fractures should be carefully considered. For these reasons the choice of an antidepressant drug in the elderly depends on side effect profiles and potential drug-drug interactions rather than therapeutic efficacy. Direct comparisons, however, between young and elderly depressed patients, in terms of tolerability, pharmacokinetics, and efficacy are seldom conducted. This should be taken into consideration when investigating antidepressant drugs in populations of mixed age. Volz and Möller recently reviewed controlled clinical trials with antidepressants in elderly patients.[147] They conclude that the progress in scientific knowledge of depression in old age only increased moderately since 1980 and that there is a great need for well-designed studies.

4 OTHER INDICATIONS

Antidepressant drugs have been investigated in a host of other CNS indications. It is now well established that antidepressants, particularly the TCAs imipramine and clomipramine, have antipanic activity.[148] Recent evidence suggests that SSRIs may also have value in the treatment of obsessive-compulsive disorder and eating and personality disorders.[149] In chronic pain, however, controlled studies do not support the use of antidepressants.[150]

5 ANTIDEPRESSANT DRUGS OF THE FUTURE

The introduction of many new antidepressants over the last 15 years has improved the benefit-risk ratio for many patients by improving the tolerability. However, new-generation drugs like the SSRIs also have adverse effects, including gastrointestinal discomfort, restlessness, and drug-drug interactions.[151]

5.1 Ideal Antidepressant Drug Profile

An ideal antidepressant would effectively treat all forms of depression. Besides this broad spectrum of activity the drug would have a greater overall efficacy than currently used antidepressant drugs, in that it is effective in considerably more than 70% of the patients treated. A very important feature concerns the speed of onset in therapeutic response. A reliable antidepressant effect within one week after initiation of drug therapy would constitute a remarkable progress in the treatment of depression. It could preclude the long-term treatment with antidepressants which is today thought to be necessary to avoid relapses in depression. Theoretically, it seems possible to devise antidepressant strategies with a rapid onset of action in analogy to the acute (but short-lasting) antidepressant effect of a one-night sleep deprivation.[152] An ideal drug would exert these effects with a side effect profile that is virtually indistinguishable from that of placebo. Currently there are approximately 125 antidepressants in varying states of development.[153]

5.2 New Mechanisms of Action

A wealth of information has become available on the heterogeneity of serotonin receptors and the involvement of the serotonin system both in the pathophysiology of depression and in the mechanism and action of antidepressant drug treatment.[154] Thus far, however, this has not led to the introduction of new antidepressant drugs. It is thought that 5-HT1A and 5-HT2 receptors may be involved in the etiology of major depression and the therapeutic effects of antidepressant treatment.[155] Several agonists and antagonists for various serotonin receptor subtypes are currently in clinical testing for multiple psychiatric disorders.[156] The effects of drugs on 5-HT1A receptor sensitivity can be investigated in healthy volunteers using a buspirone neuroendocrine challenge paradigm.[157] Also the neuroendocrine effects induced by the 5-HT releaser fenfluramine have been used in clarifying the role of serotonin receptors in the mode of action of antidepressant drugs.[158]

It is important that both in the preclinical and clinical development of new antidepressant drugs there is room for serendipity.[159] In the evaluation of potentially new antidepressant drugs attention should be devoted to both novel animal models of depression and as yet not fully explored mechanisms of drug action.[160] The new generation of antidepressant drugs may be developed based on their ability to modify signal transductors (G proteins), or possibly to act at sites distal to receptors, such as second messenger complexes.[135]

In a recent article Katz and Maas emphasized that the adherence to a unitary model of depression and, as a consequence thereof, the overreliance on diagnosis and the use of global measures in clinical drug trials tend to obscure the action of drugs.[8] Creative new drug designs and trial methodology are encouraged as rational drug development is not just following a recipe.

6 CONCLUSIONS

It is well known that phase III development, in which the drug is given to large numbers of patients, is the most resource-intensive part of drug development. Therefore, it is of utmost importance that the first two phases provide unequivocal data on the tolerability and efficacy of the new antidepressant. The pharmacokinetic and pharmacodynamic characteristics, as studied in phase I, should give clear guidelines as to what dose range should be explored in phase II. After the completion of phase II clear dose recommendations for phase III should be possible.

ACKNOWLEDGMENTS

The contributions of Drs. S. Appel, Sandoz, Basel, Switzerland, and I.M. van Vliet, Department of Biological Psychiatry, University of Utrecht, The Netherlands are highly appreciated.

REFERENCES

1. Angst, J., Epidemiology of depression, *Psychopharmacology,* 106, S71, 1992.
2. Angst, J., Bech, P., Boyer, P., Bruinvels, J., Engel, R., Helmchen, H., Hippius, H., Lingjaerde, O., Racagni, G., Saletu, B., Sedvall, G., Silverstone, J. T., Stefanis, C. N., Stoll, K. and Woggon, B., Consensus conference on the methodology of clinical trials of antidepressants, Zurich, March 1988: Report of the Consensus Committee, *Pharmacopsychiatry,* 22, 3, 1989.
3. ECSC-EEC-EAEC, Guidelines on psychotropic drugs for the EC, *Eur. Neuropsychopharmacol.*, 4, 61, 1994.
4. Baldessarini, R. J., Current status of antidepressants: clinical pharmacology and comments, *J. Clin. Psychiatry,* 50, 117, 1989.
5. Cesura, A. M. and Pletscher, A., The new generation of monoamine oxidase inhibitors, in *Progress in Drug Research,* Jucker E., Ed., Birkhäuser Verlag, Basel, 1992, 174.
6. Rudorfer, M. V. and Potter, W. Z., Antidepressants — A comparative review of the clinical pharmacology and therapeutic use of the "newer" versus the "older" drugs, *Drugs,* 37, 713, 1989.
7. Quitkin, F. M. and Rabkin, J. G., Methodological problems in studies of depressive disorder: Utility of the discontinuation design, *J. Clin. Psychopharmacol.*, 1, 283, 1981.
8. Katz, M. M. and Maas, J. W., Psychopharmacology and the etiology of psychopathologic states: are we looking in the right way?, *Neuropsychopharmacology,* 10, 139, 1994.
9. Leonard, B. E., The comparative pharmacology of new antidepressants, *J. Clin. Psychiatry,* 54, 3, 1993.
10. Kapur, S. and Mann, J. J., Role of the dopaminergic system in depression, *Biol. Psychiatry,* 32, 1, 1992.
11. Williams, R. L., Dosage regimen design: Pharmacodynamic considerations, *J. Clin. Pharmacol.*, 32, 597, 1992.
12. Kroboth, P. D., Schmith, V. D. and Smith, R. B., Pharmacodynamic modeling — Application to new drug development, *Clin. Pharmacokinet.*, 20, 91, 1991.
13. Houston, J. B., Commentary — Utility of *in vitro* drug metabolism data in predicting *in vivo* metabolic clearance, *Biochem. Pharmacol.*, 47, 1469, 1994.
14. Furlanut, M., Benetello, P. and Spina, E., Pharmacokinetic optimisation of tricyclic antidepressant therapy, *Clin. Pharmacokinet.*, 24, 301, 1993.
15. Spina, E. and Caputi, A. P., Pharmacogenetic aspects in the metabolism of psychotropic drugs: Pharmacokinetic and clinical implications, *Pharmacol. Res.*, 29, 121, 1994.

16. Alvan, G., Clinical consequences of polymorphic drug oxidation, *Fundam. Clin. Pharmacol.*, 5, 209, 1991.
17. Meyer J. W., Woggon, B. and Kupfer, A., Importance of oxidative polymorphism on clinical efficacy and side-effects of imipramine: a retrospective study, *Pharmacopsychiatry*, 21, 365, 1988.
18. Brosen, K., The pharmacogenetics of the selective serotonin reuptake inhibitors, *Clin. Investig.*, 71, 1002, 1993.
19. van Harten, J., Clinical pharmacokinetics of selective serotonin reuptake inhibitors, *Clin. Pharmacokinet.*, 24, 203, 1993.
20. Caccia, S. and Garattini, S., Formation of active metabolites of psychotropic drugs — An updated review of their significance, *Clin. Pharmacokinet.*, 18, 434, 1990.
21. Caccia, S. and Garattini, S., Pharmacokinetic and pharmacodynamic significance of antidepressant drug metabolites, *Pharmacol. Res.*, 26, 317, 1992.
22. Bertilsson, L., Nordin, C., Otani, K., Resul, B., Scheinin, M., Siwers, B. and Sjöqvist, F., Disposition of single oral doses of E-10-hydroxynortriptyline in healthy subjects, with some observations on pharmacodynamic effects, *Clin. Pharmacol. Ther.*, 40, 261, 1986.
23. Koulu, M., Scheinin, M., Kaarttinen, A., Kallio, J., Pyykkö, K., Vuorinen, J. and Zimmer, R.H., Inhibition of monoamine oxidase by moclobemide: effects on monoamine metabolism and secretion of anterior pituitary hormones and cortisol in healthy volunteers, *Br. J. Clin. Pharmacol.*, 27, 243, 1989.
24. Ghose, K., Biochemical assessment of antidepressive drugs, *Br. J. Clin. Pharmacol.*, 10, 539, 1980.
25. Kerr, F.A. and Szabadi, E., Comparison of the effects of chronic administration of ciclazindol and desipramine on pupillary responses to tyramine, methoxamine and pilocarpine in healthy volunteers, *Br. J. Clin. Pharmacol.*, 19, 639, 1985.
26. Low, P. A. and Opfer-Gehrking, T. L., Differential effects of amitriptyline on sudomotor, cardiovagal, and adrenergic function in human subjects, *Muscle Nerv.*, 15, 1340, 1992.
27. Szabadi, E. and Bradshaw, C. M., Antidepressant drugs and the autonomic nervous system, in *The Biology of Depression*, Deakin, J. F. W., Ed., Royal College of Psychiatrists/Gaskell, London, 1986, 190.
28. Allain, H., Lieury, A., Brunet-Bourgin, F., Mirabaud, Ch., Trebon, P., Le-Coz, F. and Gandon, J.M., Antidepressants and cognition: comparative effects of moclobemide, viloxazine, and maprotiline. *Psychopharmacology,* 106 (Suppl.), S56, 1992.
29. Hindmarch, I., Relevant psychometric tests for antidepressants and anxiolytics, *Int. Clin. Psychopharmacol.*, 9, Suppl. 1, 27, 1994.
30. Thompson, P. J., Antidepressants and memory: A review, *Hum. Psychopharmacol.*, 6, 79, 1991.
31. Hindmarch, I., A pharmacological profile of fluoxetine and other antidepressants on aspects of skilled performance and car handling ability, *Br. J. Psychiatry*, 153, Suppl. 3, 99, 1988.
32. O'Hanlon, J. F., Brookhuis, K. A., Louwerens, J. W. and Volkerts, E. R., Performance testing as part of drug registration, in *Drugs and Driving*, O'Hanlon, J. F. and De Gier, J. J., Eds., Taylor & Francis, London, 1986.
33. Ramaekers, J. G., Swijgman, H. F. and O'Hanlon, J. F. Effects of moclobemide and mianserin on highway driving, psychometric performance and subjective parameters, relative to placebo, *Psychopharmacology,* 106, S62, 1992.
34. Dingemanse, J., Kinetics and dynamics of drug effects on the nervous system, in *The In Vivo Study of Drug Action. Principles and Applications of Kinetic-Dynamic Modeling,* Van Boxtel, C. J., Holford, N. H. G. and Danhof, M., Eds., Elsevier, Amsterdam, 1992, 113.
35. Spring, B., Gelenberg, A. J., Garvin, R. and Thompson, S., Amitriptyline, clovoxamine and cognitive function: a placebo-controlled comparison in depressed outpatients, *Psychopharmacology*, 108, 327, 1992.
36. Hobi, V., Gastpar, M., Gastpar, G., Gilsdorf, U., Kielholz, P. and Schwarz, E., Driving ability of depressive patients under antidepressants, *J. Int. Med. Res.*, 10, 65, 1982.
37. Tiller, J. W. G., Antidepressants, alcohol and psychomotor performance, *Acta Psychiatr. Scand.*, Suppl. 360, 13, 1990.
38. Saletu, B., Pharmaco-EEG profiles of typical and atypical antidepressants, in *Typical and Atypical Antidepressants: Clinical Practice*, Costa, E. and Racagni, G., Eds., Raven Press, New York, 1982, 257.
39. Herrmann, W. M., Schärer, E. and Delini-Stula, A., Predictive value of pharmaco-electroencephalography in early human-pharmacological evaluations of psychoactive drugs, *Pharmacopsychiatry*, 24, 196, 1991.
40. Herrmann, W. M., Schärer, E., Wendt, G. and Delini-Stula, A., Pharmaco-EEG profile of levoprotiline: Second example to discuss the predictive value of pharmaco-electroencephalography in early human pharmacological evaluations of psychoactive drugs, *Pharmacopsychiatry*, 24, 206, 1991.
41. Herrmann, W. M., Schärer, E., Wendt, G. and Delini-Stula, A., Pharmaco-EEG profile of maroxepine: Third example to discuss the predictive value of pharmaco-electroencephalography in early human pharmacological evaluations of psychoactive drugs, *Pharmacopsychiatry*, 24, 214, 1991.
42. Keshavan, M. S., Kapur, S. and Pettegrew, J. W., Magnetic resonance spectroscopy in psychiatry: potential, pitfalls, and promise, *Am. J. Psychiatry*, 148, 976, 1991.
43. Boles Ponto, L. L. and Ponto, J. A., Uses and limitations of positron emission tomography in clinical pharmacokinetics/dynamics (Part I), *Clin. Pharmacokinet.*, 22, 211, 1992.
44. Boles Ponto, L. L. and Ponto, J. A., Uses and limitations of positron emission tomography in clinical pharmacokinetics/dynamics (Part II), *Clin. Pharmacokinet.*, 22, 274, 1992.
45. Dingemanse, J., Danhof, M. and Breimer, D. D., Pharmacokinetic — pharmacodynamic modeling of CNS drug effects. An overview. *Pharmacol. Ther.*, 38, 1, 1988.

46. Greenblatt, D. J. and Harmatz, J. S., Kinetic-dynamic modeling in clinical psychopharmacology, *J. Clin. Psychopharmacol.*, 13, 231, 1993.
47. van Peer, A., Snoeck, E., Huang, M.-L. and Heykants, J., Pharmacokinetic-pharmacodynamic relationships in phase I/phase II of drug development, *Eur. J. Drug Metab. Pharmacokinet.*, 18, 49, 1993.
48. Rosholm, J.-U., Hallas, J. and Gram, L. F., Concurrent use of more than one major psychotropic drug (polypsychopharmacy) in out-patients — A prescription database study, *Br. J. Clin. Pharmacol.*, 37, 533, 1994.
49. Cousins, D. H. and Crow, T. J., Drug interactions involving antidepressants (including bicyclic, tricyclic and tetracyclic agents, excluding MAOIs) and lithium, in *Nervous System, Endocrine System and Infusion Therapy*, Petrie, Ed., Elsevier Science Publishers, Amsterdam, 1984, 53.
50. Feighner, J. P., Boyer, W. F., Tyler, D. L. and Neborsky, R. J., Adverse consequences of fluoxetine-MAOI combination therapy, *J. Clin. Psychiatry*, 51, 222, 1990.
51. Dingemanse, J., An update of recent moclobemide interaction data, *Int. Clin. Psychopharmacol.*, 7, 167, 1993.
52. Jerling, M., Bertilsson, L. and Sjoqvist, F., The use of therapeutic drug monitoring data to document kinetic drug interactions: an example with amitriptyline and nortriptyline, *Ther. Drug Monit.*, 16, 1, 1994.
53. Preskorn, S. H., Alderman, J., Chung, M., Harrison, W., Messig, M. and Harris, S., Pharmacokinetics of desipramine coadministered with sertraline or fluoxetine, *J. Clin. Psychopharmacol.*, 14, 90, 1994.
54. Bergstrom, R. F., Peyton, A. L. and Lemberger, L., Quantification and mechanism of the fluoxetine and tricyclic antidepressant interaction, *Clin. Pharmacol. Ther.*, 51, 239, 1992.
55. Korn, A., Da Prada, M., Raffesberg, W., Allen, S. and Gasic, S., Tyramine pressor effect in man: studies with moclobemide, a novel, reversible monoamine oxidase inhibitor, *J. Neural Transm.*, 26, Suppl., 57, 1988.
56. Shoaf, S. E. and Linnoila, M., Interaction of ethanol and smoking on the pharmacokinetics and pharmacodynamics of psychotropic medications, *Psychopharmacol. Bull.*, 27, 577, 1991.
57. Reimann, I. W., Firkusny, L., Antonin, K. H. and Bieck, P. R., Oxaprotiline: enantioselective noradrenaline uptake inhibition indicated by intravenous amine pressor tests but not α_2-adrenoceptor binding to intact platelets in man, *Eur. J. Clin. Pharmacol.*, 44, 93, 1993.
58. Ariëns, E. J. and Wuis, E. W., Bias in pharmacokinetics and clinical pharmacology, *Clin. Pharmacol. Ther.*, 42, 361, 1987.
59. Laughren, T. P., The review of clinical safety data in a new drug application, *Psychopharmacol. Bull.*, 25, 5, 1989.
60. Smith, A., Traganza, E. and Harrison, G., Studies on the effectiveness of antidepressant drugs, *Psychopharmacol. Bull.*, 5, 1, 1969.
61. Food and Drug Administration, Guidelines for the clinical evaluation of antidepressant drugs (FDA 77 - 3042), Washington, D.C., 1977.
62. World Health Organization, Regional Office for Europe, *The Clinical Investigation of Antidepressant Drugs*, 2nd ed., 1988.
63. Woggon, B., Methodology of measuring the efficacy of antidepressants — European viewpoint, *Psychopharmacology*, 106, S90, 1992.
64. Eisenberg, L., Treating depression and anxiety in primary care, *N. Engl. J. Med.*, 326, 1080, 1992.
65. Perez-Stable, E. J., Miranda, J., Munoz, R. F. and Ying, Y. W., Depression in medical outpatients. Underrecognition and misdiagnosis, *Arch. Int. Med.*, 150, 1083, 1990.
66. American Psychiatric Association, *Diagnostic and Statistical Manual of Mental Disorders*, 4th ed., Washington D.C., 1994.
67. Carroll, B. J., Problems with diagnostic criteria for depression, *J. Clin. Psychiatry*, 45, 14, 1984.
68. Overall, J. E., Donachie, N. D. and Faillace, L. A., Implications of restrictive diagnosis for compliance to antidepressant drug therapy: alprazolam versus imipramine, *J. Clin. Psychiatry*, 48, 51, 1987.
69. Burrows, G. D., Judd, F. K. and Norman, T. R., Differential diagnosis and drug treatment of panic disorder, anxiety and depression, *CNS Drugs*, 1, 119, 1994.
70. Prien, R. F. and Levine, J., Research and methodological issues for evaluating the therapeutic effectiveness of antidepressant drugs, *Psychopharmacol. Bull.*, 20, 250, 1984.
71. Steckler, T., Hosten, K. and Müller-Oerlinghausen, B., Feasibility of phase II or III antidepressant studies under consideration of today's demands for inclusion and exclusion criteria, *Nervenarzt*, 64, 204, 1993.
72. Hamilton, M., Development of a rating scale for primary depressive illness, *Br. J. Soc. Clin. Psychol.*, 6, 278, 1967.
73. Montgomery, S. A. and Asberg, M., A new depression scale designed to be sensitive to change, *Br. J. Psychiatry*, 134, 382, 1979.
74. Lambert, M. J., Hatch, D. R., Kingston, M. D., et al. Zung, Beck and Hamilton rating scales as measures of treatment outcome; a meta-analytic comparison, *J. Consult. Clin. Psychol.*, 54, 54, 1986.
75. Prien, R. F., Carpenter, L. L. and Kupfer, D. J., The definition and operational criteria for treatment outcome of major depressive disorder. A review of the current research literature, *Arch. Gen. Psychiatry*, 48, 796, 1991.
76. Angst, J., Delini-Stula, A., Stabl, M. and Stassen, H. H., Is a cut-off score a suitable measure of treatment outcome in short-term trials in depression? A methodological meta-analysis, *Hum. Psychopharmacol.*, 8, 311, 1993.
77. Quitkin, F. M., Methodology of measuring the efficacy of antidepressants, *Psychopharmacology*, 106, S87, 1992.
78. Benkert, O. and Maier, W., Commentary — The necessity of placebo application in psychotropic drug trials, *Pharmacopsychiatry*, 23, 203, 1990.

79. D'Amico, M. F., Roberts, D. L., Robinson, D. S., Schwiderski, U. E. and Copp, J., Placebo-controlled dose-ranging trial designs in phase II development of nefazodone, *Psychopharmacol. Bull.*, 26, 147, 1990.
80. Temple, R., Dose-response and registration of new drugs, in *Dose-Response Relationships in Clinical Pharmacology*, Lasagna, L., Erill, S. and Naranjo, C. A., Eds., Elsevier Science Publishers, Amsterdam, 1989, 145.
81. Klimt, C. R., The conduct and principles of randomized clinical trials, *Controlled Clin. Trials*, 1, 283, 1981.
82. Hsu, P.-H. and Laddu, A. R., Analysis of adverse events in a dose titration study, *J. Clin. Pharmacol.*, 34, 136, 1994.
83. Leber, P. D., Hazards of inference: the active control investigation, *Epilepsia*, 30, Suppl. 1, S57, 1989.
84. Ferner, U. and Neumann, N., Active control equivalence trials: some methodological aspects, *Psychopharmacology*, 106, S93, 1992.
85. Bridges, P. K., Point of view, *Br. J. Psychiatry*, 142, 676, 1983.
86. Gram, L. F., Dose-effect relationships for tricyclic antidepressants: The basis for rational clinical testing of new antidepressants, *Psychopharmacol. Ser.*, 10, 163, 1993.
87. Khan, A., Cohen, S., Dager, S., Avery, D. H. and Dunner, D. L., Onset of response in relation to outcome in depressed outpatients with placebo and imipramine, *J. Affect. Disord.*, 17, 33, 1989.
88. Quitkin, F. M., Rabkin, J. G., Ross, D. and McGrath, P. J., Duration of antidepressant drug treatment, *Arch. Gen. Psychiatry*, 41, 238, 1984.
89. Quitkin, F. M., Rabkin, J. G., Stewart, J., McGrath, P. J. and Harrison, W. J., Study duration in antidepressant research: advantages of a 12 week trial, *J. Psychiatry Res.*, 20, 211, 1986.
90. Howland, R. H., Chronic depression, *Hosp. Commun. Psychiatry*, 44, 633, 1993.
91. Angst, J., Bech, P., Bruinvels, J., Engel, R. R., Ferner, U., Guelfi, J. D., Lingjaerde, O., Müller-Oerlinghausen, B., Paes de Sousa, M., Paykel, E., Rimon, R., Rzewuska, M., Saletu, B., Spiegel, R., Stassen, H. H., Stoll, K. D., Wiesel, F. A., Woggon, B. and Zvolsky, P., Report on the fifth consensus conference: Methodology of long-term clinical trials in psychiatry, *Pharmacopsychiatry*, 27, 101, 1994.
92. Stassen, H. H., Delini-Stula, A. and Angst, J., Time course of improvement under antidepressant treatment: A survival-analytical approach, *Eur. Neuropsychopharmacol.*, 3, 127, 1993.
93. Dunlop, S. R., Dornseif, B. E. and Wernicke, J. F., Pattern analysis shows beneficial effect of fluoxetine treatment of mild depression, *Psychopharmacol. Bull.*, 26, 173, 1990.
94. Mueller-Oerlinghausen, B. and Renfordt, E., Time-blind analysis and other video-strategies in phase II trials of psychotropic drugs, *Int. J. Clin. Pharmacol. Ther. Toxicol.*, 18, 99, 1980.
95. Byrne, M. M., Meta-analysis of early phase II studies with paroxetine in hospitalized depressed patients, *Acta Psychiatr. Scand.*, 80, Suppl. 350, 138, 1989.
96. Thacker, S. B., Meta-analysis: A quantitative approach to research integration, *JAMA*, 259, 1685, 1988.
97. Schmauss, M. and Erfurth, A., Predicting antidepressive treatment success. Critical review and perspectives, *Fortsch. Neurol. Psychiatry*, 61, 274, 1993.
98. Davidson, J. R. T., Giller, E. L., Zisook, S. and Helms, M. J., Predictors of response to monoamine oxidase inhibitors: do they exist?, *Eur. Arch. Psychiatry Clin. Neurosci.*, 241, 181, 1991.
99. Balon, R., Monoamine specificity of antidepressants and prediction of therapeutic response, *Encephale*, 17, 121, 1991.
100. Asberg, M. and Wagner, A., Biochemical effects of antidepressant treatment — studies of monoamine metabolites in cerebrospinal fluid and platelet (3H)imipramine binding, *Ciba Found. Symp.*, 123, 57, 1986.
101. Davis, B. A. and Boulton, A. A., The trace amines and their acidic metabolites in depression — An Overview, *Prog. Neuro-Psychopharmacol. Biol. Psychiatry*, 18, 17, 1994.
102. Møller, S. E. and Danish University Antidepressant Group, Plasma amino acid profiles in relation to clinical response to moclobemide in patients with major depression, *J. Affect. Disord.*, 27, 225, 1993.
103. Da Prada, M., Cesura, A. M., Launay, J. M. and Richards, J. G., Platelets as a model for neurones?, *Experientia*, 44, 115, 1988.
104. Wood, K. and Coppen, A., Psychiatry and platelets, in *Progress in Pharmacology*, Gustav Fischer Verlag, Stuttgart/New York, 1982, 4/4, 147.
105. Robinson, D. S. and Kurtz, N. M., Monoamine oxidase inhibiting drugs: pharmacologic and therapeutic issues, in *Psychopharmacology: The Third Generation of Progress*, Meltzer, Ed., Raven Press, New York, 1987, 1297.
106. Langer, S. Z., Galzin, A. M., Lee, C. R. and Schoemaker, H., Antidepressant-binding sites in brain and platelets, *Ciba Found. Symp.*, 123, 3, 1986.
107. Gronier, B., Azorin, J. M., Dassa, D. and Jeanningros, R., Lack of association between platelet tritiated imipramine binding and clinical status of depressed patients on chronic antidepressant treatment, *Eur. Neuropsychopharmacol.*, 4, 7, 1994.
108. Gronier, B., Azorin, J. M., Dassa, D. and Jeanningros, R., Evidence for a defective platelet L-tryptophan transport in depressed patients, *Int. Clin. Psychopharmacol.*, 8, 87, 1993.
109. Carroll, B. J., Feinberg, M., Greden, J. F., Tarika, J., Albala, A. A., Haskett, R. F., James, N. McI., Kronfol, Z., Lohr, N., Steiner, M., de Vigne, J. P. and Young, E., A specific laboratory test for the diagnosis of melancholia — Standardization, validation, and clinical utility, *Arch. Gen. Psychiatry*, 38, 15, 1981.
110. Langer, G., Koinig, G., Hatzinger, R., Schönbeck, G., Resch, F., Aschauer, H., Keshavan, M. S. and Sieghart, W., Response of thyrotropin to thyrotropin-releasing hormone as predictor of treatment outcome — Prediction of recovery and relapse in treatment with antidepressants and neuroleptics, *Arch. Gen. Psychiatry*, 43, 861, 1986.

111. Loosen, P. T., The TRH-induced TSH response in psychiatric patients: a possible neuroendocrine marker, *Psychoneuroendocrinology*, 10, 237, 1985.
112. Brown, G. M., Neuroendocrine probes as biological markers of affective disorders: new directions, *Can. J. Psychiatry*, 34, 819, 1989.
113. Srinivasan, V., Psychoactive drugs, pineal gland and affective disorders, *Prog. Neuropsychopharmacol. Biol. Psychiatry*, 13, 653, 1989.
114. Mendlewicz, J., Sleep-related chronobiological markers of affective illness, *Int. J. Psychophysiol.*, 10, 245, 1991.
115. Steiger, A., von Bardeleben, U., Guldner, J., Lauer, C., Rothe, B. and Holsboer, F., The sleep EEG and nocturnal hormonal secretion studies on changes during the course of depression and on effects of CNS-active drugs, *Prog. Neuropsychopharmacol. Biol. Psychiatry*, 17, 125, 1993.
116. Dawkins, K. and Potter, W. Z., Gender differences in pharmacokinetics and pharmacodynamics of psychotropics: Focus on women, *Psychopharmacol. Bull.*, 27, 417, 1991.
117. Kupfer, D. J., REM latency: a psychobiologic marker for primary depressive disease, *Biol. Psychiatry*, 11, 159, 1976.
118. Buchsbaum, M. S., Brain imaging in the search for biological markers in affective disorder, *J. Clin. Psychiatry*, 47, 7, 1986.
119. Poirier, M. F., Recovery from depression. Psychobiologic criteria of recovery, *Encephale*, 19, 451, 1993.
120. American Psychiatric Association, Tricyclic antidepressants — Blood level measurements and clinical outcome: An APA task force report, *Am. J. Psychiatry*, 142, 155, 1985.
121. Fritze, J., Becker, T., Ziegler, V., Laux, G. and Riederer, P., Brofaromine (CGP 11 305 A) in treatment of depression: biological estimation of plasma concentrations, *Pharmacopsychiatry*, 23, 131, 1990.
122. Noguchi, T., Shimoda, K. and Takahashi, S., Clinical significance of plasma levels of clomipramine, its hydroxylated and desmethylated metabolites: prediction of clinical outcome in mood disorders using discriminant analysis of therapeutic drug monitoring data, *J. Affect. Disord.*, 29, 267, 1993.
123. Kehoe, W. A., Harralson, A. F., Kwentus, J. A., Jacisin, J. J., Sheffel, W. B. and Hetnal, M. J., Early individualization of tricyclic antidepressant dosing using a Bayesian pharmacokinetic model, *DICP, Ann. Pharmacother.*, 25, 1368, 1991.
124. Hashimoto, Y. and Sheiner, L. B., Designs for population pharmacodynamics: value of pharmacokinetic data and population analysis, *J. Pharmacokin. Biopharmaceutics*, 19, 333, 1991.
125. Rowland, M. and Aarons, L., Eds., *New Strategies in Drug Development and Clinical Evaluation: The Population Approach*, Commission of the European Communities, Brussels, 1992.
126. Sanathanan, L. P., Peck, C., Temple, R., Lieberman, R. and Pledger, G., Randomization, PK-controlled dosing, and titration: an integrated approach for designing clinical trials, *Drug Inform. J.*, 25, 425, 1991.
127. Greenberg, R. N., Overview of patient compliance with medication dosing: a literature review, *Clin. Ther.*, 65, 590, 1984.
128. Babiker, I. E., Non-compliance in schizophrenia, *Psychiat. Dev.*, 4, 329, 1986.
129. Crome, P., Drug compliance in the elderly, in: *Psychopharmacology of Old Age*, Wheatley, D., Ed., Oxford University Press, Oxford, 1982, 55.
130. Urquhart, J., Ascertaining how much compliance is enough with outpatient antibiotic regimens, *Postgrad. Med. J.*, 68, Suppl. 3, S49, 1992.
131. Selai, C. E. and Trimble, M. R., The role of quality of life measures in psychopharmacoloy, *Hum. Psychopharmacol.*, 9, 211, 1994.
132. Jonsson, B. and Bebbington, P., Economic studies of the treatment of depressive illness, in *Health Economics of Depression*, Jonsson, B. and Rosenbaum, J., Eds., Chichester, Wiley, 1993, 35.
133. Pedersen, O. L., Gram, L. F., Kristensen, C. B., Møller, M., Thayssen, P., Bjerre, M., Kragh-Sørensen, P., Klitgaard, N. A., Sindrup, E., Hole, P. and Brinkløv, M., Overdosage of antidepressants: Clinical and pharmacokinetic aspects, *Eur. J. Clin. Pharmacol*, 239, 513, 1982.
134. Henry, J. A. and Antao, C. A., Suicide and fatal antidepressant poisoning, *Eur. J. Med.*, 1, 343, 1992.
135. Leonard, B. E., Biochemical strategies for the development of antidepressants, *CNS Drugs*, 1, 285, 1994.
136. Freemantle, N., House, A., Song, F., Mason, J. M. and Sheldon, T. A., Prescribing selective serotonin reuptake inhibitors as strategy for prevention of suicide, *BMJ*, 309, 249, 1994.
137. Neuvonen, P. J., Pohjola-Sintonen, S., Tacke, U. and Vuori, E., Five fatal cases of serotonin syndrome after moclobemide-citalopram or moclobemide-clomipramine overdoses, *Lancet*, 342, 1419, 1993.
138. Cafferata, G. L., Kasper, J. and Bernstein, A., Family roles, structure, and stressors in relation to sex differences in obtaining psychotropic drugs, *J. Health Soc. Behav.*, 24, 132, 1983.
139. Yonkers, K. A., Kando, J. C., Cole, J. O. and Blumenthal, S., Gender differences in pharmacokinetics and pharmacodynamics of psychotropic medication, *Am. J. Psychiatry*, 149, 587, 1992.
140. Wilson, K., Sex-related differences in drug disposition in man, *Clin. Pharmacokinet.*, 9, 189, 1984.
141. Food and Drug Administration, Guideline for the study and evaluation of gender differences in the clinical evaluation of drugs, *Fed. Reg.*, 58, no. 139, 1993.
142. Marchetti, F., Romero, M., Bonati, M. and Tognoni, G., Use of psychotropic drugs during pregnancy. A report of the international cooperative drug use in pregnancy (DUP) study. Collaborative Group on Drug Use in Pregnancy (CGDUP), *Eur. J. Clin. Pharmacol.*, 45, 495, 1993.

143. Blazer, D., Depression in the elderly, *N. Engl. J. Med.*, 320, 164, 1989.
144. Bressler, R. and Katz, M. D., Drug therapy for geriatric depression, *Drugs Aging*, 3, 195, 1993.
145. von Moltke, L. L., Greenblatt, D. J. and Shader, R. I., Clinical pharmacokinetics of antidepressants in the elderly — Therapeutic implications, *Clin. Pharmacokinet.*, 24, 141, 1993.
146. Nolan, L. and O'Malley, K., Adverse effects of antidepressants in the elderly, *Drugs Aging*, 2, 450, 1992.
147. Volz, H.-P. and Möller, H.-J., Antidepressant drug therapy in the elderly — A critical review of the controlled clinical trials conducted since 1980, *Pharmacopsychiatry*, 27, 93, 1994.
148. Nutt, D. J. and Glue, P., Clinical pharmacology of anxiolytics and antidepressants: A psychopharmacological perspective, *Pharmac. Ther.*, 44, 309, 1989.
149. Kasper, S., Fuger, J. and Möller, H.-J., Comparative efficacy of antidepressants, *Drugs*, 43, Suppl. 2, 11, 1992.
150. Walsh, T. D., Antidepressants in chronic pain, *Clin. Neuropharmacol.*, 6, 271, 1983.
151. Rudorfer, M. V., Manji, H. K. and Potter, W. Z., Comparative tolerability profiles of the newer versus older antidepressants, *Drug Safety*, 10, 18, 1994.
152. Blier, P. and de Montigny, C., Current advances and trends in the treatment of depression, *TIPS*, 15, 220, 1994.
153. Editorial, Antidepressants in clinical development, *Scrip*, 10, 1659, 1991.
154. Risch, S. C. and Nemeroff, C. B., Neurochemical alterations of serotonergic neuronal systems in depression, *J. Clin. Psychiatry*, 53, 3, 1992.
155. Cowen, P.J., Serotonin receptor subtypes: implications for psychopharmacology, *Br. J. Psychiatry*, Suppl. 12, 7, 1991.
156. Stahl, S. M., Editorial — Serotonergic mechanisms and the new antidepressants, *Psychol. Med.*, 23, 281, 1993.
157. Herdman, J. R., Cowen, P. J., Campling, G. M., Hockney, R. A., Laver, D. and Sharpley, A. L., Effect of lofepramine on 5-HT function and sleep, *J. Affect. Disord.*, 29, 63, 1993.
158. Stahl, S. M., Hauger, R. L., Rausch, J. L., Fleishaker, J. C. and Hubbell-Alberts, E., Downregulation of serotonin receptor subtypes by nortriptyline and adinazolam in major depressive disorder: neuroendocrine and platelet markers, *Clin. Neuropharmacol.*, 16, Suppl. 3, S19, 1993.
159. Pletscher, A., The discovery of antidepressants: A winding path, *Experientia*, 47, 4, 1991.
160. Moreau, J.-L., Borgulya, J., Jenck, F. and Martin, J. R., Tolcapone: a potential new antidepressant detected in a novel animal model of depression, *Behav. Pharmacol.*, 5, 344, 1994.

Chapter 25

Antipsychotic Agents

Christopher G. G. Link and Christopher G. Jones

CONTENTS

1 Introduction ... 347
2 Healthy Volunteers ... 348
  2.1 Selection Criteria ... 348
  2.2 Safety Considerations ... 348
  2.3 Methods ... 349
    2.3.1 General Trial Design ... 349
    2.3.2 Pharmacokinetic Issues ... 349
    2.3.3 Pharmacodynamic Issues ... 349
3 Patient Studies ... 349
  3.1 Suitability ... 349
  3.2 Selection Criteria ... 349
  3.3 Safety Considerations ... 350
  3.4 Methods ... 350
    3.4.1 Pharmacokinetics ... 350
    3.4.2 Surrogate Markers ... 350
  3.5 Placebo or Active Control ... 351
  3.6 Informed Consent ... 351
  3.7 Size and Duration of Trials ... 352
4 Decision Making ... 352
References ... 353

1 INTRODUCTION

There are several distinct chemical groups of antipsychotics. The phenothiazine derivatives group consists of three subgroups: group 1 (e.g., chlorpromazine); group 2 (e.g., thioridazine); and group 3 (e.g., fluphenazine) based on their sedative, antimuscarinic, and extrapyramidal side effects. Other groups include the butyrophenones (e.g., haloperidol); the diphenylbutylpiperidines (e.g., pimozide); the thioxanthines (e.g., flupenthixol); the substituted benzamides (e.g., remoxipride); oxypertine; loxapine; the benzisoxazole derivatives (e.g., risperidone); and the atypical dibenzodiazepines (e.g., clozapine) and atypical dibenzothiazepines (e.g., Quetiapine™).* (Editor's note: generic name required.)

Antipsychotic agents or neuroleptics are used to treat a variety of psychiatric disorders, which range from minor behavioral disturbances in elderly patients, to the major functional psychoses such as mania and schizophrenia. To illustrate the rationale behind the use of antipsychotic agents in CNS diseases, this chapter will focus on phase I and II trials in schizophrenia.

Schizophrenia is the most difficult of the major psychiatric syndromes to define and describe. Essentially, in acute schizophrenia the predominant clinical features are "positive" symptoms: delusions, hallucinations, and abnormal thought processes. By contrast, the main features of chronic schizophrenia are "negative" symptoms: apathy, lack of drive, slowness, and social withdrawal. The latter can be primary (arising from the disease process itself), or secondary, e.g., antipsychotic medication.

Over the last 4 decades the effectiveness of antipsychotic medication in the treatment of acute schizophrenia has been established by several controlled, double-blind studies (Cole et al., 1964). Regardless of which antipsychotic is studied, approximately 70% of patients receiving antipsychotic medication improve clinically. The main effects are on the positive symptoms, with little effect on the

* Quetiapine is a trademark, the property of Zeneca Pharmaceuticals.

0-8493-9230-6/97/$0.00+$.50
© 1997 by CRC Press, Inc.

negative symptoms. There is also good evidence that continued therapy prevents relapse. However, not all patients respond to currently available drugs. Neither standard antipsychotics, nor the newer atypical agents, ameliorate positive symptoms in all chronic schizophrenics. This treatment-resistant patient population still represents a significant medical need. In addition, the safety profile of the currently available antipsychotic agents is unacceptably poor. Common side effects of these drugs include: effects on the CNS (e.g., sedation, lowered fit threshold) and cardiovascular systems (e.g., postural hypotension, tachycardia, ECG changes and cardiac arrhythmias), and anticholinergic effects (e.g., dry mouth, blurred vision, constipation and impaired micturition). Extrapyramidal side effects (EPS) such as acute dystonia, parkinsonism, akathisia, and tardive dyskinesia can be distressing to the patient and limit acceptability and compliance. Other less common side effects, such as agranulocytosis and neuroleptic malignant syndrome (NMS) are potentially fatal.

In routine practice, clinical judgement is employed to make diagnoses and assess efficacy. However, for research purposes, operationalized criteria such as those found in ICD 10 (World Health Organization, 1994) and DSM IV (American Psychiatric Association, 1994) are to be preferred as they offer a structured approach to diagnosis, allowing definition of a homogeneous subject population for clinical research. Similarly, clinical improvements during experimental treatment may be assessed using observer rating scales such as BPRS (Overall and Gorham, 1962), CGI (*ECDU Assessment Manual for Psychopharmacology*, 1976), PANSS (Kay et al., 1986), SANS (Andreasen, 1984), SAPS (Andreasen, 1984).* Safety may be assessed using standard clinical measures (e.g., physical examination, vital signs, clinical laboratory monitoring, spontaneously elicited adverse events) as well as specific rating scales such as Simpson Scale (Simpson and Angus, 1970), AIMS (*ECDU Assessment Manual for Psychopharmacology*, 1976)** and Barnes Akathisia Scale (Barnes, 1989).

In the following sections practical considerations in undertaking a phase I and II development program for a new antipsychotic drug for the indication of schizophrenia will be discussed.

2 HEALTHY VOLUNTEERS

Healthy volunteers may be used to assess the safety, tolerance, pharmacokinetics, and pharmacodynamics of the experimental compound. An initial limited single-dose volunteer program may provide data on whether the putative antipsychotic penetrates the blood-brain barrier (e.g., by use of quantitative EEG techniques), the likely safety profile, the dose range (maximum tolerated dose), and duration of action which will assist choice of dosing regimen (o.d., b.d. or t.i.d. dosing). However, healthy volunteers are often exquisitely sensitive to the sedative effects of the classical antipsychotics and therefore the dose range which can be studied may be severely limited. Multiple dose studies in healthy volunteers are unlikely to add any useful additional safety data and should be considered superfluous. Multiple dose studies in patients are more appropriate in providing an assessment of safety, efficacy, and pharmacokinetics in the clinical setting.

2.1 Selection Criteria

The standard selection criteria for healthy volunteers should be applied.

2.2 Safety Considerations

As mentioned already, the use of healthy volunteers in assessing antipsychotic medications is of limited value with respect to both safety and efficacy. At best, studies on healthy volunteers will provide a preliminary evaluation of the general side effect and safety profiles with specific reference to CNS effects (sedation, acute dystonic reactions, EPS, akathisia) and hematological effects (particularly white blood cell counts). Although valuable information can be obtained on these safety parameters, information on the likely dose range to be employed in patients may be unobtainable in healthy volunteers. For example, the sedative effects of chlorpromazine preclude dosing of volunteers to clinically relevant doses.

* Brief Psychiatric Rating Scale (BPRS), Clinical Global Impressions (CGI), Positive and Negative Syndrome scale (PANSS), Scale for the Assessment of Negative Symptoms (SANS), Scale for the Assessment of Positive Symptoms (SAPS).

** Abnormal Involuntary Movement Scale (AIMS).

2.3 Methods

2.3.1 General Trial Design

The objectives of an initial healthy volunteer study can include: the assessment of safety and tolerance of single doses of the compound; generation of preliminary pharmacokinetic data; assessment of the duration of action and pharmacodynamic effects of the compound using, for example, quantitative EEG.

The standard considerations in terms of a safe starting dose and a single ascending dose apply to the investigation of antipsychotic agents.

2.3.2 Pharmacokinetic Issues

The standard pharmacokinetic parameters can be determined during the initial single dose volunteer trial. However, the pharmacodynamic effects of the drug in healthy volunteers may bear no relationship to its kinetic profile (e.g., a short pharmacokinetic half-life will not necessarily predict a short pharmacodynamic duration of action at the brain receptor site). This is different from many other therapeutic areas of clinical research.

2.3.3 Pharmacodynamic Issues

The importance of well-designed studies to investigate the pharmacodynamics of the compound cannot be overstated. The ability of modern brain imaging techniques to visualize brain activity *in vivo* affords a unique opportunity to correlate pharmacokinetic and pharmacodynamic effects of centrally active drugs.

Following on from the first single-dose trial, volunteer studies should be limited to pharmacodynamic evaluations such as positron-emission tomography (PET) to confirm the receptor pharmacology of the compound in man. Studies of this type provide invaluable information regarding penetration of the compound into the human brain, brain receptor occupancy (D_1, D_2, and $5HT_2$ receptors are of particular interest and may be visualized *in vivo* using this technique), and the time-course of receptor occupancy. These pharmacodynamic data can be viewed as "surrogate" clinical endpoints.

An appropriate design for a PET volunteer study is an open label, single-dose trial in up to 15 volunteers, using doses of compound based on the information obtained from the first volunteer study. Repeated PET scans, using appropriate ligands, will evaluate percentage occupancy of D_1, D_2, and $5HT_2$ receptors at various timepoints post dosing. These data will provide an estimate of the likely treatment regimen for subsequent patient studies.

3 PATIENT STUDIES

3.1 Suitability

As already explained, studies in the target patient population, rather than volunteers, should commence early to evaluate the antipsychotic potential of new compounds, since the questions which can be addressed using models in volunteers are limited.

3.2 Selection Criteria

The following should be considered as reasonable minimum requirements for studies in schizophrenic patients:

Inclusion criteria — Prospective patients should be expected to meet the following criteria:

- Male and female patients aged over 18 years old
- DSM IV diagnostic criteria for the chosen categories of schizophrenia, e.g., chronic or subchronic schizophrenia with acute exacerbation
- Clinical Global Impressions (CGI) Severity of Illness score ≥4 (moderate)
- Brief Psychiatric Rating Scale (BPRS) total item score ≥27, using the 0 to 6 point scoring system
- BPRS item score ≥3 (moderate) on two or more of the following:
  - Item 4 conceptual disorganization
  - Item 11 suspiciousness
  - Item 12 hallucinatory behavior
  - Item 15 unusual thought content
- Those subjects receiving long-acting, depot antipsychotic medication should receive their last injection not less than one dosing interval before the start of randomized treatment
- Provision of informed consent

Exclusion criteria — Prospective patients should be excluded if any of the following apply:

- Pregnant (as demonstrated by a positive serum HCG test) or lactating females
- Female patients who, in the opinion of the investigator, are at risk of becoming pregnant
- Participation in an investigational drug trial within 4 weeks of screening
- Evidence of any clinical disorder, laboratory, or ECG finding which makes the patient unsuitable to receive an investigation new drug in the opinion of the researcher

3.3 Safety Considerations

During the pretrial screen the following should be undertaken:

- Physical examination
- Medical history
- Diagnosis/psychiatric history
- Clinical chemistry (including prolactin)
- Hematology
- Pregnancy test (serum HCG)
- ECG
- Vital signs
- Weight

During randomized treatment, the following safety assessments should be evaluated on a regular basis:

1. Spontaneously elicited adverse events at each visit. These are defined as any detrimental change in the patient's condition, other than those recognized as signs and symptoms of schizophrenia.
2. Physical examination at the end of the trial (or withdrawal from the study) to assess any change from baseline.

The following should be performed weekly for the first 6 weeks, and weekly thereafter:

1. Clinical chemistry (urea and electrolytes, liver function tests, thyroid function tests, and prolactin)
2. Hematology (hemoglobin, platelets, total white cell count, differential white count)
3. Vital signs (erect and supine pulse and blood pressure) measured at T_{max}

Careful consideration needs to be given to concomitant medication. For example, a maximum daily dose of diazepam for agitation/insomnia should be specified in the protocol, and concomitant dopamine receptor antagonists are to be avoided. Inappropriate use of benzodiazepines and/or other CNS active drugs as concurrent or "escape" medications may invalidate any efficacy or safety conclusions due to their effects on some of the symptoms of schizophrenia.

3.4 Methods

3.4.1 Pharmacokinetics

Pharmacokinetic parameters should be established in the target patient population. The fate of the compound and its metabolites in different schizophrenic "special" patient groups can also be addressed (e.g., renally/hepatically impaired, the elderly). At this stage of development, studies using radiolabeled compound in patients are unlikely to provide any information which cannot be obtained from similar studies in healthy volunteers provided the radiolabeled drug can be administered at therapeutically relevant doses.

These data would not be gathered from pharmacokinetic-specific studies, rather these would be secondary data collected as population data from broader based studies with clinical efficacy and safety as their primary endpoints. Thus, for example, the majority of patients participating in a fixed dose-range finding study would have peak and trough blood samples drawn for estimation and calculation of the relevant pharmacokinetic parameters, while a minority would have extensive plasma sampling undertaken to provide clear definition of the pharmacokinetic profile relative to healthy volunteers.

3.4.2 Surrogate Markers

Markers by which different aspects of schizophrenia and antipsychotic drug effects can be measured have been described in Section 1. By repeated application, these scales afford a means by which various indices of the patient's condition can be measured over time. There are differences between the scales. However, the general principle governing each of these is that the patient is assessed by a standardized set of questions which cover a broad spectrum of psychopathological states. For example, the BPRS elicits responses from the patient by which information the assessor is able to evaluate positive, negative, and general psychopathology.

It is important to realize that all clinical assessments of efficacy in schizophrenia trials may be considered as essentially surrogate markers. They can be viewed as semi-quantitative at best, and at worst extremely qualitative, relying extensively upon rating scales which attempt to measure changes in the underlying disease process by recording symptoms reported verbally by the patient, and signs of the patient's behavior, speech, and thought patterns observed by the clinician. For example, an observer rating scale such as the BPRS can include up to 21 items, each requiring a response from the observer based upon his or her observation of the patient's mental state. These responses are gleaned from personal interview with the patient which can take the form of an hour long unstructured interview. In contrast, rating scales such as the PANSS can be used in a more organized way by employing a semi-structured interview, such as the SCIPANSS (Structured Clinical Interview for the PANSS), the advantage of which purports to be improved interrater reliability.

In an attempt to minimize the variance of scores between different observers, it is advisable to provide training to all participating investigators prior to initiating recruitment into the study. This training should use case studies in the form of videotaped interviews, which each assessor attempts to score. Open discussion of the ratings given by each assessor to the individual items allows comparison to be made with standard assessments and experience in using the rating scales is gained by each observer. While consistency across centers is desirable, it is not essential. Rather it is the intrarater reliability which is of paramount importance since each patient is assessed relative to a baseline score and it is the change from baseline which provides the clinical measure of efficacy. Thus, the absolute scores are less important than the relative change from baseline over time, for example, a reduction in BPRS total score of 48 to 33 over a 6-week treatment period is equivalent in relative change to a reduction from 53 to 38 — both are an absolute reduction of 15 units from baseline; however, these figures obviously relate to a different *percent* reduction in total scores, and hence the particular strategy adopted for statistical analysis and sample size calculations must also be borne in mind. For this reason it is vitally important that the baseline assessment, and that rating undertaken at the timepoint for the primary analysis of efficacy, should always be undertaken by the same rater.

3.5 Placebo or Active Control

The choice between placebo and an "active" control in studies with antipsychotic agents presents a dilemma for the investigator, as there are difficulties in the choice of an active control. Schizophrenia is a debilitating, life-long condition, and there is no general agreement either within the psychiatric profession itself, or across different countries, as to which treatment is to be preferred. Thus, for example, any study employing haloperidol as comparator will be criticized just because a haloperidol arm is included; on the dosage regimen of haloperidol; on the use of previous medication (as most patients entering any clinical trial are those deemed poorly responsive to "standard" therapy); on the clinical relevance of the magnitude of the effect observed compared to the test drug; and because the study is not placebo controlled.

An alternative is to design a trial which incorporates both an active- and placebo-control arm to provide evidence of absolute and comparative efficacy. However, although feasible, careful thought needs to be given to the choice of comparator agent and treatment regimen for the reasons stated above.

3.6 Informed Consent

Perhaps the most difficult aspect of designing studies in schizophrenia is the ethical aspects of informed consent, especially where placebo-control is deemed necessary. In practical terms, this would mean each "patient volunteer" would provide informed consent to be washed out from all prestudy medications, with the possibility of being randomized to placebo throughout the study, and the inherent potential of psychotic relapse. For this reason, many investigators deem it unethical to treat floridly ill psychotic patients for longer than 8 weeks with placebo.

The question as to whether true informed consent can ever be obtained from schizophrenic patients is a moot one. Schizophrenics are by no means alone in this respect, as severely ill patients, unconscious patients, mentally handicapped patients, and minors are all required to give informed consent to participate in clinical research. It is advisable to seek guidance from the relevant ethics committees and regulatory authorities as to what procedures they require for such consent to be obtained properly. Our own practical experience suggests that the patient should be given a clearly written patient information sheet, a face-to-face interview with the responsible clinician, plenty of time (at least 24 h) to consider the proposal, and the opportunity to discuss possible participation in the trial with relatives or close friends.

3.7 Size and Duration of Trials

The primary objectives of the phase II program for a novel antipsychotic should include:

- A preliminary safety and tolerance profile for the drug in patients
- Delineation of the dose response curve for the chosen indication
- A preliminary estimate of the efficacy of the drug over the dose range
- Generation of pharmacokinetic data at steady state over the dose range in the chosen patient population

Secondary objectives could include:

- Evaluation of efficacy in selected patient subgroups, for example, treatment resistant schizophrenia or patients with the deficit syndrome
- Possible variations in response between different gender and ethnic groups
- Specific pharmacodynamic data - for example, PET studies to determine the profile of receptor binding and duration of receptor occupancy in patients
- Comparative safety and efficacy data vs a standard antipsychotic such as haloperidol or chlorpromazine

To meet all these objectives a number of studies will be necessary. All of the primary objectives may be met by a single, well-designed placebo-controlled study. For example, an 8-week, 6-arm study in a total of 300 patients with acute exacerbation of schizophrenia (50 patients per group), incorporating 4 fixed doses of the compound, a single fixed dose of active comparator, and a placebo arm will allow pairwise comparisons between groups of primary endpoint measures in a trial with more than 90% statistical power. Data generated from such a trial will provide pivotal efficacy data for a regulatory submission. This approach is to be preferred to a program of smaller trials aiming for the same endpoints.

The secondary objectives are in part met by the trial outlined above. However, additional studies, if conducted at this early stage, in subgroups of patients will broaden the understanding of the range of clinical efficacy and possible differential advantages of the compound providing valuable information for internal decision making and negotiation with regulatory agencies.

4 DECISION MAKING

Figure 1 outlines an example of an antipsychotic phase I and phase II development paradigm incorporating several go/no go decision points at which the merits of progressing further studies are evaluated.

The phase I and II development program for Drug CLCJ includes the following:

1 A single study (Study 1) in normal volunteers to assess the safety, tolerance, and pharmacokinetics of the compound. This trial should utilize quantitative EEG as a pharmacodynamic endpoint to assess duration of action and quantitative effects and should generate data on the maximum tolerated dose and single-dose kinetics.

2 A multiple dose safety and tolerance study (Study 2) in schizophrenic patients to generate pharmacokinetic data in patients following multiple doses of Drug CLCJ with and without food. This study would include the evaluation of efficacy parameters and should provide the preliminary evidence of efficacy required by the FDA to permit dosing of 12-16 weeks duration in the U.S.

3. Two PET studies (Studies 3 and 4) which will provide data on absolute receptor occupancy for D_1, D_2, and $5HT_2$ receptors and a comparison of the time-course of occupancy of these same receptors with plasma levels of Drug CLCJ. Study 3 should confirm the receptor pharmacology in man, while the second PET trial assesses duration of receptor occupancy in man.

4. A study to delineate the dose-response curve (Study 5) in acute exacerbation of schizophrenia and a study to evaluate the absorption, distribution, metabolism, and excretion of the test compound.

5. A single dose study to characterize the absorption, distribution, metabolism, and excretion (ADME) of the compound (Study 6).

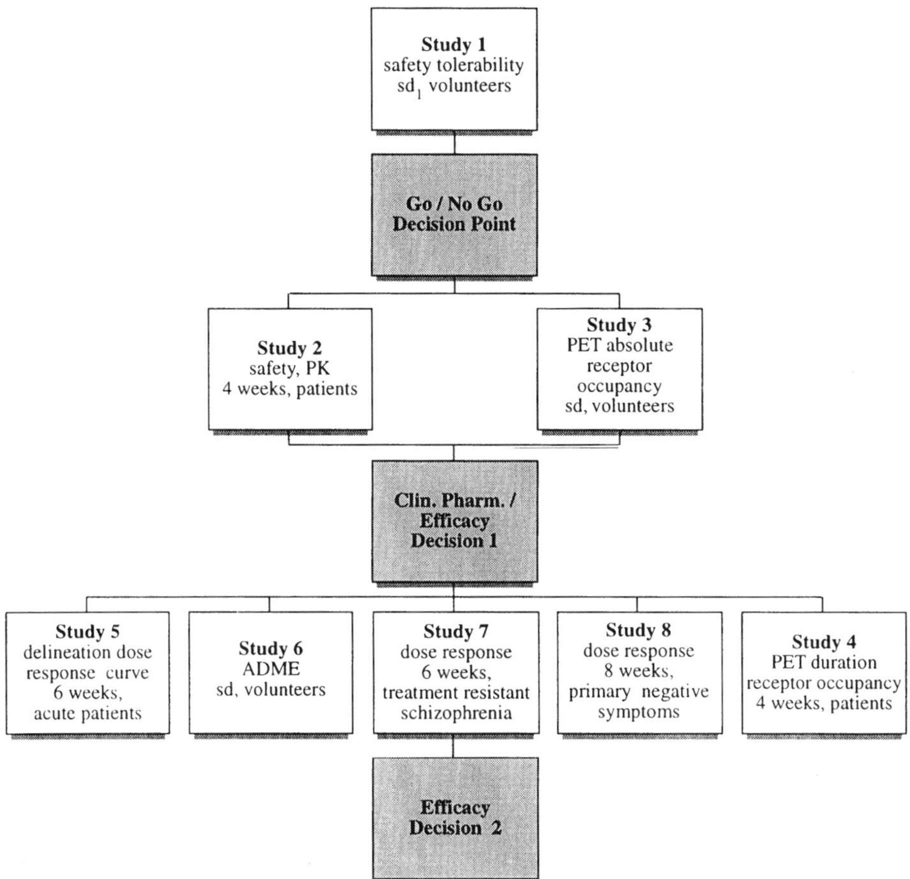

Figure 1 Example of an antipsychotic phase 1 and phase 2 development paradigm.

REFERENCES

AIMS: Abnormal Involuntary Movement Scale (1976) In: *ECDU Assessment Manual for Psychopharmacology* (Revised edition). Editor: Guy W. U.S. Department of Health, Education and Welfare.

American Psychiatric Association (1994) *Diagnostic and Statistical Manual of Mental Disorders,* 4th ed. APA, Washington D.C.

Andreasen N (1984) The Scale for the Assessment of Negative Symptoms (SANS). Iowa City, IA: the University of Iowa.

Andreasen N (1984) The Scale for the Assessment of Positive Symptoms (SAPS). Iowa City, IA: the University of Iowa.

Barnes TRE (1989) A rating scale for drug-induced akathisia. *Br. J. Psychiatry* 154, 672-676.

CGI: Clinical Global Impression (1976) In: *ECDU Assessment Manual for Psychopharmacology* (Revised Edition). Editor Guy W. U.S. Department of Health, Education and Welfare.

Cole JD, Goldberg SC, Klerman GL (1964) Phenothiazine treatment in acute schizophrenia. *Arch. Gen. Psychiatry* 10: 246-261.

Kay SR, Fiszbein A, Opler LA (1986) the positive and negative Syndrome scale (PANSS) for schizophrenia. *Schizophrenia Bull.* 13, 261-276.

Overall JE, Gorham DR (1962) The brief psychiatric rating scale. *Psychol. Rep.* 10, 799-812.

Simpson GM, Angus JWS (1979) A rating scale for extrapyramidal side effects. *Acta Psychiatr. Scand.* 45 (Suppl. 212), 11-19.

World Health Organization (1994) *International Statistical Classification of Diseases and Related Health Problems,* Tenth revision, Geneva, WHO.

Chapter 26

Alzheimer's Disease and Other Dementias

Robert L. Holland and Keith A. Wesnes

CONTENTS

1 Introduction 355
2 Healthy Volunteers 356
  2.1 Selection Criteria 357
    2.1.1 Tolerance 357
    2.1.2 Kinetics 357
    2.1.3 Dynamics 357
  2.2 Safety Considerations 358
  2.3 Methods 358
    2.3.1 General Trial Design 358
    2.3.2 Pharmacokinetic Issues 358
    2.3.3 Pharmacodynamic Issues 358
      2.3.3.1 Direct Measures of Cognition and Memory 359
      2.3.3.2 Changes in Brain Physiology (Other than Cognition and Memory) 360
      2.3.3.3 Neuroendocrine Tests 361
      2.3.3.4 Non-CNS Pharmacological Effects 361
3 Patient Studies 362
  3.1 Suitability 363
  3.2 Selection Criteria 363
  3.3 Safety Considerations 364
  3.4 Methods 364
    3.4.1 Pharmacokinetics 364
    3.4.2 Pharmacodynamic Endpoints 364
  3.5 Placebo or Active Control 366
  3.6 Design, Size, and Duration of Trials 367
4 Decision Making 368
5 Key Literature Examples 368
References 369

1 INTRODUCTION

The gradual demographic changes in the developed world are lending a sharp stimulus to the development of medications for diseases of the elderly. Cognitive decline and dementia are quintessentially such diseases. Dementia may become the most important medical condition facing the Western world in the next century. There will be an enormous social and economic burden placed on the family and society in general to provide appropriate care for demented elderly patients. Alzheimer's disease (AD) affects at least 3% of the population aged over 65 in the West[3,7,18] with an incidence rate which increases dramatically with increasing age — perhaps doubling in every five-year cohort. The other major type of dementia, vascular dementia (VaD), is clearly less common in the West.[7,18] It is, however, apparently the diagnosis of the majority of cases of dementia in Japan[75] and China.[68] Further, as our ability to measure cognitive and memory performance has improved, and perhaps as personal expectations have changed, less marked impairments than dementia are increasingly considered as illnesses suitable for treatment; e.g., age-associated memory impairment (AAMI).[9]

These dementias are characterized by the development of multiple cognitive deficits, including both memory impairment and at least one of aphasia, apraxia, agnosia, or disturbance in executive function (DSM-IV).[14] The key clinical difference between AD and VaD lies in the gradual onset and progression

0-8493-9230-6/97/$0.00+$.50
© 1997 by CRC Press, Inc.

of the former and the step-wise progression with focal neurological signs of the latter. AAMI, or more recent alternatives; e.g., age-related cognitive decline (Code 780.9; DSM-IV) and age-associated cognitive decline,[39] are operationally defined as cognitive and memory performance scores, in an otherwise healthy older person, which fall below certain preset norms. Unequivocally, the core symptoms for these illnesses are memory and cognitive impairments. This chapter will focus on the strategies available for the development of drugs to treat these key symptoms. Its focus will be on AD and other dementias, though many of the procedures recommended for phases I and II will have relevance for less severe conditions such as the cognitive deficits associated with normal aging. However, it should be borne in mind that dementia is clearly also complicated by affective symptoms (e.g., depression) and behavioral symptoms (e.g., aggression). These symptom classes are also valid treatment objectives in the wider context of helping the demented patient.[28]

The pathophysiology of AD and VaD have been extensively researched. The basic lesions in AD, neurofibrillary tangles and amyloid plaques, are well-known, but the mechanisms leading to their formation and the associated synaptic loss and cell death remain poorly understood.[6,26,41] However, recent exciting results have identified the apolipoprotein E (ApoE) genetic locus as a site where different alleles can be inherited conferring increased risks for developing the disease;[58] presumably delineating the role ApoE plays in neuronal physiology may lead to an understanding of the pathogenesis of AD. VaD, representing the consequences of multiple small infarcts, strokes, and also arteriosclerosis,[34] has a well-defined microscopic pathology of microinfarcts and lacunae.[53] Modern scanning techniques have confirmed a patchy diminution in cerebral blood flow and metabolism in these patients.[37,52]

In terms of therapy two approaches can be distinguished. One would be the treatment of the symptoms of the diseases, the second would be a treatment of the underlying pathophysiology — either to stop or slow disease progression or best of all to repair the damage (disease modification). At the moment, most success has been found with the symptomatic approach, both in AD and VaD. Therefore most of this chapter will address the issues of attaining improvements in cognitive and memory function. However, in the future as the disease processes become better understood, valid disease modifying treatments may well become available. Only two significant classes of drugs are currently available worldwide for the treatment of dementia — both were developed with the symptomatic approach.

For AD, tacrine (THA) is the lead example of cholinesterase inhibitors, and amid much controversy it is now approved in the U.S. and other countries including France. Tacrine clearly has demonstrable (but small) cognitive enhancing effects in AD patients.[19] Other procholinergic drugs including other cholinesterase inhibitors and selective muscarinic agonists are in late stages of development and may appear on the market in the next few years. The development of these drugs has stemmed from cholinergic theories of memory and AD,[48] and is an example of wider "neurotransmitter replacement" strategies for AD, analogous to the use of L-DOPA or bromocriptine in Parkinson's disease patients.

A large number of drugs are available for the treatment of VaD, from the class known as "nootropics." These drugs are thought of as cerebral metabolic enhancers. This class of drug includes piracetam[24] and its analog, e.g., oxiracetam[78] and hydergine.[44] Nootropics are widely prescribed in Japan, Germany, and Italy, but their efficacy is regarded as suspect in many other countries. Interestingly, deterioration of VaD may well be slowed using a straightforward approach to disease modification like control of risk factors and antiplatelet/anticoagulant therapy.[52]

In summary, then, though the pathophysiology of VaD is reasonably well understood, that of AD remains obscure, but exciting developments are on the horizon. Some drugs are available for both AD and VaD; however all appear at best marginally effective and are symptomatic rather than disease modifying agents. Thus, the development of a new drug is, to some extent, handicapped by the lack of a gold standard comparator and the fact that clear-cut efficacy endpoints are difficult to find. Furthermore, the target patients are elderly. Clearly, they are a difficult population requiring extensive safety monitoring and specific safety studies.

2 HEALTHY VOLUNTEERS

There are two quite separate needs to fulfill (objectives) early in the development of an antidementia drug: safety and kinetics and dose-related pharmacodynamics. With regard to the first objective, the target patients in efficacy studies are elderly, often frail, and often taking other medications. It is a *sine qua non* of safe patient studies that we should at an early stage gain experience of the pharmacokinetics of the drug and how they change with age. Furthermore, we must obtain sufficient and appropriate drug interaction data, as well as establish the tolerability and general safety of the drug in the elderly.

An understanding of the dose-pharmacodynamic relationship is fundamental to the choice of doses for phase II. It is difficult, though clearly not impossible, to show cognitive enhancement in healthy volunteers (e.g., References 73, 79, 84, 92, and 93). Furthermore, there are human models of induced cognitive deficit which can be pharmacologically reversed. Other surrogate endpoints can also be helpful, for example dose-related alerting effects in the EEG or metabolic changes on positron-emission tomography (PET) scans. Finally, other specific aspects of the drug's pharmacology can be explored, such as blockade of 5HT induced skin wheal and flare by $5HT_3$ antagonists, or changes in urinary monoamine metabolites by selective monoamine oxidase inhibitors. While these latter endpoints seem somewhat divorced from cognitive enhancement, they can at least show doses and plasma levels producing (wished for) pharmacological effects.

Is it appropriate to study drugs in this phase in healthy volunteers or should only patients be studied? The answer to this question is definitely that both types of studies are needed. We would always advocate exploring the fundamental biological characteristics of a drug in healthy volunteers, and would suggest that healthy volunteer models can help expedite patient studies. However, studies in patients at an early stage are equally necessary.

2.1 Selection Criteria

The selection criteria for volunteers and patients for any given study are, of course, strongly dependent upon the design and objectives of that study. However, if the volunteer studies are divided by type, certain recommendations are reasonable.

2.1.1 Tolerance

The experience with velnacrine[12] showed early tolerance studies in patients are vital. Tolerance studies in young, fit healthy males is the usual way to begin. However, the target patient is typically elderly, female, and rather frail. Clearly, tolerance studies (single and multiple dose) should also be performed in healthy elderly volunteers, including reasonable numbers of individuals aged at least 75 years and a reasonable number of females. An early tolerance and safety study in actual demented patients is, however, absolutely mandatory. AD patients were distinctly more sensitive to the adverse effects of velnacrine than comparable healthy elderly volunteers.[12] However, the converse has also been described for other CNS active drugs.

2.1.2 Kinetics

The influences of age and sex on the pharmacokinetics of a potential drug can be usefully explored in the tolerance studies in healthy elderly and demented patients noted above. However, another key issue is the potential for a drug to show pharmacokinetic/dynamic interactions with potential co-medications. Given that the target patients will often be taking other medications, even in early clinical trials, the issue is really one of being able to write a safe protocol for such a clinical study which does not exclude too many patients. Drug interaction studies can most easily be performed in young, fit healthy volunteers; an efficient design which gives information about the likelihood of different interactions is the so-called "cocktail" study.[5]

2.1.3 Dynamics

Certain pharmacodynamic models have been optimized in young fit, usually male, healthy volunteers (see below). When undertaking cognitive testing, nicotine and caffeine use have clear influences upon outcome.[71,92,93] A reasonable policy is to exclude smokers, and heavy users of caffeine, and to restrict caffeine use during a study.

A gray area with antidementia drugs concerns the use of nondemented older individuals with self-reported cognitive and memory decline. One strategy is to regard these individuals as patients and to devise "efficacy" studies with the intention of registering a treatment for their condition.[10] However, another strategy is to regard these individuals as having a condition representing a model of dementia. Hence, these individuals can be seen as a test bed for an antidementia product. Such an approach has been used in the early studies of a number of drugs,[10,29,45] the selection criteria for test subjects being the diagnostic criteria for AAMI.[9] Both approaches have some advantages. Very few antidementia drugs have mechanisms of action which would limit their utility solely to dementia. Thus if a compound shows some capability of improving cognitive function in these trials, the information gained would be helpful in planning future phase II trials with demented patients. Further, if the population was well defined, e.g., using the criteria of Levy et al.,[39] and regulatory authorities sympathetic to the indication, such positive findings might well be the stimulus to develop the compound for this indication, instead of, or as well as, for dementia.

2.2 Safety Considerations

In general three kinds of safety issue can be identified in volunteer studies: intrinsic properties of the drug; idiosyncratic reactions to the drug; and differences between patients and volunteers.

The intrinsic effects of a drug, pharmacological and toxicological, should be fully explored with appropriate animal safety testing, and it makes sense to perform some of these studies in elderly animals. However, some adverse experiences will always remain because they are part of the pharmacology of the drug. For example, cholinesterase inhibitors produce dose-related side effects such as nausea, vomiting, and diarrhea which are simply peripheral manifestations of the wanted CNS pharmacology.[19] The best way of dealing with this type of concomitant adverse experience is to design it out of the drug in the preclinical phase, by finding molecules which have selectivity for centrally located receptors or enzymes.[16] However, in multiple dose studies, slow upward titration of the dose can be helpful in reducing this kind of intolerance.

Idiosyncratic reactions to a drug are, of course, much more difficult to deal with. Here again, tacrine is a good example. As many as 7% of treated patients develop serum transaminase levels more than ten times the upper limit of normal, in a reaction which may not be dose dependent.[19] However, it is fair to say that the majority of idiosyncratic reactions occur at a low frequency and are not a major issue at this early stage of drug development.

The issue of patients being unexpectedly more sensitive to a drug than even elderly healthy volunteers has been alluded to before. Once again this phenomenon has been seen with a cholinesterase inhibitor (velnacrine).[12]

2.3 Methods

2.3.1 General Trial Design

Volunteer studies, especially when single-dose or short (1-2 weeks) multiple-dose studies, are almost always best done with a cross-over design. This can increase the statistical power of a pharmacodynamic study, especially a study of cognitive performance, very substantially. It is important to keep the duration of dosing in these studies as short as possible, in the first instance. This allows multiple within subject crossovers of wide ranges of doses, which can be very important in identifying potentially therapeutically effective and well-tolerated dose ranges. However, the dosing periods must be short enough so that the study duration does not become too unwieldy or too burdensome for the volunteers. Maintenance of the effect can be confirmed in later parallel group studies.

2.3.2 Pharmacokinetic Issues

Antidementia drugs are, almost by definition, drugs to be used for prolonged periods of time. Therefore, oral administration will be the route of choice. It is conceivable that potential therapies will be developed which are effective but not orally bioavailable (e.g., peptides). This would pose major technical problems as formulations will have to be developed for other routes suitable for long-term administration.

Potentially interesting specific pharmacokinetic issues include the question of how readily the compound gets into the brain and how long it stays there. Theoretically, measuring drug levels in CSF would answer this question.[76] However, practically this is not always possible at this stage of drug development. A realistic, if rather expensive option is to measure brain levels by PET scanning. This technique can show the kinetics of drugs in specific regions of the brain (if the molecule is chemically appropriate).[35]

An alternative approach is to use the brain as a sort of bioassay of central drug levels; for example, changes in the EEG power spectrum and regional blood flow can show, at least, that the drug is getting into the brain in active concentrations and, possibly, the duration of activity of differing doses of the compound.[30]

2.3.3 Pharmacodynamic Issues

There are four types of pharmacodynamic markers to be considered; first and most relevant for this field and perhaps most interesting are direct measures of cognition and memory. Second are central pharmacological effects on brain physiology which may or may not be related to therapeutic effects. Third, are anticipated peripheral pharmacological effects of the compound as it interacts with receptors, enzymes, or other targets located on both sides of the blood-brain barrier. Fourth, are unanticipated or unwanted peripheral pharmacological effects. These can occur with molecules which have only a relative selectivity for a particular target receptor; as dosages are increased the additional pharmacology of a molecule can become apparent.

2.3.3.1 Direct Measures of Cognition and Memory

Mental performance testing has a long history, and a huge variety of tests and test systems are available. Measures typically include attention, speed, and accuracy of information processing, short-term or working memory, and long-term memory storage and retrieval.[31] These measures each tap fairly discrete aspects of mental functioning which contribute to everyday behavioral competence. These aspects of functioning are known to act independently and can be differentially affected by various stressors such as trauma and drugs. Tests should ideally be as specific to one function as possible in order to facilitate interpretation of the changes on that test for the nature of the alteration of everyday behavior. No test covers all aspects of cognitive function nor simulates all aspects of everyday cognitive function, and thus the most satisfactory approach is to combine a variety of tests, each reflecting different aspects of mental function, in order that the nature of any changes can be pinpointed. The reader should therefore avoid using a single test of mental function in any study because of the limitations in what that test can reveal. Either the test will measure several aspects of functioning, so that in the end it will not be possible to decide what was actually affected, or the test will be so specific to one particular aspect of functioning that any changes will have dubious relevance for the complexities of everyday cognitive performance.

Even then, great care should be taken in selecting collections of tests (test batteries, test systems) for measuring improvements in cognitive efficiency. The relative difficulty in improving human cognition over impairing it makes the sensitivity of the procedures of paramount importance. Despite the long history of testing, there is no safety to be sought by choosing traditional measures. Automated test systems, once properly developed and validated, are gradually becoming recognized to provide better instruments than their pencil and paper predecessors (e.g., Reference 11). By controlling all aspects of stimulus presentation and, for most tasks, recording the speed of every response, microcomputerized tests enable not only a comprehensive evaluation in which speed is measured in direct relation to accuracy, but in some cases allow the only definitive assessment of aspects of attention and information processing. Over and above the considerable advantages which accrue from standardization of administration and automation of capturing responses, and subsequently scoring and analyzing them, computerization allows assessments to be made with greater sensitivity and to cover functions which were previously unequivocally unassessable.

In choosing a selection of tests, or more ideally a test system, a number of general requirements must be satisfied. All tests should have a difficulty level appropriate to the subjects, who should have the possibility of showing both improvement or deterioration (i.e., no floor or ceiling effects). The tests should be relatively easy to learn; after around four practice trials subjects should be performing at about their maximum level. There should be a large number of alternative versions of a test so that multiple experimental trials within a subject are feasible. The tests should have a known sensitivity; by this it is meant that active drugs should produce reliable dose-related changes in performance detectable with statistical significance in a certain (perhaps 12 to 24) defined number of subjects. The tests should be easy to administer and score and generate data which are easy to analyze. The test system should also have a reasonable duration (15 to 45 min) allowing multiple daily tests. Other important requirements are to confirm the utility, reliability, and validity of the test procedures. However, we would **not** recommend the adoption of new and untried or personalized versions of tests. The reader must realize that unless the system under evaluation has all the above requirements, the test system as well as the drug will be under trial. If the primary purpose of the study is to measure pharmacodynamic effects, it is not ethically justified to utilize an unproven test system unless it is used in parallel with one of known sensitivity and reliability. It is not the role of clinical development programs to help develop tests at the expense of identifying the efficacy of the compound. Without the use of a known and validated test battery, how can current results be compared to the results of previous studies with other drugs? This is important in terms of predictability. What kind of therapeutic value can be expected from a product with a particular effect size in a standardized test battery? Does the absence of a detectable effect predict lack of therapeutic efficacy? As a further consideration, it is an advantage if the test system has parallel versions which can be used with elderly and demented populations, as this will increase continuity throughout the development program.

As has been mentioned already, it is possible to detect improvements in cognitive function in healthy unimpaired young[73,79,92,93] and elderly[84] volunteers. The latter trial, for example, was a rising dose safety and tolerance trial, and demonstrates that useful information can be determined very early in the development process. Cognitive testing need not add to the number of volunteers required, nor increase the study duration, and it can be fitted around safety and other assessments. It is thus a useful addition to the early safety and tolerability trials of a novel antidementia drug.

As an alternative to seeking improvements in unimpaired healthy volunteers, over and above what can be achieved in trials with unimpaired volunteers, there are two models in which impairments to various cognitive processes are induced and drugs evaluated for the ability to either prevent or counteract these effects. These two models are the hypoxia model and the scopolamine model.

Hypoxia — Conceptually the simplest of the two models, this model can be based on one of two techniques, normobaric hypoxic hypoxidosis or hyperbaric hypoxia. Both have the same consequence, to lower the oxygen content of the blood, making less oxygen available for the CNS, resulting in cognitive impairment. This is likened to the situation in VaD, and interestingly in the early 1970s several studies placed senile patients in hyperbaric chambers to increase the oxygen getting to the brain and improve cognitive function, though the results were mixed.[1] The hypoxia model has been used to evaluate drugs in volunteer trials, and positive effects have been found, for example, with the classic nootropic, piracetam, in the hypoxic hypoxidosis version.[65] While this model has relevance for VaD, the etiology of AD is quite different. Thus a compound might be able to reverse the effects of hypoxia via a mechanism which had no relevance for treating the symptoms of AD. Nonetheless, this is an interesting model and, though not widely used, is worthy of attention, particularly for drugs aimed at VaD, and possibly other types of age-related deficits.

The scopolamine model of dementia — A more commonly used paradigm is based on scopolamine-induced impairments in healthy young or healthy elderly volunteers. This study design stemmed from the "cholinergic" theory of AD in which it was noted that centrally active anticholinergic drugs could produce cognitive and memory impairments which were not unlike those found in AD. The validity of this model therefore stemmed from both directions; on the one side its deficits were produced by blocking a system known to be crucially involved in the cognitive deficits seen in dementia, and on the other side the deficits stood scrutiny for their ability to mimic some of the core deficits exhibited by AD patients. The single-dose model has been used quite widely and has shown itself sensitive to procholinergic drugs such as nicotine,[85] as well as the anticholinesterases velnacrine and physostigmine.[25,65,91] Furthermore, and very interestingly, the model is sensitive to noncholinergic compounds including the nootropics piracetam, aniracetam, tenilsetam,[82,89] pramiracetam,[43] and oxiracetam;[56] D-cycloserine, a glycine agonist;[83] moclobemide, a monoamine oxidase-A inhibitor;[81] and a $5HT_3$ antagonist.[57] The technicalities of performing these induced impairment studies are by no means straightforward. The test battery in use must be well-characterized and known to be usable (i.e., not be at floor or ceiling) when the volunteers are showing impairment, and the degree of impairment has to be carefully controlled by, for example, using carefully chosen doses of scopolamine. It has been shown that the model is predictive for the anticholinesterase, velnacrine, a confirmatory trial using the same test system in AD patients showing improvements on some of the same measures as in the young impaired volunteers.[69] Similarly, the experience with physostigmine in the model[91] of clear but temporary effectiveness, mirrors the clinical experience with the drug.[50] However, many nootropics have only marginal mean efficacy in patients with dementia, despite showing some actions in the scopolamine model. This would suggest the use of anticholinesterases as internal controls in future studies with the scopolamine model, yielding a measure of the sensitivity of the model and also allowing the relative magnitude of the effects discovered to be considered from the clinical perspective. As tacrine is now registered and the sensitivity of the scopolamine model to anticholinesterases is established, this gives an ideal opportunity for future anticholinesterases to be modeled directly against physostigmine or tacrine in the model, and also will enable dose-response relationships to be determined and permit different candidates to be directly compared for potency. Overall the scopolamine model has considerable utility in identifying potential efficacy and delineating dose-response relationships and relative potencies and is a must for any novel anticholinesterase. Its speed might make it a valuable stage in the development of any compound, though currently not as a no-go stage, with the exception of anticholinesterases and other drugs known to act directly on the cholinergic system. Future enhancements would be to combine the cholinergic deficits with those of other neurotransmitters.

2.3.3.2 Changes in Brain Physiology (Other than Cognition and Memory)

There are a number of techniques now available which allow the detection of the effects of drugs in the brain. These effects may or may not represent a manifestation of a therapeutic drug action. At worst, it can be argued that they show that the drug is getting into the brain and "doing something;" and some of the techniques allow measurement of the duration of that effect.

Pharmaco-EEG — Effects of psychotropic drugs on the EEG have been well described.[33] It is now a relatively simple matter to digitize, and store electronically, the EEG waveforms from multiple leads. The digitized waveforms can then be subjected to a number of analytical techniques, usually a Fast Fourier Transform is used to produce a power spectrum, i.e., a description of the relative and absolute proportions of EEG activity in specific frequency bands. The capture of EEG signal typically takes place under two conditions (resting and alert) and through multiple leads. The combination of using several leads, two conditions, many frequency bands, several doses of drug and several timepoints for assessment, can lead to huge numbers of potential statistical comparisons. Therefore, the pattern and consistency of effects is perhaps as important as the presence or absence of a few statistically significant differences. Several putative antidementia products have been found to have effects on the EEG in clinical pharmacology studies (for examples, see References 62 and 63). In fact, the pharmaco-EEG is so effective in demonstrating drug activity that it was recommended as a technique for detecting drug-induced changes in vigilance by the 1989 consensus conference on the methodology of clinical trials of nootropics.[2] However, it is important to reiterate that we would not see pharmaco-EEG changes as indicative of efficacy, though much published literature in the dementia field has treated EEG effects as though they were surrogate endpoints for antidementia efficacy. Rather we would regard EEG changes as evidence that the administered dose of drug was getting into the brain and having pharmacological effects.

Evoked Potentials and Other Neurophysiological Tests — Drug effects on evoked potentials are less well established but there have been some reports of effects with antidementia compounds.[66] Other neurophysiological parameters which could be used to show drug-induced effects include sleep EEG[16] and EEG brain mapping.[62] However, experience with these techniques with antidementia compounds remains limited.

Functional Brain Imaging Studies — The rapid development of new scanning techniques offers new ways to study drug action. One such technique is PET. Either oxygen consumption rate or glucose utilization rate are measurable using PET (see Reference 4 for review) and this would allow direct observation of drug-induced changes. In practice, experience with this technique with antidementia drugs remains very limited. However, studies have been performed with single photon-emission computer tomography (SPECT). With this technique, it is possible to image brain perfusion patterns before and after treatment and effects have been found in short-term clinical pharmacology studies with velnacrine[15] and physostigmine.[30] Similarly, magnetic resonance spectroscopy (which requires a higher intensity field than imaging) will also eventually allow direct measurement of local brain metabolism and could therefore represent a method for demonstrating that drug had entered the brain and was producing the desired functional effect. However, there are currently very few machines available in the world capable of generating the intense magnetic fields required, and routine use of this technology in phase I may be a decade or more away.

2.3.3.3 Neuroendocrine Tests

Hormonal responses to single-doses of administered drug can be helpful markers of central activity (e.g., Reference 8). For example, cholinesterase inhibitors release growth hormone.[13] Drugs thought to be active at serotoninergic or dopaminergic receptors will also have effects on prolactin, growth hormone, and ACTH/cortisol.[32] Again, this approach does not necessarily indicate therapeutic action but can demonstrate the presence in the brain of pharmacologically active amounts of the drug. These neuroendocrine challenge studies are usually performed as single-dose cross-over studies, comparing several doses and placebo, and they do require relatively careful control of the experimental conditions, as plasma hormone levels are notoriously unstable in stressful conditions and are subject to large diurnal variations. Another, presumably centrally mediated, drug action which can be measured conveniently in neuroendocrine challenge studies is body temperature, which is lowered by some compounds acting on serotoninergic and dopaminergic receptors.[32]

2.3.3.4 Non-CNS Pharmacological Effects

Any pharmacologically active drug is likely to have effects peripherally as well as centrally **unless** the drug is completely selective for central targets. Thus, cholinergic drugs are likely to have effects on: the cardiovascular system; gastrointestinal secretion and motility; the pupil; sweating; and salivation. All of these effects are readily measurable using standard published techniques and will be helpful in at least defining pharmacologically active doses and setting limits to phase II dosing. Other real examples of physiological effects produced by antidementia drugs in development are the inhibition of 5HT induced skin wheal and flare reactions by $5HT_3$ antagonists,[47] and the inhibition of peripheral cholinesterases by anticholinesterases.

3 PATIENT STUDIES

As discussed in Section 2, although we feel most antidementia drugs should initially be studied in healthy volunteers, it is also necessary to study the tolerance and bioavailability in the patient population to detect any differences which quite possibly may exist. For one or two rare classes of compounds with mechanisms of action which would only benefit AD patients, such as drugs to block the toxicity of β-amyloid protein or lower brain aluminum levels, there might be a case for using a patient population from the outset, but for the vast majority of antidementia drugs aimed at symptomatic treatment, healthy volunteers should first receive the drug. However, we strongly feel that, as in phase I, safety and bioavailability should not be the sole interest at this stage of development. Traditionally though, many phase II programs of antidementia drugs have simply been exercises to measure the safety, tolerability, and pharmacokinetics of the treatments in patients, prior to large phase III trials to determine the efficacy of the compounds. This is in stark contrast to guidelines for the clinical evaluation of antidementia drugs prepared by Dr. Paul Leber of the FDA in 1990, in which he writes "phase 3 is envisioned as a period of expanded testing during which a product whose efficacy has been established definitively in rigorously controlled phase 2 studies is evaluated under conditions more typical of those likely to prevail once the drug is marketed" (Reference 38; page 31). Also there is no evidence that this trend is changing, Leon Thal[74] writing on clinical trials in AD states; "In recent years, there has been a trend to combine phases two and three into a single study" (page 434). It is the thesis of this chapter that there is little justification for such an approach. No pharmaceutical company, no matter how large and no matter what resources are at its disposal, should enter a phase III program without possessing all of the following:

1. Evidence that the drug possesses the desired effect in man
2. Knowledge of the effective dose range
3. Knowledge of the dose-response relationship
4. Knowledge of the time-course of the effects with repeated dosing

To enter into a phase III trial without such evidence is inviting disaster. How can a trial be conducted when the effective dose range is unknown? While this would be true in almost any field, it is particularly relevant for drugs designed to improve cognitive function, as it has long been known that such compounds rarely show linear dose-response relationships, and many show inverted-U effects.[72] This practice is not simply a waste of money, with the resulting implications for the stockholders and employees of the company, it is also ethically and scientifically wrong. Patients and their families enter into such trials in the hope that the symptoms of the disease will be treated. They put their faith in physicians that they might benefit from taking part, and are willing to be exposed to the risk of side effects, discomfort, and inconvenience on that basis. Many "efficacy trials" are in fact acts of faith, based on evidence that the drug has some beneficial effects in animal models and the doses selected because they can be more or less tolerated. In such cases, which are not infrequent, the hopes of the patients, families, and also physicians are mostly in vain, and further, the families are being put to great inconvenience and the patients also to risk, all most likely, for no tangible benefit. Further, they may have missed out on another trial which had a greater likelihood of success. Furthermore, the drug may have been effective if studied at the appropriate dose range with the correct dosing regimen, and thus a potentially effective treatment may have been overlooked.

Scientifically, progress is being hampered because it is not possible to determine retrospectively which of the scores of drugs thus far studied were genuinely ineffective, or instead whether the design of the trials and/or the measures of efficacy were inappropriate. Thus after 30 years of trials with antidementia drugs, anticholinesterases aside, we still do not have a good idea about which compounds and mechanisms of action are likely to prove useful, nor which are the optimum designs and assessments.

It is the firm belief of the authors that the majority of efficacy trials of antidementia compounds have been conducted without sufficient (or often any) evidence of efficacy from phases I and II. In some cases the efficacy trials probably failed due to the wrong dose range or dosing regimen being utilized, and many failed probably because the drugs were genuinely ineffective. In either case though, these compounds should not have been entered into efficacy trials. The only reason a phase III trial should fail is due to factors which cannot be identified until a trial of that size is conducted, for example, because the actual amount of improvement is smaller than that predicted from phase I and II, or because it fades after an extended period of treatment, or because some safety issue emerges which could only have been identified from exposing such a large number of patients to the drug. Clearly such a position depends on having the tools available to identify the potential efficacy of antidementia drugs. In Section 2 of this chapter such tools and methodologies which are available in phase I were described, and in this section the ideal strategy for evaluating antidementia drugs in phase II will be outlined.

As mentioned above, it will always be necessary to measure the safety, tolerability, and pharmacokinetics of antidementia compounds in patients. Equally, it was emphasized that the potential efficacy of the drug must be assessed in phase II. Many traditional researchers prefer to evaluate efficacy independently of safety, tolerability and pharmacokinetics. However, such a dualistic approach will inevitably slow drug development and would only be justified if the measurement of efficacy somehow interfered with the various other aims of the trial or vice versa. It will be argued in the following sections that efficacy measures can satisfactorily coexist with the other essential requirements of drug evaluation, and thus that efficacy evaluations are an integral aspect of all stages of phase II.

3.1 Suitability

Safety, tolerability, and pharmacokinetic trials need to be conducted in demented patient populations whether or not they have also been conducted in volunteers. There will be the usual extra difficulty encountered in conducting trials with the elderly or finding patients who are not on medication, probably more so in the demented, but this will not be a major problem.

Concerning the inclusion of efficacy testing in phase II, the obvious question which must be addressed is whether or not treatments can produce improvements in the symptoms of dementia in such trials. The two issues here are whether or not improvements in cognitive function can be identified in the relative short term (i.e., over days or weeks as opposed to months), and whether measures are available which can identify such improvements in the smaller populations which are used in phase II. Naturally, the answer to the first question lies in the intended mechanism of action of the study compound. Drugs with direct effects upon synaptic function, such as anticholinesterases, would be expected to produce fairly rapid responses, whereas drugs which act via more circuitous routes, such as desferrioxamine, which reduces brain aluminium levels, would not be expected to show a rapid onset of efficacy. However, as the vast majority of cognition enhancers under development[64] have either direct actions on neurotransmitters or actions which would be expected to take effect fairly quickly (e.g., calcium channel blockade), effects should be measurable in the short term.

The issue of informed consent is clearly a thorny one in dementia research. As the nature of the disease is an impairment of cognitive function, and as even the classification of mild AD involves what would be a severe cognitive impairment in a normal individual, it is unlikely that many of the patients are properly cognizant of the risks involved in the trial or the commitment they are undertaking. Often caretakers are asked to give consent, but these are often the children of the patients, and the law in most countries does not hold children responsible for the actions of their parents. On the other hand, AD is a fatal illness without a known cure, and would it be ethical to withhold a potentially effective treatment simply because the patient is unlikely to fully comprehend the risks involved? One possibility which has occurred to the authors is for individuals at risk, or individuals simply concerned that they might develop the disease, to give prospective consent should they go on to develop the disease. Alternatively they might nominate somebody to give informed consent should the need arise. For VaD, which has a sudden onset, this might be particularly appropriate. In this field, the absence of a cure currently outweighs the requirement of truly informed consent, but in ten years or more, when one or more fairly effective symptomatic treatments are available, this issue could become highly controversial, and prospective consent or nomination might go a little way toward allaying public concerns.

3.2 Selection Criteria

It cannot be overemphasized that a major purpose of phase II trials is to detect evidence of efficacy. Patient selection is crucial to this end; the more homogenous the population, the more likely it is that any positive effects of the drug will be detected in the small trials typical of phase II. The first thing to do is to ensure the diagnosis of the particular type of dementia is as accurate as possible, mainly in order to increase the likelihood that the patients will have the underlying pathology which the compound is intended to ameliorate, making them more likely to respond. Secondly, the severity of the illness should be identified. In many fields, the more severe the illness the more likely it is to respond to treatment, though this is almost certainly not the case for symptomatic treatment of dementia. The authors recommend using mild or moderately demented patients in phase II trials. Severely demented patients should be avoided in phase II for two reasons. First, they are by definition close to vegetative, and thus untestable using the sensitive procedures required to identify change. Secondly, the neuronal damage is so extensive that there is little hope that the fairly subtle manipulations of neurotransmitter functioning will have any detectable effect.

For AD, the safest option is to base the diagnosis on either the criteria in the Diagnostic and Statistical Manual of Mental Disorders (DSM-IV)[14] or the joint National Institute of Neurological and Communicative Disorders and Stroke and Alzheimer's Disease and Related Disorders Association criteria (abbreviated, though not enough, to NINCDS-ADRDA).[46] The dichotomization into "possible" and "probable" AD should be made and patients in the probable category selected for use in phase II, thereby increasing the homogeneity of the patients. Care must be taken to rule out confounding diseases such as pseudodementia, depression, hypothyroidism, pernicious anemia, and other forms of dementia including VaD, progressive supranuclear palsy, Picks's disease, Creutzfeldt-Jakobs disease, Huntington's disease, Lewy body dementia, and AIDS dementia.

Staging is then necessary to select the appropriate population for phase II trials. As mentioned earlier, severe patients should be avoided. A variety of instruments are available for staging including the Global Deterioration Scale and the Clinical Dementia Rating. "Mild" and "moderate" AD are stages 4 and 5, respectively, on the Global Deterioration Scale, and stages 1 and 2, respectively, on the Clinical Dementia Rating.

3.3 Safety Considerations

Patients in phase II should receive the same rigorous medical care to ensure their safety that is employed to protect healthy volunteers in phase I. "The goal of the assessment is to document that the patient suffered no ill effect during exposure" (Reference 38; p. 29, 30). To achieve this it is necessary to evaluate fully each patient with a comprehensive physical and neurological examination, in combination with thorough plasma and urine analyses and electrocardiographs. The absolute minimum is for these evaluations to take place immediately prior to dosing and on discontinuation. During dosing, medical status should be monitored regularly, though whether the entire procedure is repeated or a subselection of assessments conducted will be decided by the responsible physician, in the light of the known actions of the drug. Besides ensuring the safety of the patients, such a procedure in phase II yields a clear picture of what effects might be attributable to the drug in patients, and may prove important in helping interpret effects detected in phase III.

3.4 Methods

The core symptoms of AD and VaD are impairments to memory and other cognitive functions essential for the conduct of the activities of daily life. A range of cognitive test procedures are able to detect these impairments in demented patients and many of them are sensitive to ameliorations of these deficits produced by antidementia drugs, mainly anticholinesterases. A variety of these procedures are entirely suitable as "surrogate endpoints" in phase II trials and would also form part of the essential outcome criteria in phase III efficacy trials.

3.4.1 Pharmacokinetics

Knowledge of the pharmacokinetics of an antidementia drug is crucial in phase II. We need as much information as possible to explain the variability of our outcome measures. First we need to identify interindividual differences in plasma levels, seek any possible explanations, and consider the pharmacokinetics in the individuals in relation to the changes in their pharmacodynamic measures. Secondly, factors which influence pharmacokinetics need to be identified, such as food, age, repeated dosing, etc. The need for this information is particularly relevant for the current lead class of compounds, the anticholinesterases, where sustained release formulations of physostigmine have, for example, been necessitated by its short pharmacokinetic/pharmacodynamic half-life.

3.4.2 Pharmacodynamic Endpoints

The core symptoms of AD and other dementias are disruptions to cognitive efficiency. The cognitive impairment most commonly associated with AD is memory loss. However, more recent investigations of Alzheimer's patients using various cognitive tests have identified a wide range of impairments to other important cognitive processes including the abilities to maintain attention and to process information (e.g., References 27 and 70). Further, the impairments to these latter functions are generally as great as the deficits to memory.[70] The reason that these other decrements have traditionally been relatively underrecognized is that memory loss is a very obvious, striking, and easy to detect deficit, whereas lapses of concentration and impaired information processing are much more difficult to detect, both in clinical interviews and with cognitive tasks.

Together, these various deficits result in the reduced capacity to function in everyday life which is the early symptom of AD. As the ability to conduct the activities of daily living becomes more and more compromised, so the patient passes from the DSM-IV stage of mild dementia severity to moderate severity. There are concomitant emotional changes, including anxiety, depression, and aggression, which are partly produced by the degeneration of various neurotransmitter systems and partly an understandable response to the slow but inexorable decline in the ability to function and the resulting loss in dignity, independence, and self-esteem.

In drug development, various assessments of cognitive function, traditionally termed psychomotor tests, have long been used to identify the cognitive impairment produced by various drugs. Few procedures though had been developed for identifying improvements in mental performance, mostly due to the paucity of compounds which possessed such effects. The explosion of interest in Alzheimer's research in the late 1970s, following the discovery of central cholinergic deficits in AD patients, found psychologists ill prepared to provide appropriate measures to detect the benefits of antidementia drugs. Not only were there few measures capable of detecting improvements, but there was also very little experience available for applying tests of mental functioning to demented patients. One result was that scales which had been used to identify the presence of dementia were pressed into service to detect ameliorations of the symptoms. An example is the Mini-Mental State Examination (MMSE),[22] an excellent tool developed by Marshall Folstein and others to permit relatively inexperienced physicians to identify cognitive impairment in elderly patients. This tool rapidly became a major outcome measure in many Alzheimer's trials, something it was never designed to do and a task it was ill equipped to perform. All of the requirements for developing and validating psychometric instruments for use in clinical research were overlooked, even the most basic such as providing parallel forms for repeated testing. Thus, the outcome of multimillion dollar drug development programs, many of which involved from the outset the latest Nobel prize-winning techniques of drug synthesis, depended in the final efficacy trials, upon the sensitivity, reliability, and suitability of scales such as the MMSE. Let us emphasize that this is not a criticism of the MMSE itself, but rather the use to which it was put. The result of many of the trials may not have been affected, many of the compounds may indeed have been ineffective, but a number of now forgotten compounds would probably have shown evidence of efficacy if more appropriate procedures had been used in their evaluation.

Over the last decade a number of test systems have been developed to remedy this unfortunate situation. These are presented in Table 1. The Alzheimer's Disease Assessment Scale (ADAS)[49] is divided into two sections, an 11-item cognitive subscale with scores ranging from 0 to 70, and a 10-item noncognitive subscale that rates mood, vegetative functions, agitation, delusions, hallucinations, and concentration-distractibility. The reader may notice with interest, in view of the comments earlier in this section, that the assessment of the ability of the patient to concentrate is not included in the cognitive subscale,[23] which is unfortunate as it is only the cognitive subscale which is generally used as a primary outcome variable in clinical trials. This is a widely used scale which importantly was used to identify the efficacy of tacrine. The Dementia Rating Scale (DRS)[42] evaluates a wide range of cognitive functions including attention, praxis, verbal, and nonverbal recent memory and perseveration. The test takes about 45 min in demented patients and the score ranges from 0 to 144 (perfect performance). The CAMCOG is part of the CAMDEX[59] and contains a range of measures of cognitive efficiency. It bases some of its questions on the MMSE, though the items are much more comprehensive than the MMSE. The SKT[17] is an exciting nonautomated set of cognitive tests designed for use with impaired populations. It is brief (around 15 min), easy to administer, and, unusually for such tests, requires involvement and positive encouragement from the administrator. The system has been extensively validated and is drug sensitive.[36,55]

The other systems listed in Table 1 are computer based. Computerized systems have a number of advantages over nonautomated procedures. The most generally acknowledged advantages are the standardization these procedures bring to these assessments and the great reduction in intersite variability. Of equal importance is the extra precision of assessment which is brought by the measurement of response speed in addition to accuracy and the resulting ability to identify when motivation or strategy shifts have occurred. Furthermore, some aspects of vigilance and attention can only be definitively measured by tests properly installed on computers.[87] The four computerized systems in Table 1 all include a range of tests including assessments of attention and memory. They are all microcomputer controlled,

Table 1 Test Systems Widely Used for Identifying Change in Cognitive Efficiency in Demented Populations

Non-Computerized
Alzheimer's Disease Assessment Scale (ADAS; Mohs and Cohen, 1988)
Dementia Rating Scale (Mattis, 1988)
CAMCOG (Roth et al., 1986)
Syndrome Kurztest battery (SKT; Erzigkeit, 1989)
Computerized
Cambridge Neuropsychological Test Assessment Battery (Morris et al., 1987)
Cognitive Drug Research Computerized Assessment System (Wesnes, 1985)
Computerized Neuropsychological Test Battery (Veroff et al., 1991)
New York University Test Battery (Ferris et al., 1988)

present the task information on monitors, and use the microprocessor to record the accuracy and speed of all responses. There are large differences between the systems in the nature and implementation of the tasks, techniques for measuring responses, operator requirements, etc. Importantly, most of the systems are sensitive to the effects of scopolamine in volunteers,[21,67,82,83,88,91] indicating that the various measures have relevance for Alzheimer's deficits. Most of the systems have also published data on reliability and validity in AD patients.[20,54,61,70] Computerized tests are sensitive to cognitive improvements produced by anticholinesterases in phase II AD trials. Velnacrine was found to show improvements on computerized testing in a 12-day, 2-period cross-over trial in 34 Alzheimer's patients.[69] Importantly, these effects were consistent with a previous trial in which the effects of velnacrine were studied in the scopolamine model of dementia.[88] Tacrine was found to show improvements on computerized cognitive testing in two 12 week, 2-period cross-over trials, one involving 65 patients[60] and the other 32 patients.[86]

Understandably there has been a reluctance in many quarters to accept computers in Alzheimer's trials. It does appear at first sight strange that an elderly patient with severe cognitive disabilities would be capable of performing a computerized test, but there has now been enough experience with several systems to lay these doubts to rest. A typical impression from researchers who have newly become familiar with a computerized system is that if patients can meaningfully be tested with any sort of test, then they can also be assessed on the computerized tests.[70]

For phase II research, the tests listed in Table 1 are the ideal pharmacodynamic measures to include in phase II research projects. The recommended strategy here is to take the cognitive subscale of the ADAS as one measure, and support it with the SKT and/or one of the computerized test systems. This will give researchers an opportunity to evaluate both types of testing in the same population, and besides providing a sensitive set of assessments for the trials, will allow the relative sensitivity to be identified. Computerized tests have shown sensitivity in phase II where other assessments have failed,[86] and thus it is both necessary and appropriate to include both types of test. Although clinical global impressions and quality of life ratings should also be made, these are blunter tools of secondary importance at this stage of development. It is not until the final efficacy trials in phase III that these assessments achieve equal status to direct assessment of cognitive function.

3.5 Placebo or Active Control

In phase II trials of antidementia products there is no alternative to using placebo controls. It may also be useful to include a positive internal control at some stage, and tacrine would be the obvious first choice at the moment. This would enable the drug to be compared directly to the only drug currently approved by the FDA, and would be a useful yardstick for assessing the relative potency of the compounds. However, tacrine could not be used as an active control, the design of the study simply requiring the experimental drug to show comparable effects to tacrine. This is because negative findings with tacrine in Alzheimer's patients are still reaching the literature,[40] and thus we could not be sure without a placebo condition that the patients had actually benefited from treatment. An alternative to using a placebo that is sometimes adopted is of using a very low dose of the study compound. This is sometimes employed as a cosmetic exercise in order to prevent patients from not participating due to the fear of being randomized to placebo. It is clearly unethical when the expectation in the design of the trials is that the dose will act as a placebo. In phase II the best way to overcome this problem is to use cross-over designs where all patients receive active treatment for one period and placebo for another. Such designs are sometimes avoided due to the fear of carry-over effects, though this is largely unfounded.

If there are carry-over effects, this is in itself evidence of efficacy, and besides, the data can still be analyzed using only the first period of treatment as if it were a parallel group design.

The problem in studying a degenerative disease is that having a predosing assessment of abilities is insufficient alone to determine whether or not subsequent changes reflect improvement. Leaving aside practice or training effects, which anyway should be avoided by using appropriate measures (see Section 3.4.2), we do not know if we are simply stopping further deterioration or are actually improving over the predosing level. Thus no change from baseline over three months may be a positive finding with the drug, while equally 15% improvement may be a negative finding if the change were due to a "placebo-type" reaction due to participation in the trial as opposed to an effect of the drug. Most of the current therapies under investigation have the potential to improve performance over baseline and/or prevent further deterioration, and thus to evaluate properly antidementia drugs in phase II requires a placebo control. Further, as mentioned earlier, many of the trials in phase II could have a cross-over element, permitting placebo conditions to be included without potentially compromising patient participation.

3.6 Design, Size, and Duration of Trials

As described in the preceding section, assessment tools are available to determine efficacy in phase II, and we recommend the following design strategy utilizing such measures to achieve this. The strategy has two major stages. In the first (early phase II), the maximum tolerated dose is established, safety and pharmacokinetic assessments are conducted, and evidence of efficacy sought. If, after looking at a range of doses, no evidence of efficacy is obtained, development is stopped. Otherwise, in the second stage, the most effective dose and one or two others are tested intensively over a period of several months to confirm the effects and establish the stability of response profile over time. A successful outcome leads to phase III trials, a failure to identify any efficacy stops further development, and a promising initial response which is not maintained over time may be studied further with different dosing regimens.

Initially, a small study is conducted to identify the maximal tolerated dose in patients, starting near to the highest dose established in phase I. Depending on the speed of possible action of the drug, some cognitive testing might be included at this stage; for example, dose titration has been a feature of many tacrine trials (e.g., Reference 40). A model example of combining cognitive testing with dose-ranging designs has recently been published for the cholinergic muscarinic agonist arecoline.[72] Once a highest tolerated dose (or most potentially effective) is identified, a range of doses is tested for the minimum dosing duration in which effects might be expected to be found, based on knowledge of the drug's mode of action and also from any results obtained in phase I. This might be as brief as a few days or as long as three months. Although crossing all patients over with placebo lengthens the trial, it does greatly increase the power of the trial and is strongly recommended. Side effects should be monitored throughout and regular assessments of plasma levels made. Depending on the mechanism of action, one or more postdrug cognitive testing assessments should be included on the first day of dosing. Drugs such as anticholinesterases have previously been shown to have acute effects in carefully controlled conditions (e.g., Reference 50) and this will make the trial a single dose exercise for safety, tolerability, pharmacokinetics and pharmacodynamics as well as a multiple dose study with very little extra experimental effort. After the first dosing day, cognitive testing should be included as frequently as possible. This will enable the precise onset of any beneficial effects to be determined, and also permit an evaluation of the stability of any improvements. The size of the groups will depend on the sensitivity of the cognitive test system selected, but a minimum of 25 is likely. The number of doses tested is the major issue in such research. Three is the absolute minimum, though five or six would be better. If resources are more of an issue than development speed, three doses could be studied first, and the data analyzed to determine whether or not to test more doses. Another advantage of using a cross-over design is that each dosing group can be analyzed separately when completed.

The next decision stage is whether to proceed further or not. No evidence of efficacy on one or more sensitive instrument(s), over a range of doses, administered over a reasonable duration should be enough to stop development, particularly if no positive evidence was seen in phase I. If one or more doses show promising effects which then fade, then altering the dosing regimen (amount, frequency, or regularity) should be considered. This change might be made on the basis of the pharmacokinetics, or from considerations or concepts such as changes in receptor sensitivity. If one dose looks promising (or possibly more), a late phase II trial is the next stage, unless the effects are particularly marked (possibly extending from cognitive testing to clinical global impressions of change).

The purpose of late phase II projects is to confirm that the effects seen earlier persist over a longer dosing period, probably three months or more. One or more doses should be selected and run in parallel to a placebo group. Testing should be frequent to identify any tachyphylaxis. The group sizes should be at least 50% greater than in the first stage.

It has been stressed throughout this chapter, that evidence of efficacy should be obtained as soon as possible in the development of drugs to treat the symptoms of AD. The approach has been to include many different types of assessment and to make these assessments frequently. The researcher should not be swayed from this course by statisticians warning of an increased likelihood of making type I errors. For these trials we want the sensitivity levels to be as high as possible, and must accept the concomitant risk of making false-positive conclusions. The best defense against making such conclusions at this stage is not to reduce the number of measures or to increase the significance level we will adopt, but instead to seek patterns of results to support conclusions and avoid isolated effects, no matter how significant they might be. Phases I and II are primarily phases of discovery, when the needs of research overcome statistical caution. During phase III the reverse becomes true, and the need is to demonstrate beyond reasonable doubt that an effect can be identified at the end of the treatment period.

4 DECISION MAKING

The recommendations in this chapter for evaluating antidementia drugs in phases I and II can be encapsulated in the philosophy of learning as much about the compound as is necessary as quickly as possible. It is consistent with the two keys to successful drug development; the fastest possible development time and the expenditure of resources on successful products (avoiding the waste of resources on products destined to be failures). These recommendations are designed equally for small companies with a single compound as they are for large companies with many compounds. Cash-limited companies need as much information as possible at each stage of development prior to committing further expenditure. Large companies may wish to compare various candidates and develop only those showing most promise. For any company, however, the decision to proceed to phase III must be made on the basis of evidence not hope. Rushing ahead without proper information may get a compound into phase III in record time, but it is highly unlikely it will proceed further. In phase I, a failure in, for example, the scopolamine model can result in a no-go decision, especially for an anticholinesterase, whereas other compounds might be cautiously taken to early phase II. However, in phase II, no news is definitely bad news, and properly conducted phase II programs should yield clear go/no-go decisions.

5 KEY LITERATURE EXAMPLES

In a field without an approved widely effective medication, "model and key trials" are clearly rare, though two examples are selected which reflect the recommendations of this chapter.

The study of Soncrant et al.[72] illustrates admirably how tolerability assessments can be combined with cognitive assessment in a dose-ranging trial using only nine AD patients. The drug was the classical muscarinic agonist, arecoline, which was studied at a range of intravenous infusions. In an open phase of dose escalation, up to ten rising doses were administered over a period of 11-16 days. The optimal dose was then put into a double-blind, cross-over replication in which the optimal dose and placebo were administered each for 5 days separated by a week. This study found clear evidence of efficacy, at a lower dose than previously studied, and also showed an inverted-U dose-response function. The clear messages from such a study are that small intensively monitored trials can detect clear evidence of efficacy and identify effective doses which have previously been overlooked. This study admirably demonstrates the potential folly of basing dosing in efficacy trials solely upon tolerability data.

The phase I and II development of the anticholinesterase, velnacrine, encapsulated many of the general recommendations made in this chapter. The reader is referred to the review of Goa and Fitton.[25] The drug was first tested in the scopolamine model of dementia and found to be effective on a number of computerized assessments. The drug was then tested in a small cross-over study with 35 patients dosed on active and placebo medication for 10 days. The two studies used the same computerized assessment system, and the drug was found to affect favorably some of the same measures in AD patients as were affected in the scopolamine model. These effects were supported by changes in the ADAS. In a further small trial with 12 AD patients velnacrine was found to improve word recognition. The drug was then entered into large efficacy trials.

These two examples illustrate how drugs should be evaluated prior to being entered into efficacy trials.

REFERENCES

1. Altman H.J., Normile H.J., Gershon S. (1987) Non-cholinergic pharmacology in human cognitive disorders. In (S.M. Stall, S.D. Iverson, E.C. Goodman Eds.) *Cognitive Neurochemistry,* Oxford: Oxford University Press, pp. 346-371.
2. Amaducci L., Angst J., Bech P. et al (1990) Consensus conference on the methodology of clinical trials of "nootropics." *Pharmacopsychiatry* 23: 171-175.
3. Bachman D.L., Wolf P.A., Linn R.T., Knoefel J.E., Cobb J.L., Belanger A.J., White L.R., Agostino R.B. Incidence of dementia and probable Alzheimer's disease in a general population: the Framingham Study. *Neurology* 43: 515-519.
4. Baron J.C. Functional Metabolic Assessment Using Positron Emission Tomography. In (N. Canal, V.C. Hachinski, G. McKahann, M. Franceschi Eds.) *Guidelines for Drug Trials in Memory Disorders,* Raven Press, New York.
5. Breimer D.D., Schellens J.H.M. (1990) A "cocktail" strategy to assess *in vivo* oxidative drug metabolism in humans. *TIPS* 11: 223-225.
6. Castano E.M., Frangione B. (1991) Alzheimer's disease from the perspective of the systemic and localized forms of amyloidosis. *Brain Pathol.* 1: 263-71.
7. Copeland J.R., Davidson I.A., Dewey M.E., Gimore C., Larkin B.A., Mc William C., Saunders P.A., Scott A., Sharma V., Sullivan C. (1992). Alzheimer's disease, other dementias, depression and pseudodementia: prevalence, incidence and three year outcome in Liverpool. *Br. J. Psychiatry* 161: 230-239.
8. Cowen P.J., Anderson I.M., Graham-Smith D.F. Neuroendocrine effects of azaspirones. *J. Clin. Psychopharmacol.* 10: 21-255.
9. Crook T., Bartus R.T., Ferris S., Whitehouse P., Cohen G.D., Gershon S. (1986). Age-Associated Memory Impairment: Proposed diagnostic criteria and measures of clinical change — Report of a National Institute of Mental Health Work Group. *Dev. Neuropsychol.* 2: 261-276.
10. Crook T.H., Tinkleberg J., Yesavage J., Petrie W., Nuzi M.G., Massari D.C. (1991) Effects of phosphatidylserine in age-associated memory impairment. *Neurology* 41: 644-649.
11. Cull C., Trimble M. (1987) Automated testing in Psychopharmacology. In I. Hindmarch, P.D. Stonier (Eds.) *Human Psychopharmacology: Measures and Methods Volume 1.* Chichester, Wiley, pp 113-154.
12. Cutler N.R., Sramek J.K., Murphy M.F., Nash R.J. (1992). Implications of the study population in the early evaluation of anticholinesterase inhibitors for Alzheimer's disease. *Ann. Pharmacother.* 26:1118-1122.
13. Dinan T.G., O'Keane V., Thakore J. (1994). Pyridostigmine induced growth hormone release in mania: focus on the cholinergic/somatostatin system. *Clin. Endocrinol.* 40: 93-96.
14. DSM IV. Diagnostic and Statistical Manual of Mental Disorders — Fourth Edition (1995). The American Psychiatric Association, Washington, D.C.
15. Ebmeier K.P., Hunter R., Curran S.M., Dougal N.J., Murray C.L., Wyper D.J., Patterson J., Hanson M.T., Siegfried K., Goodwin G.M. (1992) Effects of a single-dose of the acetylcholinesterase inhibitor velnacrine on recognition memory and regional cerebral blood flow in Alzheimer's disease. *Psychopharmacology* 108: 103-109.
16. Enz A., Amstutz R., Boddeke H., Gmelin G., Malanowski J. (1993) Brain selective inhibition of acetylcholinesterase: a novel approach to therapy for Alzheimer's disease. *Prog. Brain Res.* 98: 431-8.
17. Erzigkeit H. (1988) The SKT — a short cognitive performance test as an instrument for the assessment of clinical efficacy of cognition enhancers. In (M. Bergener, B. Reisberg Eds.) *Diagnosis and Treatment of Senile Dementia.* Berlin: Springer-Verlag pp. 164-174.
18. Evans D.A., Funkenstein H.H., Albert M.S., Scherr P.A., Cook N.R., Chown M.J. Hebert L.E., Hennekens C.H., Taylor J.O. (1989). Prevalence of Alzheimer's disease in a community population of older persons. Higher than previously reported. *JAMA* 262: 2551-2556.
19. Farlow M., Gracon S.I., Hershey L.A., Lewis K.W., Sadowsky C.H., Dolan-Ureno J. (1992) A controlled trial of tacrine in Alzheimer's Disease. *JAMA* 263: 2525-2529.
20. Ferris S.H., Flicker C., Reisberg B. (1988) NYU computerized test battery for assessing cognition in aging and dementia. *Psychopharm. Bull.* 24: 699-702.
21. Flicker C., Serby M., Ferris S.H. (1990) Scopolamine effects on memory, language, visuospatial praxis and psychomotor speed. *Psychopharmacology* 100: 243-250.
22. Folstein, M.F., Folstein M.E., McHugh P.R. (1975) Mini-mental state: a practical method for grading the cognitive state of patients for the clinician. *J. Psychiatry Res.* 12: 189-198.
23. Gershon S., Ferris S.H., Kennedy J.S., Kurtz N.M., Overall J.E., Pollock B.G., Reisberg B., Whitehouse P.J. (1994). Methods for the evaluation of pharmacologic agents in the treatment of cognitive and other deficits in dementia. In (R.F. Prien, D.S. Robinson Eds.) *Clinical Evaluation of Psychotropic Drugs: Principles and Guidelines,* Raven Press, New York, pp. 467-500.
24. Giurgea C. (1980) *Fundamentals to a Pharmacology of the Mind.* Springfield IL: Charles C Thomas.
25. Goa K.L., Fitton A. (1994). Velnacrine in Alzheimer's disease: An initial appraisal of its clinical potential. *CNS Drugs* 1: 232-240.
26. Goedert M. (1993) Tau protein and the neurofibrillary pathology of Alzheimer's disease. *Trends Neurosci.* 16: 460-465.
27. Gordon B. and Carson K. (1990) The basis for choice reaction time slowing in Alzheimer's disease. *Brain Cognition* 13: 148-166.

28. Gottfries C.G., Karlsson I., Nyth A.L., (1992) Treatment of depression in elderly patients with and without dementia disorders. *Int. Clin. Psychopharmacol.* 6: 55-64.
29. Guez D. (1990) Long-term effects and safety of almitrine-raubasine in age-associated cognitive decline. *Clin. Neuropharmacol.* 13: S109-S116.
30. Gustafson K. (1993) Physostigmine and tetrahydroaminoacridine treatment of Alzheimer's disease. *Acta Neurol. Scand.* 149: 39-41.
31. Hindmarch I., Stonier P.D. (eds) (1987) *Human Psychopharmacology: Measures and Methods,* Vol. 1, Wiley, Chichester.
32. Holland R.L., Wesnes K., Dietrich B. (1994) Single-dose human pharmacology of umespirone. *Eur. J. Clin. Pharmacol.* 46: 461-469.
33. Itil T.M., Itil K.Z. (1986) The significance of pharmacodynamic measurements in the assessment of bioavailability and bioequivalence of psychotropic drugs using CEEG and dynamic brain mapping. *J. Clin. Psychiatry* 47: 20-27.
34. Kase C.S. (1991) Epidemiology of multi-infarct dementia. *Alzheimer Dis. Assoc. Disord.* 5: 71-76.
35. Kilbourn M.R., DaSilva J.N., Frey K.A., Koeppe R.A., Kuhl D.E. (1993) *In vivo* imaging of vesicular monoamine transporters in human brain using (11C) tetrabenazine and positron emission tomography. *J. Neurochem.* 60: 2315-2318.
36. Kim Y.S., Nibbelink D.W., Overall J.E. Factor Structure and Scoring of the SKT test battery. *J. Clin. Psychol.* 49: 61-71.
37. Kumar A. (1993) Functional brain imaging in late-life depression and dementia. *J. Clin. Psychiatry* 54: 21-25.
38. Leber, P. (1990) Guidelines for the clinical evaluation of antidementia drugs, First Draft. November 8, 1990. Division of Neuropharmacological Drug Products, Office of Drug Evaluation I, Food and Drug Administration, Bethesda, M.D.
39. Levy R., Howard R.J., Richards M. et al (1994) Age-Associated Cognitive Decline. *Inter. Psychogeriatr.* 6: 63-68.
40. Maltby N., Broe G.A., Creasey H., Jorm A.F., Christensen H., Brooks W.S. (1994). Efficacy of tacrine and lecithin in mild to moderate Alzheimer's disease: double blind trial. *BMJ* 308: 879-883.
41. Masliah E., Miller A., Terry R.D. (1993). The synaptic organization of the neocortex in Alzheimer's disease. *Med. Hypotheses* 41: 334-340.
42. Mattis S. (1988) Dementia rating scale professional manual. Odessa, Florida: Psychological Resources Inc.
43. Mauri M., Sinforiani E., Reverberi F., Merlo P., Bono G. (1994) Pramiracetam effects on scopolamine-induced amnesia in healthy volunteers. *Arch. Gerontol. Geriatr.* 18: 133-139.
44. McDonald R. (1979) Hydergine: a review of 26 clinical studies. *Pharmacopsychiatr. Neuropsychopharm.* 12: 407-422.
45. McEntee W.J., Crook T.H., Jenkyn L.R., Petrie W., Larrabee G.J., Coffey D.J. (1991) Treatment of age-associated memory impairment with guanfacine. *Psychopharmacol. Bull.* 27: 41-46.
46. McKhann G., Drachmann D., Folstein M., Katzman R., Price D., Stadlan E.M. (1984). Clinical diagnosis of Alzheimer's disease: report on the NINCDS-ADRDA work group under the auspices of the Department of Health & Human Services Task Force on Alzheimer's disease. *Neurology* 34: 939-944.
47. Millson D., Sohail S., Lettis S., Fenwick S. (1992) Duration of inhibition of the flare response to intradermal 5-hydroxytryptamine in man by GR 68755, a novel specific 5-HT_3 receptor antagonist. *Br. J. Clin. Pharmacol.* 33: 546P-547P.
48. Mohr E., Mendis T., Rusk I.N., Grimes J.D. (1994) Neurotransmitter replacement therapy in Alzheimer's disease *J. Psychiatry. Neurosci.* 19: 17-23.
49. Mohs R.C. and Cohen L. Alzheimer's disease assessment scale (ADAS).(1988) *Psychopharmacol. Bull.* 24: 627-628.
50. Mohs R.C., Davis K.L. (1987): The experimental pharmacology of Alzheimer's disease and related dementias. In (H. Meltzer Ed.) *Psychopharmacology: The Third Generation of Progress.* Raven Press: New York. pp. 921-928.
51. Morris R.G., Evenden J.L., Sahakian B.J., Robbins T.W. (1987) Computer-aided assessment of dementia: comparative studies of neuropsychological deficits in Alzheimer-type dementia and Parkinson's Disease. In (S.M. Stahl, S.D. Iverson, E.C. Goodman Eds.) *Cognitive Neurochemistry,* Oxford: Oxford University Press, pp 21-36.
52. Mortel K.F., Pavol M.A., Wood S., Meyer J.S., Terayama Y., Rexter J.L., Herod B. (1994) Prospective studies of cerebral perfusion and cognitive testing among elderly normal volunteers and patients with ischemic vascular dementia and Alzheimer's disease. *Angiology* 45: 171-180.
53. Munoz D.G. (1991) The pathological basis of multi-infarct dementia. *Alzheimer Dis. Assoc. Disord.* 5: 77-90.
54. Nicholl C.G., Lynch S., Kelly C.A., White L., Simpson L., Simpson P.M., Wesnes K., Pitt B.M.N. (1995). The Cognitive Drug Research computerized assessment system in the evaluation of early dementia — is speed of the essence? *Int. J. Geriatr. Psychiatry,* in press.
55. Overall J.E., Schaltenbrand R. (1991) The SKT neuropsychological test battery. *J. Geriatr. Psychiatry Neurol.*
56. Preda L., Alberoni M., Bressi S., Cattaneo C., Parini J., Canal N., Franceschi M. (1993) Effects of acute doses of oxiracetam in the scopolamine model of human amnesia. *Psychopharmacology* 110: 421-426.
57. Preston G.C., Millson D.S., Ceuppens P.R., Warburton D.M. (1992) Effects of the 5-HT3 receptor antagonist GR68755 on a scopolamine induced cognitive deficit in healthy volunteers. *Br. J Clin. Pharmacol.* 33: 546P.
58. Roses A.D. (1994) Apolipoprotem E is a genetic locus that affects the rate of Alzheimer Disease expression. *Neuropsychopharmacology* 10: 55-75.
59. Roth M., Tym E., Mountjoy C.Q., Huppert F.A., Hendrie H., Verma S., Goddard R. (1986) A standardised instrument for the diagnosis of mental disorder in the elderly with special reference to the early detection of dementia. *Br. J. Psychiatry,* 149: 698-709.

60. Sahakian B.J., Coull J.T. (1994). Nicotine and tetrahydroaminoacridine: evidence for improved attention in patients with dementia of the Alzheimer type. *Drug Dev. Res.* 31: 80-88.
61. Sahakian B.J., Morris R.G., Evenden J.L., Heald A., Levy R., Philpot M., Robbins T.W. (1988) A comparative study of visuospatial memory and learning in Alzheimer-type dementia and Parkinson's disease. *Brain* 111: 695-718.
62. Saletu B. (1993) *Neurophysiological Assessment of Efficacy in Drug Trials with Memory Disorders in Guidelines for Drug Trials in Memory Disorders* (N. Canal, V.C. Hachinski, G. McKhann, M. Frankest, Eds.) Raven Press, New York.
63. Saletu B., Grunberger J., Linzmayer L., Anderer P., Semlitsch H.V. (1990) EEG brain mapping and psychometry in age-associated memory impairment after acute and 2-week infusions with the hemoderivative Actovegin: double-blind, placebo-controlled trials. *Neuropsychobiology* 24: 135-148.
64. Sarter M. (1991). Taking stock of cognition enhancers. *TIPS Rev.* 12: 456-461.
65. Schaffler K., Klausmitzer W. (1988) Randomised placebo-controlled double-blind cross-over study on antihypoxidotic effects of piracetam using psychophysiological measures in healthy volunteers. *Arzneimittelforschung* 38: 288-291.
66. Semlitsch H.V., Anderer P., Saletu B., Hochmayer I. (1990) Topographic mapping of cognitive event-related potentials in a double-blind, placebo controlled study with the hemoderivative Actovegin in age-associated memory impairment. *Neuropsychobiology* 24: 49-56.
67. Semple J., Kumar R., Truman M.I., Shorter J. (1992) The effects of scopolamine hydrobromide upon performance of the CANTAB battery. British Association for Psychopharmacology, August 1992, Cambridge.
68. Shen U.C., Li G., Li Y.T., Chen C.H., Li S.R., Zhao Y.W., Zhang W.X. (1994) Epidemiology of age-related dementia in China. *Chin. Med. J.* (Engl) 107: 60-64.
69. Siegfried K.R. (1993) Pharmacodynamic and early clinical studies with velnacrine. *Acta Neurol. Scand.* 149: 26-28.
70. Simpson P.M., Surmon D.J., Wesnes K.A. and Wilcock G.R. (1991). The cognitive drug research computerized assessment system for demented patients: A validation study. *Int. J. Geriatr. Psychiatry,* 6: 95-102.
71. Smith A.P., Kendrick A.M., Maben A.L. (1992). Effects of breakfast and caffeine on performances and mood in the late morning and after lunch. *Neuropsychobiology* 26: 198-204.
72. Soncrant T.T., Raffaele K.C., Asthana S., Berardi A., Morris P.P., Haxby J.V. (1993) Memory improvement without toxicity during chronic, low dose intravenous arecoline in Alzheimer's disease. *Psychopharmacology* 112: 421-427.
73. Subhan Z., Hindmarch I. (1984) The psychopharmacological effects of ginkgo biloba extract in normal healthy volunteers. *Int. J. Clin. Res.* 4: 89-93.
74. Thal L.J. Clinical trials in Alzheimer's disease (1994) In (R.D. Terry Ed.) *Alzheimer Disease*, Raven Press, New York, pp. 431-443.
75. Ueda K., Kawano H., Hasuo Y., Fujishima M. (1992) Prevalence and etiology of dementia in a Japanese community. *Stroke* 23: 798-803.
76. Urakami K., Shimomura T., Ohshima T., Okada A., Adachi Y., Takahashi K., Asakura M., Matsumura R. (1993). Clinical effect of WEB 1881 (nebracetam fumarate) on patients with dementia of the Alzheimer type and study of its clinical pharmacology. *Clin. Neuropharmacol.* 16: 347-358.
77. Veroff A.E., Cutler N.R., Sramek J.J., Prior P.L., Mickelson W., Hartman J.K. (1991). A new assessment tool for neuropsychopharmacologic research: The computerized neuropsychological test battery. *J. Geriatr. Psychoneurol.* 2: 211-217.
78. Villardita C., Grioli S., Lomeo C., Cattaneo C., Parini J. (1992). Clinical studies with oxiracetam in patients with dementia of Alzheimer type and multi-infarct dementia of mild to moderate degree. *Neuropsychobiology* 25: 24-28.
79. Wallnöfer A., Prescott J., Malek N., Dingemanse J., Wesnes K., McClelland G. Physostigmine improves cognitive performance and alters EEG in healthy volunteers. An approach to study central cholinergic effects. XIXth C.I.N.P. Congress, Washington D.C., June 27-July 1st, 1994.
80. Wesnes K. A fully automated psychometric test battery for human psychopharmacology. IVth World Congress of Biological Psychiatry, Philadelphia, September 1985.
81. Wesnes K., Anand R., Lorscheid T. (1990). Potential of moclobemide to improve cerebral insufficiency identified using a scopolamine model of ageing and dementia. *Acta Psychiatr. Scand.* 82: 71-72.
82. Wesnes K., Anand R., Simpson P.M., Christmas L. (1990). The use of a scopolamine model to study the potential nootropic effects of aniracetam and piracetam in healthy volunteers. *Psychopharmacology* 4: 219-232.
83. Wesnes K., Jones R.W., Kirby J. (1991). The effects of D-cycloserine, a glycine agonist, in a human model of the cognitive deficits associated with ageing and dementia. *Br. J. Clin. Pharmacol.* 31: 577P-578P.
84. Wesnes K., Neuman E., de Wilde H.J.G., Malbezin M., Castagné I., Crijns H.J.M.J., Jonkman J.H.G., Guez D. (1994). Pharmacodynamic effects of a repeated oral administration of 4 dose levels of S 12024-2 in 36 elderly volunteers. *Neurobiol. Aging* 15: S100.
85. Wesnes, K., Revell, A. (1984). The separate and combined effects of scopolamine and nicotine on human information processing. *Psychopharmacology* 84: 5-11.
86. Wesnes K., Scott M., Boyle M., Surmon D.J., Wilcock G.K. (1994). Use of the Cognitive Drug Research computerized assessment system to measure the efficacy of THA and galanthamine in Alzheimer's disease. *Psychopharmacol. Bull.* 30: 139.
87. Wesnes K., Simpson P.M., Christmas L. (1987). The assessment of human information processing abilities in psychopharmacology. In I. Hindmarch, P.D. Stonier (Eds.) *Human Psychopharmacology: Measures and Methods Volume 1.* Chichester, Wiley, pp. 79-92.

88. Wesnes K., Simpson P., Christmas L., Siegfried K. (1990) Effects of HP 029 in a scopolamine model of ageing and dementia. 17th Congress of Collegium Internationale Neuro-Psychopharmacologicum, September 10-14, 1990, Kyoto, Japan. (Abstracts Vol. II, Page 235).
89. Wesnes K., Simpson P.M., Kidd, A.G. (1987). The use of a scopolamine model to study the nootropic effects of tenilsetam (CAS 997) in man. *Med. Sci. Res.* 15: 1063-1064.
90. Wesnes K., Simpson P.M., Kidd A.G. (1988). An investigation of the range of cognitive impairments induced by scopolamine 0.6 mg. *Hum. Psychopharmacol.* 3: 27-43.
91. Wesnes K., Simpson P.M., White L., Pinker S., Jertz G., Murphy M. and Siegfried K. (1991). Cholinesterase inhibition in the scopolamine model of dementia. *N.Y. Acad. Sci.,* 640: 268-271.
92. Wesnes, K., Warburton, D.M. (1984). Effects of scopolamine and nicotine on human rapid information processing performance. *Psychopharmacology* 82: 147-150.
93. Wesnes, K., Warburton, D.M. (1984). The effects of cigarettes of varying yield on rapid information processing performance. *Psychopharmacology* 82: 338-342.

Chapter 27

Antiparkinsonian Agents

J. L. Montastruc, O. Rascol, J. M. Senard, O. Blin, and C. Thalamas

CONTENTS

1 Introduction 373
2 Healthy Volunteers 374
2.1 Selection Criteria 374
2.2 Safety Considerations 374
2.3 Methods 374
2.3.1 General Trial Design 374
2.3.2 Pharmacokinetic Issues 375
2.3.3 Pharmacodynamic Issues 375
2.4 Controls 375
3 Patient Studies 375
3.1 Suitability 375
3.2 Selection Criteria 376
3.3 Safety Considerations 376
3.4 Methods 377
3.4.1 Pharmacokinetics 378
3.4.2 Surrogate Markers 378
3.5 Placebo or Active Control 379
3.6 Size and Duration of the Trial 380
4 Decision Making 380
Acknowledgments 380
References 380

1 INTRODUCTION

Parkinson's disease, one of the most common causes of disability among the elderly, is usually defined clinically as a syndrome with three main well-defined symptoms: bradykinesia plus resting tremor, rigidity or postural instability, and pathologically by degeneration of the dopaminergic nigrostriatal pathway, decreases in the striatal concentration of dopamine (and other related amines and neuropeptides) and the presence of inclusions (Lewy bodies) in neurons of the substantia nigra.[1-4] These observations have led to the classical pharmacological approach to the treatment of Parkinson's disease; namely restoring the disturbed neurotransmitter balance either by (1) inhibiting acetylcholine output with anticholinergic (antimuscarinic) drugs (since the terminals of the cholinergic axons located in the striatum remain fully active), or (2) countering the dopamine deficiency through direct or indirect supplementation.

Levodopa therapy remains the "gold standard" of treatment. Levodopa (which in contrast to dopamine crosses the blood-brain barrier) is decarboxylated into dopamine in the brain, increasing the level of dopamine in the nigrostriatal synaptic cleft. However, the initial therapeutic success of levodopa is blunted by the development of motor side effects, such as abnormal movements or fluctuations in performance and adverse mental effects after a few years of treatment.[2,5]

Due to the limitations of levodopa therapy, the pharmacological treatment of patients with Parkinson's disease has been recently expanded to incorporate four different research approaches: (1) the development of dopamine agonists and drugs which could potentiate the effect of levodopa; (2) the search for agents which may prevent or slow the underlying pathological process (e.g., selegiline);[6] (3) studies of the feasibility of brain tissue transplants; and (4) new routes of administration of old drugs (Table 1). Because of their major side effects and their relatively low efficacy, anticholinergic drugs are considered as old drugs and no new anticholinergic agents are currently under development.

0-8493-9230-6/97/$0.00+$.50
© 1997 by CRC Press, Inc.

Table 1 Current Research in Antiparkinsonian Therapy

Type of Research	Example
New drugs	
Long-acting dopamine agonists	Cabergoline
Non-ergoline dopamine agonists	Ropinirole
Partial dopamine agonists	Terguride
Monoaminooxidase inhibitors	Lazabemide
Catechol-*O*-methyl transferase inhibitors	Tolcapone
N-methyl-D-aspartate receptor antagonist	Dextromethorphan
Trophic agonists	GM1 ganglioside
Protective therapy	
Monoaminooxidase inhibitors	Selegiline
Scavenger of free radicals	Vitamine E
Tissue transplants	Fetal tissue
	Cultured tissues
New routes of administration of old drugs (levodopa, apomorphine...)	Controlled release
	Subcutaneous, transdermal, sublingual, transnasal

2 HEALTHY VOLUNTEERS

As indicated above, the development of levodopa and its introduction in clinical practice was performed more than 25 years ago following pathophysiological observations. No studies in healthy volunteers were performed before levodopa was first administered to parkinsonian patients. The development of dopamine agonists and especially the first one (bromocriptine) was the first to be done more closely in accordance with modern concepts of clinical pharmacology, and for the past 15 years, new antiparkinsonian drugs (especially dopamine agonists) have been investigated in phase I studies on healthy volunteers.

2.1 Selection Criteria

For phase I study of new antiparkinsonian drugs there are no selection criteria specific to antiparkinsonian drugs. As in other studies, women are usually excluded. Since the relationship between smoking, enzymatic induction, and Parkinson's disease is not well understood, it would be better to avoid heavy smokers, although no clear consensus exists on this point.

Doing studies in elderly, healthy volunteers should be considered because Parkinson's disease usually occurs after the age of 50. Most of the phase I studies are, however, currently performed in young volunteers (aged from 18 to 30 years).

2.2 Safety Considerations

Phase I studies with new antiparkinsonian drugs should be performed in clinical pharmacological units or clinical research centers with trained personnel. There are no specific safety aspects. Blood pressure and heart rate, in particular, must be carefully monitored.

2.3 Methods

2.3.1 General Trial Design

The first phase I studies should investigate the effect of a single dose, whereas subsequent trials should be multiple dose studies. There is no specific trial design that is preferable for antiparkinsonian drugs. Early dose-ranging studies, and determination of a maximum tolerated dose, appear to be important since dopaminergic drugs often induce major gastrointestinal effects (nausea and vomiting), postural dizziness and/or cardiovascular side effects (hypotension) in healthy volunteers at relatively low dosages. These side effects appear to be more pronounced in healthy volunteers than in patients. The reason is unknown. These side effects are subject to the development of tolerance, which usually develops and becomes evident after two to four administrations. Dopaminergic agonists (bromocriptine) were first developed at low dosages (10-20 mg daily) which were not fully active. It was only in phase IV studies that the effects of relative high doses (30-60 mg daily of bromocriptine) were demonstrated.[7] Thus, one can recommend the development of dose-ranging studies in phase I using increasing doses during a short period of time (e.g., 5 to 15 days, for example). On the other hand, these studies could be performed with concomitant domperidone treatment, in order to decrease these peripheral side effects and allow the administration of higher dosages to healthy volunteers (domperidone is a peripheral dopamine antagonist which does not cross the blood-brain barrier and thus does not interfere with the antiparkinsonian effect of dopaminergic drugs).[7]

2.3.2 Pharmacokinetic Issues

An important pharmacokinetic problem with new antiparkinsonian drugs concerns the development of an appropriate formulation and establishing a reliable assay. These drugs (and especially dopamine agonists) are usually relatively large molecules. No specific analytic method, for example, was developed for pergolide during its clinical development, and there are relatively few pharmacokinetic studies in healthy volunteers (or in patients) with dopamine agonists.[7] Pharmacokinetic studies must be performed with both single intravenous injections and oral regimens (single-dose followed by multiple-dose studies). Although pharmacokinetics parameters are usually investigated in blood and urine, it would be better to measure central concentrations of the drugs but, unfortunately, no simple methods are available. Since antiparkinsonian drugs must be taken several times a day, the interaction with food should be investigated. Food, and especially protein content are known to interfere with the antiparkinsonian effect of levodopa.[8] Since most of the new antiparkinsonian drugs are usually given in addition to levodopa, interaction studies with different levodopa formulations are mandatory.

The positron-emission tomography (PET) scan technique permits the *in vivo* study of central levodopa pharmacokinetics. An increase in plasma amino acid levels reduces [18F] fluorodopa capture by nigrostriatal neurons, illustrating the competition between amino acids and levodopa for transport across the blood-brain barrier.[9] It could also be useful to investigate central penetration of new drugs other than dopamine agonists like, for example, monoaminooxidase (MAO) or catechol-*O*-methyl-transferase (COMT) inhibitors.[10] However, PET studies are very expensive and their use for pharmacokinetic phase I studies is not widely established.[11,12]

As indicated in Table 1, new MAO and COMT inhibitors are currently being developed as levodopa adjuncts. Phase I studies must also investigate changes in plasma levodopa and metabolite concentrations. For example, COMT inhibitors totally suppress 3-*O*-methyl-dopa levels.

2.3.3 Pharmacodynamic Issues

Most of the currently developed new antiparkinsonian drugs are dopamine agonists. One of the major pharmacological effects of a dopamine agonist is a decrease in serum prolactin which can be explained by an action on hypothalamic D2 receptors.[13,14] The prolactin suppression test is relatively difficult to perform. It requires trained centers since nonspecific variations in plasma prolactin levels may occur like, for example, due to stress in the volunteers. Basal prolactin levels must be measured after 10 a.m. in order to avoid stress-induced increase in plasma prolactin levels.

Due to the difficulties of such classical neuropharmacological tests, several groups are currently trying to investigate new tests predictive of dopaminergic functions. Blinking and yawning behaviors,[15,16] and other objective assessment methods such as quantitative analysis of gait parameters,[17] spatiotemporal contrast sensitivity,[18] and eye movements[19,20] have been proposed. However, further studies are needed to establish their definite value in clinical pharmacology.

Phase I studies of MAO-B and new COMT inhibitors usually include additional biochemical determinations of the kinetics of platelet MAO-B or erythrocyte COMT inhibition in order to determine the future dose regimen. For MAO-B inhibitors, a pharmacodynamic interaction with orally administered tyramine must also be investigated using the classical tyramine test.

2.4 Controls

As in other phase I studies, the trials of new antiparkinsonian drugs in healthy volunteers must be performed against placebo. There is no specific gold standard for comparison of safety, tolerability, and pharmacodynamic effects.

3 PATIENT STUDIES

3.1 Suitability

The first studies in patients can be performed after full completion of both pharmacokinetic and pharmacodynamic studies in healthy volunteers. It is not ethical to perform the first entry-into-man study in patients. The first phase II studies are usually acute studies, i.e., investigations with no potential therapeutic benefits.

Later, according to the results of toxicological studies in animals, the phase II trials can lead to an open follow-up study providing possible therapeutic benefit for the patient. Signed informed consent is necessary and there is no major problem since patients with dementia are usually excluded from these studies.

3.2 Selection Criteria

The main problem of current antiparkinsonian trials concerns patient selection. The clinical features of parkinsonism are well known. However, although two different patients can be very similar in clinical terms especially during the first few years of the disease, they can suffer from a different form of parkinsonism. In fact, symptoms of parkinsonism can also be associated with several other clinical conditions, for example, dementia, depression, autonomic dysfunction, or cerebellar symptoms. Thus, classifications of parkinsonism usually differentiate between primary and secondary parkinsonism and Multiple System Atrophy (MSA; Table 2).[21,22] Among the secondary parkinsonisms, the most frequently observed clinical entity is drug-induced parkinsonism. Several drugs can induce parkinsonism like neuroleptic agents, methyldopa, flunarizine, cinnarizine, and lithium.[23] Currently used antiparkinsonian drugs (levodopa, dopamine agonists, and anticholinergic agents) are only fully active in idiopathic Parkinson's disease. There are at present no universally accepted pathognomonic diagnostic criteria; indeed, as in Alzheimer's disease and other dementias, the diagnosis of idiopathic Parkinson's disease can be only made *post mortem* with the detection of Lewy bodies. Brain-bank studies[24] have identified some useful criteria for making a more accurate diagnosis of idiopathic Parkinson's disease and these should be applied in studies with a new antiparkinsonian drug. Table 3 summarizes the clinical diagnostic and exclusion criteria of the U.K. Parkinson's Disease Society Brain Bank.[24] Patients included in phase II studies are usually older than 30 years (in order to exclude juvenile parkinsonism which could respond to levodopa in a different way than idiopathic Parkinson's disease) and younger than 75-80 years. There are male or female and if female, they will be postmenopausal, surgically sterilized, or have undergone hysterectomy. Exclusion criteria for the diagnosis of idiopathic Parkinson's disease are also listed in Table 3. Of course, patients with a history of cardiovascular (arterial hypertension, myocardial infarction, unstable angina, cardiac failure or arrhythmias, vaso-occlusive disease, or cardiomyopathy) hepatic, renal, and psychiatric (schizophrenia, depression, current alcoholism, or drug dependence) disorders will be excluded from the study. Since dopaminergic drugs are known to decrease blood pressure,[14] other concomitant antihypertensive or vasoactive drug treatments must remain stable during the month preceeding the entry into the study.

Pharmacological tests could be useful in predicting the dopa-responsiveness of patients and the likely efficacy of treatment. However, they do not predict the etiology itself because some MSA patients could respond to dopaminergic drugs. These acute tests include the "levodopa test"[25,26] and the "apomorphine test":[27] an improvement after the acute administration of levodopa and/or apomorphine is predictive of a good response to long-term dopaminergic therapy.[27,28] Analysis of eye movements can also be useful to differentiate idiopathic Parkinson's disease from Parkinson-plus syndromes.[19,20] Finally, apomorphine might be useful as a predictive indicator of levodopa responsiveness and may help to differentiate idiopathic Parkinson's disease from other extrapyramidal syndromes (which do not usually respond to dopaminergic stimulation).[27] We also observed that the apomorphine test can also be performed without stopping levodopa and is especially useful in nonfluctuating patients insufficiently improved by their current treatment. In these cases, a positive response predicts that an increase in the levodopa dosage or an additionnal drug should be beneficial while a negative response suggests the contrary.[28]

3.3 Safety Considerations

The major expected side effects of dopaminergic drugs are nausea, vomiting, and arterial hypotension[7] which can be prevented by domperidone. However, as discussed above for healthy volunteers, domperidone is not usually used as a systematic preventive treatment since tolerance to these side effects usually develops and domperidone is not available in U.S. Domperidone is sometimes allowed for the treatment of side effects of peripheral origin. In other trials, the occurence of dopaminergic side effects may lead to modifications of the dosing regimen. The dose could be kept constant or if necessary reduced. Another well-known side effect of dopaminergic drugs is sedation. It cannot be corrected by domperidone since it is of central origin.

Side effects can be assessed using either an open or a closed questionnaire.

The major central side effects of currently used dopaminergic drugs are including psychosis and/or hallucinations. Future phase II trials could establish the occurrence of these side effects in comparison to old drugs (levodopa, bromocriptine).

Table 2 Classification of Parkinsonism

- **I. Primary Parkinson's diseases**
  - A. Idiopathic — dominated by:
    1. Tremor
    2. Postural instability and gait difficulty (PIGD)
    3. Akinesia (freezing)
    4. Dementia
    5. Depression
    6. Sensory disturbance
    7. Autonomic dysfunction
  - B. Inherited — associated with essential tremor, dystonia, or peripheral neuropathy
  - C. Young onset — associated with dystonia or essential tremor
  - D. Juvenile Parkinson's disease
- **II. Secondary parkinsonisms**
  - A. Drugs
  - B. Toxins (manganese, mercury, carbon monoxide, cyanide, carbon disulfide, methanol, ethanol, MPTP)
  - C. Metabolic (parathyroid, acquired hepatocerebral degeneration, GM1, gangliosidosis, Gaucher's disease)
  - D. Postencephalitic and slow virus
  - E. Vascular (multi-infarct, Binswanger's disease)
  - F. Brain tumor
  - G. Trauma and pugilistic encephalopathy
  - H. Hydrocephalus (normal and high pressure)
  - J. Syringomesencephalia
- **III. Multiple system atrophies**
  - A. Sporadic
    1. Progressive supranuclear palsy (ophtalmoparesis)
    2. Shy-Drager syndrome (dysautonomia)
    3. Olivopontocerebellar atrophy (ataxia)
    4. Parkinsonism-dementia-ALS complex (motor neuron disease)
    5. Striatonigral degeneration
    6. Corticodentatonigral degeneration with neuronal achromasia
    7. Alzheimer's disease
  - B. Inherited
    1. Huntington's disease
    2. Wilson's disease
    3. Hallervorden-Spatz disease
    4. Familial parkinsonism-dementia syndrome
    5. Familial basal ganglia calcification
    6. Neuroacanthocytosis
    7. Spinocerebellar-nigral degeneration and Joseph disease
    8. GDH deficiency

From Jankovic J. in: *Drug for Treatment of Parkinson's Disease* (DB Calne ed). *Handb. Exp. Pharmacol.*, 1989, 88: 227-270. With permission.

3.4 Methods

During phase II A, small early studies usually investigate the acute pharmacodynamic (motor effects) and pharmacokinetic properties of the new drug. For example, ropinirole, a new non-ergoline dopamine agonist, was found to acutely improve parkinsonian symptoms in 8 male patients aged from 50 to 66 years in a double-blind, placebo-controlled dose-escalation study. Before the study, the patients were taken off their current antiparkinsonian therapy and received single doses of ropinirole with concommitant domperidone treatment.[29] Acute studies can also demonstrate that new COMT inhibitors are able to potentiate both levodopa pharmacodynamic effects (intensity and duration of the antiparkinsonian effect) and the pharmacokinetics (bioavailability).[30]

During phase II B, multiple-dose studies are performed. Most of the studies are add-on trials, i.e., the new drug is given in addition to the previous unchanged antiparkinsonian treatment in patients requiring additional treatment because of a secondary waning efficacy of levodopa (or dopamine agonist) leading to the reappearance of functional motor disability.[31] If the objective is to decrease levodopa-induced dyskinesias, the drug can also be added to the previously unchanged drug regimen.[32]

Table 3 U.K. Parkinson's Disease Society Brain Bank Clinical Diagnostic Criteria

STEP 1. Diagnosis of Parkinsonian Syndrome

Bradykinesia (slowness of initiation of voluntary movement with progressive reduction in speed and amplitude of repetitive actions).

And at least one of following:

a. Muscular rigidity
b. 4-6 Hz rest tremor
c. Postural instability not caused by primary visual, vestibular, cerebellar, or proprioceptive dysfunction

STEP 2. Exclusion Criteria for Parkinson's Disease

History of repeated strokes with step-wise progression of parkinsonian features
History of definite encephalitis
Oculogyric crises
Neuroleptic treatment at onset of symptoms
More than one affected relative
Sustained remission
Strictly unilateral features after three years
Supranuclear gaze palsy
Cerebellar signs
Early severe autonomic involvement
Early severe dementia with disturbances of memory, language, and praxis
Babinski sign
Presence of cerebral tumor or communicating hydrocephalus on CT scan
Negative response to large doses of levodopa (if malabsorption excluded)
Toxin exposure (including MPTP)

STEP 3. Supportive Prospective Positive Criteria for Parkinson's Disease

Three or more required for diagnosis of definite Parkinson's disease:
Unilateral onset
Rest tremor present
Progressive disorder
Persistent asymmetry affecting the side of onset most excellent response (70-100%) to levodopa
Severe levodopa-induced chorea
Levodopa response for 5 years or more
Clinical course of 10 years or more

From Gibb W.R.G., Lees A.J. *J. Neurol. Neurosurg. Psychiatry,* 1988, 51, 745-752. With permission.

Several recent investigations have discussed the putative "neuroprotective" effect of new drugs, and especially for selegiline following the Datatop study.[33] This point is currently under investigation but does not concern phase II studies. This interesting but not yet proven hypothesis can only be investigated in large phase III trials, the methodology of which still needs to be established.

3.4.1 *Pharmacokinetics*

Pharmacokinetics studies in patients with Parkinson's disease must be performed to confirm the data obtained in healthy volunteers. Drug levels (or levodopa levels in case of adjunct therapy) are usually measured in both plasma and urine. In the future, PET studies could offer new opportunities to directly investigate central pharmacokinetics of new drugs.

3.4.2 *Surrogate Markers*

Several papers have summarized and discussed the methods available for evaluation of new antiparkinsonian drugs,[34,35] as well as the special features of clinical trials for Parkinson's disease.[36,37] Two general approaches have been employed:

1. **Objective quantification** is based on electrophysiological techniques which have the advantage of being quantifiable. However, because of the marked fluctuations in the symptoms, this objectivity can only be exploited when recordings are made for very long periods ("tremor Holter"). Moreover, these techniques which require complex and expensive equipment are generally available in only a few centers and are restricted to small groups of patients for the investigation of the effect of a new drug on specific symptoms (e.g., tremor).

2. **Subjective assessment** requires the quantification of clinical neurological symptoms. The usual method is the assignment of scores from 0 (normal) to 4 (maximal impairment). Several scales have been proposed but the Unified Parkinson Disease Rating scale (UPDRS) has now been developed.[38] UPDRS gives an overall score for motor function (items 8 to 31), as well as cores for the three main levodopa-responsive symptoms of the disease, e.g., rest tremor (item 20), akinesia (sum of items 19, 23-27, 31), and rigidity (item 22) and for the other symptoms (e.g., freezing [item 14], falling [item 13], speech [item 30]), which are less responsive to levodopa. UPDRS allows the measurement not only of motor status but also of complications of therapy and neuropsychological impairment. The advantages and limits of UPDRS have recently been discussed. UPDRS is a combination of preexisting scales (Columbia, Webster, Schab and England, Hoehn and Yahr, etc.) and its precision is not better or worse than its individual components. Both dopa-dependent and -independent symptoms can be assessed. However, it suffers from several weaknesses such as the global assessment of cognitive functions and behavior, lack of evaluation of intra- and interobserver variations, evaluations in five items of some clinical symptoms which are not linear, insufficient quantification of motor fluctuations, etc. But despite these limitationss, UPDRS is the most comprehensive scale yet established.

The ability to improve motor fluctuations related to levodopa is a major goal for any new antiparkinsonian drug. Studies with regard to a drug's simple antiparkinsonian effects can rely on validated physical examination scales (e.g., UPDRS)[38] or objective assessment methods (for example, finger tapping or walking tests)[39] as basic efficacy measures. However, these methods are inappropriate for patients with on-off fluctuations where the motor state can alternate from minute to minute. Twenty four-hour tremor EMG recordings and ambulatory wrist activity monitoring have been proposed as an objective way of assessing on-off responses,[40-42] but recordings from many patients cannot be evaluated and the traces are sometimes difficult to interpret. Subjective self-scoring,[43] observed-scoring,[44] or patient interview data[45] have also been used, but at present diary cards appear to be the most reliable way to demonstrate the efficacy of a treatment in improving motor fluctuations. This approach has been previously used in clinical trials assessing the effect of selegiline,[46,47] subcutaneous apomorphine,[48] and grafting[49,50] but, to our knowledge, no clinical trial has yet demonstrated with this method that any oral dopamine agonist treatment improves motor fluctuations. The use of diaries requires selection of intelligent and observant patients with cooperative spouses if reliable information is to be obtained. Semantic agreement and cross-checking between investigator and patient are essential.

The clinical global evaluation (CGE) is widely used as a secondary evaluation criterion. However, it has never been validated before in Parkinson's disease. We recently found that its sensitivity was relatively comparable to that of diary cards, and that the placebo effect had nearly the same magnitude in both methods. The CGE was much easier and quicker to use than the diary cards, but the diary entries probably influenced the way the CGE was answered.[51]

Due to the subjective parameters evaluated in UPDRS, the magnitude of the placebo effect in phase II trials needs to be considered. As far as we know, this point has never been clearly investigated. In a recent trial,[51] we found that placebo reduced the baseline percentage in awake "off-time" by 24% in the intention-to-treat population. Thirty-five percent of the patients were considered as "improved" by placebo according to the CGE. This proportion rose to a maximum of 55% at week 6. These data demonstrate that the placebo effect is important even in relatively advanced stages of Parkinson's disease and even after 3 months of treatment. In addition to pharmacokinetic and pharmacodynamic factors related to levodopa, on-off fluctuations may be triggered by dietary and emotional factors, so the high placebo response is not entirely surprising. We also found large variations in the placebo response (27%) between centers. No adequate explanation for this discrepancy was found.[51]

3.5 Placebo or Active Control

According to the kind of study, the control group is usually treated by placebo (especially in phase II A and in short-term studies) or active drugs (in phase II B studies and in long-term studies since it is unethical to treat for several weeks with placebo alone). These drugs must include either levodopa (which remains the gold standard) or dopamine agonists. Among dopamine agonists, although bromocriptine has been around the longest, pergolide has tended to become the reference drug in international trials. Anticholinergic drugs (or amantadine) are not used as drugs for active controls for the reasons discussed above.

3.6 Size and Duration of the Trial

As indicated above, the first acute studies are usually followed by short-term studies, lasting from 1 to 3 months. Long-term follow-up studies can be used for final analysis and preparation of phase III trials. According to the chosen major criteria, the size of each trial investigating the clinical potency and clinical spectrum of the drug is usually around 100 patients.

4 DECISION MAKING

As far as we know, there are no published guidelines for the development of new antiparkinsonian drugs. Until now, phase I and II trials differ widely according to the drugs and the companies involved (see, for example, References 7 and 52). In fact, the map of development depends on the future indication for new drugs. In spite of an extensive number of clinical studies, several questions are still unsolved: When should levodopa be started, early or late? Should the maximum dosage be introduced from the onset? What are the role and place of adjuvant drugs (dopamine agonists, MAO or COMT inhibitors)? Is there a place for monotherapy or polypharmacy? In whom and when? Are there some drugs with protective effects? Future trials must respond to these important questions.

ACKNOWLEDGMENTS

The authors acknowledge the preparation of the manuscript by Mrs. P. Bontemps.

REFERENCES

1. Agid Y., Cervera P., Hirsch E. et al. Biochemistry of Parkinson's disease 28 years later: a critical review. *Mov. Disord.*, 1989, 4, (Suppl. 1): S126-144.
2. Montastruc J.L. Recent advances in the clinical pharmacology of Parkinson's disease. *Thérapie,* 1991, 46, 293-303.
3. Calne D.B. Treatment of Parkinson's disease. *N. Engl. J. Med.*, 1993, 329, 1021-1027.
4. Marsden C.D. Parkinson's disease. *J. Neurol. Neurosurg. Psychiatry,* 1994, 57, 672-681.
5. Obeso J.A., Grandas F., Vaamonde J., Luquin M.R., Artieda J. et al. Motor complications associated with chronic levodopa therapy in Parkinson's disease. *Neurology,* 1989, 39 (Suppl. 2), 11-19.
6. Chrisp P., Mammen G.J., Sorkin E.M. Selegiline: a review of its pharmacology, symptomatic benefits and protective potential in Parkinson's disease. *Drugs Aging,* 1991, 1, 228-248.
7. Montastruc J.L., Rascol O., Senard J.M. Current status of dopamine agonists in the Parkinson's disease management. *Drugs,* 1993, 46, 384-393.
8. Tsui J.K., Ross S., Paulin K. et al. The effect of dietary protein on the efficacy of L-dopa: a double blind study. *Neurology,* 1989, 39, 549-552.
9. Leenders K.E., Poewe W.E., Palmer A.J. et al. Inhibition of L-[18F] Fluorodopa uptake into human brain by amino acids demonstrated by positron emission tomography. *Ann. Neurol.* 1986, 20, 258-262.
10. Sawle G.V., Burn D.J., Morrish P.K., Lammerstma A.A., Show B.J., Luthra S., Osman S., Brooks D.J. The effect of entacapone (OR-611) on brain [18F]-6-L-fluorodopa metabolism: implications for levodopa therapy of Parkinson's disease. *Neurology,* 1994, 44, 1292-1297.
11. Salmon E., Frackowiak R.S.J. Neuro-imagerie fonctionnelle métabolique par émission de positrons chez l'homme. *Rev. Neurol. (Paris),* 1990, 146, 459-477.
12. Playford E.D. Positron emission tomography: applications to the investigation of movement disorders. *Eur. J. Clin. Invest.*, 1994, 24, 433-440.
13. Thorner M.O. Dopamine is an important neurotransmitter in the autonomic nervous system. *Lancet,* 1974, 1, 662-665.
14. Willems J.L., Buylaert W.A., Lefevre R.A., Bogaert M.G. Neuronal dopamine receptors on autonomic ganglia and sympathetic nerves and dopamine receptors in the gastrointestinal system. *Pharmacol. Rev.*, 1985, 37, 165-210.
15. Blin O., Masson G., Azulay J.P., Fondarai J., Serratrice G. Apomorphine-induced blinking and yawning in healthy volunteers. *Br. J. Clin. Pharmacol.*, 1990a, 30, 769-773.
16. Blin O., Durup M., Pailhous J., Serratrice G. Akathisia, mobility and locomotion in healthy volunteers. *Clin. Neuropharmacol.*, 1990b, 13, 426-435.
17. Blin O., Ferrandez A.M., Pailhous J., Serratrice G. Dopa-sensitive and dopa-resistant gait parameters in Parkinson's disease. *J. Neurol. Sci.*, 1991a, 103, 51-54.
18. Blin O., Mestre D., Masson G., Serratrice G. Selective effect of low doses of apomorphine on spatiotemporal contrast sensitivity in healthy volunteers: a double blind placebo-controlled study. *Br. J. Clin. Pharmacol.*, 1991b, 32, 551-556.
19. Rascol O., Clanet M., Montastruc J.L., Simonetta M., Soulier-Estèbe M.J., Doyon B., Rascol A. Abnormal ocular movements in Parkinson's disease. Evidence for involvement of dopaminergic systems. *Brain,* 1989, 1193-1214.
20. Rascol O., Sabatini U., Simonetta-Moreau M., Montastruc J.L., Rascol A., Clanet M. Square wave jerks in parkinsonian syndromes. *J. Neurol. Neurosurg. Psychiatry,* 1991, 54, 599-602.

21. Jankovic J. The relationship between Parkinson's disease and other Movement Disorders. In: *Drug for the Treatment of Parkinson's Disease* (Calne DB ed). *Handb. Exp. Pharmacol.*, 1989, 88: 227-270.
22. Quinn N. Multiple system atrophy. The nature of the beast. *J. Neurol. Neurosurg. Psychiatry*, 1989, Special Suppl., 78-89.
23. Montastruc J.L., Llau M.E., Rascol O., Senard J.M. Drug-induced parkinsonism: a review. *Fundam. Clin. Pharmacol.*, 1994, 8, 293-303.
24. Gibb W.R.G, Lees A.J. The relevance of Lewy body to the pathogenesis of idiopathic Parkinson's disease. *J. Neurol. Neurosurg. Psychiatry*, 1988, 51, 745-752.
25. Esteguy M., Bonnet A.M., Kefalos J., Chermitte F., Agid Y. Le Test à la L-dopa dans la maladie de Parkinson. *Rev. Neurol. (Paris)*, 1985, 141, 413-415.
26. Rascol O., Montastruc J.L., Senard J.M. et al. Two weeks of treatment with deprenyl (selegiline) does not prolong L-Dopa effect in parkinsonian patients: a double blind cross-over placebo-controlled trial. *Neurology*, 1988, 38, 1387-1391.
27. Hughes A.J., Lees A.J., Stern G.M. Apomorphine test to predict dopaminergic responsiveness in parkinsonian syndromes. *Lancet*, 1990, 2, 32-34.
28. Rascol O., Senard J.M., Rascol A., Montastruc J.L. Apomorphine test in parkinsonian syndromes. *Lancet*, 1990c, 2, 518.
29. Vidailhet M.J., Bonnet A.M., Belal S., Dubois B., Marle C., Agid Y. Ropinirole without levodopa in Parkinson's disease. *Lancet*, 1990, 335, 316-317.
30. Limousin P., Pollak P., Gervason-Tournier C.L., Hommel M., Perret J.E. RO 40-7592, a COMT inhibitor plus levodopa in Parkinson's disease. *Lancet*, 1993, 341, 1605.
31. Montastruc J.L., Fabre N., Rascol O., Senard J.M., Blin O. *N*-Methyl-D-aspartate (NMDA) antagonist and Parkinson's disease: a pilot study with dextromethorphan. *Mov. Disord.*, 1994, 9, 242.
32. Rascol O., Fabre N., Blin O., Poulik J., Sabatini U., Senard J.M., Ané M., Montastruc J.L., Rascol A. Naltrexone, an opiate antagonist, fails to modify motor symptoms in patients with Parkinson's disease. *Mov. Disord.*, 1994, 9, 437-440.
33. The Parkinson Study Group: effects of tocopherol and Deprenyl on the progression of disability in early Parkinson's disease. *N. Engl. J. Med.*, 1993, 328, 176-183.
34. Marsden C.D., Schachter M. Assessment of extrapyramidal disorders. In: *Methods in Clinical Pharmacology*, Macmillan, 1981, 89-111.
35. Teräväinen H., Tsui J. Calne D.B. Evaluation of Parkinson's disease. In: *Drugs for the Treatment of Parkinson's Disease*. (Calne DB ed.) *Handb. Exp. Pharmacol.*, Berlin: Springer-Verlag, 1989, 88, 271-279.
36. Findley L.J., Lataste X. Methodology of clinical trials in Parkinson's disease. Part II: Future trials, recommandations. In: *Methods in Clinical Trials in Neurology*. (Capildeo R, Orgogozo JM, eds.) London: Macmillan Press, 1988, 257-258.
37. Tsui J.K., Teräväinen H., Calne D.B. Clinical trials for Parkinson's disease. In: *Drugs for the Treatment of Parkinson's Disease*. (Calne DB, ed.) *Handb. Exp. Pharmacol.*, Berlin: Springer-Verlag, 1989, 88, 281-288.
38. Fahn S., Elton R.L. and members of the UPDRS Development Committee. Unified Parkinson's Disease Rating scale. In: (Fahn S., Marsden C.D., Goldstein M., Calne D.B. eds.) *Recent Development in Parkinson's Disease*. Vol. 2, New York, Macmillan 1987, 153-163.
39. Montastruc J.L., Rascol O., Senard J.M., Gualano V., Bagheri H., Houin G., Lees A.J., Rascol A. Sublingual apomorphine in Parkinson's disease: a clinical and pharmacokinetic study. *Clin. Neuropharmacol.*, 1991, 14, 432-437.
40. Scholz E., Bacher M., Dichans J. Twenty-four-hour tremor recording in the evaluation of the treatment of Parkinson's disease. *J. Neurol.*, 1988, 235, 475-484.
41. Van Hilten J.J., Kabel J.F., Middlekoop H.A., Kramer C.G., Kerkhof G.A., Roos R.A. Assessment of response fluctuations in Parkinson's disease by ambulatory wrist activity monitoring. *Acta Neurol. Scand.*, 1993, 87, 71-77.
42. Van Hilten J.J., Hoogland G., Van der Velde E.A., Van Dijk J.G., Kerkhof G.A., Roos R.A. Quantitative assessment of parkinsonian patients by continuous wrist activity monitoring. *Clin. Neuropharmacol.*, 1993, 16, 36-45.
43. Stern G.M., Lees A.J., Sandler M. Recent observations on the clinical pharmacology of (-) deprenyl. *J. Neural Transm.*, 1978, 43, 245-251.
44. Schatcher M., Marsden C.D., Parkes J.D., Jenner P., Testa B. Deprenyl in the management of response fluctuations in patients with Parkinson's disease on levodopa. *J. Neurol. Neurosurg. Psychiatry*, 1980, 43, 1016-1021.
45. Brodersen P., Philibert A., Gulliksen G., Stigard A. The effect of L-deprenyl on on-off phenomena in Parkinson's disease. *Acta Neurol. Scand.*, 1985, 71, 494-497.
46. Lees A.J., Kohout L.J., Shaw K.M., Stern G.M., Elsworth J.D., Sandler M., Youdim M. Deprenyl in Parkinson's disease. *Lancet*, 1977, 2, 291-295.
47. Golbe L.I., Lieberman A.N., Muenter M.D., Ahlskog J.E., Gopithan G., Neophytides A.N., Foo S-H., Duvoisin R. Deprenyl in the treatment of symptom fluctuations in advanced Parkinson's disease. *Clin. Neuropharmacol.*, 1988, 11, 45-55.
48. Stibe C.M., Lees A.J., Kempster P.A., Stern G.M. Subcutaneous apomorphine in parkinsonian on-off oscillations. *Lancet*, 1988, ii, 404-406.

49. Goetz C.G., Olanow C.W., Koller W., Penn R.D., Cahill D., Morantz R., Stebbins G., Tanner C.M., Klawans H.L., Shannon K.M., Comella C.L., Witt T., Cox C., Waxman M., Gaauger L. Multicenter study of autologous adrenal medullary transplantation to the corpus striatum in patients with advanced Parkinson's disease. *N. Engl. J. Med.*, 1989, 320, 337-341.
50. Lindvall O., Rehncrona S., Brundin P., Gustavii B., Astedt B., Widner H., Lindholm T., Bjorklund A., Leenders K.L., Rothwell J.C., Frackowiak R., Marsden C.D., Johnels B., Steg G., Freedman R., Hoffer B.J,. Seiger A., Bygdeman M., Stromberg I., Olson L. Human fetal dopamine neurons grafted into the striatum in two patients with severe Parkinson's disease. A detailed account of methodology and a 6-month follow-up. *Arch. Neurol.*, 1989, 46, 615-631.
51. Rascol O., Lees A.J., Senard J.M., Pirtosek Z., Montastruc J.L., Fuell D. Ropinirole in the treatment of levodopa-induced motor fluctuations with Parkinson's disease. *Clin. Neuropharmacol.*, 1996.
52. Wiseman L.R., Fitton A. Cabergoline: a review of its clinical potential in Parkinson's disease. *CNS Drugs*, 1994, 2, in press.

Part VIII. Assessment of Drug Effects on the Gastrointestinal System

Chapter 28

Gastrointestinal Effects

K. H. Antonin and P. R. Bieck

CONTENTS

1. Introduction 386
2. Motility 386
   2.1 Esophagus 386
   2.2 Stomach 386
   2.3 Biliary Tract 387
   2.4 Small Intestine, Large Bowel, and Rectum 388
   2.5 Transit Time in the Upper Intestinal Tract 388
   2.6 Colonic Transit Time 389
   2.7 Total Transit Time 389
   2.8 Conclusion 389
3 Secretion 389
   3.1 Small Intestine 389
   3.2 Bile 389
   3.3 Conclusion 390
4 Drug Absorption 390
   4.1 Intubation Techniques 390
   4.2 HF Capsule 390
   4.3 Application of Drugs into the Large Bowel During Colonoscopy 391
   4.4 Patients with Artificial Stoma 391
   4.5 Buccal Absorption 391
   4.6 Conclusion 391
5 Drug-Induced Gastrointestinal Damage 391
   5.1 Gastric Electrical Transmural Potential Difference 392
   5.2 DNA Content of Cellular Exfoliation 392
   5.3 Secretion of Bicarbonate 392
   5.4 Mucosal Blood Flow — Laser Doppler Flowmetry 392
   5.5 Gastroscopy 393
   5.6 Colonoscopy 393
   5.7 Fecal Blood Loss 393
   5.8 [^{51}Cr]-EDTA Excretion in Urine 393
   5.9 Pepsinogen in Blood 394
   5.10 Buccal Assay 394
   5.11 Conclusion 394
6 Other Methods 394
   6.1 Collection of Saliva 394
   6.2 Induced Diarrhea 394
   6.3 Biopsies 394
   6.4 Gastrointestinal Hormones 395
7 Inflammatory Bowel Diseases 395
   7.1 Clinical Assessment 395
   7.2 Laboratory Parameters 395
   7.3 Endoscopic Assessment 395
   7.4 Histological Assessment 395

0-8493-9230-6/97/$0.00+$.50
© 1997 by CRC Press, Inc.

7.5 Radiography 395
7.6 Scintigraphy 395
7.7 Conclusion......... 396
References......... 396

1 INTRODUCTION

Most drugs are administered orally, and the gastrointestinal tract is frequently exposed to high concentrations of substances given with the aim of acting at low concentrations elsewhere in the body. It is known that a number of drugs influence physiological and morphological patterns, and may lead to clinically important problems. Drugs may alter gastrointestinal motility and secretion, and cause mucosal lesions throughout the alimentary tract. Absorption of drugs is a complex process influenced by the type of formulation, by the origin and surface of gastrointestinal mucosal membranes, and by physicochemical properties of the luminal contents. For the measurement of drug effects on the gastrointestinal tract, a wide variety of methods is used which originate from different specialities, such as anatomy, physiology, chemistry, biochemistry, clinical medicine, and radiology. These methods are summarized in this chapter with regard to the measurement of motility, secretion, drug absorption, drug safety, and assessment of drug efficacy in diseases.

2 MOTILITY

Highly sensitive and well-standardized techniques are available for the recording and quantification of motility and for the measurement of passage of liquid and solid substances through the gastrointestinal tract.

2.1 Esophagus

Fluoroscopy — The effect of size and shape of tablets or capsules on esophageal transit time can be measured with barium sulfate-containing formulations visualized by fluoroscopy. The time needed for the formulations to reach the stomach is measured with a stopwatch (Channer and Virjee, 1986).

Scintigraphy — The transit of swallowed materials through the esophagus can be quantified with radionuclides. The subject is positioned under a gamma scintillation camera coupled to a computer system. Fluid mixed with [^{99m}Tc]-sulfur colloid as radioactive marker or drug formulations impregnated with the same marker are swallowed. From time-activity curves, the transit time through the esophagus is calculated. These methods provide an objective parameter for the evaluation of treatment effects (Stacher, 1985; Horowitz et al., 1987).

Manometry — Effects of drugs on esophageal motility can be assessed by manometry. Multilumen catheter systems are used with side holes continuously perfused and filled with water. The manometric catheter is attached to an external transducer, an infusion pump, a preamplifier/amplifier, and, finally, a polygraph recorder (Soffer et al., 1988). The system is introduced into the stomach and then slowly withdrawn until the pressure of the lower esophageal sphincter can be recorded.

Direct pressure measurements are also done by strain gauge probes connected directly to the preamplifier.

Long-Term pH Monitoring — Documentation of gastroesophageal reflux with long-term pH monitoring has been shown to be of considerable value, not only in diagnosis and management of this disease, but also for evaluation of drug effects. Several types of pH-sensitive electrodes, such as glass, antimony, plastic, and iridium or tethered radiotelemetric pills, are available. Computerized replay units with visual display and printout facilities are used for recording and calculation of the number of reflux episodes and cumulative duration of high acidity (Branicki et al., 1982; Atkinson, 1987; Emde et al., 1987).

2.2 Stomach

Fluoroscopy — The use of liquid barium sulfate or other radioopaque markers gives only qualitative estimates of the time needed for nearly complete emptying of liquids and subjective impressions on contractility. Barium meals are emptied similarly to liquids with an emptying half-time of 15-20 min. The generally accepted 6-h limit of normal emptying from the stomach gives only an approximate estimation of motility (Smith and Feldman, 1986).

Scintigraphy — Radionuclear methods are very useful to assess gastrointestinal motility. ^{99m}Tc is the most commonly used isotope. Technetium meals consist of chicken liver, egg preparations, and cereals. Indigestible solids have been studied with ^{131}I bound to cellulose. The ^{111}In and ^{113}In isotopes, bound to diethylenetriaminepentaacetic acid (DPTA), can be used as liquid markers in dual liquid and/or solid gastric emptying measurements. The gastric emptying of liquids or solids is expressed as the fraction of radioactivity remaining in the stomach plotted against time. Half-time ($t^1/_2$) of emptying is calculated from such emptying curves (Trotman and Misiewicz, 1982; Malagelada et al., 1984; Minami and McCallum, 1984; Santander et al., 1988). Indium and technetium are not well absorbed by the gastric mucosa. They emit gamma rays at different frequencies. The use of a gamma camera and a computer enables simultaneous analysis and monitoring of liquid and solid phase emptying (Collins et al., 1983; Horowitz et al., 1987). This method does not take into account gastric secretion or duodeno-gastric reflux. Therefore, residual stomach volumes or the quantity emptied from the stomach cannot be assessed.

Abdominal Ultrasound — Gastric emptying can be measured accurately with ultrasound techniques. However, measurement is technically difficult and time-consuming and cannot be used in obese subjects or in the presence of excessive air in the stomach. These limitations and the fact that ultrasound techniques are only suitable for measurement of liquid emptying, have prevented widespread acceptance (Bateman and Whittingham, 1982; Holt et al., 1986).

Impedance Techniques — The measurement of changes of electrical impedance in the epigastric region after ingestion of liquids of low conductivity allows an accurate determination of liquid emptying. Four electrodes are used, two on the anterior and two on the posterior trunk. One pair of electrodes measures current flow and the second pair is used for recording. The subjects lie flat on their backs and a liquid of low electrical conductivity (e.g., orange-flavored Quosh) is administered. As gastric emptying proceeds, transabdominal impedance alters. The changes are plotted and give an index of emptying rate. Comparison with scintigraphy demonstrated a close correlation, indicating that the method is a valid measurement of gastric emptying. The impedance techniques are inexpensive and well reproducible and might gain wider acceptance as experience increases (McClelland and Sutton, 1985).

Electrogastrography — With the electrogastrogram, abnormalities of gastric electrical rhythm can be monitored. Silver-silver chloride electrodes are placed on the skin of the epigastrium and on a limb as reference lead (Stern et al., 1987). An excellent correlation with surgically placed electrodes has been shown (Hamilton et al., 1986).

Manometry — Intraluminal pressure changes in the stomach are measured either with perfused catheters or with probes containing transducers. Each method has advantages and disadvantages. Perfusion catheters are cheaper, but thicker and less well tolerated. The constant infusion of fluid into the lumen may affect motility. Transducers are more expensive, but thinner and better tolerated. They also cause fewer perturbations of the luminal environment. Pressure wave activity is quantified by a motility index based on amplitude and frequency of the phasic pressure waves (Trotman and Misiewicz, 1982; Santander et al., 1988). During fasting, the different phases of the migrating motor complex are recorded. Phase I is characterized by the absence of any spike activity, phase II by a period of irregular contractile activity followed by a characteristic propagated burst of contractions (phase III). To ensure registration of an adequate number of migrating motor complexes, as well as postprandial activity, the monitoring time should be at least 6 h or longer.

2.3 Biliary Tract

Fluoroscopy — Fluoroscopy is a standard method of visualizing the gallbladder and biliary duct after oral or intravenous administration of a contrast medium. The contrast medium is concentrated in the gallbladder and produces an image that can be quantified as an accurate estimation of gallbladder volume. The kinetics of bile duct flow can be studied with cholangiography. Motility of the bile duct and of the sphincter of Oddi can be visualized by cineradiography. However, fluoroscopy in healthy subjects is rarely used, because of considerable radiation exposure.

Scintigraphy — Gallbladder emptying in response to cholagogic stimuli is measured in volunteers and patients with scintigraphy. ^{99m}Tc-labeled diethyl phenylcarbamomethyl iminodiacetate ([^{99m}Tc]-HIDA) is injected intravenously. The gallbladder area is identified and mapped on control scans. Gallbladder activity in subsequent views is expressed as a percentage of the initial values. Activity is plotted against time to obtain a gallbladder emptying curve (Lanzini et al., 1987; Mackie et al., 1987).

Ultrasonography — Ultrasonography is commonly used to study effects of drugs or hormones on gallbladder or bile duct function. Gallbladder volume is determined from a series of cross-sectional images. Volume is calculated as sum of a series of cylinders (Marzio et al., 1987). Volume can also be derived from measurements of gallbladder length and diameter (Hansen and Felgenträger, 1987).

Manometry — The effects of drugs or hormones on intraluminal pressure changes or motor activity of the bile duct are assessed in patients with T-tube drains (McFarland et al., 1984). In healthy subjects a duodenoscope with side view is used. During endoscopy a manometric catheter or a strain gauge probe is passed through the biopsy channel of the endoscope and inserted into the bile duct. Manometric examinations are done before and after administration of the test drug or hormones (Funch-Jensen et al., 1987).

2.4 Small Intestine, Large Bowel, and Rectum

Manometry — The technique of pressure measurement in the small intestine with perfused tubes is essentially that of esophageal or stomach manometry (Santander et al., 1988). To measure motor activity of the colon, a manometric catheter is introduced by advancing it together with a colonoscope (Narducci et al., 1987). Prolonged manometric studies of small and large bowel motility are an important tool in the investigation of drug effects in intestinal motility disorders (Camilleri et al., 1986).

Telemetry — Bowel motility can be assessed by ingestible radiotelemetric pills for long periods of time. Pressure changes can be measured with a pressure-sensitive radiotelemetric pill. It consists of a capsule with pressor sensor, a miniature battery, and a transmitting coil. The signals are transmitted as pulses at very low power and are detected by aerials placed on the body surface of the subject. The radiotelemetric pill is tethered with a fine thread and attached to the mouth. It can be located in any area and stationed at a fixed location in the gastrointestinal tract. It has been shown that radiotelemetric pills give information comparable with that provided by intubation systems (Thompson et al., 1980; Trotman and Misiewicz, 1982).

2.5 Transit Time in the Upper Intestinal Tract

Fluoroscopy — The transit of nondisintegrating solid dosage forms containing a radiopaque compound, such as barium sulfate or small steel balls, can be followed by X-ray examinations. However, the necessity of simultaneous administration of barium sulfate suspension, in order to visualize the intestinal tract, may cause difficulties in locating radiopaque bodies against the background.

Scintigraphy — Detailed information about transit through stomach and small intestine is provided by labeling a meal or solid dosage forms with a gamma-emitting isotope (Davis et al., 1984; Malagelada et al., 1984; Camilleri et al., 1986). The passage through the gastrointestinal tract is monitored with a gamma camera linked to a computer. ^{99m}Tc is the most commonly used isotope. If, in addition, another isotope such as ^{111}In is used, the passage of solids and liquids, or of two drug formulations, can be measured simultaneously. Images of the distribution of radioactivity in the abdominal regions are collected over time and stored in the computer. The stomach is identified first and the colon last. Radioactive counts outside of stomach and colon are assumed to be in the small intestine. The proportion of total radioactivity present in the stomach, small intestine, and colon is determined at any given time during the study. Profiles of gastric emptying, colonic filling, and small bowel residence can be constructed from the data (Davis et al., 1986; Read et al., 1986).

Salicylazosulfapyridine — Mouth-to-cecum transit time can be measured by the use of salicylazosulfapyridine. This drug practically is not absorbed in the upper part of the gastrointestinal tract. It is metabolized by the microbial flora in the large bowel to sulfapyridine, which is rapidly absorbed. The time lag until detection of sulfapyridine in plasma or saliva gives an estimate of the transit time from mouth to cecum. In normal fasting subjects this is around 3.5-5 h (Kellow et al., 1986; Antonin et al., 1988).

Hydrogen Breath Test — The appearance of hydrogen in expired air after ingestion of a nonabsorbable carbohydrate is the basis for measurement of small bowel transit time. In humans H_2 is produced by bacterial fermentation of carbohydrates in the gastrointestinal tract. In healthy subjects this occurs only in the colon (Bond and Levitt, 1975). H_2 diffuses from bowel to blood at a constant rate and is eliminated from the body by exhalation. A standard dose (10-20 g in 100 ml water) of a nonabsorbable carbohydrate, usually lactulose, is given orally. Lactulose is a disaccharide consisting of fructose and galactose, which is not split by brush border disaccharidases. H_2 production occurs almost entirely in the colon by fermentation by colonic bacterial flora. End-expiratory samples of air are collected at 10-min intervals and hydrogen concentrations are determined by gas chromatography or selective and sensitive electrochemical cells. Transit time is defined as time from ingestion of lactulose to a rise in breath H_2 concentration of at least 20 ppm (Trotman and Misiewicz, 1982; van Wyk et al., 1985). Lactulose is an osmotic purgative and will interfere with intestinal motility. It cannot be regarded as a physiological marker of transit. Therefore, test meals rich in carbohydrates are provided as alternatives (Read et al., 1985).

2.6 Colonic Transit Time

Colonic motility and transit time are measured by scintigraphic methods. Through a thin tube, positioned in the cecum, a nonabsorbable radionuclide ([^{111}In]-DTPA) is instilled. Passage through the colon is monitored by a gamma camera (Krevsky et al., 1986).

2.7 Total Transit Time

Fluoroscopy — In this test 20 radiopaque ring-shaped markers are ingested on day 1, 20 rod-shaped pellets on day 2, and 20 plastic rods containing metal balls on day 3. On day 4 the abdomen is X-rayed and the markers that are retained in the gastrointestinal tract are counted. The number is plotted against the time elapsed from ingestion to visualization. The intersection with the time axis is defined as gastrointestinal transit time (Jaup et al., 1985; Hallerback et al., 1988). Transit time through the gut can also be measured by collecting and analyzing one stool specimen. Twenty radiopaque markers are given with breakfast to a subject on three consecutive days. Different, but comparable, markers are used each day. The first stool specimen on day 4 is collected and the markers are counted fluoroscopically. The average transit time can be calculated from the number of each type of marker found and the time of ingestion to defecation (Cummings and Wiggins, 1976).

Scintigraphy — Scintigraphic methods, as described above, are used to measure total gastrointestinal transit time of meals or controlled-release dosage forms (Davis et al., 1984, 1986; Malagelada et al., 1984).

2.8 Conclusion

Carefully designed scintigraphic studies are the most accurate and sophisticated methods to measure transit through the gastrointestinal tract. The SASP test and radiopaque marker studies are simple and inexpensive methods. Scintigraphic techniques allow accurate measurements of the gastrointestinal transit, dispersion, and dissolution of oral drugs (Spiller, 1986). The currently available instrumentation for gastrointestinal manometry provides an effective means for the clinical investigation of motor function in health and disease and for the measurement of drug effects. Radiotelemetric probes allow a greater degree of mobility and comfort for the subjects studied. Long-term pH recording of esophagus or stomach increased knowledge of the pathology of gastroesophageal reflux and gastroduodenal ulcer disease and is useful in the evaluation of new treatments for these disorders.

3 SECRETION

In addition to the transport of materials through the gastrointestinal tract, water and electrolyte fluxes due to secretion and/or reabsorption in the different regions may be significantly influenced by drugs. On the other hand, water flux may also facilitate dissolution and absorption of drugs.

3.1 Small Intestine

Intubation techniques are used to investigate the effects of drugs on water and electrolyte transport in the human small intestine. Double-lumen or multilumen perfusion tubes with occluding balloons and infusion and collection holes are swallowed and positioned fluoroscopically. A glucose electrolyte solution is infused with a peristaltic pump through the infusion hole and aspirated through the collection hole (Moriarty et al., 1986).

3.2 Bile

Quantification of biliary excretion and enterohepatic circulation of drugs and their metabolites in man is difficult, as the biliary tract is not readily accessible.

T-tube Drainage or Nasobiliary Tubes in Patients — Most biliary excretion studies have been performed in patients with T-tube drainage following cholecystectomy or other biliary tract surgery (Rollins and Klaassen, 1979; Terhaag and Hermann, 1986). They can also be performed in patients with nasobiliary tubes. However, these patients are not ideal for such studies. They usually have hepatobiliary disease, with or without extrahepatic cholestasis. Bile flow and bile salt output are diminished for 2-4 weeks after surgery. Most biliary drainage tubes are not designed to totally divert bile flow. Therefore, it is not known whether bile collection is complete or not. Interruption of normal enterohepatic circulation of bile and bile constituents markedly alters bile output and composition (Rollins and Klaassen, 1979).

Intubation Techniques in Healthy Subjects — In order to overcome the difficulties encountered in patients, healthy human volunteers are studied by use of gastrointestinal tubes. Single- or double-lumen nasoduodenal tubes are positioned with the aspiration site just distal to the ampulla of Vater. Bile samples are obtained by continuous or intermittent aspiration of duodenal fluid, which is rich in bile (Lind et al., 1987).

Multiluminal tubes are positioned in the duodenum and perfused with a liquid lipid diet in order to keep the gallbladder contracted and a nonabsorbable marker to quantify bile collection. This procedure appears to be more reliable for quantification than the T-tube drainage technique. However, enterohepatic circulation cannot be interrupted completely, when needed, and bile collection is difficult if the drug being studied is administered orally (Dujovne et al., 1982).

A balloon-occludable multiluminal duodenal tube has been used successfully for studying biliary excretion of drugs. The tube is passed into the duodenum and a balloon is inflated distal to the ampulla of Vater. It allows proximal aspiration and distal reinfusion of bile. With this method enterohepatic circulation can be maintained at the desired level, as the amount of aspirated bile can be reinfused into the intestine (Askin et al., 1978).

3.3 Conclusion

Intubation techniques for the study of drug effects on fluid or electrolyte secretion in the intestine or on bile flow are not widely used. They are complicated, costly, and time-consuming. Investigations in patients with T-tubes can give qualitative indications of biliary drug excretion.

4 DRUG ABSORPTION

Most orally administered drugs are designed to be absorbed from the upper gastrointestinal tract. However, absorption of drugs is a complex process. There are several physiological and pathological factors affecting absorption, such as motility, gastrointestinal diseases, certain foods, or the formulation of a drug. On the other hand, development of new dosage formulations that release drug slowly through the entire length of the gastrointestinal tract requires systematic studies of the absorptive capacity of all parts of the gastrointestinal tract (Antonin, 1993).

4.1 Intubation Techniques

Drug absorption in man can be investigated by intubation techniques. Absorption rates are estimated from the rate of disappearance of drug from the gut lumen. Nonabsorbable markers such as polyethylene glycol (PEG) are used to enable corrections for changing volumes due to fluid fluxes. Thin flexible tubes are swallowed by the subjects and placed in different levels of the gastrointestinal tract. After administration of the test drug and the markers, gastric and intestinal contents are collected at frequent intervals (Hirtz, 1987).

Gastric absorption of drugs is studied after occlusion of the pylorus with two balloons. Absorption from the ileum is examined with multiluminal tubes and with an occlusive balloon. The balloon is inflated after intubation to isolate the intestinal segment to be studied. Secretions from the proximal intestine are aspirated continuously by a tube above the balloon. The drug is infused together with the marker just below the balloon and luminal fluid is aspirated 30 cm distal from this side (Hirtz, 1987).

To study drug absorption in the colon, a tube is swallowed and its distal end is positioned into the cecum under radiological control. Drug is administered through the tube, and the rate of absorption is calculated from plasma concentration profiles (Hirtz, 1987). With intubation techniques it is possible to characterize the absorption of drugs in all segments of the gastrointestinal tract. However, it is complicated, costly, and time-consuming, and, therefore, cannot be used extensively.

4.2 HF Capsule

A high-frequency capsule (HF capsule) has been developed to study absorption characteristics in man. With the HF capsule extent and rate of drug absorption from all sites of the gastrointestinal tract can be investigated. A smooth plastic capsule (12 × 8 mm) contains a small latex balloon (1 ml) filled with drug and the release mechanism. The capsule is taken together with a small oral dose of contrast medium to enable the radiological localization in the intestines. The release mechanism is triggered with a short impulse from a high-frequency generator to release the drug in a defined segment of the gastrointestinal tract. From plasma concentration profiles, the rate of absorption can be calculated (Staib et al., 1986; Schuster and Hugemann, 1987; Antonin, 1993).

4.3 Application of Drugs into the Large Bowel During Colonoscopy

Colonoscopy has become a routine procedure in diagnosis and treatment of colonic diseases. Development of instruments that are easier to handle made the procedure shorter and more acceptable. Dissolved drug can be placed into distinct areas under visual and fluoroscopic control through instrumental channels in the colonoscope, within 5-20 min (Antonin and Bieck, 1987; Antonin, 1993).

The large intestine must be very well cleaned prior to endoscopy. This led to criticism of the assessment of absorption capacity of the large bowel under "nonphysiological" conditions. However, colonoscopy proved to be a simple, well-tolerated, and suitable method for phase I studies with new compounds or drug formulations. Colonoscopy allows quantification of relative colonic bioavailability of a drug. Disadvantages are discomfort to the volunteers, the necessity of a clean colon, and exposure to X-rays. Colonoscopy should only be performed by skilled endoscopists.

4.4 Patients with Artificial Stoma

Drug absorption by the colonic mucosa can be investigated in patients with intestinal stoma, if no stenosis is present. Stomas can be used in two ways to study drug absorption. First, intestinal contents of the upper parts of the gastrointestinal tract can be collected from end stomas. After oral drug intake, the portion of the dose not absorbed can be recovered. This gives an indication of the extent of absorption occurring between mouth and stoma. Studying patients with end stomas at different levels of the gastrointestinal tract may give hints toward location and extent of absorption. With this method it is possible to obtain information on effective bactericidal intracolonic concentrations after oral antimicrobial drug application (Antonin and Bieck, 1987; Antonin, 1993) or on therapeutic intracolonic drug concentrations with new oral formulations of 5-amino salicylic acid (Riley et al., 1988). Second, drugs can be introduced into the distal gastrointestinal tract in patients with a loop stoma. The absorptive capacity between stoma and anus can be assessed by measurements of drug concentrations in body fluids (Antonin and Bieck, 1987). Investigations with artificial stomas must be performed in hospitalized patients. They are not inconvenient to the patients. However, the absorptive capacity of only one part of the gastrointestinal tract can be assessed.

4.5 Buccal Absorption

To quantify buccal absorption of drugs, an external closed-perfusion cell design can be used (Barsuhn et al., 1988). The flow cell, which allows perfusion of a 1.8 cm^2 area, is placed against the buccal mucosa and fixed with an extended clamp. Drug solutions are recirculated through the perfusion apparatus by use of a reciprocating pump.

4.6 Conclusion

The development of a dosage formulation with extended drug release requires basic knowledge of the absorption of compounds throughout the entire gastrointestinal tract. Intubation techniques are highly sophisticated and permit exact characterization of the absorption processes in all segments of the gastrointestinal tract. However, intubation techniques are complicated, costly, time-consuming, and a burden for the study subject. Therefore, they cannot be used routinely. HF capsules may become the most useful method for the investigation of rate and extent of drug absorption from all regions of the gastrointestinal tract. However, at present this technique is not generally available. Limits of this method lie in repeated X-ray controls, the sometimes difficult placement of a drug into the capsule, and the fact that the capsule can be used only one time. Colonoscopic application of drugs in healthy volunteers seems to be a simple, well-tolerated, and suitable method for studying drug absorption from the colon. Investigation of drug absorption in patients with artificial stomas can give a qualitative impression of the absorptive capacity of the part of the gastrointestinal tract investigated.

5 DRUG-INDUCED GASTROINTESTINAL DAMAGE

Many drugs can induce gastrointestinal lesions. These may be related to the pharmacological mechanism of action or to direct toxicity due to high local drug concentrations. More than 20 drugs or classes of drugs associated with gastrointestinal toxicity are known (Dukes, 1992). The need to understand the problems and to estimate the risks of drug treatment stimulated development of human models of gastric mucosal injury (Hawkey et al., 1987).

5.1 Gastric Electrical Transmural Potential Difference

The concept of a gastric mucosal barrier emerged from animal studies showing that the mucosa is relatively impermeable to back-diffusion of hydrogen ions, and that permeability increases after response to aspirin and other nonsteroidal antiphlogistic drugs (NSAIDs), ethanol, or bile salts. This is followed by a fall in potential difference across the mucosa. Gastric potential difference is measured most frequently by the method of Andersson and Grossman (1965). The potentials are measured from electrolyte bridges (1.5% agar; 3 mol/l KCl) between gastric mucosa — luminal or gastric electrode — peripheral vein — reference electrode. The luminal electrode is a double-luminal gastric tube, the reference electrode an infusion tube with a butterfly needle placed into a forearm vein. Both tubes are filled with KCl-agar. The luminal and the reference electrodes are attached to separate Erlenmeyer flasks, containing 3 mol/l KCl solution and two calibrated calomel electrodes. The potential differences are monitored continuously with an analog recorder until a stable baseline potential has been established. After the test substances are instilled, measurements are made until potentials return to baseline. During examination, the volunteers lie in a stable left lateral position. The tip of the luminal tube should be positioned in gastric juice (Laule et al., 1982; Fimmel et al., 1984; Hogan, 1988).

Measurement During Gastroscopy — The electrical potential difference can be measured under visual guidance between a stomach microelectrode and an intravenous reference electrode connected to a millivoltmeter during gastroscopic examinations. pH is measured by an intragastric microelectrode and the junction potential is calculated by the Henderson-Hasselbach equation, taking into account the measured pH. This junction potential is subtracted from the potential difference. The corrected potential difference values can be used to evaluate drug effects in different parts of the stomach (Højgaard et al., 1987).

5.2 DNA Content of Cellular Exfoliation

Injuries causing loss of epithelial cells can be quantified by measuring cellular exfoliation in gastric washings. Cells differ in their lysing properties and cannot be reliably quantified by counting alone. Therefore, the DNA content in gastric washings has been used as an index of cellular exfoliation. DNA can be quantified by a modification of the diphenylamine method, which is not affected by the presence of sialic acid (Ruppin et al., 1981; Fimmel et al., 1984). The method is relatively time-consuming and insensitive. Prolonged periods of storage at low temperatures are necessary for the precipitation of DNA.

An alternative approach is a radioimmunoassay that is sensitive and quickly done. Serum from patients with systemic lupus erythematosus is used as the source for anti-DNA antibodies (Hurst et al., 1984).

With such techniques, signs of increased cellular exfoliation can be found in patients with atrophic gastritis or gastric ulcerations and in volunteers challenged with ethanol, bile, or aspirin. Cellular exfoliation is reduced after treatment with carbenoxolone and prostaglandin E. This technique does not distinguish between increased loss and increased production of epithelial cells. It seems likely that the higher DNA content of gastric washings observed after single acute challenges with aspirin or taurocholate is due to enhanced loss of epithelial cells, but the higher DNA content of washings after chronic dosing may reflect also increased production of DNA.

5.3 Secretion of Bicarbonate

Human gastric and/or duodenal bicarbonate secretion is an important protective factor, preventing gastroduodenal damage. Therefore, bicarbonate is measured to determine the influence of drugs on its secretion (Feldman et al., 1984; Isenberg et al., 1986; Selling et al., 1987). A double-luminal gastroduodenal tube is positioned under fluoroscopic control, and the pylorus is occluded with two balloons. This prevents any escape of gastric juices into the duodenum and reflux of duodenal contents into the stomach. The duodenum is occluded by a distal balloon creating an isolated duodenal segment. Duodenal secretions are aspirated and bicarbonate secretion is measured by a back-titration method (Isenberg et al., 1986).

5.4 Mucosal Blood Flow — Laser Doppler Flowmetry

Endoscopic laser Doppler flowmetry is used to evaluate the effects of drugs or hormones on gastric blood circulation in man. During gastroscopy, a fiberoptic probe is introduced through the biopsy channel of the instrument. The probe contains optic fibers for transmission of laser light to the gastric wall and fibers for collecting the reflected light. Recordings are made from specifically defined areas of the stomach and plotted with a linear recorder. Laser Doppler flowmetry measures relative flow, and the flow values are expressed in units of relative flux (Kvernebo et al., 1986; Lunde et al., 1988).

5.5 Gastroscopy

Gastroscopic studies are performed in healthy subjects (Lanza, 1984; Hogan, 1988) or in patients who are treated with drugs that damage the mucosa (Caruso and Bianchi Porro, 1980; Larkai et al., 1987). Before start of the trial, a baseline examination is performed. An absolute exclusion criterion is the presence of any esophageal, gastric, or duodenal lesions. Endoscopic examinations are performed at the end of each treatment period (no later than 24 h after the last drug administration). They are repeated when severe gastrointestinal symptoms or severe lesions occur. The procedure for this is standardized. After fasting for 10-12 h, the volunteers receive local anesthesia of the faucet and posterior pharyngeal wall with Xylocaine spray. Gastroscopy is done with the volunteer lying in the left lateral position.

All lesions are described at each stage of the examination and are documented by photography or film or using a video camera. Television, together with tape recording, permits not only documentation, but also instant analysis. Lesions are graded according to scales (Lanza, 1984). Artifacts caused by the endoscope are not recorded. It is advantageous if the same investigator performs all endoscopic examinations in a study.

Advantages of endoscopy are the directness of visualization and the possibility of obtaining biopsies. Some open questions about the use of gastroscopy are:

1. In about 15-30% of healthy, asymptomatic volunteers gastric lesions are observed during the initial examination (Akdamar et al., 1986). However, in the literature pretreatment data are often not given. Placebo-treated subjects have low gastric injury scores in these studies. It is suggested, therefore, that all volunteers are endoscopically examined before inclusion into such a study. The design should be cross-over and placebo-controlled. This would lead to the necessary sound database of results from healthy asymptomatic volunteers.
2. The treatment period is frequently too short to reveal changes that might appear with chronic administration.
3. There is no universally accepted scale for quantification of mucosal damage. Therefore, studies cannot be easily compared. Most often used are estimates of macroscopic changes. Most rating scales attempt to assess the size of the lesions. However, how many small lesions are equivalent to a large one? Or how should petechiae be scored?
4. Endoscopic studies are usually performed in young and healthy subjects. This population is different from that in which peptic ulcers and complications caused by NSAIDs occur.

5.6 Colonoscopy

Colonoscopy, probably because of discomfort, is not widely used for the evaluation of possible harmful effects of drugs on the large bowel. In the past, relatively little attention has been given to the question of side effects of drugs in this segment of human gut (Somerville and Hawkey, 1986; Rampton, 1987). The reason is that most drugs are completely absorbed in the upper intestinal tract after oral administration. They will not reach the large bowel. However, the development of dosage forms that release drug over extended periods of time raises the question as to whether, and to what extent, the mucosa of the large bowel can be damaged.

5.7 Fecal Blood Loss

Red blood cells are tagged with radiolabeled sodium chromate (Na[^{51}Cr]O_4) and the blood is injected back to the same subject. Gastrointestinal micro-bleeding (ml/day) is determined by the amount of radioactive chromium in three successive 24-h stool specimens collected thereafter (Lussier et al., 1983).

5.8 [^{51}Cr]-EDTA Excretion in Urine

Changes in intestinal permeability caused by diseases or NSAIDs in healthy subjects and patients is assessed by measuring the radioactivity in 24-h urines after oral administration of [^{51}Cr]-EDTA. After an overnight fast, the test solution of [^{51}Cr]-EDTA is administered. Urine is collected for 24 h after ingestion and aliquots are assayed in a scintillation counter (Bjarnason et al., 1983, 1986).

5.9 Pepsinogen in Blood

Changes in gastric permeability caused by diseases or drugs can be assessed by measuring concentrations of pepsinogen I and pepsinogen II in serum of healthy subjects and patients (Chuong et al., 1986; Hengels, 1987). Serum pepsinogen concentrations are measured by use of radioimmunoassays. A positive correlation between the increase of pepsinogen concentrations and incidence and severity of gastric lesions has been reported (Hengels, 1987). The author concludes that serum pepsinogen determination may be a useful noninvasive technique for early detection of drug-induced gastric side effects.

5.10 Buccal Assay

A new method for studying the potential of drugs to irritate the gastrointestinal tract has recently been reported. Drugs in aqueous gels are applied to the buccal mucosa in small disposable cups. The open face of the cup is in contact with the buccal mucosa of the lip for 1 h. At defined intervals during and after application, subjective sensations and changes in the mucosal surface are recorded. Scales are used for scoring and an irritation index is calculated (Place et al., 1988). The buccal assay is useful only in examining the contact irritation potential of drugs and formulations under most unfavorable conditions, as in cases of adherence of drugs to the esophageal mucosa.

5.11 Conclusion

The gastrointestinal tract is most prone to serious side effects of drugs. Therefore, human models of gastrointestinal injury are needed in early phases of drug development. For basic research on mucosal damage, measurements of mucosal blood flow or bicarbonate secretion are useful. First data on the development of clinically significant signs of toxicity are obtained by endoscopy. Macroscopic lesions can be detected and may be used as predictors for the risk of major adverse effects during long-term treatment in patients. Measurement of mucosal potential difference is an indirect method and seems useful in the assessment of acute injury. However, after multiple dosage there is no correlation between changes of potential difference and gastroscopic findings (Antonin et al., 1985). Cellular desquamation as measured by DNA content in gastric washings, fecal blood loss as measured by ^{51}Cr labeling, changes of intestinal permeability as measured by urinary excretion of [^{51}Cr]-EDTA, or analysis of pepsinogen in serum are not widely used.

6 OTHER METHODS

6.1 Collection of Saliva

To determine anticholinergic effects of drugs, salivary secretion rate can be measured. Basal and stimulated saliva can be collected with cups occluding the orifices of distinct salivary ducts (von Knorring and Mörnstad, 1986). The secretion rate is expressed in ml/min. Mixed salivary secretion from all glands can be quantified with rolls of cotton wool between lips and gingiva and under the tongue. The rolls are weighed before and one or two minutes after application. Salivation can be stimulated by having the subjects chew on a small ball of Parafilm. Drug concentrations in saliva are often proportional to concentrations in plasma. This led to the use of saliva for therapeutic drug monitoring or pharmacokinetic studies (Graham, 1982). Measuring saliva concentrations of drugs can prevent unnecessary blood loss, especially during pharmacokinetic studies in patients. A prerequisite for the use of saliva is a constant range of concentrations between saliva and plasma.

6.2 Induced Diarrhea

For the evaluation of antidiarrheal drugs in healthy volunteers, diarrhea can be induced by castor oil (LaCorte et al., 1982), by synthetic prostaglandin analogs such as misoprostol, or by prolonged infusion of vasoactive intestinal polypeptide (Kane et al., 1983). The number and character (formed, soft, or watery) of bowel movements are noted. The stool is weighed and analyzed for sodium, potassium, chloride, bicarbonate, and osmolality. Subjective side effects such as flatulence or abdominal cramps are rated for severity (mild, moderate, or severe).

6.3 Biopsies

NSAIDs inhibit cyclooxygenase activity. Suppression of endogenous prostaglandin synthesis in gastric mucosa has been implicated as a possible mechanism of NSAID-induced gastric lesions. Therefore, the effect of NSAIDs on gastric mucosal prostaglandin synthesis was measured and a correlation with effects on the mucosa was sought. During gastroscopy, biopsies were obtained and prostaglandin concentrations of the mucosal biopsy specimens were measured by radioimmunoassay (Goldin et al., 1988; Levine et al., 1988). NSAIDs reduce gastric prostaglandin synthesis without regard to presence or absence of mucosal damage. There was no correlation between degree of suppression of prostaglandin concentrations and endoscopic evidence of mucosal damage.

6.4 Gastrointestinal Hormones

Gastrointestinal functions are modulated by complex hormonal and neural interrelationships. The gastrointestinal hormones are a family of polypeptides produced by endocrine cells in the gastrointestinal tract. These hormones regulate specific biological functions of stomach, small and large intestine, endocrine and exocrine pancreas, liver, and biliary system, in order to optimize physiological conditions for digestion, absorption, and motility (Norman and Litwack, 1987). Measurement of hormones, such as gastrin or pancreatic polypeptide, is used to assess the effects of nutrients or drugs. As radioimmunoassays for most gastrointestinal hormones are not yet generally available, such measurements are mostly used for diagnostic purposes in specialized centers.

7 INFLAMMATORY BOWEL DISEASES

The etiology of ulcerative colitis and Crohn's disease remains unknown, and no specific therapy exists. Palliative therapy with several nonspecific agents has evolved. However, advances in drug therapy should be evaluated critically (Korelitz, 1980; Riis, 1980). Clear criteria for diagnosis and judgment of therapeutic efficacy are needed (Hodgson, 1982).

7.1 Clinical Assessment

The diagnosis of inflammatory bowel disease is usually made on the basis of clinical symptoms. In order to assess clinical activity, indices were developed (Hodgson, 1982). Recently, a new index including morphological alterations has been reported (Maier et al., 1988).

7.2 Laboratory Parameters

Laboratory findings are very helpful in diagnosis and control of treatment. Acute-phase proteins or orosomucoid concentrations correlate well with disease activity. Hypoproteinemia and hypalbuminemia are often present, resulting from excessive enteric protein loss. [^{51}Cr]-EDTA excretion in urine, as described above (Bjarnason et al., 1986) and ^{111}In autologous leukocyte scanning in feces (Saverymuttu et al., 1983b) have been used to assess disease activity. Identification and quantification of leukotrienes and prostaglandins in tissue, feces, and urine have also been used (Rampton and Hawkey, 1984; Lauritsen et al., 1988).

7.3 Endoscopic Assessment

Endoscopy is the most accurately diagnostic tool in inflammatory bowel disease. Inspection of the altered mucosa allows a direct judgment about severity and extent of the inflammatory processes.

7.4 Histological Assessment

Biopsies during endoscopy can offer an objective assessment of the severity of the inflammatory process and will confirm the diagnosis.

7.5 Radiography

Radiographic examinations may be useful in confirming diagnosis, extent of disease, and complications such as strictures or fistulas. However, there is a poor correlation between clinical indices and radiographic images.

7.6 Scintigraphy

^{111}In autologous leukocyte scanning is used for the assessment of extent of the disease as well as therapeutic efficacy. White blood cells are separated from venous blood and incubated with ^{111}In. The labeled cells are reinjected intravenously. Radioactivity over the abdomen is scanned with a gamma camera (Saverymuttu et al., 1983a). However, there is poor correlation between scan scores and other indices of disease activity (Park et al., 1988).

7.7 Conclusion

For therapeutic trials in inflammatory bowel diseases, the quality of test methods is of crucial importance. Clinically specific symptoms should be assessed and graded by use of standardized indices together with laboratory parameters. Endoscopic and histological findings are useful for the demonstration of an effective treatment regimen.

REFERENCES

Akdamar, K., Ertan, A., Agrawal, N., McMahon, F. G. and Ryan, J. (1986). Upper gastrointestinal endoscopy in normal asymptomatic volunteers. *Gastrointest. Endosc.*, 32, 78-80.

Andersson, S. and Grossman, M. J. (1965). Profile of pH, pressure and potential difference at gastroduodenal junction in man. *Gastroenterology,* 49, 364-71.

Antonin, K. H. and Bieck, P. (1987). Evaluation of the colonic drug absorption in patients with an artificial intestinal stoma and by colonoscopy in normal volunteers. In Rietbrock, N., Woodcock, B. G., Staib, A. H. and Loew, D. (Eds.), *Methods in Clinical Pharmacology,* No. 7. Vieweg-Verlag, Braunschweig, pp. 39-51.

Antonin, K. H., Britzelmeier, C. and Kohlstetter, K. (1985). Gastric potential difference: A method to establish gastric mucosal integrity in man after longterm treatment with gastric irritants. *Naunyn-Schmiedeberg's Arch. Pharmacol.*, 329 (Suppl.), R100.

Antonin, K. H., Jedrychowski, M. and Bieck, P. R. (1988). Effects of codeine phosphate on gastric motility and mouth-to-cecum transit-time in humans measured by sulfapyridine appearance in saliva after oral salicylazosulfapyridine. *Hepatogastroenterology,* 35, 186.

Antonin, K. H. (1993). Other methods in studying colonic drug absorption. In P. R. Bieck (Ed.), *Colonic Drug Absorption and Metabolism,* Marcel Dekker, New York, Basel, pp. 89-107.

Askin, J. R., Lyon, D. I., Shull, S. D., Wagner, C. I. and Soloway, R. D. (1978). Factors affecting delivery of bile to the duodenum in man. *Gastroenterology,* 74, 560-5.

Atkinson, M. (1987). Monitoring esophageal pH. *Gut,* 28, 509-14.

Barsuhn, C. L., Olanoff, L. S., Gleason, D. D., Adkins, E. L. and Ho, N. F. H. (1988). Human buccal absorption of flurbiprofen. *Clin. Pharmacol. Ther.,* 44, 225-31.

Bateman, D. N. and Whittingham, T. A. (1982). Measurement of gastric emptying by real-time ultrasound. *Gut,* 23, 524-7.

Bjarnason, I., O'Morain, C., Levi, A. J. and Peters, T. J. (1983). Absorption of ^{51}chromium-labeled ethylenediaminetetraacetate in inflammatory bowel disease. *Gastroenterology* 85, 318-22.

Bjarnason, J., Williams, P., Smethurst, P., Peters, T. J. and Levi, A. J. (1986). Effect of nonsteroidal anti-inflammatory drugs and prostaglandins on the permeability of the human small intestine. *Gut,* 27, 1292-7.

Bond, J. H. and Levitt, M.D. (1975). Investigation of small bowel transit time in man utilizing pulmonary hydrogen (H_2) measurements. *J. Lab. Clin. Med.*, 85, 546-55.

Branicki, F. J., Evans, D. F., Ogilvie, A. L., Atkinson, M. and Hardcastle, J. D. (1982). Ambulatory monitoring of esophageal pH in reflux oesophagitis using a portable radiotelemetry system. *Gut,* 23, 992-8.

Camilleri, M., Brown, M. L. and Malagelada, J. R. (1986). Impaired transit of chyme in chronic intestinal pseudoobstruction. Correction by cisapride. *Gastroenterology,* 91, 619-26.

Caruso, I. and Bianchi Porro, G. (1980). Gastroscopic evaluation of anti-inflammatory agents. *Br. Med. J.,* 280, 75-8.

Channer, K. S. and Virjee, J. P. (1986). The effect of size and shape of tablets on their esophageal transit. *J. Clin. Pharmacol.,* 26, 141-6.

Chuong, J. J. H., Fisher, R. L., Chuong, R. L. B. and Spiro, H. M. (1986). Duodenal ulcer — incidence, risk factors, and predictive value of plasma pepsinogen. *Dig. Dis. Sci.,* 31, 1178-84.

Collins, P. J., Horowitz, M., Cook, D. J., Harding, P. E. and Shearman, D. J. C. (1983). Gastric emptying in normal subjects — a reproducible technique using a single scintillation camera and computer system. *Gut,* 24, 1117-25.

Cummings, J. H. and Wiggins, H. S. (1976). Transit through the gut measured by analysis of a single stool. *Gut,* 17, 219-23.

Davis, S. S., Hardy, J. G. and Fara, J. W. (1986). Transit of pharmaceutical dosage forms through the small intestine. *Gut,* 27, 886-92.

Davis, S. S., Hardy, J. G., Taylor, M. J., Whalley, D. R. and Wilson, C. G. (1984). A comparative study of the gastrointestinal transit of a pellet and tablet formulation. *Int. J. Pharmacol.,* 21, 167-77.

Dujovne, C. A., Gustafson, J. H. and Dickey, R. A. (1982). Quantitation of biliary excretion of drugs in man. *Clin. Pharmacol. Ther.,* 31, 187-94.

Dukes, M. N. G. (Ed.) (1992). *Side Effects of Drugs, Annual 12.* Elsevier, Amsterdam, New York, Oxford.

Emde, C., Garner, A. and Blum, A. L. (1987). Technical aspects of intraluminal pH-metry in man: current status and recommendations. *Gut,* 28, 1177-88.

Feldman, M. and Colturi, T. J. (1984). Effect of indomethacin on gastric acid and bicarbonate secretion in humans. *Gastroenterology,* 87, 1339-43.

Fimmel, C. J., Müller-Lissner, S. A. and Blum, A. L. (1984). Bile salt induced, acute gastric mucosal damage in man: Time course and effect of misoprostol, a PGE analogue. *Scand. J. Gastroenterol.,* 19 (Suppl. 92), 184-8.

Funch-Jensen, P., Kruse, A. and Ravnsbaek, J. (1987). Endoscopic sphincter of Oddi manometry in healthy volunteers. *Scand. J. Gastroenterol.*, 22, 243-9.

Goldin, E., Stalnikowicz, R., Wengrower, D., Eliakim, R., Fich, A., Ligumsky, M., Karmeli, F. and Rachmilewitz, D. (1988). No correlation between indomethacin-induced gastroduodenal damage and inhibition of gastric prostanoid synthesis. *Aliment. Pharmacol. Ther.*, 2, 369-75.

Graham, G. G. (1982). Noninvasive chemical methods of estimating pharmacokinetic parameters. *Pharm. Ther.*, 18, 333-49.

Hallerbäick, B., Glise, H., Karlsson, F. and Tegnebjer, M. (1988). Beta-adrenoceptor blockade does not modify gastrointestinal transit time in healthy volunteers. *Scand. J. Gastroenterol.*, 23, 817-20.

Hamilton, J. W., Bellahsene, B. E., Reichedefer, M., Webster, J. G. and Bass, P. (1986). Human electrogastrograms. Comparison of surface and mucosal recordings. *Dig. Dis. Sci.*, 31, 33-9.

Hansen, W. E. and Felgenträger, B. (1987). Bestimmung der Gallenblasengrösse mit Ultraschall-Methoden und Ergebnisse. *Leber Magen Darm*, 166-72.

Hawkey, C. J. (1987). Review: acute human models of gastric mucosal injury. *Aliment. Pharm. Ther.*, 1, 593-606.

Hengels, K. J. (1987). Eignet sich die Serum-Pepsinogen-Bestimmung zur Früherkennung gastraler Nebenwirkungen nichtsteroidalder Antirheumatika? In Simon, B. (Ed.), *Nichtsteroidale Antirheumatika und Gastrointestinaltrakt.* Schattauer Vetlag, Stuttgart, New York, pp. 35-40.

Hirtz, J. (1987). Intubation techniques for the study of the absorption of drugs in man. In Rietbrock, N., Woodcock, B. G., Staib, A. H. and Loew, D. (Eds.), *Methods in Clinical Pharmacology*, No. 7. Vieweg-Verlag, Braunschweig, pp. 3-11.

Hodgson, H. J. F. (1982). Assessment of drug therapy in inflammatory bowel disease. *Br. J. Clin. Pharmacol.*, 14, 159-70.

Hogan, D. L. (1988). Damage and protection of the gastric mucosa. A multiparameter assessment. *Am. J. Med.*, 84 (Suppl. 2A), 35-40.

Højgaard, L., Andersen, J. R. and Krag, E. (1987). A new method for measurement of electrical potential difference across the stomach wall. Clinical evaluation of the gastric mucosal integrity. *Scand. J. Gastroenterol.*, 22, 847-58.

Holt, S., Cervantes, J., Wilkinson, A. A. and Wallace, K. J. H. (1986). Measurement of gastric emptying rate in humans by real-time ultrasound. *Gastroenterology*, 90, 918-23.

Horowitz, M., Maddox, A., Harding, P. E., Maddern, G. J., Chatterton, B. E., Wishart, J. and Shearman, D. (1987). Effect of cisapride on gastric and esophageal emptying in insulin-dependent diabetes mellitus. *Gastroenterology*, 92, 1899-907.

Hurst, B.C., Rees, W. D. W. and Garner, A. (1984). Cell loss from human, canine, and guinea pig gastric mucosa measured by DNA radioimmunoassay. *Clin. Sci.*, 66, 701-8.

Isenberg, J. I., Hogan, D. L., Koss, M. A. and Selling, J. A. (1986). Human duodenal mucosal bicarbonate secretion. Evidence for basal secretion and stimulation by hydrochloric acid and a synthetic prostaglandin E_1 analogue. *Gastroenterology*, 91, 370-8.

Jaup, B. H., Abrahamsson, H., Stockbruegger, R. W., Rosengren, K. and Dotevail, G. (1985). Effect of selective and nonselective antimuscarinics on rectosigmoid motility and gastrointestinal transit. *Scand. J. Gastroenterol.*, 20, 1101-9.

Kane, M. G., O'Dorisio, T. M. and Krejs, G. J. (1983). Production of secretory diarrhea by intravenous infusion of vasoactive intestinal polypeptide. *N. Engl. J. Med.*, 309, 1482-5.

Kellow, J. E., Borody, T. J., Phillips, S. F., Haddad, A. C. and Brown, M. L. (1986). Sulfapyridine appearance in plasma after salicylazosulfapyridine. Another simple measure of intestinal transit. *Gastroenterology*, 91, 396-400.

Korelitz, B. I. (1980). Therapy of inflammatory bowel disease including use of immunosuppressive agents. *Clin. Gastroenterol.*, 9 (2), 331-49.

Krevsky, B., Malmud, L. S., D'Ercole, F., Maurer, A. H. and Fisher, R. S. (1986). Colonic transit scintigraphy. A physiologic approach to the quantitative measurement of colonic transit in humans. *Gastroenterology*, 91, 1102-12.

Kvernebo, K., Lunde, O. C., Stranden, E. and Larsen, S. (1986). Human gastric blood circulation evaluated by endoscopic laser Doppler flowmetry. *Scand. J. Gastroenterol.*, 21, 685-92.

LaCorte, W. S. J., McMurtrey, J. J., Chapman, J., Gotzkowsky, S., Chang-Chien, S., Ryan, J. R. and McMahon, F. G. (1982). A simple controlled method for the clinical evaluation of antidiarrheal drugs. *Clin. Pharmacol. Ther.*, 31, 766-9.

Lanza, F. L. (1984). Endoscopic studies of gastric and duodenal injury after the use of ibuprofen, aspirin and other nonsteroidal anti-inflammatory agents. *Am. J. Med.*, 77 (Suppl. 1A), 19-24.

Lanzini, A., Jazrawi, R. P. and Northfield, T. C. (1987). Simultaneous quantitative measurements of absolute gallbladder storage and emptying during fasting and eating in humans. *Gastroenterology*, 92, 852-61.

Larkai, E. N., Smith, J. L., Lidsky, M.D. and Graham, D. Y. (1987). Gastroduodenal mucosa and dyspeptic symptoms in arthritic patients during chronic nonsteroidal anti-inflammatory drug use. *Am. J. Gastroenterol.*, 82, 1153-8.

Laule, H., Luecker, P. W., Altmayer, P. and Eldon, M. A. (1982). Gastric potential difference as a model in clinical pharmacology: assessment of gastric mucosal response to aspirin. *Eur. J. Clin. Pharmacol.*, 22, 147-51.

Lauritsen, K., Laursen, L. S., Bukhave, K. and Rask-Madsen, J. (1988). *In vivo* profiles of eicosanoids in ulcerative colitis, Crohn's colitis, and *Clostridium difficile* colitis. *Gastroenterology*, 95, 11-17.

Levine, R. A., Petokas, S., Nandi, J. and Enthoven, D. (1988). Effects of nonsteroidal, antiinflammatory drugs on gastrointestinal injury and prostanoid generation in healthy volunteers. *Dig. Dis. Sci.*, 33, 660-6.

Lind, T., Andersson, T., Skanberg, I. and Olbe, L. (1987). Biliary excretion of intravenous [^{14}C]omeprazole in humans. *Clin. Pharmacol. Ther.*, 42, 504-8.

Lunde, O. C., Kvernebo, K. and Larsen, S. (1988). Evaluation of endoscopic laser Doppler flowmetry for measurement of human gastric blood flow. Methodologic aspects. *Scand. J. Gastroenterol.*, 23, 1072-8.

Lussier, A., Tétreault, L. and Lebel, E. (1983). Comparative study of gastrointestinal microbleeding caused by aspirin, fenbufen, and placebo. *Am. J. Med.*, 75, 80-3.

McClelland, G. R. and Sutton, J. A. (1985). Epigastric impedance: a non-invasive method for the assessment of gastric emptying and motility. *Gut,* 26, 607-14.

McFarland, R. J., Corbett, C. R. R., Taylor, P. and Nash, A. G. (1984). The relaxant action of hymecromone and lignocaine on induced spasm of the bile duct sphincter. *Br. J. Clin. Pharmacol.*, 17, 766-8.

Mackie, C. R., Baxter, J. N., Grime, J. S., Hulks, G. and Cuschieri, A. (1987). Gall bladder emptying in normal subjects — a data base for clinical cholescintigraphy. *Gut,* 28, 137-41.

Maier, K., von Gaisberg, U. and Kraus, B. (1988). Colitis ulcerosa — Aktivitätsindex zur klinischen und histologischen Klassifikation der Entzindungsaktivität. *Schweiz. Med. Wschr.*, 118, 763-6.

Malagelada, J. R., Robertson, J. S., Brown, M. L., Remington, M., Duenes, J. A., Thomforde, G. M. and Carryer, P. W. (1984). Intestinal transit of solid and liquid components of a meal in health. *Gastroenterology,* 87, 1255-63.

Marzio, L., Capone, F., Neff, M., di Felice, F., Celiberti, V., Mezzetti, A., Giorgi, D. and Cuccurullo, F. (1987). Effect of cholinergic agonists and antagonists on gallbladder volume in fasting man. *Eur. J. Clin. Pharmacol.,* 33, 151-3.

Minami, H. and McCallum, R. W. (1984). The physiology and pathophysiology of gastric emptying in humans. *Gastroenterology,* 86, 1592-610.

Moriarty, K. J., O'Grady, J., Rolston, D. D. K., Kelly, M. J. and Clark, M. L. (1986). Effect of prostacyclin (PGIs) on water and solute transport in the human jejunum. *Gut,* 27, 158-63.

Narducci, F., Bassotti, G., Gaburri, M. and Morelli, A. (1987). Twenty-four hour manometric recording of colonic motor activity in healthy man. *Gut,* 28, 17-26.

Norman, A. W. and Litwack, G. (1987). *Hormones.* Academic Press, Orlando, pp. 322-54.

Park, R. H. R., McKillop, J. H., Duncan, A., MacKenzie, J. F. and Russell, R. I. (1988). Can ^{111}-indium autologous mixed leucocyte scanning accurately assess disease extent and activity in Crohn's disease? *Gut,* 29, 821-5.

Place, V., Darley, P., Baricevic, K., Ramans, A., Pruitt, B. and Guittard, G. (1988). Human buccal assay for evaluation of the mucosal irritation potential of drugs. *Clin. Pharmacol. Ther.*, 43, 233-41.

Rampton, D. S. (1987). Non-steroidal anti-inflammatory drugs and the lower gastrointestinal tract. *Scand. J. Gastroenterol.,* 22, 1-4.

Rampton, D. S. and Hawkey, S. J. (1984). Prostaglandins and ulcerative colitis. *Gut,* 25, 1399-413.

Read, N. W., Al-Janabi, M. N., Bates, T. E., Holgate, A. M., Cann, P. A., Kinsman, R. I., McFarlane, A. and Brown, C. (1985). Interpretation of the breath hydrogen profile obtained after ingesting a solid meal containing unabsorbable carbohydrate. *Gut,* 26, 834-42.

Read, N. W., Al-Janabi, M. N., Holgate, A. M., Barber, D.C. and Edwards, C. A. (1986). Simultaneous measurement of gastric emptying, small bowel residence and colonic filling of a solid meal by the use of the gamma camera. *Gut,* 27, 300-8.

Redfern, J. S., Lee, E. and Feldman, M. (1987). Effect of indomethacin on gastric mucosal prostaglandins in humans. Correlation with mucosal damage. *Gastroenterology,* 92, 969-77.

Riis, P. (1980). A critical survey of controlled studies in the treatment of ulcerative colitis and Crohn's disease. *Clin. Gastroenterol.,* 9 (2), 351-69.

Riley, S. A., Tavares, I. A., Bennett, A. and Mani, V. (1988). Delayed-release mesalazine (5-aminosalicylic acid): coat dissolution and excretion in ileostomy subjects. *Br. J. Clin. Pharmacol.,* 26, 173-7.

Rollins, D. E. and Klaassen, C. D. (1979). Biliary excretion of drugs in man. *Clin. Pharmacokin.*, 4, 368-79.

Ruppin, H., Person, B., Robert, A. and Domschke, W. (1981). Gastric cytoprotection in man by prostaglandin E_2. *Scand. J. Gastroenterol.,* 16, 647-52.

Santander, R., Mena, I., Gramisu, M. and Valenzuela, J. E. (1988). Effect of nifedipine on gastric emptying and gastrointestinal motility in man. *Dig. Dis. Sci.,* 33, 535-9.

Saverymuttu, S. H., Lavender, J. P., Hodgson, H. J. F. and Chadwick, V. S. (1983a). Assessment of disease activity in inflammatory bowel disease: a new approach using ^{111}-In granulocyte scanning. *Br. Med. J.,* 287, 1751-3.

Saverymuttu, S. H., Peters, A. M., Lavender, J. P., Pepys, M. B., Hodgson, H. J. F. and Chadwick, V. S. (1983b). Quantitative fecal indium 111-labeled leukocyte excretion in the assessment of disease in Crohn's disease. *Gastroenterology,* 85, 1333-9.

Schuster, O. and Hugemann, B. (1987). Course of development of the HF-capsule — variations and method-related typical findings. In Rietbrock, N., Woodcock, B. G., Staib, A. H. and Loew, D. (Eds.), *Methods in Clinical Pharmacology,* No. 7. Vieweg-Verlag, Braunschweig, pp. 28-37.

Selling, J. A., Hogan, D. L., Aly, A., Koss, M. A. and Isenberg, J. I. (1987). Indomethacin inhibits duodenal mucosal bicarbonate secretion and endogenous prostaglandin E_2 output in human subjects. *Ann. Int. Med.,* 106, 368-71.

Smith, H. J. and Feldman, M. (1986). Influence of food and marker length on gastric emptying of indigestible radiopaque markers in healthy humans. *Gastroenterology,* 91, 1452-5.

Soffer, E. E., Kumar, D., Mridha, K., Das-Gupta, A., Britto, J. and Wingate, D. L. (1988). Effect of pirenzepine on esophageal, gastric, and enteric motor function in man. *Scand. J. Gastroenterol.,* 23, 146-50.

Somerville, K. W. and Hawkey, C. J. (1986). Non-steroidal anti-inflammatory agents and the gastrointestinal tract. *Postgrad. Med. J.,* 62, 23-8.

Spiller, R. C. (1986). Where do all the tablets go in 1986? *Gut,* 27, 879-85.

Stacher, G. (1985). Esophageal motility, esophageal transit, and gastro-esophageal reflux — a methodological overview. *Hepatogastroenterology,* 32, 299-304.

Staib, A. H., Loew, D., Harder, S., Graul, E. H. and Pfab, R. (1986). Measurement of theophylline absorption from different regions of the gastrointestinal tract using a remote controlled drug delivery device. *Eur. J. Clin. Pharmacol.,* 30, 691-7.

Stern, R. M., Koch, K. L., Stewart, W. R. and Vasey, M. W. (1987). Electrogastrography: current issues in validation and methodology. *Psychophysiology,* 24, 55-64.

Terhaag, B. and Hermann, U. (1986). Biliary elimination of indomethacin in man. *Eur. J. Clin. Pharmacol.,* 29, 691-5.

Thompson, D. G., Wingate, D. L., Archer, L., Benson, M. J., Green, W. J. and Hardy, R. J. (1980). Normal patterns of human upper small bowel motor activity recorded by prolonged radiotelemetry. *Gut,* 21, 500-6.

Trotman, I. and Misiewicz, G. (1982). Methods in human alimentary motility. *Br. J. Clin. Pharmacol.,* 14, 757-63.

Van Wyk, M., De Sommers, K. and Steyn, A. G. W. (1985). Evaluation of gastrointestinal motility using the hydrogen breath test. *Br. J. Clin. Pharmacol.,* 20, 479-81.

Von Knorring, L. and Mörnstad, H. (1986). Saliva secretion rate and saliva composition as a model to determine the effect of antidepressant drugs on cholinergic and noradrenergic transmission. *Neuropsychobiology,* 15, 146-54.

Chapter 29

Anti-Ulcer Drugs

Colin Broom

CONTENTS

1 Introduction ... 401
2 Healthy Volunteers ... 402
2.1 Selection Criteria ... 402
2.2 Safety Considerations ... 402
2.3 Methods ... 403
2.3.1 General Trial Design ... 403
2.3.2 Pharmacokinetic Issues ... 403
2.3.3 Pharmacodynamic Issues ... 403
2.3.3.1 Aspiration of Gastric Secretion ... 403
2.3.3.2 Continuous Intragastric pH Monitoring ... 405
2.3.3.3 Cytoprotective Agents ... 406
2.4 Controls ... 406
3 Patient Studies ... 406
3.1 Suitability ... 407
3.2 Selection Criteria ... 407
3.3 Safety Considerations ... 407
3.4 Methods ... 407
3.4.1 Pharmacokinetics ... 407
3.4.2 Surrogate Markers ... 407
3.4.2.1 Presentation and Interpretation of Antisecretory Data ... 407
3.4.2.2 Aspiration or pH Monitoring ... 409
3.4.2.3 Correlation Between Antisecretory Activity and Therapeutic Effect ... 409
3.5 Activity Against *H. pylori* ... 409
3.6 Placebo or Active Control ... 409
3.7 Size and Duration of Trial ... 409
4 Decision Making ... 410
5 Key Literature Example ... 410
References ... 410

1 INTRODUCTION

Ulceration of the upper gastrointestinal tract includes ulceration of the duodenum and stomach, in addition to reflux esophagitis. All these disorders present with similar symptoms of upper abdominal or retrosternal pain and tend to be chronic. The main class of drugs used in the treatment of these disorders are the antisecretory agents. Alternative therapies include cytoprotective and prokinetic agents. Chronic duodenal ulceration is being increasingly treated with drugs active against the bacterium *Helicobacter pylori*. The therapeutic activity of all these agents are conventionally studied by endoscopic evaluation of the upper gastrointestinal tract during and following therapy.

The development of the antisecretory H_2 receptor antagonist cimetidine represented a major therapeutic advance. Other H_2 receptor antagonists include ranitidine, famotidine, roxatidine, and the shorter elimination half-life drug nizatidine. Anticholinergic drugs such as pirenzepine are also available but have moderate antisecretory activity. The subsequent development of gastric H^+/K^+ ATPase inhibitors or proton pump inhibitors such as omeprazole, lansoprazole, and pantoprazole have allowed more profound and long-lasting inhibition of acid secretion. These drugs are useful in treating patients who do not respond to conventional or high doses of H_2 receptor antagonists, particularly patients with reflux

0-8493-9230-6/97/$0.00+$.50
© 1997 by CRC Press, Inc.

esophagitis. The inhibition of acid secretion produced by these drugs can be readily measured either by aspiration of gastric acid secretion or by continuous intragastric pH monitoring. The pharmacological activity of these drugs has been correlated with their therapeutic effect.

Anti-ulcer drugs with mucosal protective activity include the prostaglandin analog misoprostil and other agents claiming to have cytoprotective properties such as sucralfate. The methodology of their early phase evaluation is less well established. Prokinetic agents such as cisapride, metoclopramide, and domperidone have limited therapeutic success in reflux disease and will not be discussed. Drugs with therapeutic activity against *H. pylori* include the bismuthate compounds, however, without the addition of antibiotics such as amoxicillin or erythromycin in addition to metronidazole (triple therapy) the bacterium is suppressed rather than eradicated. The combination of antisecretory agents and antibiotics are also effective against *H. pylori*, and novel agents with greater activity against this bacterium are being sought. The presence and subsequent eradication of *H. Pylori* can be measured noninvasively using a simple breath test.

2 HEALTHY VOLUNTEERS

Healthy volunteers have frequently been used to study the effect of antisecretory agents. The findings in healthy volunteers usually hold true for the patient population, although ulcer patients, on average, secrete more acid than do a control population.[1-3] The methodologies involved in the assessment of antisecretory drugs are well established, but invasive and inconvenient. Because of this, studies are usually completed quicker when healthy volunteers can be studied. Alternatively, patients in remission from their disease may be used. Antisecretory data from volunteers or patients in remission are considered applicable to patients with active duodenal ulceration, as well as to patients with reflux esophagitis and gastric ulceration. The measurement of reflux of gastric acid into the esophagus can only be studied in patients.

Definitive methodology for the assessment of cytoprotective agents is not available. Studies of these agents and methodologies of potential relevance have used both healthy volunteers and ulcer patients in remission.

Healthy volunteers may also be used to evaluate the effect of drugs active against *H. pylori*. The incidence of infection in a healthy population is proportional to age. In the developed world, approximately 50% of healthy individuals are infected at the age of 50 years. The incidence is much higher in the developing world, particularly in children, probably because of differences in standards of hygiene. The incidence in relatively young healthy volunteers is low and screening would be required to identify individuals with asymptomatic infection. Eradication of *H. pylori* in volunteers may provide some longer term benefit, due to the possible association between infection and the development of gastric cancer. The benefit to patients in remission from duodenal ulceration is clearer, in that eradication reduces the risk of recurrence. The potential adverse effects of the antibacterial agents used against *H. pylori* and the low incidence of infection argue against the evaluation of such drugs in healthy volunteers.

2.1 Selection Criteria

Healthy volunteers with high acid outputs are the most relevant group for study of antisecretory agents. Gastric acid output is correlated with size[4] and therefore larger volunteers, and males have the highest outputs. It is not unusual to find otherwise healthy individuals who have very low acid outputs or who are anacidic, particularly in older age groups. The reason for this is often not apparent, in spite of investigation. Some individuals have anaciditiy in the morning, but respond normally to subsequent stimulation with food. It is therefore important to measure acid secretion on a control day before entering healthy volunteers into studies.

2.2 Safety Considerations

In addition to the general safety considerations involved in early studies, it is important to use volunteers who are familiar with the procedures involved in measuring gastric acid secretion. The passage of a nasogastric tube or electrode can cause considerable anxiety in new volunteers, particularly if the procedure has been traumatic. To avoid the disruption of safety monitoring, in particular cardiovascular measurements, it is best to use experienced volunteers on whom the procedure has been accomplished previously. It is even possible to use experienced volunteers to measure antisecretory effect in first administration studies, since it can be argued that measurement of pharmacological effect allows an early indication that pharmacologically active doses have been reached and reduces the chances of excessively high doses being administered. Less experienced subjects can be used in later studies of antisecretory effect when it is no longer necessary to measure cardiovascular effect. Even in the most experienced volunteers it is important to allow subjects to relax after placement so that cardiovascular parameters return to normal.

2.3 Methods

2.3.1 General Trial Design

Most early studies of the H_2 receptor antagonists tended to look at the activity of single doses, mainly because they had relatively short elimination half-lives with no pharmacokinetic accumulation on repeat dosing. It has subsequently been shown that the antisecretory effect of H_2 receptor antagonists diminishes on repeat dosing, perhaps as early as after the second dose.[5-9] The presence of a short lasting hypersecretory state has also been reported after stopping H_2 receptor antagonists.[10] Irreversible ATPase inhibitors, such as omeprazole, lanzoprazole, and pantoprazole have a different mechanism of action from that of H_2 receptor antagonists. They bind irreversibly to actively secreting gastric parietal cell H^+/K^+ ATPase enzymes. Because not all the enzyme is active at any one time, repeat dosing with these rapidly eliminated drugs is required for at least one week before pharmacodynamic steady state is attained.[11] Consequently, repeat doses are necessary to assess the pharmacodynamics of both H_2 receptor antagonists and H^+/K^+ ATPase inhibitors, even in the absence of pharmacokinetic accumulation of drug.

Because of the large between subject variability in acid secretion and the variability in individual response to antisecretory agents, it is imperative that each subject should act as his/her own control. Cross-over designs should be used whenever possible.

2.3.2 Pharmacokinetic Issues

Studies involving 24-h intragastric pH measurement usually utilize food as a stimulant of acid secretion. The presence or absence of a food interaction and its relevance needs to have been assessed early in the development program. It is possible to measure drug concentration in gastric secretion if an aspiration technique is being used, although the relevance of this data is dubious. Urinary concentrations should be taken if considered important. If an aspiration technique is being used to assess gastric secretory function it is important to give intravenous fluid replacement to ensure adequate hydration and urinary flow.

2.3.3 Pharmacodynamic Issues

The antisecretory effect of drugs can be assessed by a number of different methodologies. Several noninvasive tests have been described, although none have been widely accepted. The two major methods of determining antisecretory effect are by the aspiration of gastric contents or by the continuous monitoring of intragastric pH using an intragastric electrode.

2.3.3.1 Aspiration of Gastric Secretion

The technique of aspiration of gastric secretion has long been established in clinical use.[4] A nasogastric tube needs to be positioned in the antrum of the stomach, either under fluoroscopic control or using the water recovery test.[12,13] Aspiration may be performed manually with a syringe or using continuous or intermittent aspiration with a low pressure suction pump.

Basal gastric acid secretory rate is variable[14] and has a circadian rhythm in both healthy subjects and patients.[15,16] Aspiration is often technically difficult because of the relatively small volumes secreted, especially after antisecretory drugs have been administered. However, it is possible to demonstrate pharmacological activity of very low doses of drug on basal gastric acid secretion.[17] The variability in basal secretory rate can be overcome by using a stimulant of gastric acid secretion. A number of stimulants have been used in the past, including histamine, histamine analogs, and the H_2 receptor agonist impromidine; however, these have significant disadvantages in terms of tolerability. Pentagastrin (Peptavlon, ICI), which is a synthetic peptide incorporating the active C terminal tetrapeptide sequence of gastrin, is the most widely used and acceptable stimulant, especially when used in low dose by continuous i.v. infusion. An infusion rate of 0.6 $\mu g\ kg^{-1}h^{-1}$ is a near-maximal stimulatory dose for the majority of healthy subjects, although a higher dose level may be required in ulcer patients.[18,19] Steady-state stimulation of secretion normally takes 30 min to attain. Early experience with pentagastrin, predominantly at higher dose levels, indicated fading of secretory response with time. Fading of response is less likely to occur with lower doses, perhaps over periods as long as seven hours.[20,21] Maintaining the hydration of subjects with i.v. fluids during extended aspiration is important, to replace the fluid lost from the stomach.

Aspirated secretion is normally collected into 15-min. collection periods and the pH and volume are noted before an aliquot is titrated to pH 7 with 0.1 *M* sodium hydroxide to determine hydrogen ion concentration. The volume of secretion is multiplied by the hydrogen ion concentration to determine the total acid output during each period.

Other technical aspects associated with aspiration methods include whether to correct for contamination of gastric secretion by saliva or duodenal fluids, and whether to allow for loss of secretion through the pylorus. Although methods of correction are available,[22] they are rarely used.

The onset and peak effect of i.v. administered drugs on pentagastrin-stimulated acid output can be clearly seen and followed for a period of a few hours (Figure 1). Corresponding effects on pH can also be presented (Figure 2). When drug is given orally, time must be allowed for it to leave the stomach before stimulation and aspiration can begin. The effect of drug is usually compared with a placebo study day and the percentage inhibition of acid secretion is presented. Alternatively, the pretreatment peak level of stimulated secretion can be used as the baseline, although this is less satisfactory than using a placebo study day as a control.

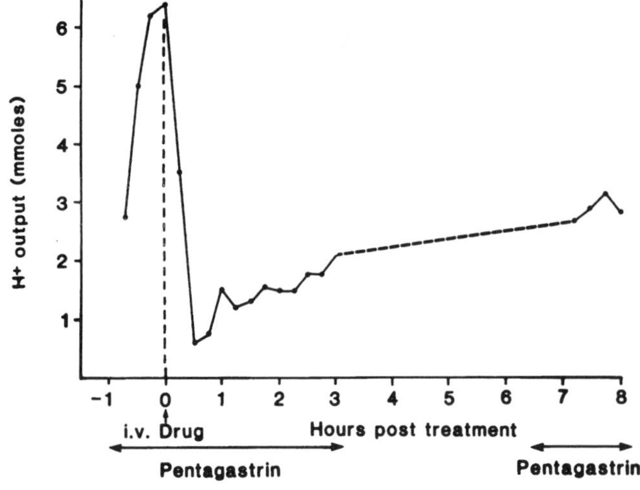

Figure 1 Inhibition of pentagastrin stimulated acid output following an i.v. antisecretory agent.

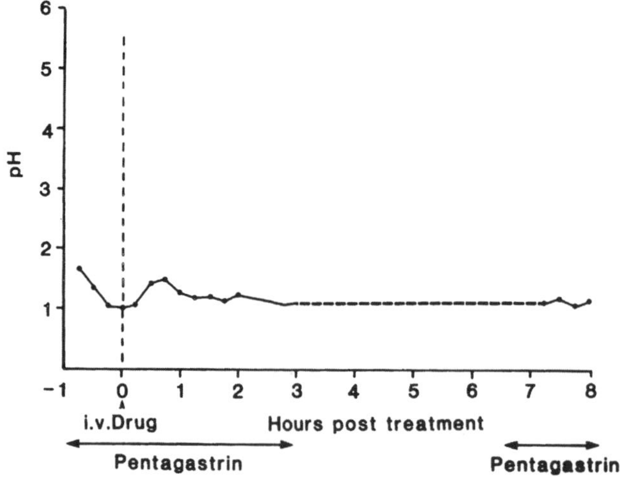

Figure 2 Inhibition of pentagastrin stimulated acid secretion measured by pH.

There are other techniques to measure gastric secretion, including the "spit and chew" technique, which measures cephalic, vagally mediated stimulation of gastric secretion caused by chewing and tasting food. Ingested food, usually as a standardized homogenized meal, or a peptone meal, can also be used. These stimuli are more difficult to standardize, and with the aspiration method blocking of the tube with food particles can occur.

Total acid output may be calculated following food stimulation if an intragastric titration technique is used.[23] In this method and subsequent variants, intragastric pH is maintained at an arbitrary pH of around 5 units by the instillation of 0.1 *M* sodium hydroxide down a nasogastric tube. The acid output of the stomach can be calculated from the amount of sodium hydroxide required. There are potential problems with this methodology since it takes away any negative feedback caused by low intragastric acidity.

Aspiration techniques also allow the measurement of other constituents of gastric secretion, such as pepsin and intrinsic factor.

2.3.3.2 Continuous Intragastric pH Monitoring

Although measurement of pH can be made on aspirated samples of gastric secretion, pH may be more conveniently monitored by means of a nasogastric pH electrode. A small glass electrode is usually used, although other types, such as antimony electrodes are available. The electrode is connected to a recording device by means of an insulated and protected wire. Radiotelemetry has also been used to relay the signals from the electrode to a recording device. The electrode tip is positioned in the body of the stomach under fluoroscopic control or simply positioned by advancing the pH electrode by approximately 8 cm from the point at which an acid pH was first registered (the region of the gastroesophageal sphincter). The length that the electrode is inserted is noted and used on future study days.

Gastric pH data obtained by this technique may be considered to be closer to physiological reality, since the intragastric contents are not interfered with by aspiration or by instillation of alkali. Subjects can be ambulatory and food and drink may be taken which cause temporary increases of intragastric pH, as illustrated in Figure 3. The antisecretory activity and duration of effect of two agents can be compared over a 24-h period. There is considerable experience with this methodology.[24] It has been compared with established methods[25] and appears to have good sensitivity and reproducibility when prolonged pH monitoring is required.[26]

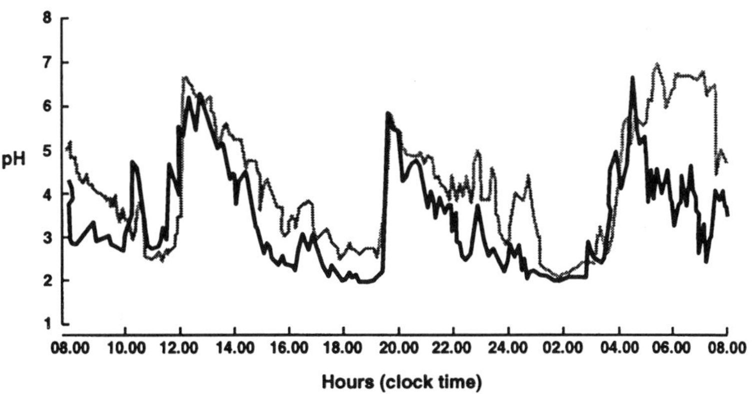

Figure 3 Comparison of the effect of two potent oral antisecretory agents on 24-h intragastric pH.

The pH data measured by the intragastric electrode can be collected either onto magnetic tape or by a solid state recording system. The advantage of the latter system is that the electronically stored data can be transferred more rapidly to a computer, but the disadvantage is that data are more easily lost than with a tape-based system. There are now a number of commercially available systems for continuous pH monitoring, and although originally intended for clinical use in the diagnosis of gastroesophageal reflux, most are applicable, although not necessarily ideal, for the continuous monitoring of intragastric pH. Important aspects to be considered are the reliability of the electrodes and recording devices and, in the case of solid state memory systems, whether data can be inadvertently lost because of technical problems such as battery failure and poor connections. Computer software is available to allow the collected data to be presented and analyzed.

The major disadvantage of continuous pH recording is the inability to measure changes in volume of secretion. Also, there is more marked intersubject and intrasubject variability in pH measurements, and larger numbers of subjects, i.e., greater than 12, are often required to determine an effect on pH. With this number of subjects the technique may be sensitive enough to detect consistent changes in pH of greater than 0.11 pH units over a 24-h period, although the sensitivity may be considerably less over shorter periods of time.[26]

2.3.3.3 Cytoprotective Agents

Some controversy surrounds the use of the term "cytoprotection." In animal studies, drugs such as prostaglandin analogs protect the gastric mucosa from the injury inflicted by noxious stimuli, and this protective effect is independent of any inhibition of acid secretion. In man the results of therapeutic studies conducted with prostaglandin analogs are generally disappointing. The ulcer healing rate in most studies appears to be consistent with the antisecretory effects of these drugs, with little evidence of an addictive effect due to a cytoprotective mechanism.

The mechanism of cytoprotection is unclear; however, there are probably a number of factors that contribute to the resistance of the mucosa to noxious agents. These include the properties of the mucus layer, the alkaline nonacid secretion of the mucosa, and rapid regeneration of mucosa. There has been considerable interest in this type of drug, particularly for the prevention of nonsteroidal anti-inflammatory induced ulceration.

Demonstration of a protective effect of drugs on the gastric mucosa has been attempted in man by a number of techniques. These include the inhibition of aspirin-induced gastric bleeding, the assessment of the endoscopic appearance of the mucosa, and inhibition of changes in mucosal potential difference.[27] In addition, a number of techniques have been described measuring the production of alkaline secretion in the stomach or duodenum.[28,29] The defective secretion of bicarbonate in the duodenum of ulcer patients has been suggested.[30] All these methodologies could, theoretically, be adapted to test the effect of drugs. Indeed, misoprostil, has been shown to stimulate mucus secretion[31] and duodenal bicarbonate secretion in man.[32]

If antisecretory activity of a cytoprotective drug can be identified, those dose levels producing minimal or slight acid inhibition may be taken forward for clinical evaluation in patients. Drugs with no antisecretory effect are clearly more difficult to evaluate in early studies, which will primarily need to establish tolerability before therapeutic studies in patients.

2.4 Controls

Because of the marked interindividual differences in gastric secretion and antisecretory effect between different populations of volunteers, it is important to use a comparator agent in all studies of new antisecretory drugs. The use of a placebo or control study day when no drug is given is also required to demonstrate the secretory status of the individual. The most desirable active comparator agents are either one of the "standard" H_2 receptor antagonists or omeprazole because of the amount of pharmacological data available on these drugs.

3 PATIENT STUDIES

It is possible to assess antisecretory effect in patients in remission from their disease before initiating therapeutic studies, however the doses to take forward into therapeutic studies can be determined with some confidence from antisecretory studies in volunteers. Longer term studies of antisecretory agents are more appropriately performed in patients. Additionally, studies of intraesophageal pH monitoring can only be studied in patients with acid reflux disease. In phase II studies patients may be studied for up to eight weeks and the response to therapy determined from regular endoscopy. The assessment of cytoprotective agents is less clearly defined and conventional phase II studies of ulcer healing properties need to be carried out.

In the development of agents active against *H. pylori* there is little to be gained in assessing the drug initially in healthy volunteers other than the generation of initial safety information. *H. pylori* is a Gram-negative bacillus which may be found beneath the mucus layer of the human stomach. Although similar organisms have been previously described, and mostly ignored, recent interest has been stimulated by the demonstration of an association with duodenal ulceration. Drugs that have been available for a number of years, with known anti-ulcer effect, e.g., colloidal bismuth subcitrate, have received a resurgence of interest with the finding that they eradicate, at least temporarily, *H. pylori* from the gastric mucosa of ulcer patients. The mechanism by which *H. pylori* contributes to peptic ulcer disease is currently unclear; however, it is likely that further drugs will be developed with antibacterial properties in the hope that they will be effective in healing ulcers and will reduce the relapse rate that occurs following the cessation of treatment with antisecretory agents.

3.1 Suitability

The evaluation of antisecretory or cytoprotective drugs in patients is identical to that already described in the healthy volunteer population. The evaluation of drugs with activity against *H. pylori* can be assessed in patients with a history of chronic duodenal ulceration who are currently in remission and not on any medication. There is a near 100% incidence of infection in this population.

3.2 Selection Criteria

Patients selected for participation in longer term studies of antisecretory or cytoprotective agents need to be in remission from their disease and not on other potentially confounding medications. Only patients with known gastroesophageal reflux are suitable for studies involving esophageal pH measurements. Studies of *H. pylori* can be performed in patients in remission from duodenal ulceration. Infection can be confirmed by serological markers or by performing a simple breath test (see below).

3.3 Safety Considerations

The usual safety considerations need to be employed in studies utilizing patients. In addition, the risk of recurrence of ulcer disease has to be considered and patients taken off study to receive alternative therapy if relapse occurs and therapeutic benefit has not been derived. The adverse-event profile associated with most antisecretory agents is excellent. However, potential longer term effects are related to anacidity in the stomach. This includes overgrowth of bacteria within the anacidic stomach and also the stimulation of gastrin release. It has been debated whether both these factors could, in the longer term, lead to the development of tumors in man, particularly enterochromaffin-cell hyperplasia and gastric carcinoids. Such tumors are rarely seen in patients suffering from pernicious anemia, which is associated with anacidity, increased bacterial growth within the stomach, and high plasma gastrin levels (far higher than have been seen with treatment using antisecretory agents). The clinical use of more potent and longer acting antisecretory agents such as the irreversible ATPase inhibitors has led to higher gastrin levels than those seen with conventional doses of H_2 receptor antagonists, although there has been no data to substantiate a concern. Following short-term treatment with the ATPase inhibitor omeprazole, the elevation of gastrin is modest in comparison with those in pernicious anemia.[33]

3.4 Methods

3.4.1 Pharmacokinetics

The same principles apply to patient studies of antisecretory agents as apply to volunteer studies. There are no known clinically important differences in the pharmacokinetics of antisecretory agents in patients compared to healthy volunteers. The pharmacokinetics of drugs active against *H. pylori* can be performed in early studies, however the relevance of systemic levels in what is a local infection is questionable. Assessment of the local concentration of drug may be obtained using biopsies during endoscopic evaluation of the patient.

3.4.2 Surrogate Markers

3.4.2.1 Presentation and Interpretation of Antisecretory Data

The data from different methodologies can be presented in a number of ways. However, first it is important to understand the meaning of the following parameters of gastric acid secretion.

Gastric acid output: The total acid output measured over a given time, which is the volume of secretion multiplied by the H^+ ion concentration.

H^+ concentration: Usually determined by titration to pH 7 with alkali. This is greater than the H^+ activity in gastric secretion, due to the buffering of some H^+ ions by intragastric contents.

pH or H^+ ion activity: In biological fluids the pH is negatively related to the log of the H^+ ion activity (effective concentration of H^+ ions at the surface of the measuring electrode). $pH = -\log[H^+ \text{ activity}]$

Figures 1 and 2 illustrate the differences in presenting antisecretory data and the potential for misinterpretation. An apparently large effect on acid output (Figure 1) is virtually undetectable if presented as changes in pH (Figure 2). This is particularly evident at the 7- to 8-h post-treatment timepoint where an approximate 50% inhibition of acid output is still present but is not apparent by looking at the pH data. Presentation of data in terms of hydrogen ion activity would give results apparently intermediate to the extremes of Figures 1 and 2. When inhibition of acid output is increased to greater than 95%, as shown in Figure 4, it becomes more difficult to differentiate between doses by measurement of acid output. Figure 5 illustrates the same data measured by pH, where a clear demarcation between the two doses can be seen.

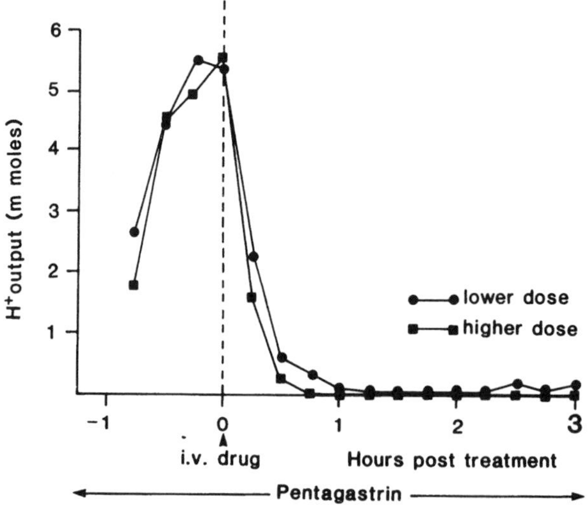

Figure 4 Inhibition of pentagastrin stimulated acid output following i.v. administration of two antisecretory agents.

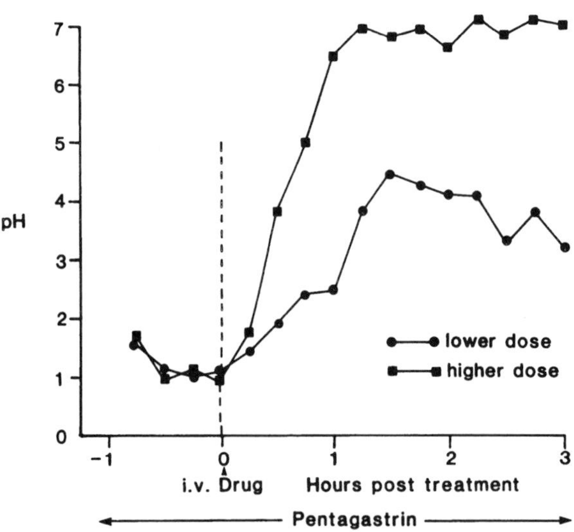

Figure 5 Inhibition of pentagastrin stimulated acid secretion, as measured by pH, following i.v. administration of two antisecretory agents.

3.4.2.2 Aspiration or pH Monitoring

Low levels of antisecretory effect, particularly if mediated predominantly through changes in volume of secretion, can be more easily detected from methodologies using aspiration to determine acid output. At higher doses of drug, where near-abolition of gastric secretion occurs, pH monitoring allows the clear separation of activity between two potent drugs. The implications of this for drug development is that it is often easier to initially evaluate an antisecretory agent in a small number of subjects by measuring stimulated acid output, before choosing a clinically relevant and relatively high antisecretory dose to evaluate further using pH monitoring.

3.4.2.3 Correlation between Antisecretory Activity and Therapeutic Effect

The relationship between antisecretory effect and ulcer healing has been elaborated for duodenal ulceration using meta-analysis.[34-36] The duration of treatment and the time intragastic pH is maintained above pH 3 appear to be the critical factors. Maintaining intragastric pH above 3 for about 16 h per day is associated with a healing rate of nearly 100% at four weeks. Achieving higher pH threshold does not appear to confer any additional benefit. Similar relationships have also been identified for gastric ulceration,[37] where the duration of treatment appears to be a more critical factor related to ulcer healing. The relationship between the healing of reflux esophagitis and inhibition of acid secretion has also been elaborated.[38] The strongest condition is between the time that intragastric pH is maintained above 4 and the healing rate observed after eight weeks of therapy. Intraesophageal pH monitoring may be performed in these patients using similar methodology to that already described for intragastric monitoring. The data derived from this technique is more variable than for intragastric pH monitoring because small differences in electrode placement can have considerable impact on the data. Also there is marked day-to-day variation in the degree of acid reflux. Despite this variability, healing rates can be shown to be inversely proportional to the degree of acid exposure of the esophagus.

3.5 Activity Against *H. pylori*

The *in vitro* effects of drugs active against *H. pylori* do not seem to correlate well with *in vivo* activity. Therefore it is necessary to assess the activity of promising agents or combinations *in vivo*. A number of techniques are available including the use of endoscopic biopsy techniques.[39] Noninvasive methods are also available to detect the urea splitting properties of the bacteria. These noninvasive tests involve drinking a solution of urea in which carbon atoms are labeled with an isotope and measuring the amount of labeled carbon dioxide exhaled by the subject. Techniques are available utilizing nonradioactive ^{13}C isotope[40] and the radioactive ^{14}C isotope.[41,42] Although the eradication of *H. pylori* is associated with a reduced relapse rate of duodenal ulceration, confirmatory data is still likely to be required in larger scale studies which will also assess safety.

3.6 Placebo or Active Control

The study of antisecretory and cytoprotective agents in patients should follow the same principles as those already outlined for healthy volunteers. For drugs active against *H. pylori* the use of a placebo is not mandatory because the spontaneous rate of eradication of *H. pylori* is very low,[43] however, the use of a placebo treatment provides more objective data for a number of reasons including the assessment of safety. The use of an active comparator regimen is appropriate for more exhaustive studies. Triple therapy, with a bismuth salt, metronidazole and erythromycin or amoxicillin, has become the standard although the combination of antisecretory agents and antibiotics are becoming more commonly used.

3.7 Size and Duration of Trial

Studies of antisecretory agents can be performed with relatively few patients, typically 12 to 18, to demonstrate the difference or similarity between two agents. Patients are usually treated for at least one week to confidently assess antisecretory effect. Subsequent phase II studies to measure healing rates need to be conducted in larger groups of patients with around 100 patients per treatment arm, depending on the expected healing rates of the therapies under study.

At least two weeks of treatment should be used to demonstrate the activity of drugs against *H. pylori*. These studies can be relatively small, with as few as 20 patients, if presence or absence of effect is the primary objective. Larger studies will be required if a dose-response or active comparator study is being performed, the size will be dependent on the anticipated response rates. Subsequent studies of the rate of recurrence of ulceration need to be performed in phase III studies.

4 DECISION MAKING

The development of a new antisecretory drug is now a well-trodden path. The relationship between antisecretory effect and healing of upper gastrointestinal ulceration has been well established and may obviate the need to perform conventional dose ranging studies in phase IIB. The antisecretory activity can be assessed from the early studies in phase I/IIA and a single dose chosen for phase III studies. This strategy would need to be discussed with regulatory bodies but represents a feasible "fast track" development for an antisecretory agent. Similarly if an agent is not capable of attaining similar antisecretory activity to currently available agents in a comparative phase I/IIA study there is no reason to develop that drug further. Because there are not such well-developed models correlating cytoprotective activity and ulcer healing, studies of this category of drug need to be restricted to confirming tolerability and safety, and elaborating possible mechanism of action. These studies may identify the dose range likely to be of interest in therapeutic studies.

Drugs active against *H. pylori* can be identified in relatively small studies using the methodologies already outlined. There is no reason to pursue development of a drug shown to be inactive in these early studies. A dose-response relationship against *H. pylori* can be identified in these early studies before progressing to larger studies that will confirm efficacy, safety, and rate of ulcer recurrence. A specific issue here is that many therapies are combinations. It would be necessary to establish eradication of the bacterium and an additive or synergistic effect of each of the components using the eradication of *H. pylori* as the endpoint. The confirmation that this translates into a reduced recurrence rate of healing may still need to be established in large phase III studies.

5 KEY LITERATURE EXAMPLES

A number of meta-analyses of the correlation of antisecretory activity and ulcer healing have been cited in the text. The papers by Jones[34] and Burget[35] were the first to link the extent of antisecretory activity required to heal duodenal ulceration. The subsequent papers by Howden[37] and Bell[38] provide a correlation between antisecretory effect and healing of stomach ulcers and reflux esophagitis, respectively.

REFERENCES

1. Howden, C. W., Jones, D. B., Burget D. W. and Hunt, R. H., Comparison of the effects of gastric antisecretory agents in healthy volunteers and patients with duodenal ulcer, *Gut*, 27, 1058, 1986.
2. Merki, H. S., Fimmel, C. J., Walt, R. P. et al., Pattern of 24 hour intragastric acidity in active duodenal ulcer disease and in healthy controls, *Gut*, 29, 1583, (1988a).
3. Savarino, V., Mela, G. S., Scalabrini, P. et al., 24-Hour study of intragastric acidity in duodenal ulcer patients and normal subjects using continuous intraluminal pH-metry, *Dig. Dis. Sci.*, 33, No. 9, 1077, 1988.
4. Baron, J. H., *Clinical Tests of Gastric Secretion*, Macmillan, London, 1978.
5. Wilder-Smith, C., Halter, F, Ernst, T., Gennoni, M., et al., Loss of acid suppression during dosing with H_2-receptor antagonists. *Aliment. Pharmacol. Ther.*, 4 (S1), 15, 1990.
6. Nwokolo, C. U., Smith, J. T. L., Gavey, C., Sawyerr, A. and Pounder, R. E., Tolerance during 29 days of conventional dosing with cimetidine, nizatidine, famotidine or ranitidine. *Aliment. Pharmacol. Ther.*, 4 (S1), 29, 1990.
7. Smith, J. T. L., Gavey, C., Nwokolo, C. U. and Pounder, R. E., Tolerance during 8 days of high-dose H_2-blockade: placebo-controlled studies of 24-h acidity and gastrin. *Aliment. Pharmacol. Ther.*, 4 (S1), 47, 1990.
8. Rogers, M. J., Holmfield, J. H. M., Primrose, J. N. and Johnston, D. J., The effects of 15 days of dosing with placebo, sufotidine 600 mg nocte or sufotidine 600 mg twice daily upon 24-h intragastric acidity and 24-h plasma gastrin. *Aliment. Pharmacol. Ther.*, 4 (S1), 65, 1990.
9. Broom, C., Eagle, S., Pue, M. and Laroche, J., Comparison of the antisecretory activity of the reversible proton pump inhibitor SK&F 96067 and rantitidine, *Gastroenterology*, Vol 104, 4, A46, 1993.
10. Prewett, E. J., Hudson, M., Nwokolo, C. U., Sawyerr, A. F. M. and Pounder, R. E., Nocturnal intragastric acidity during and after a period of dosing with either ranitidine or omeprazole, *Gastroenterology*, 100(4), 873, 1991.
11. Howden, C. W., Forrest, J. A. and Reid, J. L., Effect of single and repeated doses of omeprazole on gastric acid and pepsin secretion in man, *Gut*, 25, 707, 1984.
12. Hassan, M. A. and Hobsley, M., Positioning of subject and nasogastric tube during a gastric secretion study, *Br. Med. J.*, 1, 458, 1970.
13. Findlay, J. M., Prescott, R. J. and Sircus, W., Comparative evaluation of water recovery test and fluoroscopic screening in positioning a nasogastric tube during gastric secretory studies, *Br. Med. J.*, IV, 458, 1972.
14. Faber, R. G. and Hobsley, M., Basal gastric secretion, reproducibility and relationship with duodenal ulceration, *Gut*, 18, 57, 1977.
15. Moore, J. G. and Englert, E., Circadian rhythm of gastric acid secretion in man, *Nature*, 226, 1261, 1970.

16. Moore, J. G. and Halberg, F., Circadian rhythm of gastric acid secretion in man with active duodenal ulcer, *Dig. Dis. Sci.*, 31, 22, 1986.
17. Acton, G., Broom, C., Burnham, D., Friedman K., Laroche, J. and Wareham, A. K., Effects of low dose cimetidine on nocturnal acid secretion in healthy volunteers, *Aliment. Pharmacol. Ther.*, 5, 61, 1991.
18. Wormsley, K. G., Responses to pentagastrin in man, *Acta Hepatogastroenterol.*, 19, 120, 1972.
19. Petersen, H. and Myren, J., Pentagastrin dose-response in peptic ulcer disease, *Scand. J. Gastroenterology*, 10, 705, 1975.
20. Petersen, B., Christiansen, J., Kirkegaard, P. and Skov Olsen, P., The stability of gastric acid secretion during prolonged pentagastrin stimulation in man, *Clin. Sci.*, 66, 99, 1984.
21. Chin, T. W. F., MacLeod, S. M. and Mahon, W. A., Absence of tachyphylaxis in gastric acid secretion during pentagastrin infusion, *J. Clin. Pharmacol.*, 26, 281, 1986.
22. Whitefield, P. F. and Hobsley, M., A standardized technique for the performance of accurate gastric secretion studies, *Agents and Actions*, Vol. 9/4. Birkhauser Verlag, Basel, 327, 1979.
23. Fordtran, J. S. and Walsh, J. H., Gastric acid secretion rate and buffer content of the stomach after eating, *J. Clin. Invest.*, 52, 645, 1973.
24. Bumm, R. and Blum, A. L., Lessons from prolonged gastric pH monitoring, *Aliment. Pharmacol. Ther.*, 1, 518S, 1987.
25. Fimmel, C. J., Etienne, A., Cilluffo, T. et al., Long term ambulatory gastric pH monitoring; validation of a new method and effect of H_2-antagonists, *Gastroenterology*, 88, 1842, 1985.
26. Merki, H. S., Witzel, L., Walt, R. P. et al., Day to day variation of 24 hour intragastric acidity, *Gastroenterology*, 94, 887, 1988b.
27. Hogan, D. L., Thomas, F. J. and Isenberg, J. I., Cimetidine decreases aspirin-induced gastric mucosal damage in humans, *Aliment. Pharmacol. Ther.*, 1(5), 383, 1987.
28. Rees, W. D. W., Botham, D. and Turnberg, L. A., A demonstration of bicarbonate production by the normal human stomach *in vivo*, *Dig. Dis. Sci.*, 27, 961, 1982.
29. Hogan, D. L., Ainsworth, M. A. and Isenberg, J. I., Gastro duodenal bicarbonate secretion, *Aliment. Pharmacol. Ther.*, 8, 5, 1994.
30. Isenberg, J. I., Selling, J. A., Hogan, D. L. and Koss, M. A., Impaired proximal duodenal bicarbonate secretion in patients with duodenal ulcer, *N. Engl. J. Med.*, 316(7), 374, 1987.
31. Wilson, P. E., Quadros, E., Rajapaksa, T. et al., Effects of misoprostol on gastric acid and mucus secretion in man, *Dig. Dis. Sci.*, 31(2), 1265, 1986.
32. Isenberg, J. I., Hogan, D. L., Koss, A. K. and Selling, J. A., Human duodenal mucosal bicarbonate secretion, *Gastroenterology*, 91, 370, 1986.
33. Lanzon-Miller, S., Pounder, R. E., Hamilton, M. R. et al., Twenty-four hour intragastric acidity and plasma gastrin concentrations before and during treatment with either ranitidine or omeprazole, *Aliment. Pharmacol. Ther.*, 1, 239, 1987.
34. Jones, D. B., Howden, C. W., Burget, D. W. et al., Acid suppression in duodenal ulcer; a meta analysis to define optimal dosing with antisecretory drugs, *Gut*, 28, 1120, 1987.
35. Burget, D. W., Chiverton, S. G. and Hunt, R. H., Is there an optimal degree of acid suppression in healing duodenal ulcer? A model of the relationship between ulcer healing and acid suppression, *Gastroenterology*, 99, 345, 1990.
36. McIsaac, R. L., Dixon, J. S., Mills, J. G. and Wood, J. R., Ranitidine in the treatment of duodenal ulcer disease: relationship between antisecretory effect and ulcer healing rate, *Aliment. Pharmacol. Ther.*, 5, 227, 1991.
37. Howden, C. W. and Hunt, R. H., The relationship between suppression of acidity and gastric ulcer healing rates, *Aliment. Pharmacol. Ther.*, 4, 25, 1990.
38. Bell, N. J. V., Burget, D., Howeden, C. W., et al, Appropriate acid suppression for the management of gastro-oesophageal reflux disease, *Digestion*, 51 (Suppl. 1), 59, 1992.
39. Marshall, B. J., Warren, R., Francis, G. et al., Rapid urease test in the management of *Campylobacter pyloridis*-associated gastritis, *Am. J. Gastroenterol.*, 82, 200, 1987.
40. Klein, P. D. and Graham, D. Y., CáPylori detection by the ^{13}C-rea breath test in Rathbone B., Heatley, V. eds *Campylobacter Pylori and Gastroduodenal Disease*, Blackwell Science Publications, Oxford, 94, 1989.
41. Bell, G. D., Weil, J., Harrison, G. et al., ^{14}C-rea breath analysis, a non-invasive test for *Campylobacter pylori* in the stomach, *Lancet*, i, 1367, 1987.
42. Rauws, E. A., Royen, E. A. V., Langenberg, W., Woensel, J. V., Vrij, A. A. and Tytgat, G. N., ^{14}C-rea breath test in *C. pylori* gastritis, *Gut*, 30, 798, 1989.
43. Parsonnet, J., Blaser, M. J., Perez, P.G., et al., Symptoms and risk factors of *Helicobacter pylori* infection in a cohort of epidemiologists, *Gastroenterology*, 104, 41, 1992.

Part IX. Assessment of Drug Effects on the Genito-Urinary System

Chapter 30

Diuretics

J. McMurray and J. McEwen

CONTENTS

1 Introduction 415
2 Clearance 415
3 Normal Renal Water and Electrolyte Handling 415
4 Mode of Action of Diuretics 416
5 Extrarenal Activity 416
6 Pharmacokinetics 417
7 Pharmacodynamic Assessment 417
  7.1 Nephron Sites of Action 417
    7.1.1 Glomerular Filtration Rate 417
    7.1.2 Segmental Tubular Function 418
      7.1.2.1 Site I 418
      7.1.2.2 Site II 419
      7.1.2.3 Site III 419
      7.1.2.4 Site IV 419
  7.2 Potency 420
8 Protocols for Diuretic Evaluation 420
  8.1 Segmental Nephron Function Studies 420
  8.2 Dose-Ranging and Potency Studies 421
9 Investigation of Possible Adverse Effects 421
References 422

1 INTRODUCTION

Diuretics increase urine output and electrolyte excretion, and are very widely used. Many millions of prescriptions are written each year and it is estimated that diuretics are prescribed for one in four medical patients (Roberts and Daneshmend, 1981; Whelton and Watson, 1987).

2 CLEARANCE

Clearance is a concept crucial to the evaluation of diuretics (Levinsky and Levy, 1973); it is defined as the volume of plasma completely cleared of a given substance in unit time (Smith, 1956). Renal clearance is derived by dividing total urinary excretion by the plasma concentration during the collection interval; it expresses the input-output relationship for any endogenous or exogenous substance and measures renal excretory function (Maack, 1986). Clearance techniques are used to determine glomerular filtration rate (GFR), renal plasma flow (RPF), and renal tubular function. Many assumptions have to be made, however, in calculating clearance, and precautions should be taken to ensure validity (Levinsky and Levy, 1973; Seldin and Rector, 1973; Schuster and Seldin, 1985; Maack, 1986).

3 NORMAL RENAL WATER AND ELECTROLYTE HANDLING

Proper characterization of a diuretic requires an understanding of basic renal physiology (Seldin and Giebisch, 1985). Approximately 180 l of filtrate per day are produced by the kidney, of which 99% is reabsorbed by the renal tubules. Figure 1 shows the contribution of the postglomerular nephron to the reabsorption of sodium (Jacobson, 1981). Different tubular segments have quantitatively different importance, which becomes relevant when predicting the potential magnitude of effect of a given diuretic.

0-8493-9230-6/97/$0.00+$.50
© 1997 by CRC Press, Inc.

Figure 2 illustrates the factors influencing water reabsorption and excretion by the kidney (Puschett, 1981; Roy and Jamison, 1985). Any given solute or osmolar load requires an obligatory water loss. Further water loss ("free water") is determined by the presence or absence of antidiuretic hormone (ADH), also referred to as arginine vasopressin (AVP). Fluid leaving the proximal tubule is isotonic with plasma; it enters the descending limb of the loop of Henle, where solute is added and an insignificant amount of water is extracted. The ascending limb of the loop of Henle (ALH) is impermeable to water, but solute is reabsorbed in this segment, causing a relative dilution of the tubular fluid and generation of "solute-free water," measured as free water clearance CH_2O. A quantitatively much less important cortical diluting segment also operates in the early distal tubule. After this point, in the absence of ADH (Figure 2a), tubular fluid will be excreted without further reabsorption of water as dilute urine. However, when ADH is present (Figure 2b), the nephron distal to the ALH becomes highly permeable to water, which then passes from the tubular lumen into the hyperosmolar medullary interstitium. This hypertonicity is largely due to the transport of solute out of the loop of Henle; transport of solute from the cortical diluting segment does not contribute to hyperosmolality. Extraction of water from the lumen of the distal nephron in the presence of ADH results in "free water reabsorption" (denoted as TcH_2O) and the production of concentrated urine.

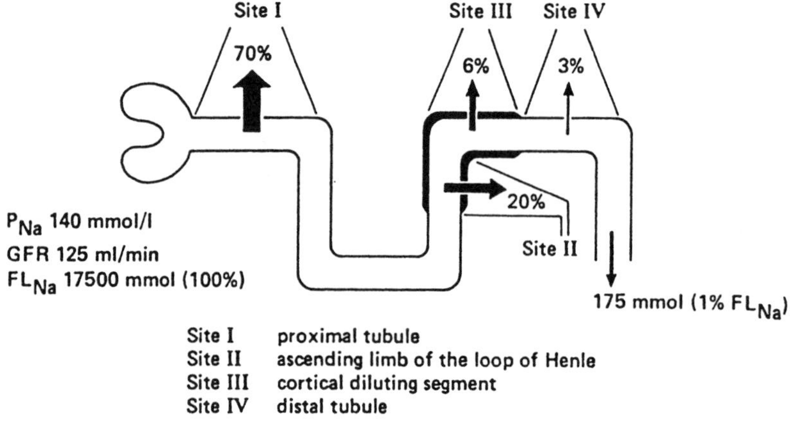

Figure 1 Principal sites of sodium reabsorption and of diuretic action in the nephron.

4 MODE OF ACTION OF DIURETICS

Diuretics in current use can be broadly classified into four groups (Hendry and Ellory, 1988). *Loop diuretics* such as frusemide act on the thick ALH, inhibiting a $Na^+/K^+/Cl^-$ cotransporter in the luminal membrane. *Thiazides* largely act on the early portion of the distal tubule, inhibiting a Na^+/Cl^- cotransporter. *Potassium-sparing diuretics* act on the later portion of the distal tubule, as aldosterone antagonists (e.g., spironolactone) or, with agents such as amiloride, inhibiting transepithelial sodium uptake; consequent hyperpolarization of apical cell membranes reduces the driving force for K^+ exit into the lumen. *Osmotic diuretics* increase the osmolality of tubular fluid, inducing additional obligatory water loss.

5 EXTRARENAL ACTIVITY

Some of the beneficial effects of diuretics in heart failure and hypertension seem to be the result of direct vasodilator activity. After frusemide treatment in acute pulmonary edema, the left atrial pressure falls before the onset of diuresis (Dikshit et al., 1973); frusemide has also been shown to increase vascular capacitance in the human forearm (Biamino et al., 1975). Evidence for a prostaglandin-induced effect of frusemide on vasculature which itself depends upon functioning kidneys has been presented by Johnston et al. (1983). In the case of thiazides, following an initial shrinkage in plasma volume, responding hypertensive patients show a fall in peripheral resistance after several weeks of treatment (van Brummelen et al., 1980).

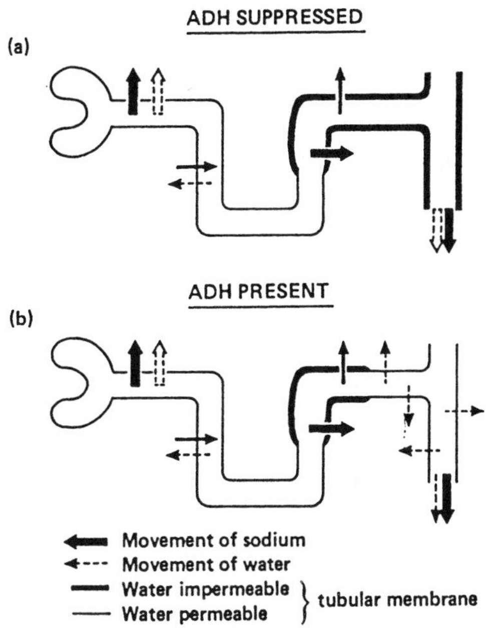

Figure 2 Water and sodium transport in the nephron in the presence (b) and absence (a) of ADH.

6 PHARMACOKINETICS

Although measurement of circulating plasma concentrations of diuretics can sometimes be necessary (for example, assessment of absorption and bioavailability), urinary drug levels are of greater pharmacodynamic significance, since most diuretics influence electrolyte transport from within the lumen of the renal tubule (Homeida et al., 1977). However, Brater (1983) has pointed out that the time-course of drug delivery to the active site is itself also a determinant of response — thus, oral doses, maintaining concentrations in urine at the low end of the dose-response curve for a longer period, can produce a greater sodium excretion rate than i.v. doses which give higher urinary levels for a shorter time. Pharmacokinetic factors can also account in part for diuretic resistance; for example, in patients with severe renal insufficiency the accumulation of endogenous organic acids can block secretion of loop diuretics into the tubular lumen (Rose et al., 1977). In severe nephrotic syndrome, substantial amounts of frusemide can be bound to the excess urinary protein appearing in this disorder, preventing drug access to the tubular epithelium (Smith et al., 1985).

Extensive "depot" binding of chlorthalidone to erythrocyte carbonic anhydrase (Fleuren et al., 1977) may contribute to its long duration of action.

7 PHARMACODYNAMIC ASSESSMENT

In order to characterize a new diuretic, it is necessary to determine its site of action in the nephron and to assess its relative potency and efficacy (Goldberg, 1973; Roberts and Daneshmend, 1981; Puschett, 1986). Effects on GFR and RPF should also be measured.

7.1 Nephron Sites of Action

7.1.1 Glomerular Filtration Rate

The extent of tubular reabsorption of sodium alters in response to changes in tubular delivery of sodium ("glomerulotubular balance"). Before ascribing any increase in urinary sodium excretion to blockade of tubular reabsorption, it is necessary to allow for any increase in the filtered load (FL) of sodium; this requires awareness of changes in GFR. Many conditions in which diuretics are indicated are themselves characterized by reduced GFR — another reason to identify drug-induced changes in GFR (McMurray and Struthers, 1987).

Although it is not ideal, only inulin (or the related substance polyfructosan) is really suitable for repeated measurements of GFR in man. This requires an i.v. infusion, stable plasma levels and, assuming no urinary catheterization, accurate bladder emptying. A protocol for inulin administration in normal subjects is shown in Table 1 (Liedtke and Duarte, 1980; Kampmann and Molholm Hansen, 1981).

Renal plasma flow and renal blood flow (RBF) should also be measured: first, because knowledge of RPF helps interpretation of changes in glomerular and tubular function; and second, because an increase in RBF is a desirable therapeutic objective in many illnesses treated by diuretics (McMurray and Struthers, 1987).

Table 1 Estimation of Inulin Clearance

Loading dose:	50 mg/kg in 100 ml of 0.9% saline over 10 min
Maintenance infusion rate:	30 mg/kg in 0.9% saline at 0.5-2 ml/min
Optimum serum concentration:	200-250 mg/I
Normal range:	Male 127-130 ml min^{-1} $(1.73\ m^2)^{-1}$
	Female 118-120 ml min^{-1} $(1.73\ m^2)^{-1}$

Para-aminohippurate (PAH) clearance is frequently used to measure RPF and RBF in man, although this again has some limitations (Schuster and Seldin, 1985; Maack, 1986). PAH clearance varies with its plasma concentration, so a constant plasma level is imperative. A protocol for PAH clearance is given in Table 2 (Liedtke and Duarte, 1980).

Table 2 Estimation of PAH Clearance

Loading dose:	8 mg kg^{-1} of stock solution (20% PAH) over 1-2 min
Maintenance infusion rate:	15 mg kg^{-1} in 0.9% saline at 0.5-2 ml min^{-1}
Optimum serum concentration:	20-25 mg l^{-1}
Normal range:	Male 650-660 ml min^{-1} $(1.73m^2)^{-1}$
	Female 585-595 ml min^{-1} $(1.73\ m^2)^{-1}$

7.1.2 Segmental Tubular Function

7.1.2.1 Site I

The proximal tubule accounts for the major part (70%) of sodium reabsorption. However, it is not easy to document inhibition of sodium reabsorption in this segment, because enhanced reabsorption in more distal segments compensates for increased sodium delivery. Two main approaches have been used to overcome this problem.

First, sodium entering the ALH in the absence of ADH is absorbed there, so increased free water clearance should be detected. If the fractional excretion of sodium in the urine (CNa/GFR) is added to fractional free water clearance (CH_2O/GFR), a rough index of fractional proximal tubular outflow is obtained. This calculation can be further refined: first, by allowing for the exchange of potassium with sodium in the more distal nephron (Seldin and Rector, 1973) and second, by substituting chloride for sodium in the original calculation.

Sodium bicarbonate represents a nonreabsorbable load to the ALH; thus, after a drug such as acetazolamide (Danovitch and Bricker, 1976),

$$\frac{C_{Cl} + CH_2O}{GFR}$$

is a truer representation of distal delivery than

$$\frac{C_{Na} + CH_2O}{GFR}$$

In the presence of ADH, increased sodium delivery to the ALH should result in increased free water reabsorption.

The second approach is to measure the excretion rate of ions cotransported with sodium in the proximal tubule (Seldin and Rector, 1973; Schuster and Seldin, 1985). Phosphate is mainly reabsorbed in the proximal tubule and is frequently used as a marker for proximal tubular sodium reabsorption (Goldberg, 1973; Roberts and Daneshmend, 1981; Puschett, 1986). More recently lithium has been proposed as a proximal marker (Thornsen, 1984), although this has not gained widespread acceptance (Navar and Schafer, 1987); lithium may itself alter proximal tubular function. Measures of a proximal effect of a diuretic are summarized in Table 3.

Table 3 Indices of Increased Proximal Tubular Outflow

(1)	$\uparrow \dfrac{C_{Na} + C_{H_2O}}{GFR}$
(2)	$\uparrow \dfrac{U_{(Na+K)}V}{P_{Na} \cdot GFR} \times 100 + \dfrac{C_{H_2O}}{GFR} \times 100$
(3)	$\uparrow \dfrac{C_{Cl} + C_{H_2O}}{GFR}$
(4)	$\uparrow \dfrac{C_{PO_4}}{GFR}$
(5)	$\uparrow \dfrac{C_{Li}}{GFR}$

Note: U = urinary concentration, P = plasma concentration, V = urine volume.

7.1.2.2 Site II

The ALH reabsorbs about 20% of FLNa (Kokko, 1984; Odlind, 1984), and complete inhibition of electrolyte transport in this segment can cause a large diuresis and natriuresis, since distal compensatory reabsorption is more limited (Anderton and Kincaid-Smith, 1971). Because of the importance of the ALH in urinary concentration and dilution, blockade of this site will cause a large reduction in free water reabsorption and usually a decrease in free water clearance; the fall in the latter may be small if the cortical diluting segment continues to function (Davies and Wilson, 1975; Lant, 1981). Since the loop of Henle also reabsorbs a significant fraction of the filtered load of magnesium and calcium, loop diuretics also increase urinary calcium and magnesium excretion.

7.1.2.3 Site III

Approximately 6% of filtered sodium is reabsorbed in the cortical diluting segment. Blockade of sodium transport in this site can, therefore, only cause a moderate saliuresis. Free water clearance is decreased but free water reabsorption does not change, as solute transport in this segment does not contribute to medullary hypertonicity (Table 4).

Table 4 Localization of Diuretic Action by Effect on Solute-Free Water Clearance and Reabsorption

Site of Action	$T^{C}_{H_2O}$	CH_2O
I	↑ ↑	↑ ↑
II	↓ ↓	— ↓
III	—	↓
IV	—	—

7.1.2.4 Site IV

As only 3% of sodium reabsorption occurs in the distal tubule and collecting duct, inhibition at this site can only cause a small diuresis and natriuresis. A proportion of sodium is reabsorbed here in exchange for potassium (under the regulation of aldosterone) and hydrogen ions (Shackleton et al., 1986). A diuretic acting proximal to this segment will increase sodium exchange with potassium and hydrogen; such diuretics cause a kaliuresis and metabolic alkalosis (Puschett, 1985). In contrast, diuretics blocking sodium transport in this segment cause hyperkalemia and metabolic acidosis (Shackleton et al., 1986).

7.2 Potency

Differences in diuretic response on a molar basis can strictly only be interpreted as differences in potency and efficacy if drugs have the same site of action. For example, an efficacy of 1 at site III will still produce less natriuresis than an efficacy of 0.5 at site II (Weiner, 1986).

A second important factor when assessing potency is the time-course of diuretic action. Loop diuretics induce a large and rapid saliuresis and diuresis within 3 h, followed by rebound sodium retention from 12 to 24-h — the so-called "undershoot" (Hamdy et al., 1984; Reyes and Leary, 1987; McMurray and Struthers, 1988). This is not a feature of thiazide diuretics. Consequently, a single 24-h urine collection underestimates the peak natriuretic effect of loop diuretics, so the net 24-h response may be less than thiazide diuresis. This underlines the importance of the time factor and re-emphasizes the difficulties of interclass comparisons. Frequent urine collection is necessary for comprehensive profiling of a diuretic agent.

A further important factor is the physiological state of the subjects studied (Roberts and Daneshmend, 1981; Wilcox, 1987). First, their pre-existing sodium and volume status will influence the magnitude of the response and second, natriuretic and diuretic effects of treatment will activate compensatory homeostatic mechanisms (McMurray and Struthers, 1988). Consequently, sodium and water should be replaced during the study to reveal the true pharmacological effect of the drug (Burke et al., 1972), particularly if repeated drug administration is planned.

8 PROTOCOLS FOR DIURETIC EVALUATION

In order to select appropriate and safe doses for efficacy studies, some form of ascending-dose design is required when first doses are given to man (McEwen, 1989), to ensure acceptable tolerability and to determine whether the pharmacokinetic profile is similar to that in laboratory animals used in pharmacology and toxicology (McEwen, 1988).

Once a dosage of a new diuretic has been selected for full evaluation, two types of study are needed: first, assessment of effects on segmental nephron function and second, evaluation of potency (Puschett, 1981; Roberts and Daneshmend, 1981). The opportunity should also be taken to define concentration-response relationships.

8.1 Segmental Nephron Function Studies

This type of study localizes the site of action following acute single doses and has two limbs: maximal hydration and dehydration. A minimum of four sessions are needed, preferably at weekly intervals — a water-loaded balanced cross-over of placebo and active drug and a similar dehydration cross-over. Responses vs. placebo are better than comparisons with predrug baseline, which is rarely a true steady state.

Subjects should receive a standardized diet for 72 h before each treatment (for example, 140 mmol sodium, 80 mmol potassium, 20 mmol calcium, and 10 mmol magnesium per day). Compliance and balance should be documented with daily 24-h urine collection. No alcohol or xanthine drinks are permitted in the 36 h preceding the study. Normal exercise and sleep patterns should be followed. Subjects should be fasted from midnight prior to the study morning. The study should take place in a temperature-controlled room (24°C), avoiding stressful noises, interruptions, or conversations. Subjects should remain seated or supine during the study, standing only to void urine. A standardized light lunch and evening meal should be given. Smoking is forbidden.

In the maximal hydration protocol, comfortable infusion lines for inulin/ PAH and saline are placed, together with a venous sampling cannula, at the beginning of each treatment morning. A 20 ml/kg oral water load is then given over 20 min, followed by voiding at 20-min intervals. Each volume of urine is measured (with an aliquot saved) and an equal volume of water, plus 1 ml/min for insensible loss, is then given orally. Alternatively, urinary sodium and water loss can be replaced i.v. After 90 min a relatively high urine flow, around 10-12 ml/min, should be obtained. At this point urine osmolality should be checked to ensure that it is below 80 mosm/kg, to check that ADH is suppressed. Venous blood should be sampled at the midpoint of each collection period for clearance calculations. The experimental drug may then be administered, with continued urine and blood collections as before. Urine collections for activity need only be continued until the peak diuretic effect has passed, although later collections may help to characterise the duration of activity and the pharmacokinetic profile of parent compound and metabolites.

The dehydration protocol is technically more difficult. Instead of water loading at the start of the study, an infusion of AVP 0.5 mU kg^{-1} min^{-1} is given, plus 3% sodium chloride solution (not mannitol) at a rate which gives a urine output of at least 4 ml min^{-1}. The experimental procedure is otherwise the same as the hydration protocol, although 30-min clearance periods (or longer) may allow more complete and accurate bladder emptying.

In both protocols, urine and blood are collected for determination of the clearance of inulin, PAH, sodium, potassium, calcium, magnesium, phosphate, urate, chloride, and osmoles. Recent examples of such protocols are given by Steinmuller and Puschett (1972); Teredesai and Puschett (1979); Brooks et al. (1984); McNabb et al. (1984); Cuvelier et al. (1986); McMurray and Struthers (1988); and McMurray et al. (1989).

8.2 Dose-Ranging and Potency Studies

These studies should have a balanced cross-over design, a placebo day, and enough active days to construct a dose-response curve, and should include one or more doses of a diuretic from the same class, ideally with 7 days between study days. Restoration of pretreatment sodium balance should be ensured by 3 days of standardized diet and confirmed by measurement of body weight and 24-h sodium excretion. Inulin and PAH clearance should be measured, at least for the first 6-8 h of each session. Following drug administration, urine should be collected: suggestions for a loop diuretic are half-hourly to 2 h, hourly to 6 h, two-hourly to 12 h, then 12-24-h; for a thiazide diuretic, 0-3, 3-6, 6-9, 9-12, and 12-24-h collections are suggested. Blood should be taken at the midpoint of each collection period as before.

Sodium and water replacement for urinary losses is important; this can be gauged either from pilot studies or by measurement of the sodium content of each urinary sample. Hourly rates of solute excretion should be tabulated, comparing placebo with each active day. Response may also be presented as percentage of filtered load excreted. Examples of studies of this type are given by Hamdy et al. (1984), Reyes and Leary (1987), and Brater et al. (1987).

9 INVESTIGATION OF POSSIBLE ADVERSE EFFECTS

Many potential adverse effects are unlikely to be detected in single-dose studies, so chronic dosing will also be necessary once an appropriate active dose has been selected. The major predictable adverse effects of nonpotassium-sparing diuretics are listed in Table 5. These are due both to the direct action of the diuretic agent (e.g., hyponatremia) and the compensatory homeostatic responses invoked by these drugs (e.g., hyperuricemia).

Table 5 Predictable Adverse Effects of Nonpotassium-Sparing Diuretics

Hyponatremia	Glucose intolerance
Hypokalemia	Metabolic alkalosis[a]
Hypomagnesemia	Allergic reactions[b]
Hyperuricemia	Ototoxicity
Hyperlipidemia	

[a] Metabolic acidosis with carbonic anhydrase inhibitors.
[b] Including skin rashes, hematological abnormalities and interstitial nephritis.

Hypokalemic potential may be predicted from the potency measurements outlined above. A plot of natriuretic effect vs. kaliuretic effect for the test drug under investigation and one or more established diuretics from the same class gives some estimation of the hypokalemic potency of the new agent (Puschett and Rastegar, 1974).

In addition to routine measurement of blood glucose, an oral glucose tolerance test should be performed before and after chronic dosing to fully assess the effect of any new diuretic on carbohydrate handling.

Measurement of urate and its handling by the body is complicated and is discussed in detail by Roberts and Daneshmend (1981) and Mejia and Steele (1986). For example, diuretics may augment urate excretion acutely, but with chronic dosing most decrease urate clearance. A strict, standardized diet is essential for any assessment of urate handling.

Ototoxicity is a rare complication of loop diuretics; high-tone audiometry should be considered in the evaluation of such agents.

To exclude direct nephrotoxic effects, screening for microalbuminuria should be performed to exclude glomerular damage; beta-microglobulin or NAG may similarly indicate tubular damage.

Since many adverse effects may occur over months or even years, careful evaluation during treatment of patients will also be a prerequisite in the safety profiling of any new agent (Roberts and Daneshmend, 1981).

REFERENCES

Anderton, J. L. and Kincaid-Smith, P. (1971). Diuretics I: Physiological and pharmacological considerations. *Drugs*, 1, 54-81.

Biamino, G., Wessel, H. J., Noring, J. and Schroder, R. (1975). Plethysmographische und *in vitro* Untersuchungen uber die vasodilatorische Wirkung von Furosemid (Lasix). *Int. J. Clin. Pharm. Biopharm.*, 12, 356-68.

Brater, D.C. (1983). Determinants of the overall response to furosemide: pharmacokinetics and pharmacodynamics. *Fed. Proc.*, 42, 1711-13.

Brater, D.C., Leinfelder, J. and Anderson, S. A. (1987). Clinical pharmacology of torasemide, a new loop diuretic. *Clin. Pharmacol. Ther.*, 42, 187-92.

Brooks, B. A., Lant, A. F., McNabb, W. R. and Noormohamed, F. H. (1984). Renal actions of a uricosuric diuretic, racemic indacrinone, in man: comparison with ethacrynic acid and hydrochlorothiazide. *Br. J. Clin. Pharmacol.*, 17, 497-512.

Burke, T. J., Robinson, R. R. and Clap, J. R. (1972). Determinants of the effect of furosemide on the proximal tubule. *Kid. Int.*, 1, 12-18.

Cuvelier, R., Pellergrin, P., Lesne, M. and Van Ypersele de Strihou, Ch. (1986). Site of action of torasemide in man. *Eur. J. Clin. Pharmacol.*, 31 (Suppl.), 15-19.

Danovitch, G. M. and Bricker, N. S. (1976). Influence of volume expansion on NaC1 reabsorption in the diluting segments of the nephron: a study using clearance methods. *Kid. Int.*, 10, 229-38.

Davies, D. L. and Wilson, G. M. (1975). Diuretics: mechanisms of action and clinical application. *Drugs*, 9, 178-226.

Dikshit, K., Vyden, J. B., Forrester, J. S., Chatterice, K., Prakesh, R. and Swan, H. J. C. (1973). Renal and extrarenal hemodynamic effects of furosemide in congestive cardiac failure after acute myocardial infarction. *N. Engl. J. Med.*, 288, 1087-90.

Fleuren, H. L. J. and van Rossum, J. M. (1977). Nonlinear relationship between plasma and red blood cell pharmacokinetics of chlorthalidone in man. *J. Pharmacokinet. Biopharm.*, 5, 359-75.

Goldberg, M. (1973). The renal physiology of diuretics. In Orloff, J., Berliner, R. W. and Geiger, S. R. (Eds.), *Handbook of Physiology: Renal Physiology.* American Physiologic Society, Washington D.C., pp. 1003-31.

Hamdy, R. C., Vinson, M., Robbins, A. D., Struthen, L. P. L., Chapman, S. F., Norris, R. J. and Shaw, H. L. (1984). Diuretic potency of loop, thiozide and potassium-sparing agents: a reappraisal of relative activity. In Puschett, J. B. and Greenberg, A. (Eds.), *Diuretics: Chemistry, Pharmacology and Clinical Applications.* Elsevier, Amsterdam, pp. 403-6.

Hendry, B. M. and Ellory, J. C. (1988). Molecular sites for diuretic action. *TIPS*, 9, 416-21.

Homeida, M., Roberts, C. and Branch, R. A. (1977). Influence of probenecid and spironolactone on furosemide kinetics and dynamics in man. *Clin. Pharmacol. Ther.*, 22, 402-8.

Jacobson, H. R. (1981). Functional segmentation of the mammalian nephron. *Am. J. Physiol.*, 241, F203-F218.

Johnston, G. D., Hiatt, W. R., Nies, A., Payne, N. A., Murphy, R. C. and Gerber, J. G. (1983). Factors influencing the early nondiuretic vascular effects of furosemide in man. *Circ. Res.*, 53, 630-5.

Kampmann, J. P. and Molholm Hansen, J. (1981). Glomerular filtration rate and creatinine clearance. *Br. J. Clin. Pharmacol.*, 12, 7-14.

Kokko, J. P. (1984). Site and mechanism of action of diuretics. *Am. J. Med.*, 77(SA), 11-17.

Lant, A. F. (1981). Modern diuretics and the kidney. *J. Clin. Pathol.*, 34, 1267-75.

Levinsky, N. G. and Levy, M. (1973). Clearance techniques. In Orloff, J., Berliner, R.W. and Geiger, S. R. (Eds.), *Handbook of Physiology: Renal Physiology.* American Physiologic Society, Washington D.C., pp. 103-17.

Liedtke, R. R. and Duarte, C. G. (1980). Laboratory protocols and methods for the measurement of glomerular filtration rate and renal plasma flow. In Duarte, C. G. (Ed.), *Renal Function Tests: Clinical Laboratory Procedures and Diagnosis.* Little Brown, Boston, pp. 49-63.

Maack, T. (1986). Renal clearance and isolated kidney perfusion techniques. *Kid. Int.*, 311, 142-51.

McEwen, J. (1988). Biochemical pharmacodynamics. *Pharm. Med.*, 3, 111-20.

McEwen, J. (1989). Studies in man with potential therapeutic agents. In Illing, H. P. A. (Ed.), *Xenobiotic Metabolism and Disposition: The Design of Disposition and Metabolism Studies on Novel Compounds*. CRC Press, Boca Raton, FL, pp. 89-97.

McMurray, J., Seidelin, P. H. and Struthers, A. D. (1989). Evidence for a proximal and distal nephron action of atrial natriuretic factor in man. *Nephron*, 51, 39-43.

McMurray, J. and Struthers, A. D. (1987). Role of neuroendocrine abnormalities in the enhanced sodium and water retention of chronic heart failure. *Pharmacol. Toxicol.*, 61, 209-14.

McMurray, J. and Struthers, A. D. (1988). Frusemide pretreatment blunts the inhibition of renal tubular sodium reabsorption by ANF in man. *Eur. J. Clin. Pharmacol.*, 35, 333-8.

McNabb, W. R., Noormohamed, F. H., Brooks, B. A. and Lant, A. F. (1984). Renal actions of piretanide and three other loop diuretics. *Clin. Pharmacol. Ther.*, 35, 328-37.

Mejia, G. and Steele, T. H. (1986). Uricosuric diuretics. In Dirks, J. H. and Sutton, R. A. L. (Eds.), *Diuretics: Physiology, Pharmacology and Clinical Use*. W. B. Saunders, Philadelphia, pp. 135-48.

Navar, L. G. and Schafer, J. A. (1987). Comments on 'Lithium clearance: a new research area'. *NIPS*, 2, 34-5.

Odlind, B. (1984). Site and mechanism of the action of diuretics. *Acta Pharm. Toxicol.*, 54 (Suppl. 1), 5-15.

Puschett, J. B. (1981). Sites and mechanisms of action of diuretics in the kidney. *J. Clin. Pharmacol.*, 21, 564-74.

Puschett, J. B. (1985). Determination of diuretic sites and mechanisms of action — an outline of the methodology employed. In Puschett, J. B. and Greenberg, A. (Eds.), *The Diuretic Manual*. Elsevier, Amsterdam, pp. 139-52.

Puschett, J. B. (1986). Clinical pharmacologic implications in diuretic selection. *Am. J. Cardiol.*, 57 (Suppl. A), 6A-13A.

Puschett, J. B. and Rastegar, A. (1974). Comparative study of the effects of metolazone and other diuretics on potassium excretion. *Clin. Pharmacol. Ther.*, 15, 397-405.

Reyes, A. J. and Leary, W. P. (1987). Natriuretic potency of various drugs. In Andreucci, V. E. and Dal Canton, A. (Eds.), *Diuretics: Basic, Pharmacological and Clinical Aspects*. Martinus Nijhoff, Boston, pp. 506-8.

Roberts, C. J. C., Daneshmend, T. K. (1981). Assessment of natriuretic drugs. *Br. J. Clin. Pharmacol.*, 12, 465-74.

Rose, H. J., O'Malley, K. and Pruitt, A. W. (1977). Depression of renal clearance of furosemide in man by azotemia. *Clin. Pharmacol. Ther.*, 21, 141-6.

Roy, D. R. and Jamison, R. L. (1985). Countercurrent system and its regulation. In Seldin, D. W. and Giebsch, G. (Eds.), *The Kidney: Physiology and Pathophysiology*. Raven Press, New York, pp. 903-32.

Schuster, V. L. and Seldin, D. W. (1985). Renal clearance. In Seidin, D. W. and Giebisch, G. (Eds.), *The Kidney: Physiology and Pathophysiology*. Raven Press, New York, pp. 365-95.

Seldin, D. W. and Giebisch, G. (1985). *The Kidney: Physiology and Pathophysiology*. Raven Press, New York.

Seldin, D. W. and Rector, F. C. (1973). Evaluation of clearance methods for localisation of site of action of diuretics. In Lant, A. F. and Wilson, G. M. (Eds.), *Modern Diuretic Therapy in the Treatment of Cardiovascular and Renal Disease*. Excerpta Medica, Amsterdam, pp. 97-110.

Shackleton, C. R., Wong, N. L. M. and Sutton, R. A. L. (1986). Distal (potassium-sparing) diuretics. In Dirks, J. H. and Sutton, R. A. L. (Eds.), *Diuretics: Physiology, Pharmacology and Clinical Use*. W. B. Saunders, Philadelphia, pp. 117-34.

Smith, D. E., Hyneck, M. L., Beradi, R. R. and Port, F. K. (1985). Urinary protein binding, kinetics and dynamics of furosemide in nephrotic patients. *J. Pharmacol. Sci.*, 74, 603-7.

Smith, H. (1956). *Principles of Renal Physiology*. Oxford University Press, New York.

Steinmuller, S. R. and Puschett, J. B. (1972). Effects of metolazone in man: comparison with chlorothiazide. *Kid. Int.*, 1, 169-81.

Teredesai, P. and Puschett, J. B. (1979). Acute effects of piretanide in normal subjects. *Clin. Pharmacol. Ther.*, 25, 331-9.

Thornsen, K. (1984). Lithium clearance: a new method for determining proximal and distal tubular reabsorption of sodium and water. *Nephron*, 37, 217-23.

van Brummelen, P., Man in 't Veld, A. J. and Schalekamp, M. A. D. H. (1980). Haemodynamic changes during long-term thiazide treatment of essential hypertension in responders and nonresponders. *Clin. Pharmacol. Ther.*, 27, 328-36.

Weiner, I. M. (1986). General pharmacological aspects of diuretics. In Dirks, J. H. and Sutton, R. A. L. (Eds.), *Diuretics: Physiology, Pharmacology and Clinical Use*. W. B. Saunders, Philadelphia, pp. 3-28.

Whelton, A. and Watson, A. J. (1987). The incidence of hypokalaemia and hyperkalaemia associated with diuretic use. In Puschett, J. B. and Greenberg, A. (Eds.), *Diuretics H: Chemistry, Pharmacology and Clinical Applications*. Elsevier, Amsterdam, pp. 677-85.

Wilcox, C. S. (1987). Roles of renin angiotensin aldosterone and autonomic nervous systems in the response to diuretic drugs in man. In Puschett, J. B. and Greenberg, A. (Eds.), *Diuretics II: Chemistry, Pharmacology and Clinical Applications*. Elsevier, Amsterdam, pp. 503-9.

Chapter 31

Renal Side Effects

Anne Dawnay

CONTENTS

1 Introduction 425
2 Drug-Induced Nephrotoxicity 426
3 General Considerations 426
4 Assessment Of Glomerular Filtration Rate 427
5 Assessment of Glomerular Permeability 427
6 Assessment of Tubular Function 428
  6.1 Electrolytes and Water 428
  6.2 Low Molecular Weight Proteins (LMWP) 428
  6.3 Enzymes 429
  6.4 Kidney-Derived Antigens 429
7 Biochemical Test Strategy 430
8 Proton NMR Spectroscopy 430
9 Summary 431
References 431

Measuring the therapeutic effects of drugs on the kidney has been dealt with elsewhere in this book and this chapter will concentrate on the methods available for detecting their adverse effects. Space does not permit a detailed critique of each analytical method but reference has been made to recent reviews.

1 INTRODUCTION

Conventionally, renal dysfunction is detected by impairment of glomerular filtration rate (GFR), reflected by elevation of the plasma creatinine or diminution of the creatinine clearance, and/or proteinuria. These tests alone are not sufficiently sensitive or specific to detect the early stages of drug-induced nephrotoxicity. Impairment of GFR often reflects late, secondary change following a primary insult of sufficient magnitude to the tubules or interstitium. Dipsticks for urine protein are predominantly sensitive to albumin and are only positive at concentrations in excess of 150 mg/l, which is approximately tenfold higher than the normal urine albumin output. Quantitative methods for urine total protein are insensitive and highly imprecise at low (normal) concentrations, and give no indication of the origin of the protein and therefore the possible underlying pathology. The differentiation of glomerular and tubular proteinuria requires the measurement of specific proteins (Peterson et al., 1969).

Overt renal dysfunction due to toxins may be preceded by the appearance in urine of markers of cytotoxicity (e.g., tubular antigens and enzymes) and biochemical abnormalities (Cárdenas et al., 1993a). The heterogeneous nature of the kidney and of the mode of drug toxicity necessitates the use of several tests specific for different aspects of renal integrity. In the last 15 years numerous new tests for detecting early renal dysfunction have appeared in the literature. Many of these are of unproven value in humans and have assumed, simplistically, that the detection of a drug-associated abnormality equates with toxicity. However, increasing evidence for the potential use of such sensitive tests in detecting nephrotoxicity due to drugs may be inferred from studies of their use in workers following occupational exposure to known nephrotoxins such as perchloroethylene (Mutti et al., 1992), mercury vapor (Cárdenas et al., 1993a), lead (Cárdenas et al., 1993b), and cadmium (Roels et al., 1993).

In this chapter, I have aimed to provide recommendations for screening for adverse effects taking into account not only what is scientifically most appropriate but also what is feasible, both in terms of subject and staff compliance, analytical simplicity, speed, and cost. A discussion of what constitutes an adverse effect is outside the scope of this chapter. I believe that persistent and/or consistent abnormalities

0-8493-9230-6/97/$0.00+$.50
© 1997 by CRC Press, Inc.

in screening tests associated with drug administration warrant further investigation to determine whether such changes are innocuous or reflect reversible or irreversible damage or cell necrosis.

2 DRUG-INDUCED NEPHROTOXICITY

About two thirds of drugs are in some way dependent on the kidneys for clearance. Their concentration increases during passage through the tubules as the urine is concentrated, potentiating tubular cytotoxicity. Drug toxicity may also result from hemodynamic or immunological reactions. Up to a quarter of cases of acute renal failure may be due to drug toxicity predominantly associated with gentamicin, angiotensin converting enzyme (ACE) inhibitors and nonsteroidal anti-inflammatory drugs (NSAIDs; Cove-Smith, 1991; Davidman et al., 1991). The contribution of drug toxicity to the development of chronic, irreversible renal failure is more difficult to estimate. Chronic tubulointerstitial nephritis and nephritis of unknown origin account for 15 to 30% of the cases of endstage renal disease in the U.S. and Europe (Ronco and Flahault, 1994). The proportion of these due to nephrotoxins is unknown. There are some data to implicate occupational pollutants (Nuyts et al., 1995) but little information regarding drugs. Analgesic nephropathy due to phenacetin has long been recognized as a culprit, accounting for some 2% of cases on average, but the role of other analgesics remains highly controversial (Perneger et al., 1994 and ensuing correspondence). To date, cyclosporin and cisplatin are the only nonanalgesic drugs which have been established to cause chronic renal disease (Ronco and Flahault, 1994).

Evidence of the nephrotoxicity of new drugs should not only be sought in young healthy volunteers. Drugs are often prescribed to patients who may be predisposed to nephrotoxic effects due to age- or disease-related diminished renal functional reserve or altered pharmacokinetics and pharmacodynamics, interaction with other prescribed drugs, noncompliance, and dehydration. The elderly are at particular risk of adverse reactions to drugs (Hurwitz, 1969; Ramsay and Tucker, 1981; Gosney and Tallis, 1984; Rochon and Gurwitz, 1995) but are generally underrepresented in clinical trials (Rochon and Gurwitz, 1995). Whether such risk factors for acute renal failure may also predispose to the development of chronic renal failure is unknown. Testing for nephrotoxicity during phase I and II trials is only likely to detect those drugs which are acutely toxic due to the relatively short duration of exposure. Whether some drugs may cause chronic renal failure in the absence of detectable, albeit subclinical, effects in the short term is unknown. However, all of the drugs currently known to cause irreversible renal impairment (some analgesics, cyclosporin, cisplatin) also manifest acute effects on the kidney too.

3 GENERAL CONSIDERATIONS

Urine is a readily accessible fluid but a highly variable and relatively hostile environment. Analytes and their assay methods must be sufficiently robust to withstand the range of urine pH, ionic strength and composition, proteolytic enzymes, and contaminating bacteria without elaborate patient preparation or urine collection conditions. Timed urine collections should be avoided whenever possible because of errors due to incomplete collection of urine passed, incomplete bladder emptying, and mistakes in timing.

In most circumstances, untimed urine samples are suitable; however, the concentration of most compounds in urine is independent of, and therefore varies inversely with, urine flow rate. This will normally vary between 0.5 and 5 ml/min during the day, depending on fluid intake. Correction for flow rate is achieved most simply by also measuring urine creatinine, whose excretion rate is relatively constant (*vide infra*), and computing a ratio. Physiologically, urine creatinine output depends on muscle mass which in turn varies with age and sex. With some, but not all, analytes this necessitates the use of appropriate reference ranges. The excretion of most compounds in urine does not follow a normal distribution and reference ranges must be derived using nonparametric methods. It is worth noting that most reference ranges are based on the 95th percentile of the population and therefore, by definition, 5% will be abnormal. If 20 separate tests are carried out on 100 individuals, 64% will show one or more abnormal result (Rogers and Spector, 1986). The excretion of many proteins is not constant throughout the day due to circadian rhythms, posture, exercise, etc. Reference ranges derived from early morning urine samples (i.e., overnight urine) may not be applicable to daytime samples and vice versa. Generally, the type of sample is irrelevant provided that the same type is consistently used during the study. I have given illustrative reference ranges, but these will obviously vary depending on the method used.

Tests for specific proteins in urine, including enzymes, are notorious for high intraindividual variability and random aberrant results. Fluctuations within the reference range and sporadic abnormal results are probably of little significance (Warrington et al., 1990). Several samples, to demonstrate consistency within an individual, and/or several subjects, to demonstrate consistency of response, are necessary. This problem has been widely studied in relation to urine albumin (Feldt-Rasmussen and Mathiesen, 1984; Howey et al., 1987; Mogensen, 1987). This does not devalue their use but merits attention when designing protocols and interpreting results.

4 ASSESSMENT OF GLOMERULAR FILTRATION RATE

The only practicable means of assessing GFR is by creatinine clearance and plasma creatinine and urea. For a full discussion of this subject, I recommend the reviews by Payne (1986) and Perrone et al. (1992).

Calculation of creatinine clearance involves the collection of timed samples, usually over 24 h. Measurement of the volume, and urine and plasma concentrations of creatinine allow calculation of creatinine clearance using the formula uv/p, where u and p are the respective urine and plasma concentrations of creatinine in identical units, and v is the rate of urine flow in ml/min. As a check for inaccurate timing, two consecutive collections should always be made. Plasma creatinine and urine creatinine output are not constant over 24 h on a diet containing meat protein (Heymsfield et al., 1983; Mayersohn et al., 1983) and creatinine clearance may therefore vary considerably depending on the timing of the urine collection period and blood sample (Morrison, 1991).

Assessment of GFR is usually for two reasons (Payne, 1986): first, to determine whether it is abnormal and if so to what extent; secondly, to determine whether it has changed. To detect abnormality demands the use of appropriate reference ranges. Creatinine clearance steadily declines with age from a mean of 112 ml/min (range 78-146) in the third decade, to 78 ml/min (range 52-102) in the eighth in men (Rowe et al., 1976a). In contrast, plasma creatinine measured in the morning in men was unaffected by age (mean 88 μmol/l in the third and 90 μmol/l in the eighth decade) and averaged 10 μmol/l less in women (De Lauture et al., 1973). The constancy of plasma creatinine with increasing age, in spite of a reduction in creatinine clearance, is most likely due to a decrease in muscle mass as reflected by a decreasing urine creatinine output with age (Rowe et al., 1976b). The detection of change depends on the analytical reproducibility of the measurement and on the biological variability. Day to day coefficients of variation for morning plasma creatinine are some 8% in health (Rosano and Brown, 1982) but may be three times as high (Brochner-Mortensen and Rodbro, 1976) or worse (personal experience) for creatinine clearance even after careful instruction. It is a well-known fact that an accurately timed collection of urine is very difficult to obtain.

In nephrotoxicity studies, creatinine clearance, plasma creatinine, and urea should be measured on at least two occasions before commencing a study to establish a baseline and to gauge any necessary reduction in drug dose in elderly patients with a naturally reduced GFR if the drug depends on renal clearance. Thereafter, plasma creatinine measured on samples taken preferably in the morning after a nonmeat protein breakfast offers the most precise means of detecting change. The result should be reported the same day to enable immediate action should any increase occur. Typically, an increase of 30 μmol/l is significant, even if remaining within the reference range. Impairment of GFR due to hemodynamic factors may occur rapidly, e.g., in some forms of nephrotoxicity associated with NSAIDs (Garella and Matarese, 1984) or cyclosporin (Walker and Duggin, 1988).

Of all the tests for detecting renal dysfunction, creatinine is most prone to interference. Ketones, especially acetoacetate, cause positive interference with the Jaffe colorimetric assay and prolonged fasting, to an extent that ketones are readily detectable in urine, may be sufficient to cause significant error, especially in a dilute urine sample (Harrison, 1987). Drugs may interfere with creatinine analysis (e.g., cephalosporin antibiotics) or compete for tubular secretion (e.g., cimetidine; Narayanan and Appleton, 1980; Payne, 1986). In either case this can cause misleading increases in plasma creatinine and therefore it is advisable to also measure plasma urea. Enzymatic assays for creatinine are less susceptible to interference than the Jaffe reaction. Parent drugs can be tested for analytical interference but their metabolites are not often available. Although comparatively rare, the interference of drugs in laboratory tests should always be borne in mind. The use of serum creatinine as an index of renal function has recently been reviewed (Perrone et al., 1992).

5 ASSESSMENT OF GLOMERULAR PERMEABILITY

Glomerular proteinuria can only be accurately assessed by specific immunoassays for proteins of high Mr (>60,000). In practice, urine albumin (Mr 66,000) is stable, easy to measure, and has been widely studied; there is no evidence that any other protein of high Mr gives more useful information unless an index of selectivity is required. Since results may not be available the same day, urine samples should be checked for protein using dipsticks during the course of drug trials to detect gross damage requiring immediate action.

Urine albumin is readily detected by most types of immunoassay, be they of the unlabeled (e.g., nephelometry, turbidimetry, rocket electrophoresis) or labeled (e.g., isotopic, fluorescent, enzyme) type. The recent recognition that diabetic nephropathy can now be predicted from the early detection of small elevations of albumin (Mogensen, 1987) years in advance of the appearance of clinical proteinuria, has resulted in a proliferation of commercial kits and published inhouse assays for urine albumin. Many of these methods are easily automated (Watts et al., 1986; Elving et al., 1989) or are manually so simple (Silver et al., 1986) as to allow the processing of several hundred samples per day. A comprehensive review of the analytical goals and conditions of urine collection and storage is available (Rowe et al., 1990). Normal urine output is <20 mg/24 h (Feldt-Rasmussen and Mathiesen, 1984) or <2.8 mg/mmol creatinine (Silver et al., 1986) and is typically lower in samples collected while recumbent compared with ambulant and in males than in females (Silver et al 1986; Howey et al., 1987). Clinical glomerular proteinuria is known to occur following the use of many drugs, e.g., gold (Hall, 1988), and may be the presenting feature in some forms of NSAID toxicity (Garella and Matarese, 1984). However, there is a dearth of information concerning the use of sensitive urine albumin assays in the early detection of nephrotoxicity.

6 ASSESSMENT OF TUBULAR FUNCTION

Urine microscopy is a simple and rapid means of detecting gross effects due to inflammatory reactions and tubular cell damage before laboratory results are available.

6.1 Electrolytes and Water

The measurement of plasma electrolytes (sodium, potassium, calcium, bicarbonate, chloride) and clinical evaluation of the patient provides the most practicable means of screening for drug-induced abnormalities of water and electrolyte homeostasis. Magnesium wasting, resulting in hypomagnesemia, has been reported with aminoglycosides (Davey and Harpur, 1987) and cisplatin (Litterst and Weiss, 1987) but usually occurs in conjunction with hypocalcemia. The 24-h excretion of electrolytes and dynamic tests for urine acidification and concentration are cumbersome and should only be considered if other evidence suggests they are necessary. However, an increase in the fractional excretion of sodium (FENa) is a simple indicator of tubular dysfunction which can be readily measured by assaying sodium and creatinine in plasma and a random sample of urine (FENa = [urine Na plasma creatinine/plasma Na urine creatinine] × 100). Urine concentrating ability is also a good indicator of general tubular integrity and can be most simply monitored on a first morning urine sample following an overnight (more than eight hours) fluid fast (Morrison, 1991).

6.2 Low Molecular Weight Proteins (LMWP)

LMWP is a term which comprises that group of plasma proteins, generally of Mr less than 35,000, which are filtered to a significant extent by the glomerulus. Some 99.95% of the filtered load is absorbed and catabolized in the proximal tubule. Increased excretion of these proteins may be due either to decreased absorption, as a consequence of proximal tubular dysfunction, or to an increase in their serum concentration and therefore a filtered load exceeding the tubular absorptive capacity (Maack et al., 1979; Beetham et al., 1987). This second mechanism is unlikely, other than in malignancy, systemic inflammatory processes, or renal dysfunction with a plasma creatinine in excess of some 180 μmol/l (Bernard et al., 1988) and will be apparent from baseline samples. Elevated urine excretion of LMWPs following exposure to drugs, chemicals, and heavy metals toxic to the proximal tubule is well proven both in healthy volunteers, industrial workers, and patients (Weise et al., 1981; Topping et al., 1986; Bernard et al 1987; Stonard, 1987). Levels may be elevated several hundredfold in the face of severe proximal tubular damage.

The most widely studied protein in this group is beta-2-microglobulin (b2m) (Schardijn and Statius van Eps, 1987). However, it is rapidly and irreversibly degraded in urine of pH less than 6 (Evrin and Wibell, 1972; Bernard et al., 1982; Davey and Gosling, 1982; Donaldson et al., 1989) and its use is no longer recommended. Either retinol-binding protein (RBP; Peterson and Berggard, 1971) or alpha-1-microglobulin (a1m; Berggard et al., 1980; Grubb, 1992), both of which are comparatively stable at pH 5 and above (Bernard et al., 1982; Yu et al., 1983; Beetham et al., 1985; Donaldson et al., 1989), are theoretically suitable alternatives and an increasing amount of empirical evidence suggests this is so (Bernard et al., 1982, 1987; Topping et al., 1986; Beetham et al., 1987). The excretion rate of LMWPs appears to be unaffected by age, sex, or water diuresis (Evrin and Wibell, 1972; Wibell and Karlsson, 1976; Beetham et al., 1985; Beetham, 1986). Normal excretion rates are typically <1.7 mg/mmol creatinine for a1m (Yu et al., 1983) and <13 μg/mmol creatinine for RBP (Beetham et al., 1985).

6.3 Enzymes

The assay of tissue-specific enzymes in serum to detect and monitor tissue damage has a long-established history in clinical chemistry. Such a proven role, together with the cheapness and relative ease of assay, undoubtedly contributed to the application of such assays to urine samples. Urine contains many enzymes whose origin can be located in a particular part of the nephron (Schmidt and Guder, 1976; Price, 1982). They are generally of high Mr and contamination with their serum counterparts is unlikely provided that glomerular permeability is normal. Their different distribution, not only along the length of the nephron but also to different cellular and subcellular locations in the same part of the nephron, suggested that measurement of a panel of enzymes would be a noninvasive means of giving highly specific information concerning the sites affected by nephrotoxins. Such ambitions have generally not been realized, partly due to difficulties experienced with enzyme stability and nonspecific effects on activity measurements, often necessitating dialysis or gel filtration of urine samples prior to analysis, and partly because of the difficulties in obtaining corroborative evidence in humans.

The only enzyme which is simple to measure and has emerged from experimental research as a serious contender for detecting subclinical toxicity is *N*-acetyl-beta-D-glucosaminidase (EC 3.2.1.30, NAG; Price, 1992). NAG is a lysosomal enzyme found in most parts of the nephron but with toxins affecting the proximal convoluted tubule being the predominant cause of increased excretion in urine. However, in the rat (Stonard, 1987) and dog (Piperno, 1981), experimental papillotoxins also increase NAG excretion. The original assay used a fluorescent substrate (Tucker et al., 1975), necessitating the inclusion of blanks for each urine sample due to their highly variable and nonspecific endogenous fluorescence. The recent advent of colorimetric substrates, with measurements made at 505 nm (Yuen et al., 1984) or 580 nm (Goren et al., 1986), has obviated the need for blanks, provided samples are not icteric or blood-stained, and are easily automated. NAG is stable over the pH range 5-8 (Lockwood and Bosmann, 1979) and no inhibitors or activators are known (Piperno, 1981; Mueller et al., 1986). Neither urine flow rate, age, or sex have appreciable effects on the urine excretion rate (Lockwood and Bosmann, 1979; Houser, 1986; Jung et al., 1986). As with all assays of enzyme activity, reference ranges are highly method-dependent.

A prospective evaluation of NAG excretion compared with plasma creatinine and urine b2m illustrate its potential use. In a study of 28 patients with normal renal function (plasma creatinine <100 μmol/l, no proteinuria, and sterile urine) treated with gentamicin, only 1 of 12 patients with an initially normal NAG excretion developed renal failure (increase in plasma creatinine of >50 μmol/l) although 7 showed a marked and persistent increase in the excretion of NAG and, later, of b2m (Gibey et al., 1981). However, 11 of 16 patients with an initially elevated NAG developed renal failure and showed a more rapid increase in NAG and b2m excretion which preceded the increase in plasma creatinine. Thus, drug-induced abnormalities in the absence of overt renal dysfunction may predict a risk of toxicity which is overt in patients with pre-existing tubular abnormalities. In clinical practice, aminoglycoside use is associated with acute renal failure in 8-26% of patients (Humes, 1988). NAG excretion can provide information on both the extent of and recovery from nephrotoxic damage (Gibey et al., 1984). Identification of the NAG isoenzymes involved may give additional information on the mechanism of nephrotoxicity (Gibey et al., 1984; Sanchez-Bernal et al., 1991).

6.4 Kidney-Derived Antigens

The measurement of kidney-derived material to detect renal pathology remains a research tool of promising but as yet, unproven use (Dawnay and Cattell, 1987 for review). Only a few of the renal antigens excreted in urine have been isolated and characterized, e.g., ligandin, urine protein-1, and BB-50 from the proximal tubule, Tamm-Horsfall glycoprotein from the thick ascending limb of the loop of Henle and early distal convoluted tubule, and various basement membrane antigens. Many assays have been developed using monoclonal antibodies reactive with specific cellular or subcellular compounds within the nephron. Their reactivity with nonrenal antigens is generally unknown and caution should be exercised in the interpretation of results using these assays. Certainly many monoclonal antibodies to B cells react with kidney antigens which share common epitopes (Fleming et al., 1989).

7 BIOCHEMICAL TEST STRATEGY

Before drug administration, tests should be carried out on at least two separate days to ensure consistency of baseline values. These tests should continue for up to a week after cessation of the drug and for longer if adverse effects have been noted to determine whether values return to baseline. The frequency of monitoring during the period of drug administration will vary depending on the trial design but should be at least thrice weekly if toxicity is unknown or if the drug is highly likely to manifest a nephrotoxic reaction. The frequency, magnitude, and reversibility of abnormal values can then be compared to determine any relationship with drug administration and dose (Mutti et al., 1992; Warrington et al., 1993). If renal function is likely to be unstable during the period of study, independent of drug administration, or when there is difficulty separating disease effects from true drug effects (Parish and Miller, 1992), a randomized, cross-over placebo-controlled study may be more appropriate.

The actual tests to be carried out should include an assessment of GFR (e.g., creatinine clearance) and urine total protein (or preferably albumin) output. Frequent monitoring of plasma creatinine, urea and electrolytes, urine protein by dipstick, and urine microscopy should be carried out and reviewed the same day during the period of the trial to allow remedial action should gross toxicity occur. For drugs of unknown toxicity, more sensitive tests to detect subclinical toxicity should also be included such as urine RBP and NAG, although samples for these may be batched for subsequent analysis. Tests to detect specific renal effects of certain drugs, e.g., hypomagnesemia with cisplatin, should be included where appropriate.

In trials designed to assess the toxicity of known nephrotoxic drugs in new formulations, e.g., cisplatin-albumin complex (Holding et al., 1992), liposomal antimicrobials (Sabra and Branch, 1990; Karlowsky and Zhanel, 1992) or to assess methods to minimize toxicity, e.g., hydration during chemotherapy (Cornelison and Reed, 1993), co-administration of sulfydryls with cisplatin (Bohm et al., 1991; Howell et al., 1991) or with different dosing regimes (Craig, 1993), appropriate tests may be selected based on prior knowledge of the manifestations of nephrotoxicity.

There are a few published studies in which a range of sensitive biochemical tests have been included when looking for nephrotoxicity in either healthy volunteers (Warrington et al., 1989, 1990, 1993) or patients (Gibey et al., 1981; Dawnay et al., 1988; Daugaard, 1990; Metz-Kurschel et al., 1990; Kurschel et al., 1991; Skinner et al., 1991; Riley et al., 1992; Wilkie et al., 1993). The absence of detectable adverse effects with such sensitive tests bodes well for their nephrotoxic potential (other than for allergic reactions), although it does little to enhance the publication value of such studies in the eyes of many editors.

8 PROTON NMR SPECTROSCOPY

The preceding sections have described the wide variety of biochemical tests available for detecting nephrotoxicity, some of which are specific for nephron segments and some not. In screening for the nephrotoxic effects of a new drug for which the site, mechanism, and severity of toxicity is unknown, it is therefore necessary to measure several different analytes, a labor-intensive and time-consuming process.

A possible solution to these problems lies in the use of high resolution proton NMR spectroscopy. Hundreds of endogenous metabolites can be detected and therefore monitored simultaneously and comparison with the NMR spectrum obtained in the absence of the drug enables ready identification of changes. The complexity of the spectra obtained necessitates the use of sophisticated computer-based pattern recognition for analysis (Gartland et al., 1990; Holmes et al., 1994). The ability of NMR to detect renal impairment due to nephrotoxicity and its relationship to more conventional biochemical markers has been confirmed in several studies (Anthony et al., 1992; Murgatroyd et al., 1992; Anthony et al., 1994a). Sequential monitoring of changes in concentration (or excretion rate) and patterns of endogenous metabolites following drug exposure yields information on the severity and location of toxic lesions and insights into the underlying molecular mechanism of toxicity (Nicholson and Wilson, 1989; Anthony et al., 1992).

From the analysis of urine samples obtained following exposure of rats to nephrotoxins with known sites of action, it has been possible to characterize the changes in concentration and pattern of endogenous metabolites (Nicholson and Wilson, 1989; Gartland et al., 1990; Anthony et al., 1994b). The site of toxicity of other compounds can subsequently be deduced by comparison. An obvious advantage is that advanced knowledge of the identity of the analyte is not necessary. Indeed NMR has been used to characterize the changes associated with exposure to medullary toxins resulting in renal papillary necrosis for which no specific analytical marker has been available. The early appearance of peaks specifically associated with papillary toxins was noted and these were subsequently identified as being due to trimethylamine *N*-oxide and dimethylamine (Gartland et al., 1989). Thus proton NMR spectroscopy can be used to identify new markers of endorgan damage for which individual quantitative analytical methods can be developed if necessary.

The detection of abnormal urine patterns does not confirm a renal toxic insult since any compound interacting with normal metabolic processes may result in an altered NMR pattern even though no toxic effect exists. Also toxicity in nonrenal organs may result in increased or altered excretion of endogenous metabolites, e.g., taurine in acute liver toxicity and creatinine in testicular toxicity (Nicholson and Wilson, 1989; Nicholson et al., 1989). Dietary composition can also affect the urinary metabolite profile (Nicholson and Wilson, 1989; Gartland et al., 1990) and interpretation of results from toxicological studies, especially isolated abnormalities in humans where strict dietary control is not generally feasible, should consider diet as a possible cause. Since abnormalities detected by proton NMR of urine cannot be considered specific for nephrotoxicity, independent confirmatory tests of the cause are required.

In summary, the proton NMR of urine combined with sophisticated data reduction has the potential to yield large amounts of information rapidly and is likely to be used increasingly in the evaluation of nephrotoxic drugs. Studies to date have generally involved only urine samples from overtly nephrotoxic cases, i.e., when plasma urea and/or creatinine increased markedly. Whether the technique will have sufficient sensitivity to find a role as a screening test to detect sub-clinical nephrotoxicity remains to be seen.

9 SUMMARY

Drug-induced nephrotoxicity occurs via numerous mechanisms and may develop acutely or chronically. Sensitive tests to detect sub-clinical abnormalities may be useful to determine the inherent toxicity of a drug; to compare the relative toxicity of different drugs with a similar therapeutic index; and to select and monitor patients for trials in order to minimize the risk of toxicity. Several samples should be obtained from each subject both before, during and after drug administration to determine whether any abnormalities are persistent or random and whether they are reversible. In the past, nephrotoxicity has often only manifested after widespread clinical use in predisposed patients. Common risk factors include dose and duration of treatment, advancing age, pre-existing renal insufficiency or hepatic disease, hypovolaemia and concurrent nephrotoxic drug administration. The use of sensitive tests to detect subclinical abnormalities during phase I and II trials should be useful in predicting the likelihood of drug-induced clinical nephrotoxicity.

REFERENCES

Anthony, M.L., Gartland, K.P.R., Beddell, C.R., Lindon, J.C., Nicholson, J.K., Cephaloridine-induced nephrotoxicity in the Fischer 344 rat: proton NMR spectroscopic studies of urine and plasma in relation to conventional clinical chemical and histopathological assessments of nephronal damage, *Arch. Toxicol.*, 66, 525, 1992.

Anthony, M.L., Gartland, K.P.R., Beddell, C.R., Lindon, J.C., Nicholson, J.K., Studies of the biochemical toxicology of uranyl nitrate in the rat, *Arch. Toxicol.*, 68, 43, 1994a.

Anthony, M.L., Sweatman, B.C., Beddell, C.R., Lindon, J.C., Nicholson, J.K., Pattern recognition classification of the site of nephrotoxicity based on metabolic data derived from proton nuclear magnetic resonance spectra of urine, *Mol. Pharmacol.*, 46, 199, 1994b.

Beetham, R., The development of immunoassays for retinol-binding protein and their application, Ph.D. thesis, London University, 1986.

Beetham, R., Dawnay, A., Landon, J., Cattell, W.R., A radioimmunosassay for retinol-binding protein in serum and urine, *Clin. Chem.*, 31, 1364, 1985.

Beetham, R., Dawnay, A., Cattell, W.R., The effect of a synthetic polypeptide on the renal handling of protein in man, *Clin. Sci.*, 72, 245, 1987.

Berggard, B., Erkstrom, B., Akerstrom, B., Alpha-1-microglobulin, *Scand. J. Clin. Lab. Invest.*, 40 (Suppl. 154), 63, 1980.

Bernard, A.M., Moreau, D., Lauwerys, R., Comparison of retinol-binding protein and beta-2-microglobulin determination in urine for the early detection of tubular proteinuria, *Clin. Chim. Acta*, 126, 1, 1982.

Bernard, A.M., Vyskocil, A.A., Mahieu, P., Lauwerys, R.R., Assessment of urinary retinol-binding protein as an index of proximal tubular injury, *Clin. Chem.*, 33, 775, 1987.

Bernard, A., Vyskocyl, A., Mahieu, P., Lauwerys, R., Effect of renal insufficiency on the concentration of free retinol-binding protein in urine and serum, *Clin. Chim. Acta*, 171, 85, 1988.

Bohm, S., Battista Spatti, G., Di Re, F. et al., A feasibility study of cisplatin administration with low-volume hydration and glutathione protection in the treatment of ovarian carcinoma, *Anticanc. Res.*, 11, 1613, 1991.

Brochner-Mortensen, I., Rodbro, P., Selection of routine method for determination of glomerular filtration rate in adult patients, *Scand. J. Clin. Lab. Invest.*, 36, 35, 1976.

Cárdenas, A., Roels, H., Bernard, A.M. et al., Markers of early renal changes induced by industrial pollutants. I. Application to workers exposed to mercury vapor, *Br. J. Ind. Med.*, 50, 17, 1993a.

Cárdenas, A., Roels, H., Bernard, A.M., Markers of early renal changes induced by industrial pollutants. II. Application to workers exposed to lead, *Br. J. Ind. Med.*, 50, 28, 1993b.

Cornelison, T.L., Reed, E., Nephrotoxicity and hydration management for cisplatin, carboplatin, and ormaplatin, *Gynecol. Oncol.*, 50, 147, 1993.

Cove-Smith, R., Drugs and the kidney, *Med. Int.*, 85, 3539, 1991.

Craig, W., Pharmacodynamics of antimicrobial agents as a basis for determining dosage regimens, *Eur. J. Clin. Microbiol. Infect. Dis.*, 12(Suppl. 1), S6, 1993.

Daugaard, G., Cisplatin nephrotoxicity: experimental and clinical studies, *Dan. Med. Bull.*, 37, 1, 1990.

Davey, P.G., Gosling, P., Beta-2-microglobulin instability in pathological urine, *Clin. Chem.*, 28, 1330, 1982.

Davey, P.G., Harpur, E.S., Antibiotics: The experimental and clinical situation, in *Nephrotoxicity in the Experimental and Clinical Situation* (Part 2), Bach, P.H. and Lock, E.A., Eds., Martinus Nijhoff, Lancaster, 1987, 643.

Davidman, M., Olson, P., Kohen, J., Leither, T., Kjellstrand, C., Iatrogenic renal disease, *Arch. Int. Med.*, 151, 1809, 1991.

Dawnay, A., Cattell, W.R., The measurement of kidney-derived immunologically reactive material in urine and plasma for studying renal integrity, in *Nephrotoxicity in the Experimental and Clinical Situation* (Part 2), Bach, P.H. and Lock, E.A., Eds., Martinus Nijhoff, Lancaster, 1987, 593.

Dawnay, A., Lucey, M.R., Thornley, C. et al., The effects of long-term, low-dose cyclosporin A on renal tubular function in humans, *Transplant. Proc.*, XX(Suppl. 3), 725, 1988.

De Lauture, H., Caces, E., Dubost, P., Tournier, M., Dolle, Y., Weill, J., Boulard, P., Rossier, J., *Reference Values in Human Chemistry*, Siest, G., Ed., Karger, Basel, 1973, 141.

Donaldson, M.D.C., Chambers, R.E., Woolridge, M.W., Whicher, J.T., Stability of alpha-1-microglobulin, beta-2-microglobulin and retinol binding protein in urine, *Clin. Chim. Acta*, 179, 73, 1989.

Elving, L.D., Bakkeren, J., Jansen, M., de Kat Angelino, C., de Nobel, E., van Munster, P., Screening for microalbuminuria in patients with diabetes mellitus: frozen storage of urine samples decreases their albumin content, *Clin. Chem.*, 35, 308, 1989.

Evrin, P.-E., Wibell, L., The serum levels and urinary excretion of beta-2-microglobulin in apparently healthy subjects, *Scand. J. Clin. Lab. Invest.*, 29, 69, 1972.

Feldt-Rasmussen, B., Mathiesen, E.R., Varability of urinary albumin excretion in incipient diabetic nephropathy, *Diab. Nephropath.*, 3, 101, 1984.

Fleming, S., Jones, D.B., Moore, K., B-cell markers in the human kidney, *Nephrol. Dial. Transplant.*, 4, 85, 1989.

Garella, S., Matarese, R.A., Renal effects of prostaglandins and clinical adverse effects of nonsteroidal anti-inflammatory agents, *Medicine*, 63, 165, 1984.

Gartland, K.P.R., Bonner, F.W., Nicholson, J.K., Investigation into the biochemical effects of region-specific nephrotoxins, *Mol. Pharmacol.*, 35, 242, 1989.

Gartland, K.P.R., Sanins, S.M., Nicholson, J.K., Sweatman, B.C., Beddell, C.R., Lindon, J.C., Pattern recognition analysis of high resolution ^{1}H NMR spectra of urine. A nonlinear mapping approach to the classification of toxicological data, *NMR Biomed.*, 3, 166, 1990.

Gibey, R., Dupond, J.-L., Albert, D., Leconte des Floris, R., Henry, J.-C., Predictive value of urinary *N*-acetyl-beta-D-glucosaminidase (NAG), alanine aminopeptidase (AAP) and beta-2-microglobulin (b2m) in evaluating nephrotoxicity of gentamicin, *Clin. Chim. Acta*, 116, 25, 1981.

Gibey, R., Dupond, J.-L., Henry, J.-C., Urinary *N*-acetyl-ß-D-glucosaminidase (NAG) isoenzyme profiles: a tool for evaluating nephrotoxicity of aminoglycosides and cephalosporins, *Clin. Chim. Acta*, 137, 1, 1984.

Goren, M.P., Wright, R.K., Osborne, S. Two automated procedures for *N*-acetyl-beta-D-glucosaminidase determination evaluated for detection of drug-induced tubular nephrotoxicity, *Clin. Chem.*, 32, 2052, 1986.

Gosney, M., Tallis, R., Prescription of contraindicated and interacting drugs in elderly patients admitted to hospital, *Lancet*, 2, 564, 1984.

Grubb, A., Diagnostic value of analysis of cystatin C and protein HC in biological fluids, *Clin. Nephrol.*, 38(Suppl.1), S20, 1992.

Hall, C.L., Gold nephropathy, *Nephron*, 50, 265, 1988.

Harrison, S.P., More on urinary albumin and creatinine (letter), *Clin. Chem.*, 33, 740, 1987.

Heymsfield, S.B., Arteaga, C., McManus, C., Measurement of muscle mass in humans: validity of the 24 hour urinary creatinine method, *Am. J. Clin. Nutr.*, 37, 478, 1983.

Holding, J.D., Lindup, W.E., van Laer, C. et al., Phase I trial of a cisplatin-albumin complex for the treatment of cancer of the head and neck, *Br. J. Clin. Pharmacol.*, 33, 75, 1992.

Holmes, E., Foxall, P.J.D., Nicholson, J.K., Neild, J.H., Brown, S.M., Beddell, S.M., Sweatman, B.C., Rahr, E., Lindon, J.C., Spraul, M., Neidig, P., Automatic data reduction and pattern recognition methods for analysis of ^{1}H nuclear magnetic resonance spectra of human urine from normal and pathological states, *Analyt. Biochem.*, 220, 284, 1994.

Houser, M.T., The effects of age and urine concentration on lysozyme and *N*-acetyl-beta-D-glucosaminidase (NAG) content in urine, *Ann. Clin. Biochem.*, 23, 297, 1986.

Howell, S.B., Kirmani, S., McClay, E.F., Kim, S., Braly, P., Plaxe, S., Intraperitoneal cisplatin-based chemotherapy for ovarian carcinoma, *Semin. Oncol.*, 18(Suppl.3), 5, 1991.

Howey, J.E.A., Browning, M.C.K., Frasser, C.G., Selecting the optimum specimen for assessing slight albuminuria, and a strategy for clinical investigation: novel uses of data on biological variation, *Clin. Chem.*, 33, 2034, 1987.

Humes, H.D., Aminoglycoside nephrotoxicity, *Kidney Int.*, 33, 900, 1988.

Hurwitz, N., Predisposing factors in adverse reactions to drugs, *Br. Med. J.*, 1, 536, 1969.

Jung, K., Schulze, G., Reinholdt, C., Different diuresis dependent excretions of urinary enzymes: *N*-acetyl-beta-D-glucosaminidase, alanine aminopeptidase, alkaline phosphatase, and gamma glutamyltransferase, *Clin. Chem.*, 32, 529, 1986.

Karlowsky, J.A., Zhanel, G.G., Concepts on the use of liposomal antimicrobial agents: applications for aminoglycosides, *Clin. Infect. Dis.*, 15, 654, 1992.

Kurschel, E., Metz-Kurschel, U., Niederle, N., Aulbert, E., Investigations on the subclinical and clinical nephrotoxicity of interferon alpha-2B in patients with myeloproliferative syndromes, *Renal Failure*, 13, 87, 1991.

Litterst, C.L. Weiss, R.B., Clinical and experimental nephrotoxicity of cancer chemotherapeutic agents, in *Nephrotoxicity in the Experimental and Clinical Situation* (Part 2), Bach, P.H. and Lock, E.A., Eds., Martinus Nijhoff, Lancaster, 1987, 771.

Lockwood, T.D., Bosmann, H.B., The use of urinary *N*-acetyl-beta-glucosaminidase in human renal toxicology, *Toxicol. Appl. Pharmacol.*, 49, 323, 1979.

Maack, T., Johnson, V., Kau, S.T. Figueiredo, J., Sigulem, D., Renal filtration, transport and metabolism of low-molecular-weight proteins: a review, *Kidney Int.*, 16, 251, 1979.

Mayersohn, M., Conrad, K.A., Achari, R., The influence of a cooked meat meal on creatinine plasma concentration and creatinine clearance, *Br. J. Clin. Pharmacol.*, 15, 227, 1983.

Metz-Kurschel, U., Kurschel, E., Niederle, N., Aulbert, E., Investigations on the acute and chronic nephrotoxicity of the new platinum analogue carboplatin, *J. Cancer Res. Clin. Oncol.*, 116, 203, 1990.

Mogensen, C.E., Microalbuminuria as a predictor of clinical diabetic nephropathy, *Kidney Int.*, 31, 673, 1987.

Morrison, B., Assessment of renal function, *Medicine Int.*, 85, 3516, 1991.

Mueller, P.W., MacNeil, M.L., Steinberg, K.K., Stabilisation of alanine aminopeptidase, gamma glutamyltranspeptidase, and *N*-acetyl-beta-D-glucosaminidase activity in normal urines, *Arch. Environ. Contam. Toxicol.*, 15, 343, 1986.

Murgatroyd, L.B., Pickford, R., Smith, I.K., Wilson, I.D., ^{1}H NMR spectroscopy as a means of monitoring nephrotoxicity as exemplified by studies with cephaloridine, *Hum. Exp. Toxicol.*, 11, 35, 1992.

Mutti, A., Alinovi, R., Bergamaschi, E. et al., Nephropathies and exposure to perchloroethylene in dry-cleaners, *Lancet*, 340, 189, 1992.

Narayanan, S., Appleton, H.D., Creatinine: a review, *Clin. Chem.* 26, 1119, 1980.

Nicholson, J.K. Wilson, I.D., High resolution proton magnetic resonance spectroscopy of biological fluids, *Prog. NMR Spectrosc.*, 21, 449, 1989.

Nicholson, J.K., Higham, D.P., Timbrell, J.A. Sadler, P.J., Quantitative high resolution ^{1}H NMR urinalysis studies on the biochemical effects of cadmium in the rat, *Mol. Pharmacol.*, 36, 398, 1989.

Nuyts, G.D., Van Vlem, E., Thys, J. et al., New occupational risk factors for chronic renal failure, *Lancet,* 346, 7, 1995.

Parish, R.C., Miller, L.J., Adverse effects of angiotensin converting enzyme (ACE) inhibitors. An update, *Drug Safety*, 7, 14, 1992.

Payne, R.B., Creatinine clearance: a redundant clinical investigation, *Ann. Clin. Biochem.*, 23, 243, 1986.

Perneger, T.V., Whelton, P.K., Klag, M.J., Risk of kidney failure associated with the use of acetaminophen, aspirin and nonsteroidal anti-inflammatory drugs, *N. Engl. J. Med.,* 331, 1675, 1994 (and ensuing correspondence on kidney failure and analgesic drugs, *ibid*, 332, 1514, 1995).

Perrone, R.D., Madias, N.E., Levey, A.S., Serum creatinine as an index of renal function: New insights into old concepts, *Clin. Chem.*, 38, 1933, 1992.

Peterson, P.A., Evrin, P.-E., Berggard, I., Differentiation of glomerular, tubular and normal proteinuria: determinations of urinary excretion of beta-2-microglobulin, albumin, and total protein, *J. Clin. Invest.*, 48, 1189, 1969.

Peterson, P.A. Berggard, I., Isolation and properties of a human retinol-transporting protein, *J. Biol. Chem.*, 246, 25, 1971.

Piperno, E., Detection of drug-induced nephrotoxicity with urinalysis and enzymuria assessment, in *Toxicology of the Kidney*, Hook, J.B., Ed., Raven Press, New York, 1981, 31.

Price, R.G., Urinary enzymes, nephrotoxicity and renal disease, *Toxicology*, 23, 99, 1982.

Price, R.G., The role of NAG (*N*-acetyl-ß-D-glucosaminidase) in the diagnosis of kidney disease including the monitoring of nephrotoxicity, *Clin. Nephrol.*, 38(Suppl.1), S14, 1992.

Ramsay, L.E., Tucker, G.T., Drugs and the elderly, in *Today's Treatment:4*, Lock, S., Ed., British Medical Association, London, 1981, 149.

Riley, S.A., Lloyd, D.R., Mani, V., Tests of renal function in patients with quiescent colitis: effects of drug treatment, *Gut*, 33, 1348, 1992.

Rochon, P.A., Gurwitz, J.H., Drug therapy, *Lancet*, 346, 32, 1995.

Roels, H., Bernard, A.M., Cárdenas, A. et al., Markers of early renal changes induced by industrial pollutants. III. Application to workers exposed to cadmium, *Br. J. Ind. Med.*, 50, 37, 1993.

Rogers, H.J., Spector, R.G., *Handbook of Clinical Drug Research*, Glenny, H. and Nelmes, P., Eds., Blackwell Scientific, Oxford, 1986, 33.

Ronco, P.M., Flahault, A., Drug-induced endstage renal disease, *N. Engl. J. Med.*, 331, 1711, 1994.

Rosano, T.G., Brown, H.H., Analytical and biological variability of serum creatinine and creatinine clearance: implications for clinical interpretation, *Clin. Chem.*, 28, 2330, 1982.

Rowe, D.J.F., Dawnay, A., Watts, G.F., Microalbuminuria in diabetes mellitus: review and recommendations for the measurement of albumin in urine, *Ann. Clin. Biochem.*, 27, 297, 1990.

Rowe, J.W., Andres, R., Tobin, J.D., Norris, A.H., Shock, N., Age-adjusted standards for creatinine clearance, *Ann. Intern. Med.*, 84, 567, 1976a.

Rowe, J.W., Andres, R., Tobin, J.D., Norris, A.H., Shock, N.W., The effect of age on creatinine clearance in men: a cross-sectional and longitudinal study, *J. Gerontol.*, 31, 155, 1976b.

Sabra, R., Branch, R.A., Amphotericin B nephrotoxicity, *Drug Safety*, 5, 94, 1990.

Sanchez-Bernal, C., Vlitos, M., Cabezas, J.A., Price, R.G., Variation in the isoenzymes of *N*-acetyl-ß-D-glucosaminidase and protein excretion in amino-glycoside nephrotoxicity in the rat, *Cell Biochem. Function*, 9, 209, 1991.

Schardijn, G.H.C., Statius van Eps, L.W., Beta-2-microglobulin: its significance in the evaluation of renal function, *Kidney Int.*, 32, 635, 1987.

Schmidt, U., Guder, W.G., Sites of enzyme activity along the nephron, *Kidney Int.*, 9, 233, 1976.

Silver, A., Dawnay, A., Landon, J., Cattell, W.R., Immunoassays for low concentrations of albumin in urine, *Clin. Chem.*, 32, 1303, 1986.

Skinner, R., Pearson, A.D., Coulthard, M.G., et al., Assessment of chemotherapy-associated nephrotoxicity in children with cancer, *Cancer Chemother. Pharmacol.*, 28, 81, 1991.

Stonard, M.D., Proteins, enzymes and cells in urine as indicators of the site of renal damage, in *Nephrotoxicity in the Experimental and Clinical Situation* (Part 2), Bach, P.H. and Lock, E.A., Eds., Martinus Nijhoff, Lancaster, 1987, 563.

Topping, M.D., Forster, H.W., Dolman, C., Luczynska, C.M., Bernard, A.M., Measurement of urinary retinol-binding protein by enzyme-linked immunosorbent assay, and its application to detection of tubular proteinuria, *Clin. Chem.*, 32, 1863, 1986.

Tucker, S.M., Boyd, P.J.R., Thompson, A.E., Price, R.G., Automated assay of *N*-acetyl-beta-glucosaminidase in normal and pathological urine, *Clin. Chim. Acta*, 62, 333, 1975.

Walker, R.J., Duggin, G.G., Drug Nephrotoxicity, *Annu. Rev. Pharmacol. Toxicol.*, 28, 331, 1988.

Warrington, S.J., Dawnay, A., Johnston, A., Saul, S., Turner, P., Ferber, H.P., Chlortenoxicam and renal function of normal human volunteers, *Hum. Toxicol.*, 8, 53, 1989.

Warrington, S.J., Lewis, Y., Dawnay, A. et al., Renal and gastrointestinal tolerability of lornoxicam, and effects on haemostasis and hepatic microsomal oxidation, *Postgrad. Med. J.*, 66(Suppl.4), S35, 1990.

Warrington, S.J., Ravic, M., Dawnay, A., Renal and general tolerability of repeated doses of nimesulide in normal subjects, *Drugs*, 46(Suppl.1), 263, 1993.

Watts, G.F., Bennett, J.F., Rowe, D.J., Morris, R.W., Gatling, W., Shaw, K.M., Polak, A., Assessment of immunochemical methods for determining low concentrations of albumin in urine, *Clin. Chem.*, 32, 1544, 1986.

Weise, M., Prufer, D., Jaques, G., Keller, M., Mondorf, A.W., Beta-2-microglobulin and other proteins as parameter for tubular function, *Contr. Nephrol.*, 24, 88, 1981.

Wibell, L., Karlsson, A., Urinary excretion of beta-2-microglobulin after the induction of a diuresis, *Nephron*, 17, 343, 1976.

Wilkie, M.E., Beer, J.C., Raftery, M.J., Dawnay, A., Barton, C., Marsh, F.P., Effect of nifedipine on renal haemodynamics and urinary protein excretion in stable renal transplant recipients, *Transplant. Proc.*, 25, 612, 1993.

Yu, H., Yanagisawa, Y., Forbes, M.A., Cooper, E.H., Crockson, R.A., Alpha-1-microglobulin: an indicator protein for renal tubular function, *J. Clin. Pathol.*, 36, 253, 1983.

Yuen, C.T., Kind, P.R.N., Price, R.G., Praill, P.F.G., Richardson, S.C., Colorimetric assay for *N*-acetyl-beta-D-glucosaminidase (NAG) in pathological urine using the w-nitrostyryl substrate: the development of a kit and the comparison of manual procedure with the automated fluorimetric method, *Ann. Clin. Biochem.*, 21, 295, 1984.

Part X. Assessment of Drug Activity in the Skin

Chapter 32

Measurement of Skin Response to Drugs

Sam Shuster, P. M. Farr, and C. M. Lawrence

CONTENTS

1 Introduction ... 438
2 Skin Structures, Functions, and Constituents ... 438
 2.1 Epidermal Cell Replication ... 438
 2.2 Stratum Corneum ... 438
  2.2.1 Structural ... 438
  2.2.2 Functional ... 438
 2.3 Skin Constituents ... 439
  2.3.1 Direct Analysis ... 439
  2.3.2 Tissue Fluids ... 439
 2.4 Skin and Lesion Thickness ... 439
  2.4.1 Harpenden Skinfold Caliper ... 439
  2.4.2 Radiographic Method ... 439
  2.4.3 Ultrasound ... 439
  2.4.4 Histology ... 439
 2.5 Physical Properties of Dermis ... 439
 2.6 Blood Vessels ... 440
  2.6.1 Visual Grading ... 440
  2.6.2 Color Comparison Charters and Optical Filters ... 440
  2.6.3 Reflectance Spectrophotometry ... 440
 2.7 Hair ... 440
 2.8 Nail ... 440
 2.9 The Sebaceous Gland ... 441
 2.10 Sweat Gland Function ... 441
 2.11 Skin Sensation ... 441
  2.11.1 Pain ... 441
  2.11.2 Itch ... 441
  2.11.3 Self-Image ... 441
3 Specific Diseases and Drugs ... 441
 3.1 Psoriasis ... 441
  3.1.1 Clinical Assessment ... 441
  3.1.2 Objective Measurements ... 442
 3.2 Adolescent Acne ... 442
  3.2.1 Clinical Response ... 442
  3.2.2 Measurement of Sebum Excretion Rate ... 442
 3.3 Dermatitis and Eczema ... 442
 3.4 Corticosteroids ... 442
  3.4.1 Potency ... 442
  3.4.2 Atrophy ... 442
 3.5 Other Drugs ... 442
4 The Response of Inflammation to Therapy ... 442
 4.1 Ultraviolet Erythema ... 443
  4.1.1 Minimal Erythema Dose ... 443
  4.1.2 Erythema Dose-Response Curves ... 443
 4.2 Wheal Reactions ... 443
  4.2.1 Measurement of Wheals ... 443
  4.2.2 Dermographic Whealing ... 443

0-8493-9230-6/97/$0.00+$.50
© 1997 by CRC Press, Inc.

4.3 Irritant Inflammation.......443
4.4 Immune Reactions.......443
4.4.1 The Immediate (Antigen-IGE) Response.......443
4.4.2 The Delayed (Lymphocyte-Born) Response.......443
Acknowledgment.......444
References.......444

Be grateful to the eye that it may see all, but be devoted to the mind that it may understand all.
De Selby

1 INTRODUCTION

The increasing use of drugs for the treatment of skin disease has exposed the poverty of traditional visual methods for assessing therapeutic response. The wider employment of good clinical trial practice has of course helped, but however good the design, the limits of detection are dictated by sensitivity of the measures of response. There are a number of objective methods available which could be more generally used, as well as several which would be better avoided. In this chapter we give a brief account of some of the more important methods and their uses and limitations. Our problem in presenting this briefly is the very nature of skin as an organ, the bland appearance of which conceals a riot of different tissues and functions. Thus our account will mostly be a series of discrete structural and functional attributes which are affected by drugs, with a few examples of the response of specific reactions which can, to some extent, be used as models of disease. For a fuller account see Greaves and Shuster (1989).

2 SKIN STRUCTURES, FUNCTIONS, AND CONSTITUENTS

2.1 Epidermal Cell Replication

Some indication can be obtained by the time to disappearance of dye applied to the stratum corneum (Baker and Blair, 1968; Roberts and Marks, 1980), but the method has never been properly validated and there are problems of avidity, penetration, and loss. Great differences are seen likewise with the various methods for measuring cell cycle events, and the mitotic index is too variable for reliability (Dover and Wright, 1989). The stathmokinetic method measures the birth rate of cells, by counting mitoses in sequential biopsies at timed intervals after the local injection of vinblastine, to ensure mitotic arrest (Duffill et al., 1976, 1977); it is very time-consuming, but it is doubtful that the other less rigorous procedures are worth doing. As with the proverbial peasant's reply, when the route to a particular destination is difficult, it is probably better to aim for somewhere else.

2.2 Stratum Corneum

2.2.1 Structural

The number and size of scales can be measured, and their ease of removal gives a measure of adhesion (Nicholls and Marks, 1977; Roberts and Marks, 1980). The surface pattern of scale can be studied by a skin-surface recording device or photography, but numerical analysis is complex. These methods are now well established but are little used in the study of drug action.

2.2.2 Function

The simplest way to study the stratum corneum barrier function is by measuring evaporative loss of water. With such methods, the magnitude of water loss is dependent on rate of flow of the collecting gas (Johnson and Shuster, 1969a); a simpler, if less informative, method uses an electrical sensing device (the Servomed Evaporimeter) to measure water vapor pressure differences, on and above the skin surface (Blichmann and Serup, 1987). Percutaneous absorption is studied *in vivo* by measurement of drug, or metabolites or a radiolabeled tracer in the blood, urine or feces, but analysis of concentration in successive cellophane-tape stripped layers of stratum corneum provides an interesting and simple way of predicting steady-state absorption (Tojo and Lee, 1989).

2.3 Skin Constituents

2.3.1 Direct Analysis

Changes in a variety of skin constituents have been measured as an index of drug action and it has proved important (1) to dissociate epidermis from dermis because of their grossly different composition and (2) to use an appropriate unit of reference. In the epidermis this is usually DNA; in the dermis, the simplest unit is surface area using a rotary punch biopsy (Shuster and Bottoms, 1963). The importance of the point of reference first became apparent when the effect was studied of aging and corticosteroids on skin collagen (Shuster and Bottoms, 1963; Shuster et al., 1967) and serious errors of interpretation were made until collagen content was related to skin surface area and not unit mass (see below and Kohn and Schnider, 1989). The former is an absolute quantity per unit of skin, the latter relative to the base unit chosen.

2.3.2 Tissue Fluids

Needle perfusion of the skin is neither pleasant nor entirely satisfactory, and suction blisters are preferred (Kistala, 1968) for analysis of tissue constituents and the kinetics of drugs in the skin.

2.4 Skin and Lesion Thickness

Measurement of skin and lesion thickness is a simple and important method of studying the cutaneous response to drugs. The normal epidermis contributes only about 5% and variation in skin thickness with site, age, and sex is due principally to differences in the dermal collagen layer (Shuster et al., 1975).

2.4.1 Harpenden Skinfold Caliper

The Harpenden skinfold caliper was designed to measure subcutaneous fat (Tanner and Whitehouse, 1955) but can be used to measure skin thickness at sites where the skin can be picked up separately from the underlying tissue. The caliper gives a resolution of 0.1 mm and measurements are reproducible with little observer bias (Lawrence and Shuster, 1985a; Cook and Shuster, 1980); it has been used to measure normal and atrophic skin (McConkey et al., 1963), skin lesions, and the response to inflammation and drugs (Marsden et al., 1983; Moss et al., 1981; Friedmann et al., 1983; Lawrence and Shuster, 1985b, 1987). It is inexpensive, portable, easy to use, and robust, but it can only be used where a fold of skin can be lifted separate from the underlying fat (Lawrence and Shuster, 1985a).

2.4.2 Radiographic Method

This was first described by Meema et al., (1964). An X-ray beam is directed tangentially through skin flattened by a wooden block, using metal plates to facilitate focusing and alignment (Black, 1969). Skin thickness is measured from the radiographic image. The technique has been used in endocrine disease and to measure corticosteroid induced dermal thinning (Black et al., 1973; Tan et al, 1982). Disadvantages are the use of ionizing radiation, the large fixed equipment, and the limitation to certain skin sites.

2.4.3 Ultrasound

See Alexander and Miller (1979) and Kirsch et al., (1984) for reviews. A transducer, offset from the skin by a water bath, detects the pulse transit time, oscillograph peaks representing the water-skin, dermis-fat, and fat-muscle interfaces. Skin thickness is calculated from the distance between the first and second peaks using a constant for the speed of sound in skin (Tan et al., 1982). Ultrasound is used to measure normal and atrophic skin thickness, but tends to underestimate it somewhat (Tan et al., 1982; Lawrence and Shuster, 1985a). The equipment is portable and the method is quick and harmless and can be used at any skin site, but it gives poor results in inflamed skin (Lawrence and Shuster, 1985a) because it fails to detect the lower limit of the dermis and because inflammation may extend beyond that interface.

2.4.4 Histology

Histology has a limited use because it is invasive, and because of distortion by elastic recoil of the tissue after removal and subsequent shrinkage during fixation (Dykes and Marks, 1977; Tan et al., 1982).

2.5 Physical Properties of Dermis

A variety of devices are now available to measure the extensile response to a linear, shear, rotational or suctional force, and can demonstrate the effects on connective tissue of drugs such as corticosteroids.

It is surprising that these methods have not been used more often in the study of drug action (see Cook, 1989 for review).

2.6 Blood Vessels

Increased skin blood flow is a feature of inflammatory dermatoses, and the response to ultraviolet radiation and chemical irritants. Measurement of vascular changes in skin may therefore be used to monitor disease severity, response to treatment, and, as in the case of topical corticosteroid-induced vasoconstriction (Barry and Woodford, 1977), as a bioassay of potency.

Cutaneous blood flow can be measured by thermal (Challoner, 1976) or radioactive isotope clearance (Tsuchida, 1979), but as the techniques are time-consuming, and the data produced can be difficult to interpret, they are not used much clinically. Laser Doppler flowmetry has been used increasingly (Tur et al., 1983; Farr and Diffey, 1986a). In this technique, a low-intensity laser beam of red light is shone onto the skin surface and the Doppler frequency shift of the remitted light is used to calculate the blood flux, a value related to the product of the number of red blood cells in the field of view and their average velocity (Nilsson et al., 1980); absolute flow cannot be calculated. By scanning the whole field change in total lesion flow can be measured (Speight et al., 1993).

Increased cutaneous blood flow is usually accompanied by dilatation of superficial vessels and several methods are used to quantify this (see Forrest and Williams, 1989).

2.6.1 Visual Grading

Small differences in erythemal intensity can be detected but the eye is poor at estimating their magnitude.

2.6.2 Color Comparison Charters and Optical Filters

The intensity of erythema can be graded using known color standards and although it is subjective, the method has advantages over visual grading because the eye performs well in the null system used in the matching of two colors. A series of filters with high transmittance for red light and decreasing transmittance for blue/green light has been used to quantify erythema by observing which of the filters just causes the erythema to disappear.

2.6.3 Reflectance Spectrophotometry

The methods are objective and quantitative. Hemoglobin in the vessels of the superficial dermis is the main cutaneous chromophore of green light. The consequent eduction in reflectance of green light re-emitted from inflamed skin has been used to quantify erythema (Farr and Diffey, 1985), and computer-controlled spectrophotometers allow reliable *in vivo* measurement of the spectral reflectance (Wan et al., 1983).

2.7 Hair

The effect of drugs on hair is complex and the main features to be measured are: (1) density (number/cm^2); (2) diameter (microscopy); (3) growth rate; (4) hair cycle; (5) color; and (6) physical properties.

Growth rate is measured after marking the hair, light hair with black dye and dark hair with bleach, and remeasuring after a timed period, the rate being 0.3-0.4 mm/day.

Hair cycle duration can usually be inferred by rate of hair growth and mean hair length and is the main determinant of the regional differences in hair appearance. Further information is obtained by examining plucked follicles; normally 5-15% of the scalp hairs are in the resting phase (anagen) and cytostatic drugs produce atrophic follicles.

Follicular analysis has developed in two main ways: (1) metabolic activity of the hair follicle can be measured in short-term incubation media and (2) follicular culture allows greater analysis of the effect of drugs (Sanders et al., 1994).

2.8 Nail

The rate of nail growth is about 0.1 mm/day and can easily be measured; it will, for example, demonstrate the effect of cytostatic drugs such as methotrexate (Dawber, 1970). The nail is marked with a file at the apex of the lunula, and the distance the scratch has traveled over a fixed period of time is measured from the proximal nailfold cuticle or the lunula; these two measurements should be the same. There is a small difference in rate of growth of the different finger nails and sequential measurements should therefore be done on the same fingers. With the new evidence that anychomysis can be cured by courses of antifungal drugs shorter than the time taken for diseased nail to grow out, it has become necessary to measure the movement of diseased nail as an index to the effect of antifungal drugs. This has been done as with the measurement of wheals (see below) but by using a soft lead pencil to mark the nail since the nail keratinocytes are not removed by cellophane tape (Munro, Rees and Shuster, 1992).

2.9 The Sebaceous Gland

The effect of drugs such as 13-*cis* retinoic acid and various hormones used for treatment of acne can be assayed by their effect on the sebaceous glands. The simplest method is to measure sebum output, most often on the forehead, over a timed period. The sebum is either collected onto absorbent paper and measured gravimetrically, or else onto ground glass and measured by light transmission. Gland function can also be studied by measuring sebaceous lipogenesis using ^{14}C glucose or acetate as substrate. This has been done in isolated glands, but it is simpler to measure total dermal lipogenesis and express in relationship to surface area (see Thody and Shuster, 1989a,b for a review of methods and the effect of drugs).

2.10 Sweat Gland Function

The effect of drugs on sweat rate or sweat constituents is best measured using chemically induced sweating either by intradermal injection of a cholinergic drug or more often by iontophoresis of 0.1% pilocarpine with 4 m for 5 min (see Johnson and Shuster, 1969b; Collins, 1989). Sweat is collected onto filter papers, in capsules stuck onto the skin or under plastic held in place with strapping, over a 15-20 min period and measured gravimetrically. Sweat, Na,K,Cl, and urea are the most frequently assayed constituents. Micropuncture of sweat glands has been used experimentally and short-term studies can also be made of glands removed from excised skin (Lee et al., 1984).

2.11 Skin Sensation

2.11.1 Pain

This is an uncommon manifestation of skin disease and is difficult to quantify (see Lynn,1989).

2.11.2 Itch

Itch can be measured subjectively by simple grading or by marking on a 10-cm scale. The most reproducible, and probably the best method, uses scratch as a measure of itch (Shuster, 1989). Scratch can be measured by needle electrodes or by amplifying discharges along nerve fibers, but is most easily measured by limb movement meters or by monitoring bed movement at night (Felix and Shuster, 1975). Both arm and leg movement are measured because itch-provoked scratch is done mostly by the arms, arm movement mostly being due to scratch whereas leg movement represents restlessness. Because of the variation from night to night, measurements are made over two consecutive nights.

2.11.3 Self-Image

The depressing effect of skin disease on self-image has been assessed subjectively by psychological questionnaires (Finlay et al., 1990) and objectively by psychometric methods (Shuster, 1981). Both methods have been used to measure the effect of treatment.

3 SPECIFIC DISEASES AND DRUGS

3.1 Psoriasis

3.1.1 Clinical Assessment

Erythema, scale palpability, and area of involvement are scored clinically. Area is seriously overestimated by most observers, e.g., using the rule of nines (Ramsay and Lawrence, 1989), especially for low areas of involvement (Tiling-Gross and Rees, 1993). The addition of the component scores to make a single overall score (as in the widely used PASI method; Fredrikson and Pettersson, 1978) is unacceptable as it presumes a numerically equivalent relationship of these components to response, and assumes a linear distribution of psoriasis extent between 0 and 100%, whereas in the majority of clinical studies most patients have less than 10% of body surface involved. Furthermore, as the PASI score has only one grade to represent up to 10% involvement changes below this value are not detected. Point counting of psoriasis lesions of a grid system may be a quick and effective method of assessing severity but has not been fully assessed (Bahmer, 1989).

3.1.2 Objective Measurements

Change in lesion thickness measured by calipers and transepidermal water loss correspond well to therapeutic response (Shuster et al., 1989) and allow calculation of a $T_{1/2}$ for plaque regression (Farr et al., 1987). There are no published studies of the use of X-ray and ultrasound techniques but our own (unpublished) evidence is that ultrasound gives variable and unsatisfactory recordings. Attempts to produce a computer image analysis system to measure the extent of psoriasis have not yet succeeded (Levell, 1994). Scanning laser-Doppler velocimetry can be used to measure area of individual plaques (Speight et al., 1993) and therapeutic response (Speight and Farr, 1994).

3.2 Adolescent Acne

Drugs act either by reducing the rate of sebum production or by antibiotic activity. Despite claims to the contrary, there is no evidence of a primary effect on duct keratinization or that duct blockage plays any part in the disease (Shuster, 1989).

3.2.1 Clinical Response

This is usually estimated by a global clinical grading or by separate grades for the different components of the disease in specific areas (Burke and Cunliffe, 1984). Less often individual lesions are counted, but it is not clear whether this offers much advantage over clinical grading. Antibiotic effect is usually studied by the clinical response.

3.2.2 Measurement of Sebum Excretion Rate

This is a simple assay of the effect of drugs which improve acne by a sebostatic effect (see Section 2.9).

3.3 Dermatitis and Eczema

This is the largest group of disease requiring study and one of the least susceptible to existing methods of measurement. The symptom of itch can be measured indirectly as scratch, but the extent and degree of dermatitis is still assessed by simple clinical grading, although lesion thickness, transepidermal water penetration, and skin blood flow could be used (see also Chapter 33).

3.4 Corticosteroids

3.4.1 Potency

The vasoconstrictor assay (Barry and Woodford, 1977) is still widely used to rank topical corticosteroids. This is surprising as the inhibitory effect on induced inflammation e.g., anthralin inflammation (Lawrence and Shuster, 1985b) or contact sensitivity (Friedmann et al., 1983) should give greater sensitivity.

3.4.2 Atrophy

Since the study of Black et al., (1973) skin thickness measurements have been widely used to assess collagen loss after corticosteroids. However, there are serious reservations because changes in skin thickness are only an indirect measure of dermal collagen content (Shuster et al., 1975). More importantly most studies of the atrophic potency of corticosteroids are concerned with the small changes which occur in the first weeks of treatment and there is no evidence that these changes are due to collagen loss. Thus, most of the published measurements of the "atrophic potency" of topical corticosteroids are of dubious relevance.

3.5 Other Drugs

Effects are usually assayed clinically on the disease process, occasionally on related models (e.g., histamine whealing and antihistamines, see below) or pharmacological properties (e.g., cytostatic drugs on nail growth).

4 THE RESPONSE OF INFLAMMATION TO THERAPY

There are few good models of skin disease, and of these the response to inflammatory agents and its modification by drugs is the most often used to study the effect of drugs. (For a review of the pharmacological agents associated with different types of inflammation see Greaves and Lawlor, 1989).

4.1 Ultraviolet Erythema

4.1.1 Minimal Erythema Dose

Adjacent areas of skin are exposed to geometrically increasing doses of radiation and the lowest dose required to achieve erythema is noted, usually at 24 h. The difficulty in judging this threshold point is compounded by the varying definitions, which range from a faint erythema (Epstein, 1962), to a uniform redness with sharp borders (Willis and Kligman, 1970). More importantly, the minimal erythema dose is a single point at the foot of the dose-response curve and cannot therefore characterize the biological event.

4.1.2 Erythema Dose-Response Curves

For these reasons full erythema dose-response curves are better than the frequently used minimal erythema dose. Reflectance measurements of erythema have allowed differences in the slope of the dose-response curve to be measured for different wavelengths of radiation (Farr and Diffey, 1985), and the erythemal action of drugs such as the photosensitizer 8-methoxypsoralen can be defined (Cox et al., 1989).

4.2 Wheal Reactions

4.2.1 Measurement of Wheals

The response to spontaneous whealing and to vasoactive agents such as histamine and its antagonists can be measured as wheal area, wheal thickness and calculated volume (Cook and Shuster, 1980). wheal area is measured at the time of maximum definition by transferring the inked outline on cellophane tape stripped stratum corneum, and computing the area on a digitizing pad (Humphreys and Shuster, 1987) or planimeter (Krause and Shuster, 1985b). Wheal thickness is measured by calipers and dose-response curves can be used to study the effect of disease and drugs. Rate constants of wheal formation and disappearance can also be used to analyze the effect of drugs and different whealing agents (Cook and Shuster, 1980; Humphreys et al., 1987).

4.2.2 Dermographic Whealing

A spring-loaded stylus is used to produce shear distortion as the stylus is moved across the skin, and wheal diameter is used to construct wheal force-response curves using a series of different forces. Site and skin frictional resistance are important (Krause and Shuster, 1985). The response to H_1 receptor antagonists can be demonstrated by a shift in the force-response curve and in dermographic threshold (Krause and Shuster, 1984, 1985a). The force-response characteristics have been recently reviewed and found to linearized by a computerized double-exponential plot using nonlinear regression (Sharpe and Shuster, 1994).

4.3 Irritant Inflammation

The effect of drugs can be studied by their action on inflammation induced by various chemicals, e.g., detergents (Berardesea and Maibach, 1988), weak acids, or anthralin. Although the response is measured as erythema, skin blood flow, edema, and transepidermal water loss, their mechanisms and response to drugs differs, and this can be used for therapeutic assay, e.g., the response to anthalin (Lawrence and Shuster, 1985b, 1986, 1987).

4.4 Immune Reactions

4.4.1 The Immediate (Antigen-IGE) Response

This is usually measured by the wheal and flare reaction to antigen introduced by pricking, but this is less satisfactory than intradermal injection which allows construction of dose-response curves and measurement of wheal kinetics (Humphreys et al., 1987). This response has been used to study the effect of antihistamines, corticosteroids, cromoglycates, cyclooxygenase inhibitors, cyclosporin and other agents. The delayed response to antigens such as house-dust mite which occurs in patients with atopy remains semi-quantitative, and dose-response curves have not yet been established.

4.4.2 The Delayed (Lymphocyte-Borne) Response

This is measured by sensitization, e.g., with dinitrochlorobenzene (DNCB; Moss et al., 1981). The capacity of a particular population to become sensitized is measured by using different sensitizing doses of the agent to be tested, and measuring the degree of sensitization 3-4 weeks later by the magnitude of the 48-h response to increasing concentrations of DNCB, measured as thickness by calipers (area does not change linearly with response). Erythema, blood flow, and transepidermal water loss have been used less extensively. These measurements have been used to study the effects of drugs such as corticosteroids and cyclosporin.

ACKNOWLEDGMENT

Professor Shuster gratefully acknowledges a Leverhulme Emeritus Fellowship.

REFERENCES

Alexander H and Miller DL (1979) Determining skin thickness with pulsed ultrasound. *J. Invest. Dermatol.* 72, 17-19.

Baker H and Blair CP (1968) Cell replacement in the stratum corneum in old age. *Br. J. Dermatol.* 80, 367-372.

Bahmer F (1989) The size of lesions or point counting as a step towards the solution of the PASI problem. *Arch. Dermatol.* 125, 1282-3.

Barry BW and Woodford R (1977) Vasoconstrictor activities and bioavailabilities of proprietary corticosteroids assessed using a non-occluded multiple dosage regimen. *Br. J. Dermatol.* 97, 555-560.

Berardesea A and Maibach HI (1988) Racial differences in sodium lauryl sulphate induced cutaneous irritation. *Contact Derm.* 18, 65-70.

Black MM (1969) A modified radiographic method of measuring skin thickness. *Br. J. Dermatol.* 81, 661-668.

Black MM, Shuster S and Bottoms E (1973) Skin collagen and thickness in Cushing's syndrome. *Arch. Dermatol. Forsch.* 246, 365-368.

Blichmann CW and Serup J (1987) Reproducibility and variability of transepidermal water loss measurement. Studies on the Servo Med evaporimeter. *Acta Derm. Venereol (Stockholm)* 678, 206-210.

Burke BM and Cunliffe WJ (1984) The assessment of acne vulgaris — the Leeds technique. *Br. J. Dermatol.* 111, 83-92.

Challoner AVJ (1976) Measurement of cutaneous blood flow by thermal, optical and radio-isotope methods. In: *Clinical Blood Flow Measurements.* Ed. JP Woodcock, Sector, London.

Collins KJ (1989) Measurement of sweating and sweat-gland function. *Pharmacology of the Skin Vol II, Handbook of Experimental Pharmacology Vol 87/II,* p. 19-22. Eds. Greaves MW and Shusters S, Springer-Verlag, Heidelberg.

Cook TH (1989) Mechanical properties of human skin. In: *Aging and the Skin.* Eds. Balin AK and Kligman AM, Raven Press, NY 205-225.

Cook LJ and Shuster S (1980) Histamine formation and absorption in man. *Br. J. Pharmacol.* 69, 579-586.

Cox NH, Farr PM and Diffey BL (1989) A comparison of the dose-response relationship for psoralen-UVA erythema and UVB erythema. *Arch Dermatol.* 125, 1653-7.

Dawber RPR (1970) The effect of methotrexate, corticosteroids and azathioprine on fingernail growth in psoriasis. *Br. J. Dermatol.* 83, 680-683.

Dover E and Wright NA (1989) Methods for the study of proliferation. *Pharmacology of the Skin Vol II, Handbook of Experimental Pharmacology* Vol 87/II, p. 3-11. Eds: Greaves MW and Shuster S, Springer-Verlag, Heidelberg.

Duffill M, Wright NA, and Shuster S (1976) The cell proliferation kinetics of psoriasis examined by three *in vivo* techniques. *Br. J. Dermatol.* 94, 355-362.

Duffill M, Appleton D, Dyson P, Shuster S, and Wright NA (1977) The measurement of cell cycle time in squamous epithelium using the metaphase arrest technique with vincristine. *Br. J. Dermatol.* 96, 493-502.

Dykes RJ and Marks R (1977) Measurement of skin thickness; a comparison of *in vivo* techniques and conventional histometric methods. *J Invest Dermatol.* 69, 275-278.

Epstein JH (1962) Polymorphous light eruptions. Wavelength dependency and energy studies. *Arch. Dermatol.* 85, 82-88.

Farr PM and Diffey BL (1985) The erythemal response of human skin to ultraviolet radiation. *Br. J. Dermatol.* 113, 65-76.

Farr PM and Diffey BL (1986a) The vascular response of human skin to ultraviolet radiation. *Photochem. Photobiol.* 44, 501-507.

Farr PM and Diffey BL (1986b) A quantitative study of the effect of topical endomethacin on cutaneous erythema induced by UVB and UVC erythema. *Br. J. Dermatol.* 115, 453-490.

Farr PM, Diffey BL and Marks JM (1987) Phototherapy and dithranol treatment of psoriasis: new lamps for old. *Br. Med. J.* 294, 205-207.

Felix and Shuster S (1975) A new method for the measurement of itch and the response to treatment. *Br. J. Dermatol.* 93, 303-312.

Finlay AY, Khan GK, Luscombe DK and Salek MS (1990) Validation of sickness impact profile and psoriasis disability index in psoriasis. *Br. J. Dermatol.* 123, 751-756.

Forrest MJ and Williams TJ (1989) Blood flow — including microcirculation. In: *Handbook of Experimental Pharmacology Vol I.* Eds: Greaves MW and Shuster S, Springer-Verlag, Heidelberg, 117-124.

Friedmann PS, Moss C, Shuster S, and Simpson JM (1983) Quantitative relationships between sensitising dose of DNCB and reactivity in normal subjects. *Clin. Exp. Immunol.* 53, 709-715.

Friedrickson T and Pettersson N (1978) Severe psoriasis - oral therapy with a new retinoid. *Dermatologica.* 157, 238-244.

Greaves MW and Lawlor F (1989) Specific acute inflammatory responses. In *Handbook of Experimental Pharmacology Vol I,* Eds: Greaves MW and Shuster S, Springer-Verlag, Heidelberg, 479-490.

Greaves MW and Shuster S (1989) *Pharmacology of the Skin Vol I and II, Handbook of Experimental Pharmacology* Vol 87, I and II. Springer-Verlag, Heidelberg.

Humphreys F and Shuster S (1987) The effect of nedocromil on wheal reactions in human skin. *Br. J. Clin. Pharmacol.* 24, 405-408.

Humphreys F, Krause LB, and Shuster S (1987) The effects of astemizole and indomethacin on wheal and flare reactions to histamine 48/80 and house dust mite antigen. *Br. J. Dermatol.* 116, 435.

Johnson C and Shuster S (1969a) The measurement of transepidermal water loss. *Br. J. Dermatol.* 81 Suppl. 4, 40-45.

Johnson C and Shuster S (1969b) Eccrine sweating in psoriasis. *Br. J. Dermatol.* 81, 119-124.

Kirsch JM, Hanson ME and Gibson JR (1984) The determination of skin thickness using conventional diagnostic ultrasound equipment. *Clin. Exp. Dermatol.* 9, 280-285.

Kistala W (1968) Suction blister device for separation of viable epidermis from dermis. *J. Invest. Dermatol.* 50, 128-137.

Kohn RR and Schnider SL (1989) Collagen changes in aging skin. p. 131-132, in *Aging and the Skin.* Ed. Balin AK and Kligman AM, Raven Press, NY.

Krause LB and Shuster S (1984) The effect of terfenadine on dermographic whealing. *Br. J. Dermatol.* 110, 73-80.

Krause LB and Shuster S (1985a) A comparison of astemizole and chlorpheniramine in dermographic urticaria. *Br. J. Dermatol.* 112, 447-453.

Krause LB and Shuster S (1985b) Enhanced wheal and flare response to histamine in chronic idiopathic urticaria. *Br. J. Clin. Pharmacol.* 20, 486-488.

Lawrence CM and Shuster S (1985a) Comparison of ultrasound and caliper measurement of normal and inflamed skin thickness. *Br. J. Dermatol.* 112, 195-200.

Lawrence CM and Shuster S (1985b) Mechanism of anthralin inflammation: 1. Dissociation of response to clobetasol and indomethacin. *Br. J. Dermatol.* 113, 107-115.

Lawrence CM, Howel D and Shuster S (1986) Site variations in anthralin inflammation on forearm skin. *Br. J. Dermatol.* 114, 609-613.

Lawrence CM and Shuster S (1987) Effect of arachidonic acid on anthralin inflammation. *Br. J. Clin. Pharmacol.* 24, 125-131.

Lee CM, Jones CJ and Keeley T (1984) Biochemical and ultrastructural studies of human eccrine sweat glands isolated by shearing and maintained for seven days. *J. Cell Sci.* 72, 259.

Levell NJ (1994) Assessment of the validity of computerised image analysis techniques to measure psoriasis extent. M.D. Thesis, University of Manchester.

Lynn B (1989) Structure, function and control: afferent nerve endings in the skin. In: *Handbook of Experimental Pharmacology Vol I.* Eds: Greaves MW and Shuster S, Springer-Verlag, Heidelberg, 117-124.

Marsden JR, Coburn PR, Marks JM, and Shuster S (1983) Measurement of the response of psoriasis to short term application of anthralin. *Br. J. Dermatol.* 109, 209-218.

McConkey B, Fraser GM, Bligh AS, and Whiteley H (1963) Transparent skin and osteoporosis. *Lancet* i, 693-695.

Meema HE, Sheppard RH and Rappoport A (1964) Roentgenographic visualisation and measurement of skin thickness and its diagnostic application in acromegaly. *Radiology* 82, 411.

Moss et al., (1981) Impaired contact hypersensitivity in untreated psoriasis and the effects of photochemotherapy and dithranol/UV-B. *Br. J. Dermatol.* 105, 503-508.

Munro CS, Rees JL and Shuster S. (1992) The unexpectedly rapid response of fungal nail infection and short duration therapy. *Acta. Derm. Venerol. (Stockholm)* 131-133.

Nicholls S and Marks R (1977) Novel techniques for the estimation of intracorneal adhesion *in vivo. Br. J. Dermatol.* 96, 595-602.

Nilsson GE, Tenland T, and Oberg PA (1980) Evaluation of a laser Doppler flowmeter for measurement of tissue blood flow. IEEE Transactions on Biomedical Engineering, BME-27, 597-604.

Ramsay B and Lawrence CM (1989) Comparison of subjective and objective methods of assessment of psoriasis plaque area. *Br. J. Dermatol.* in press.

Roberts D and Marks R (1980) The determination of regional and age variations in the rate of desquamation: a comparison of four techniques. *J. Invest. Dermatol.* 74, 13-16.

Sanders DA, Philpott MP, Nicolle FV and Kealey T (1994) The isolation and maintenance of the human pilosebaceous unit. *Br. J. Dermatol.* 131, 166-176.

Sharpe GR and Shuster S (1994) Characterisation and analysis of skin whealing by computerised nonlinear regression. *Br. J. Dermatol.* 131, 78-84.

Shuster S (1989) The blocked duct and the dying mythology of acne. In: *Acne & Related Disorders.* p. 81-86. Eds. Marks R and Plewing G.

Shuster S (1981) Reason and the rash. *Proc. R. Inst. Great Br.* 53, 136-163.

Shuster S, Black MN, and MacVitie E (1975) The influence of age and sex on skin thickness, skin collagen and density. *Br. J. Dermatol.* 93, 639-643.

Shuster S and Bottoms E (1963) Senile degeneration of skin collagen. *Clin. Sci.* 25, 487-491.

Shuster S, Rawlins MD, Rogers S, Chadirk W, Marks JM, and Comaish S (1980) Objective comparison of the response of psoriasis to treatment with PUVA and dithranol. *Proceedings of First World Conference on Clinical Pharmacology and Therapeutics.* Ed: Paul Turner. Macmillan, London, pp. 421-423.

Shuster S, Raffle EJ, and Bottoms E (1967) Skin collagen in rheumatoid arthritis and the effects of corticosteroids. *Lancet* i, 525-527.

Speight EL, Essex TJH and Farr PM (1993) The study of plaques of psoriasis using a scanning laser Doppler velocimeter. *Br. J. Dermatol.* 128, 519-24.

Speight EL and Farr PM (1994) Calcipotriol improves the response of psoriasis to PUVA. *Br. J. Dermatol.* 130, 79-82.

Tan CY, Marks R and Payne P (1981) Comparison of xeroradiographic and ultrasound detection of corticosteroid induced dermal thinning. *J. Invest. Dermatol.* 76, 657-667.

Tan CY, Statham B, Marks R and Payne PA (1982) Skin thickness measurement by pulsed ultrasound: its reproducibility, validation and variability. *Br. J. Dermatol.* 106, 657-667.

Tanner JM and Whitehouse RH (1955) The Harpenden skinfold caliper. *Am. J. Phys. Anthropol.* 13, 743-746.

Thody AJ and Shuster S (1989a) Control and function of sebaceous glands. *Physiol. Rev.* (1989) 69, 383-416.

Thody AJ and Shuster S (1989b) The sebaceous glands. *Pharmacology of the Skin I. Handbook of Experimental Pharmacology Vol 87/I.* Eds: Greaves and Shuster, Springer-Verlag, Heidelberg, 233-246.

Tiling-Gross S and Rees J (1993) Assessment of area of involvement in skin disease: a study using schematic figure outlines. *Br. J. Dermatol.* 128, 69-74.

Tojo K and Lee ARC (1989) A method for predicting steady-state rate of skin penetration *in vivo*. *J. Invest. Dermatol.* 92, 105-108.

Tsuchida Y (1979) Rate of skin blood flow in various regions of the body. *Plast. Reconstr. Surg.* 64, 505-508.

Tur E et al., (1983) Basal perfusion of the cutaneous microcirculation: measurement as a function of anatomic position. *J. Invest. Dermatol.* 81, 442-446.

Wan S, Parrish JA, Jaenicke KF (1983) Quantitative evaluation of ultraviolet induced erythema. *Photochem. Photobiol.* 37, 643-648.

Willis I and Kligman AM (1970) Aminobenzoic acid and its esters. *Arch. Dermatol.* 102, 405-417.

Chapter 33

Drugs for Eczema

John R. Gibson and Vasant K. Manna

CONTENTS

1 Introduction 447
2 Targeting Drugs in Eczema 448
3 The Evaluation of Drugs for Eczema 448
  3.1 The Population to be Studied 453
  3.2 The Model/Eczema Subtype to Study and the Experimental Design 453
  3.3 What to Measure and How to Measure It 455
4 Conclusions 456
References 456

1 INTRODUCTION

The majority of drugs used in dermatology (e.g., corticosteroids, antibiotics) were not initially developed for the skin but are spinoffs from drug development in other fields. The concept of developing an agent specifically for the treatment of eczema remains somewhat underworked. Thus, the approach that has been taken here is to present a brief overview of the issues which need to be considered rather than a finely detailed commentary on research methodologies. The latter would be premature in the case of drug development for eczema, in view of the unresolved aspects in the pathogenesis of the disease and the relatively unrefined status of most volunteer models that could be relevant to the drug development process. However, a range of measurement techniques that may be applicable to eczema research are mentioned and referenced below and are described in detail in Chapter 32. A selection of volunteer models is also briefly presented and commented upon. The major aim is to provide the reader with an overall plan for the drug development process in eczema and to stimulate him/her to further develop the range of available techniques and models in a critical and logical manner, thus helping to bring dermatopharmacology into line with the more advanced areas of drug research and development. It is hoped that, in the future, problem-oriented drug development for skin diseases will result in the production of a new generation of agents with optimized dermatological benefits.

Before considering the process of human drug evaluation in eczema, it is important to clarify a few basic issues such as the definition of the disease and the possible targets for therapeutic intervention. These points will be briefly dealt with in the first two sections of this chapter.

Although, in its stricter sense, dermatitis refers to any inflammation of the skin, it is commonly used interchangeably with eczema to denote a pruritic, papulovesicular or lichenified condition occurring as a result of the interaction of the skin with a variety of endogenous and/or exogenous factors.[1] For the purpose of this chapter these terms will be used synonymously. Eczema occurs in acute, subacute, and chronic stages, each with a wide range of severity, with corresponding clinical and histological features. In addition, eczema embraces several distinct clinical subtypes (Table 1), each being associated with various predisposing and triggering factors. While it is easy to identify certain of these (e.g., a genetic predisposition in atopic eczema, a specific allergen or irritant in contact dermatitis), in other cases such associations may be unclear and/or controversial. Broadly speaking, however, it is likely that in many situations a given genetic background predisposes to the blend of immunological, pharmacological, and anatomical features needed to prime the subject to respond to triggering factors (internal and/or external) leading to a pathway of inflammatory events which initiate and interweave with a range of secondary reactions to create the spectrum of clinical features known as eczema.

0-8493-9230-6/97/$0.00+$.50
© 1997 by CRC Press, Inc.

Table 1 Examples of Eczema Subtypes

Atopic
Contact allergic
Contact irritant
Discoid/nummular
Infective
Pompholyx
Seborrheic
Venous stasis

2 TARGETING DRUGS IN ECZEMA

The currently available therapeutic armamentarium for eczema consists of:

1. Emollient applications and soap substitutes
2. Topical, and occasionally systemic, corticosteroids
3. Topical and systemic antimicrobial agents including antibiotics, antifungals, and antivirals
4. Systemic antihistamines
5. Sedatives and tranquilizers
6. Orally administered essential fatty acids, e.g., gamma-linolenic acid
7. Orally administered immunosuppressants such as azathioprine and cyclosporin
8. Psoralens plus ultraviolet light (PUVA)

Possible targets for new agents in eczema are outlined in Figure 1. It is clear that this diagram represents an over-simplification of highly complex interrelated events in the pathogenesis of the disease. One relatively straightforward example of this is the role of *Staphylococcus aureus* in both exacerbating atopic eczema via a series of inflammatory events, possibly based on an immunological trigger,[2] and in further complicating the process by causing frank secondary infection of the diseased skin.

There are several important, interrelated aspects to be considered when targeting drugs for eczema. They are

1. The specific pathophysiological process(es) to be modified and the optimum stage (timing) for intervention
2. The choice of a broad- vs. a narrow-spectrum approach
3. The route of administration for the agent (systemic or topical)

In addition, consideration needs to be given to whether the target represents a fundamental, primary event or a secondary complication.

At one end lies a broad-spectrum, systemically administered attack on inflammatory and/or immunological events occurring early in the pathogenesis of the disease. This approach is likely to strike one or more of the important targets and be highly effective, e.g., systemic corticosteroids, but may carry with it the risk of an unacceptable level of adverse effects. Conversely, a topically administered, specifically targeted, narrow-spectrum agent given after the onset of the disease is less likely to be highly effective in the full range of eczema subtypes and may miss several key targets, but has a greater chance of avoiding unwanted effects. The ideal drug is clearly one that could be used safely, effectively, and conveniently to intervene at the earliest possible stage in the disease process. When more than 10-20% of the surface area of the skin is involved, and particularly if the distribution of the disease is patchy, oral therapy may be the preferred mode of administration.

3 THE EVALUATION OF DRUGS FOR ECZEMA

When developing a drug for the treatment of "eczema," it is likely that the condition to be focused on will be that associated with the atopic state.[3] Indeed, from a therapeutic viewpoint, all the general headings for targets normally considered in the management of eczema are relevant to this form of the disease, although the exact details concerning pathogenesis may vary from one subtype of eczema to another. These headings include psychosomatic aspects, irritant, allergic and microbial triggers, immunological and inflammatory disturbances, and anatomical and microanatomical derangement.[4,5] However, it should be remembered that differences in pathogenesis may yield one approach to therapy a viable

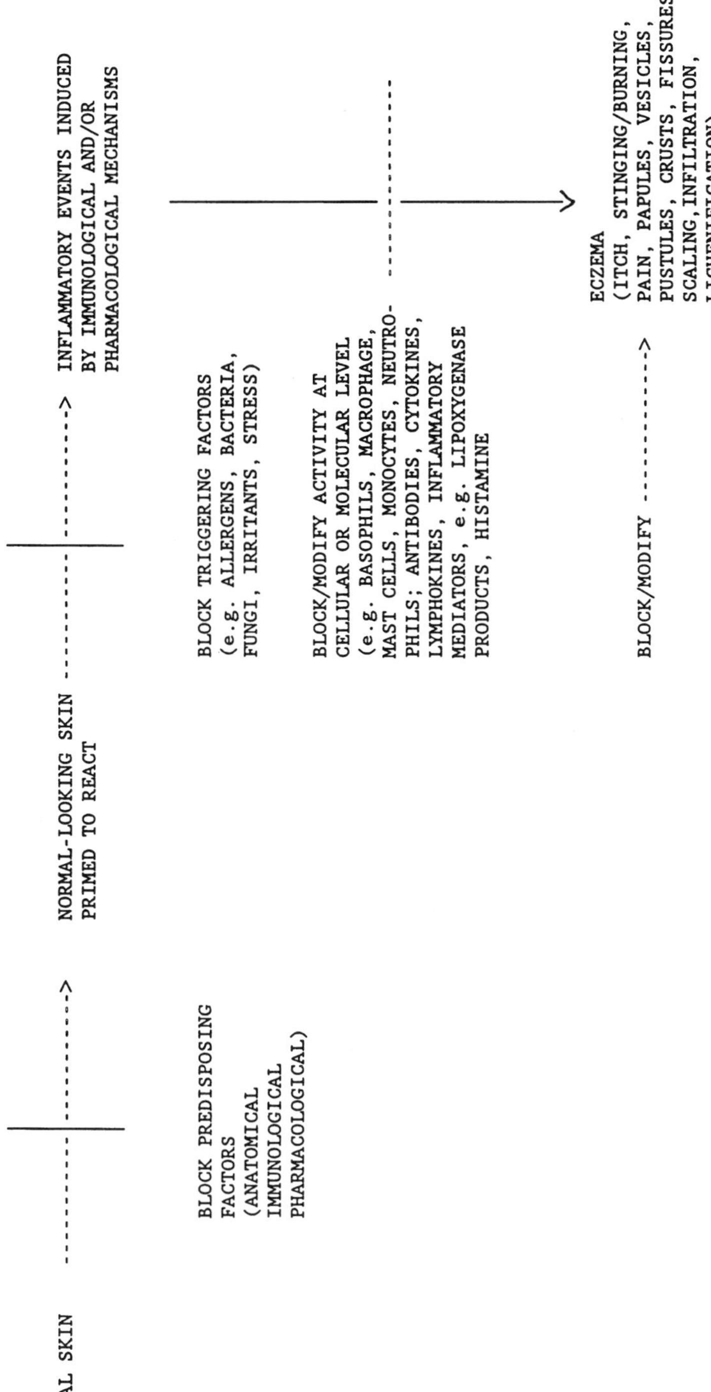

Figure 1 Drug targets in eczema.[1,4,5,73]

proposition in one eczema subtype, but not in another. Conversely, other approaches may be more broadly relevant. Compare, for example, the successful specific treatment of seborrheic dermatitis with an imidazole antifungal agent[6] vs. the use of topical corticosteroid therapy for all forms of eczema. Thus, it may be appropriate to evaluate drug effects in a range of eczema subtypes and the extent to which such exploration will be necessary in the early phases of clinical development will depend on the pharmacological profile of the agent and, in particular, the nature and specificity of its therapeutic attack. Data from such studies must be interpreted against a background of genuine understanding of important pathophysiological[4,5] and clinical[1,3] aspects of the various eczema subtypes and of exactly what one is trying to achieve.

With suitable modification and a creative, flexible approach, the general plan and specific techniques described below can be used, as appropriate, to evaluate all subtypes of eczema and the effects of all potentially useful drugs, no matter the proposed mechanism of action. Clearly some techniques will be more suitable than others in any given situation. It is appreciated that when applying a drug either topically or systemically for the treatment of skin diseases, it is important to gather information on all aspects of its effects in humans. However, for the purposes of this chapter, the focus will be on the skin. The depth to which early human exploratory work is taken will depend, in part, on what is known about the therapeutic class to which the test substance belongs. For example, in the case of a topical corticosteroid, the key questions would relate to speed and degree of efficacy vs. the risk of well-known adverse effects, e.g., skin thinning. On the other hand, the question asked of a drug based on an unproven concept would be: does it work? If so, is the mechanism of action that which was proposed? Did the agent perform as predicted pharmacodynamically at a molecular or cellular level and yet fail to benefit the disease process?

Essentially, what needs to be done in the early phase human evaluation of both topical and systemic agents is to:

1. Establish that the test substance has the potential to be effective in eczema
2. Define the optimal dosage regimen
3. Define the pharmacokinetic and pharmacodynamic profile of the drug in human skin, as well as systemically
4. Determine the likely relative efficacy of the agent vs. standard therapies, allowing preliminary judgments to be made regarding commercial viability
5. Estimate the risk/benefit profile of the agent

In the case of topical therapy, the vehicle and concentration of active agent in the formulation need to be optimized. These aims may appear logical and obvious, but it is surprising how often fundamental principles are ignored in dermatological drug development, e.g., failure to determine, at an early stage, optimal dosing regimens for topical corticosteroid therapy, failure to determine with reasonable precision the changes in corticosteroid concentration in a given vehicle needed to achieve definite changes in clinical efficacy.[7,8]

The early clinical development plans for both topical and systemic drugs are summarized in Figures 2 and 3. The exact timing of the "important associated activities" may vary from project to project, but attention should be paid to each of them at an appropriate time. It is worth recalling that some of the advantages of dermatological drug development are that clinical changes are readily visible and usually occur quickly, and, in the case of topical therapy especially over localized areas, the safety margin is generally good. In addition, the skin represents the ideal organ for exploring human tissue pharmacology in a relatively low-invasive manner and this should be exploited as fully as possible.[9]

With regard to drugs for topical application, it is sensible to gain some experience of use in normal human skin before proceeding to patients, due to the inflammatory nature of the eczema process and its propensity for exacerbation following irritation. This can be most simply done in normal human volunteers using an occlusive technique involving Finn chambers and a simple double-blind assessment evaluating epidermal and dermal changes ("dryness"/scaling, erythema, papules, vesiculation, infiltration/induration, erosion/ulceration) much like the method used in allergic contact dermatitis patch test clinics.[10,11] Alternatively, repeated application techniques with or without occlusion, can be used.[10] With regard to systemic drugs, "standard" phase I studies evaluating safety and general human pharmacology will be needed.

Table 2 details the established and potential uses of volunteer models and studies in patients. The backbone of the exercise is the treatment of patients with eczema to establish efficacy. However,

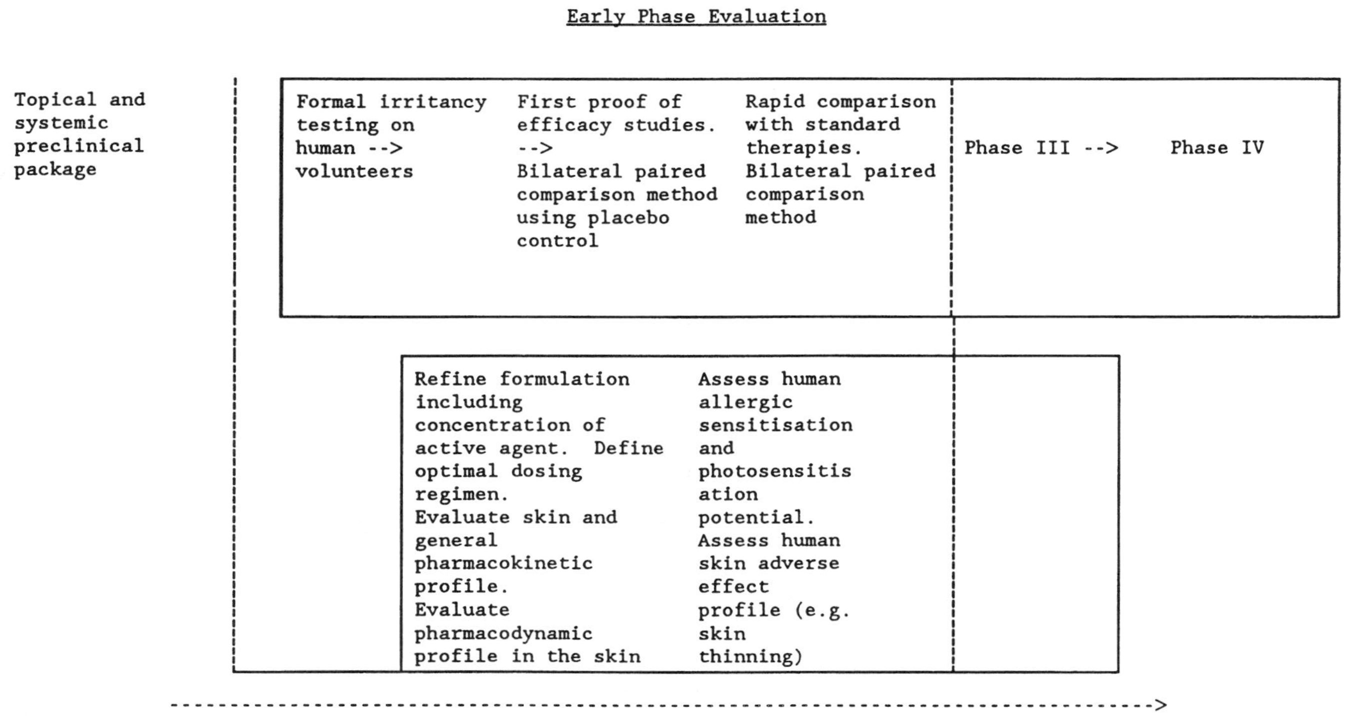

Early Phase Evaluation

Topical and systemic preclinical package

Formal irritancy testing on human --> volunteers

First proof of efficacy studies. --> Bilateral paired comparison method using placebo control

Rapid comparison with standard therapies. Bilateral paired comparison method

Phase III --> Phase IV

Refine formulation including concentration of active agent. Define optimal dosing regimen. Evaluate skin and general pharmacokinetic profile. Evaluate pharmacodynamic profile in the skin

Assess human allergic sensitisation and photosensitisation potential. Assess human skin adverse effect profile (e.g. skin thinning)

--->

Figure 2 The clinical development plan for topical eczema drugs: upper box, primary pathway; lower box, important associated activities.

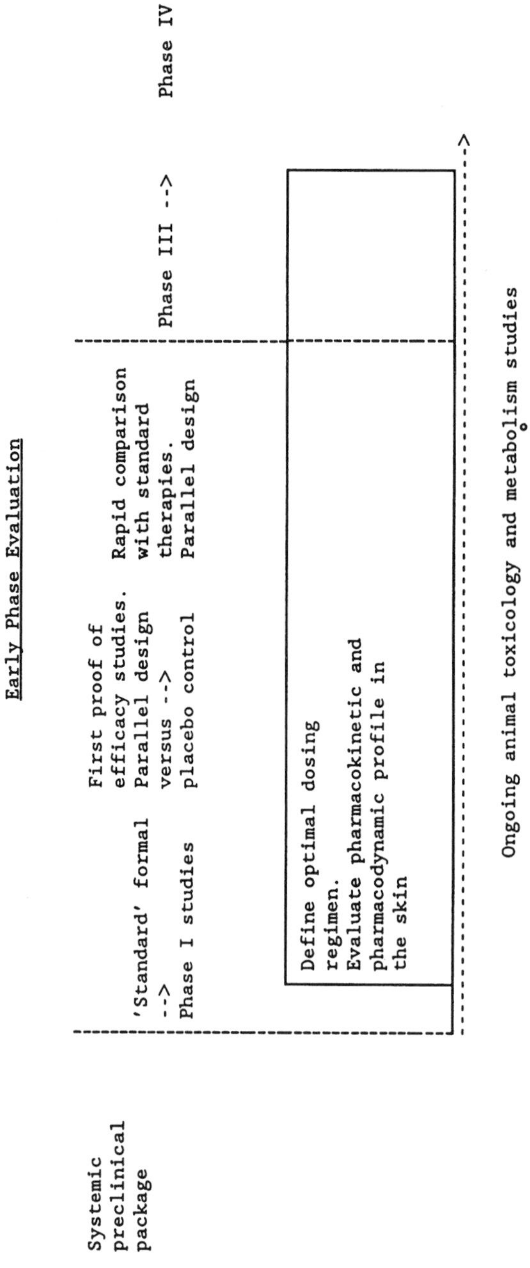

Early Phase Evaluation

Systemic preclinical package

'Standard' formal --> Phase I studies

First proof of efficacy studies. Parallel design versus --> placebo control

Rapid comparison with standard therapies. Parallel design

Phase III -->

Phase IV

Define optimal dosing regimen.
Evaluate pharmacokinetic and pharmacodynamic profile in the skin

Ongoing animal toxicology and metabolism studies

Figure 3 The clinical development plan for systemic eczema drugs.

Table 2 The Real and/or Potential Uses of Volunteer Models and Patient Studies

Volunteer Models	Patient Studies
Irritancy, allergenicity, photosensitizing, and skin thinning potential in normal skin[10,48-56]	Efficacy, safety and acceptability in various eczema subtypes[12,13]
Drug pharmacokinetics and pharmacodynamics in normal and experimentally challenged/damaged skin[8,14,16,21,43,47,58,59]	Drug pharmacokinetics and pharmacodynamics in diseased skin[57]
Refinement of topical formulation including concentration of active agent[8,14]	Refinement of topical formulation including concentration of active agent[7,8]
Definition of treatment regimen[15]	Definition of treatment regimen[60,61]

experimental volunteer models can be of value if they are used judiciously and if it is recognized that few, if any, of them have been fully refined and that in some instances their exact roles have yet to be unequivocally established.

The important issues in any given study in the early evaluation of eczema drugs are

1. The population to use — patients or volunteers?
2. The model/eczema subtype to study and the experimental design.
3. What to measure? Clinical symptoms and signs; pharmacological, immunological, and anatomical/structural parameters.
4. How to perform measurements?

The best overall assessment will most likely be obtained using data generated from creatively designed and rigorously conducted studies in both patients and volunteers. Some of the references given below relate to the evaluation of psoriasis as this disease tends to have been studied more extensively, and as some lessons learned from that field are relevant to eczema.

3.1 The Population to be Studied

The most fundamental question to be answered is: does the drug work in eczema? This obviously requires studies in patients. In assessing irritancy potential prior to use in eczema, one may choose to use healthy volunteers, volunteers with a "normal" skin but with a personal and/or family history of atopy, or the "normal" skin of patients with eczema. In practice, a screening study as discussed above in healthy volunteers should suffice, with the majority of data concerning irritancy being collected during the clinical phase of development.

3.2 The Model/Eczema Subtype to Study and the Experimental Design

Study design, with the possible exception of early dose determination work, should be double-blind and pay due regard to the need for proper controls, full randomization, and other statistically important considerations. Whenever possible, the bilateral, symmetrical, paired comparison method should be used as this reduces variability,[8,12,13] and utilizes the valuable resource of the study population in the most efficient manner, with the subject acting as his own control.[13] The theoretical objection that drug administered to one site may affect another is unlikely to be of practical significance (except in the case of antimicrobial therapy) if small amounts of drug are applied to limited areas of diseased/experimentally damaged skin.

Table 3 lists a range of models that could be considered in the evaluation and development of drugs for eczema. In many cases, further refinement would be needed to optimize their value. In some instances, e.g., presensitization and rechallenge with dinitrochlorobenzene (DNCB), the ethical status of the test system is open to question. For a variety of reasons, which include the lack of definitive knowledge concerning critical aspects of the pathogenesis of various eczema subtypes, it is most likely that the best use of models is not as a predictor of efficacy in eczema per se (that is best left to studies in patients), but rather as a set of methods for refining topical formulations[8,14] and dosing regimens[15] and for acquiring further knowledge of the agent's human dermatopharmacology.[16,17,18] Thus, if it has been established in a screening program that an agent has a "therapeutic" effect in a given human model system, it could be utilized for the purposes specified above with greater ease, efficiency, and accuracy than in a typical clinical trial setting due to the higher level of standardization and speed of subject recruitment possible when performing volunteer studies. Models need not be assumed to be mechanistically relevant to the eczema process in order to be of value, provided that they are shown to be relevant to the test agent in question. However, it is of great importance not to attempt extrapolation of results gained from model systems to the clinical situation until it has been unequivocally established that this is scientifically valid.

Table 3 Patient/Volunteer Models of Real and/or Potential Use

Challenge System/Inducer	Model Category
Dinitrochlorobenzene (DNCB)[62]	Eczema/dermatitis
Rhus[63]	Eczema/dermatitis
Sodium lauryl sulfate (SLS)[64]	Inflammation/dermatitis
Croton oil[65]	Inflammation
Dithranol[66,67]	Inflammation
Kerosene[65]	Inflammation
LTB_4[68]	Inflammation
Tetrahydrofurfuryl nicotinate[16]	Inflammation
UVB[69-71]	Inflammation
	Weal and flare mimicking
Intradermal antigen, compound 48/80,[18,21] histamine[17]	Type I allergy/inflammation
Skin stripping[20]	Epidermal disruption/inflammation/hyperemia
Intradermal histamine/trypsin[27,72]	Itch
Atopic eczema[30]	Itch
Topical corticosteroids[8,24,25]	Human vasoconstriction assay
Topical corticosteroids[7,34,42]	Skin thinning

The ideal model would be ethical, simple to use, reliable in response both to the challenge modality and the test therapies, noninvasive and nonscarring, reproducible, and clinically relevant. Of the models listed in Table 3, croton oil, tetrahydrofurfuryl nicotinate, sodium lauryl sulfate (SLS), and LTB_4 induced inflammation; adhesive tape stripping; weal and flare reactions following histamine, compound 48/80 and antigen challenge; the human vasoconstriction assay (for corticosteroids only); an itch assessment; and ultrasound for examining skin thinning would appear to represent a reasonable range of potentially useful methods. Rapid screening using small numbers of volunteers should be used to fine tune the choice of models used to assess any given agent. The four "inflammation" models simply represent a range of methods for inducing various types of inflammatory changes in the skin which may respond to certain anti-inflammatory agents. They would be considered when a novel agent with a suitable anti-inflammatory profile was being evaluated. They utilize a range of insults from both the chemical and biological ends of the spectrum.

Adhesive tape stripping may be used as an entity in itself to produce epidermal derangement[19] accompanied by hyperemia, as an adjunct to the human vasoconstriction assay for corticosteroid assessment,[20] and as a method for ensuring greater penetration of drug into skin challenged by various modalities.

Weal and flare reactions may be usefully employed in the evaluation of both systemic[21] and topical[18] agents with antihistamine effects, as well as those with an ability to modify mast cell[17,18] and/or basophil behavior. This model could readily be extended to assess drug effects on various other vasoactive substances besides histamine.[22,23]

The human vasoconstriction assay has been used with great success to screen topical corticosteroids for clinical activity,[25] for determining the bioavailability of corticosteroids from their vehicles,[47] and for predicting the relative clinical potencies of topical corticosteroid preparations.[7,8,24] An excellent review of this model has been prepared by Barry.[25] It is probably the most used and refined of all the methods outlined in Table 3, but unfortunately its use is currently limited to the evaluation of topical corticosteroids.

Volunteer models for the assessment of itching generally utilize intracutaneous injections of histamine or various proteases, e.g., trypsin, papain, or the epicutaneous application of cowhage extract.[26,27,28,72] Parameters which are usually measured are itch threshold, duration, and intensity.[26,72] It should be noted that the sensation induced by pruritogenic agents varies qualitatively depending on the depth to which the injection is given.[72] The role of available models of experimentally induced itch in predicting with accuracy that a drug will act as an antipruritic agent in eczema remains to be clarified.

Measurement of itching in patients may be performed by subjective evaluation with or without the added sophistication of the use of data loggers[29,30] or by limb meters[31,32] which evaluate scratching as a direct correlate of itching. Several important weaknesses have recently been stressed concerning the use of the latter method.[33] A simple, subjective evaluation currently appears to be the method of choice both in terms of practicality and clinical relevance.

For studies in patients, preference should be given in the early stages to evaluating subtypes of eczema which lend themselves to assessment by the bilateral paired comparison method. Thus atopic eczema, venous stasis eczema, and contact dermatitis would be appropriately selected in circumstances where a broad-spectrum, anti-inflammatory effect is anticipated.

3.3 What to Measure and How to Measure It

Techniques for evaluating drug effects on eczema and experimentally challenged skin are summarized in Table 4. These are described in detail in chapter 32. They may be usefully applied in a range of models and clinical conditions.

Table 4 Measurement Techniques of Real and/or Potential Value

Technique	Useful In
Blinded, carefully constructed, subjective scoring systems based on clinical symptoms and signs[8,13,24,34]	Patient studies and volunteer models
Measurement of area and/or volume[21]	Weal and flare studies
Laser Doppler velocimetry/flowmetry[74,76-79,84]	Volunteer models with a sufficient inflammatory component to increase skin blood flow, including weal and flare studies
Laser Doppler velocimetry/flowmetry[36]	Specially adapted forms of the human vasoconstriction assay
Measurement of transepidermal water loss (TEWL) by evaporimetry[19,37,82,83,85]	Patient studies and volunteer models which involve functional disturbance of the epidermis
Skin thickness determination, using calipers, ultrasound, or radiographically[39,41,75]	Volunteer studies to determine the skin-thinning potential of topical agents
Skin absorption of radiolabeled drug[43,44]	Studies to determine drug pharmacokinetics where the use of pharmacodynamic endpoints is not feasible
Suction blisters and skin windows[45,46,80,81]	Patient studies and volunteer models of eczema/inflammation to determine skin drug levels and effects at a molecular and cellular level

In all clinical and volunteer studies, characteristic symptoms and signs (e.g., itching, stinging/burning, pain, erythema, blanching, papules, vesicles, pustules, infiltration/induration, scaling) produced by the challenge modality or clinical condition, and modification of these by the test agent can be readily evaluated using carefully constructed scoring systems performed under blinded conditions.[13,34] The most important aspects of such evaluations are summarized in Table 5. Despite the subjective nature of these assessments, they remain of central importance in dermatological studies, they are surprisingly accurate and reproducible when performed by a trained, experienced investigator, and their value should not be underestimated. Suitable methods of eliciting the subject's opinion should be used to add to the database. Properly "educated" patients and volunteers often agree with the investigator's evaluation.

Measurement of the area of weals and flares produced by various intradermally injected challenge substances, e.g., histamine, is a simple, reliable, and reproducible method of objectively evaluating drug effects on these parameters[18,21] and has been extensively used to determine the time of onset, intensity, and duration of drug activity in man. The theoretically more appropriate measurement of weal volume is technically more difficult and does not add significantly to the usefulness of the data obtained.

Laser Doppler velocimetry/flowmetry is useful as an objective measure of cutaneous blood flow and has been utilized to study the pharmacodynamic response following application of topical vasodilators.[35] It may be used to provide objective data to supplement and expand upon subjective evaluation when

Table 5 Points to Consider in Performing Subjective Skin Evaluations

1. Experience and training is invaluable.
2. Use a double-blind, fully randomized study design with adequate controls.
3. Use the bilateral, paired comparison method or multiple lesions/challenge sites within the same subject where possible. This allows use of highly discriminating questions. Which side is better and to what degree (slightly better, better, very much better)? Or ranking of treatment effects.
4. Scoring systems for individual symptoms and signs should include the full range of possibilities, e.g., no response-intense response, using a 5 to 10 point scale with clinically meaningful and evenly separated spacing between descriptive terms. An overall "severity" score incorporating grouped signs should also be included.
5. Progress in the condition should be scored using a similarly constructed scale, e.g., very much worse-completely cleared.

assessing drug effects in skin inflammatory disease/models where the drug under test directly or indirectly has an effect on cutaneous blood flow. To date, it has been of no value in situations where blood flow is reduced below normal baseline values, e.g., corticosteroid-induced vasoconstriction.[36]

The measurement of transepidermal water loss (TEWL) by evaporimetry[37] provides a practical and objective method for determining the effect of treatment on the return to full functional integrity of the epidermis, particularly the stratum corneum. Normal functioning of the stratum corneum, as determined by its ability to restrict TEWL to a baseline level, may occur several days after the skin has returned to normal as judged by the naked eye.[38]

Several methods have been used to determine the thickness of skin. They include the use of calipers, histometric techniques, X-rays, and ultrasound.[39-42] Currently, with regard to dermatological drug development, the key purpose of such work is to determine the relative skin thinning effects of topical corticosteroid preparations and future competitors to such agents. This is probably best done using subjective assessment[34] and ultrasound.[7,41]

Methods involving the use of radiolabeled agents[43,44] to evaluate and/or predict the rate, depth, and degree of penetration of drugs into and through the skin are currently under development and may prove to be of value in the future evaluation of topically applied agents.

Suction blister[45] and skin window[46] techniques permit the sampling of biological fluids derived from the deeper epidermis/upper dermis and allow the determination of skin drug levels at or near the target site following systemic administration, as well as the study of the effects of drugs (topical and systemic) on mediators of inflammation and other parameters at a molecular or cellular level. For example, they could be used to verify whether an agent with a particular pharmacological profile, e.g., lipoxygenase blockade, does actually perform that role in human skin *in vivo*. However, due to a lack of hard pathophysiological data, such work would not necessarily accurately predict that the test agent would be effective in the treatment of eczema.

4 CONCLUSIONS

The key element in the early phase evaluation of drugs for eczema is proof of efficacy in a clinical setting as determined by the eyes and palpating fingers of a skilled clinician. However, much could be gained in terms of clarification of pathogenesis, definition of an agent's pharmacological profile, and refinement of dose and treatment schedules by more detailed study involving the use of a range of techniques in volunteer models and patients. Before this ideal can be attained, considerable work is still needed in refining, validating, and standardizing the currently available methods. Human skin has the supreme advantage of accessibility. The development of new purpose-orientated means by which dermatopharmacology may be advanced to a stage where the skin takes its place as an ideal organ for the study of human tissue pharmacology, must remain the goal of those who work in this field.

REFERENCES

1. Burton, J. L., Rook, A. and Wilkinson, D. S. Eczema, lichen simplex, erythroderma and prurigo. In: Rook, A., Wilkinson, D. S., Ebling, F. J. G., Champion, R. H. and Burton, J. L. (eds.), *Textbook of Dermatology Volume 1*, 4th edition, Blackwell Scientific Publications, Oxford, 367, 1986.

2. Dahl, M. V. *Staphylococcus aureus* and atopic dermatitis. *Arch. Dermatol.*, **119**, 840, 1983.
3. Champion, R. H. and Parish, W. E. Atopic dermatitis. In: Rook, A., Wilkinson, D. S., Ebling, F. J. G., Champion, R. H. and Burton, J. L. (eds.), *Textbook of Dermatology Volume 1*, 4th edition, Blackwell Scientific Publications, Oxford, 419, 1986.
4. Hanifin, J. M. Pharmacophysiology of atopic dermatitis. *Clin. Rev. Allergy*, **4**, 43, 1986.
5. Leung, D. Y. M. and Geha, R. S. Immunoregulatory abnormalities in atopic dermatitis. *Clin. Rev. Allergy*, **4**, 67, 1986.
6. Green, C. A., Farr, P. M. and Shuster, S. Treatment of seborrhoeic dermatitis with ketoconazole: II. Response of seborrhoeic dermatitis of the face, scalp and trunk to topical ketoconazole. *Br. J. Dermatol.*, **116**, 217, 1987.
7. Gibson, J. R., Kirsch, J. M., Darley, C. R., Harvey, S. G., Burke, C. A. and Hanson, M. E. An assessment of the relationship between vasoconstrictor assay findings, clinical efficacy and skin thinning effects of a variety of undiluted and diluted corticosteroid preparations. *Br. J. Dermatol.*, **111** (Suppl.27), 204, 1984.
8. Gibson, J. R., Hough, J. E., Marks, P. Webster A. Effect of concentration on the clinical potency of corticosteroid ointment formulations. In: Shroot, B. and Schaefer, H. (eds.), *Pharmacology and the Skin Volume 1*, Karger, Basel, 214, 1987.
9. Camp, R. D. R. and Greaves, M. W. Inflammatory mediators in the skin. *Br. Med. Bull.*, **43**, 401, 1987.
10. Bronaugh, R. L. and Maibach, H. I. Evaluation of skin irritation: correlations between animals and humans. In: Kligman, A. M. and Leyden, J. J. (eds.), *Safety and Efficacy of Topical Drugs and Cosmetics*, Grune & Stratton, New York, 51, 1982.
11. Wilkinson, J. D. and Rycroft, R. J. G. Contact dermatitis. In: Rook, A., Wilkinson, D. S., Ebling, F. J. G., Champion, R. H. and Burton, J. L. (eds.), *Textbook of Dermatology Volume 1*, 4th edition, Blackwell Scientific Publications, Oxford, 435, 1986.
12. Akers, W. A. Topical corticosteroids: proof of efficacy in skin diseases. In: Kligman, A. M. and Leyden, J. J. (eds.), *Safety and Efficacy of Topical Drugs and Cosmetics*, Grune & Stratton, New York, 1, 1982.
13. Allen, A. M. Design methodology in trials of topical drugs. In: Kligman, A. M. and Leyden, J. J. (eds.), *Safety and Efficacy of Topical Drugs and Cosmetics*, Grune & Stratton, New York, 25, 1982.
14. Malone, T., Haleblian, J. K., Poulsen, B. J. and Burdick, K. G. Development and evaluation of ointment and cream vehicles for a new topical steroid, fluclorolone acetonide. *Br. J. Dermatol.*, **90**, 187, 1974.
15. Woodford, R., Haigh, J. M. and Barry, B. W. Possible dosage regimens for topical steroids, assessed by vasoconstrictor assays using multiple applications. *Dermatologica*, **166**, 136, 1983.
16. Hensby, C. N., Maloubier, A., Civier, A. A., Shroot, B. and Ortonne, J. P. A model for studying the anti-prostaglandin activity of drugs in human skin. *Br. J. Dermatol.*, **111** (Suppl. 27), 147, 1984.
17. Stahle, M. and Hagermark, O. Effects of topically applied clobetasol-17-propionate on histamine release in human skin. *Acta Derm. Venereol.*, **64**, 239, 1984.
18. Gibson, J. R. Topically applied drugs in type I allergic reactions. In: Maibach, H. I. and Lowe, N. J. (eds.), *Models in Dermatology Volume 4*, Karger, Basel, 240, 1989.
19. Frodin, T. and Skogh, M. Measurement of transepidermal water loss using an evaporimeter to follow the restitution of the barrier layer of human epidermis after stripping the stratum corneum. *Acta Derm. Venereol.*, **64**, 537, 1984.
20. Wells, G. C. The effect of hydrocortisone on standardized skin-surface trauma. *Br. J. Dermatol.*, **69**, 11, 1957.
21. Fowle, A. S. E., Hughes, D. T. D. and Knight, G. J. The evaluation of histamine antagonists in man. *Eur. J. Clin. Pharmacol.*, **3**, 215, 1971.
22. Hagermark, O., Hokfelt, T. and Pernow, B. Flare and itch induced by substance P in human skin. *J. Invest. Dermatol.*, **71**, 233, 1978.
23. Soter, N. A., Lewis, R. A., Corey, E. J. and Austen, K. F. Local effects of synthetic leukotrienes (LTC_4, LTD_4, LTE_4 and LTB_4) in human skin. *J. Invest. Dermatol.*, **80**, 115, 1983.
24. Cornell, R. C. and Stoughton, R. B. Correlation of the vasoconstriction assay and clinical activity in psoriasis. *Arch. Dermatol.*, **121**, 63, 1985.
25. Barry, B. W. Dermatological formulations: percutaneous absorption. In: Swarbrick, J. (ed.), *Drugs and the Pharmaceutical Sciences Volume 18*, Marcel Dekker, Inc., New York, 264, 1983.
26. Hagermark, O. Influence of antihistamines, sedatives and aspirin on experimental itch. *Acta Derm. Venereol.*, **53**, 363, 1973.
27. Rajka, G. A method for evaluation of the influence on experimental itch of topically applied drugs. *Acta Derm. Venereol.*, **49**, 163, 1969.
28. Spilker, B. Clinical evaluation of topical antipruritics and antihistamines. In: Maibach, H.I. and Lowe, N.J., *Models in Dermatology Volume 3*, Karger, Basel, 55, 1987.
29. Doherty, V., Sylvester, D. G. H., Kennedy, C. T. C., Harvey, S. G., Calthrop, J. G., Gibson, J. R. Treatment of itching in atopic eczema with antihistamines with a low sedative profile. *Br. Med. J.*, **298**, 96, 1989.
30. Wahlgren, C.-F., Hagermark, O., Bergstrom, R. and Hedin, B. Evaluation of a new method of assessing pruritus and antipruritic drugs. *Skin Pharmacol.*, **1**, 3, 1988.
31. Krause, L. and Shuster, S. Mechanism of action of antipruritic drugs. *Br. Med. J.*, **287**, 1199, 1983.
32. Savin, J. A., Dow, R., Harlow, B. J., Massey, H. and Yee, K. F. The effect of a new non-sedative H_1-receptor antagonist (LN2974) on the itching and scratching of patients with atopic eczema. *Clin. Exper. Dermatol.*, **11**, 600, 1986.
33. Gibson, J. R. The use of antihistamines with a low sedative potential in the treatment of the itching of atopic eczema. *Clin. Exper. Dermatol.*, **12**, 469, 1987.

34. Wendt, H. and Frosch, P. J. *Clinico-Pharmacological Models for the Assay of Topical Corticoids*, Karger, Basel, 1982.
35. Guy, R. H., Tur, E. and Maibach, H. I. Optical techniques for monitoring cutaneous microcirculation. Recent applications. *Int. J. Dermatol.*, **24**, 88, 1985.
36. Bisgaard, H., Kristensen, J. K. and Sondergaard, J. A new technique for ranking vascular corticosteroid effects in humans using laser-Doppler velocimetry. *J. Invest. Dermatol.*, **86**, 275, 1986.
37. Blichmann, C. W. and Serup, J. Reproducibility and variability of transepidermal water loss measurement. Studies on the Servo Med evaporimeter. *Acta Derm. Venereol.*, **67**, 206, 1987.
38. Grice, K. A. Transepidermal water loss in pathological skin. In Jarret, A. (ed.), *Physiol. Pathophysiology of the Skin, Volume 6*, Academic Press, London, 2147, 1980.
39. Dykes, P. J. and Marks, R. Measurement of skin thickness: a comparison of two *in vivo* techniques with a conventional histometric method. *J. Invest. Dermatol.*, **69**, 275, 1977.
40. Kingston, T. P. and Lowe, N. J. Experimental assessment of human cutaneous irritant reactions using anthralin. In: Maibach, H. I. and Lowe, N. J., *Models in Dermatology Volume 3*, Karger, Basel, 74, 1987.
41. Tan, C. Y., Statham, B., Marks, R. and Payne, P. A. Skin thickness measurement by pulsed ultrasound: its reproducibility, validation and variability. *Br. J. Dermatol.*, **106**, 657, 1982.
42. Thomas, R. H. M. and Black, M. M. Corticosteroids: cutaneous atrophy. In: Maibach, I. H. and Lowe, N. J. (eds.), *Models in Dermatology Volume 2*, Karger, Basel, 30, 1985.
43. Guy, R. H., Bucks, D. A. W., McMaster, J. R., Villaflor, D. A., Roskos, K. V., Hinz, R. S. and Maibach, H. I. Kinetics of drug absorption across human skin *in vivo*. In: Shroot, B. and Schaefer, H. (eds.), *Pharmacology and the Skin, Volume 1*, Karger, Basel, 70, 1987.
44. Rougier, A. and Lotte, C. Correlations between horny layer concentration and percutaneous absorption. In: Shroot, B. and Schaefer, H. (eds.), *Pharmacology and the Skin, Volume 1*, Karger, Basel, 81, 1987.
45. Kobza Black, A., Greaves, M. W., Hensby, C. N., Plummer, N. A. and Eady, R. A. J. A new method for recovery of exudates from normal and inflamed human skin. *Clin. Exp. Dermatol.*, **2**, 209, 1977.
46. Cunningham, F. M. and Camp, R. D. R. New assays for inflammatory mediators in skin diseases. In: Maibach, H. I. and Lowe, N. J., *Models in Dermatology, Volume 3*, Karger, Basel, 39, 1987.
47. Barry, B. W. and Woodford, R. Activity and bioavailability of topical steroids. *In vivo/in vitro* correlations for the vasoconstrictor test. *J. Clin. Pharm.*, **3**, 43, 1978.
48. Buehler, E. V. and Ritz, H. L. Patch testing techniques for risk assessment of allergic contact dermatitis. In: Maibach, H. I. and Lowe, N. J. (eds.), *Models in Dermatology, Volume 2*, Karger, Basel, 251, 1985.
49. Epstein, J. H. Photocontact allergy in humans. In: Marzulli, F. N. and Maibach, H. I. (eds.), *Advances in Modern Toxicology, Volume 4 (Dermatotoxicology and Pharmacology)*, Halsted Press, New York, 413, 1977.
50. Frosch, P. J. Methods for quantifying the cutaneous adverse effects of topical corticosteroids. In: Kligman, A. M. and Leyden, J. J. (eds.), *Safety and Efficacy of Topical Drugs and Cosmetics*, Grune & Stratton, New York, 119, 1982.
51. Frosch, P. J. and Wendt, H. Human models for quantification of corticosteroid adverse effects. In: Maibach, H. I. and Lowe, N. J. (eds.), *Models in Dermatology, Volume 2*, Karger, Basel, 5, 1985.
52. Hjorth, N. Diagnostic patch testing. In: Marzulli, F. N. and Maibach, H. I. (eds.), *Advances in Modern Toxicology, Volume 4 (Dermatotoxicology and Pharmacology)*, Halsted Press, New York, 341, 1977.
53. Jordan, W. P. and King, S. E. Human experimental contact dermatitis. In: Kligman, A. M. and Leyden, J. J. (eds.), *Safety and Efficacy of Topical Drugs and Cosmetics*, Grune & Stratton, New York, 193, 1982.
54. Kaidbey, K. Assessment of topical photosensitizers in humans. In Kligman, A. M. and Leyden, J. J. (eds.), *Safety and Efficacy of Topical Drugs and Cosmetics*, Grune & Stratton, New York, 213, 1982.
55. Maibach, H. I. and Marzulli, F. N. Phototoxicity (photoirritation) of topical and systemic agents. In: Marzulli, F. N. and Maibach, H. I. (eds.), *Advances in Modern Toxicology, Volume 4 (Dermatotoxicology and Pharmacology)*, Halsted Press, New York, 211, 1977.
56. Marzulli, F. N. and Maibach, H. I. Contact allergy: predictive testing in humans. In: Marzulli, F. N. and Maibach, H. I. (eds.), *Advances in Modern Toxicology, Volume 4 (Dermatotoxicology and Pharmacology)*, Halsted Press, New York, 353, 1977.
57. Kobza Black, A., Greaves, M. W. and Hensby, C. N. The effect of systemic prednisolone on arachidonic acid, and prostaglandin E_2 and F_{2a} levels in human cutaneous inflammation. *Br. J. Clin. Pharmacol.*, **14**, 391, 1982.
58. Plummer, N. A., Hensby, C. N., Kobza Black, A. and Greaves, M. W. Prostaglandin activity in sustained inflammation of human skin before and after aspirin. *Clin. Sci. Mol. Med.*, **52**, 615, 1977.
59. Sussman, G. L., Petillo, J. J., Zisblatt, M., Vukovich, R. A., Neiss, E. S. and Schocket, A. L. Inhibition of compound 48/80 induced mediator release following oral administration of tiaramide hydrochloride in normal subjects. *Ann. Allergy*, **51**, 367, 1983.
60. Harst, L. C. A. V. D., de Jonge, H., Pot, F. and Polano, M. K. Comparison of two application schedules for clobetasol 17 propionate. *Acta Derm. Venereolo.*, **62**, 270, 1982.
61. Sudilovsky, A., Muir, J. G. and Bocobo, F. C. A comparison of single and multiple applications of halcinonide cream. *Int. J. Dermatol.*, **20**, 609, 1981.
62. Friedmann, P. S., Moss, C., Shuster, S. and Simpson, J. M. Quantitative relationships between sensitizing dose of DNCB and reactivity in normal subjects. *Clin. Exp. Immunol.*, **53**, 709, 1983.
63. Kaidbey, K. H. and Kligman, A. M. Assay of topical corticosteroids. Efficacy of suppression of experimental Rhus dermatitis in humans. *Arch. Dermatol.*, **112**, 808, 1976.

64. Van Neste, D., Masmoudi, M., Leroy, B., Mahmoud, G. and Lachapelle J. M. Regression patterns of transepidermal water loss and of cutaneous blood flow values in sodium lauryl sulfate induced irritation: a human model of rough dermatitic skin. *Bioengin. Skin*, **2**, 103, 1986.
65. Kaidbey, K. H. and Kligman, A. M. Assay of topical corticosteroids by suppression of experimental inflammation in humans. *J. Invest. Dermatol.*, **63**, 292, 1974.
66. Lawrence, C. M. and Shuster, S. Mechanism of anthralin inflammation. I. Dissociation of response to clobetasol and indomethacin. *Br. J. Dermatol.*, **113**, 107, 1985.
67. Lawrence, C. M. and Shuster, S. Mechanism of anthralin inflammation. II. Effect of pretreatment with glucocorticoids, anthralin and removal of stratum corneum. *Br. J. Dermatol.*, **113**, 117, 1985.
68. Camp, R., Jones, R. R., Brain, S., Woollard, P. and Greaves, M. Production of intraepidermal microabscesses by topical application of leukotriene B_4. *J. Invest. Dermatol.*, **82**, 202, 1984.
69. Rupp, W., Badian, M., Dagrosa, E., Ganshorn, F., Lucena, M., Petri, W. and Sittig, W. Kinetics of UV-erythema in normal subjects. *Br. J. Dermatol.*, **109**(Suppl.25), 111, 1983.
70. Tan, P., Flowers, F. P., Araujo, O. E. and Doering, P. Effect of topically applied flurbiprofen on ultraviolet-induced erythema. *Drug Intell. Clin. Pharm.*, **20**, 496, 1986.
71. Torrent, J., Izquierdo, I., Barbanoj, M. J., Moreno, J., Lauroba, J. and Jane, F. UV-induced erythema model: a tool in dermatopharmacology for testing the topical activity of non-steroidal anti-inflammatory agents in man. *Methods Findings Exp. Clin. Pharmacol.*, **10**, 341, 1988.
72. Woodward, D. F., Conway, J. L. and Wheeler, L. A. Cutaneous itching models. In: Maibach, H. I. and Lowe, N. J. (eds.), *Models in Dermatology, Volume 1*, Karger, Basel, 187, 1985.
73. Ring, J. and Dorsch, W. Altered releasability of vasoactive mediator secreting cells in atopic eczema. *Acta Derm. Venereol.*, Suppl. 114, 9, 1985.
74. Bisgaard, H. and Kristensen, J. K. Quantitation of microcirculatory blood flow changes in human cutaneous tissue induced by inflammatory mediators. *J. Invest. Dermatol.*, **83**, 184, 1984.
75. Black, M. M. A modified radiographic method for measuring skin thickness. *Br. J. Dermatol.*, **81**, 661, 1969.
76. Drouard, V., Wilson, D. R., Maibach, H. I. and Guy, R. H. Quantitative assessment of UV-induced changes in microcirculatory flow by laser Doppler velocimetry. *J. Invest. Dermatol.*, **83**, 188, 1984.
77. Engelhart, M. and Kristensen, J. K. Evaluation of cutaneous blood flow responses by ^{133}Xenon washout and a laser-Doppler flowmeter. *J. Invest. Dermatol.*, **80**, 12, 1983.
78. Holloway, G. A. Laser Doppler measurement of cutaneous blood flow. In: Rolfe, P., ed. *Non-invasive Measurements:2*, Academic Press Inc., London, 219, 1983.
79. Holloway, G. A. and Watkins, D. W. Laser Doppler measurement of cutaneous blood flow. *J. Invest. Dermatol.*, **69**, 306, 1977.
80. Kobza Black, A., Barr, R. M., Wong, E., Brain, S., Greaves, M. W., Dickinson, R., Shroot, B. and Hensby, C. N. Lipoxygenase products of arachidonic acid in human inflamed skin. *Bri. J. Clin. Pharmacol.*, **20**, 185, 1985.
81. Michel, L. and Dubertret, L. A simple method for studying chemotaxis, vascular permeability and histological modifications induced by mediators of inflammation *in vivo* in man. *Br. J. Dermatol.*, **113** (Suppl.28), 61, 1985.
82. Nilsson, G. E. Measurement of water exchange through skin. *Med. Biol. Eng. Computing*, **15**, 209, 1977.
83. Scott, R. C., Oliver, G. J. A., Dugard, P. H. and Singh, H. J. A comparison of techniques for the measurement of transepidermal water loss. *Arch. Dermatol.*, **274**, 57, 1982.
84. Stevenson, J. M., Maibach, H. I. and Guy, R. H. Laser Doppler and photoplethysmographic assessment of cutaneous microvasculature. In: Maibach, H. I. and Lowe, N. J., *Models in Dermatology, Volume 3*, Karger, Basel, 121, 1987.
85. Werner, Y. and Lindberg, M. Transepidermal water loss in dry and clinically normal skin in patients with atopic dermatitis. *Acta Derm. Venereol.*, **65**, 102, 1985.

Part XI. Assessment of Drugs Used for the Treatment of Metabolic Disorders

Chapter 34

Phase II Trials with Lipid-Acting Drugs

C. A. Dujovne, P. E. Krehbiel, W. S. Harris, and S. J. Held

CONTENTS

1 Introduction 463
2 Study Designs 464
3 Professional Staff Requirements 464
4 Selection of Patients 465
4.1 Dyslipidemias 465
4.2 Concomitant Medications 465
4.3 Concurrent Illnesses 465
4.4 Clinical-Biochemical Laboratory Baselines 465
4.5 Other Considerations in the Selection of Subjects-Patients 466
4.6 Ethical Issues in Testing Drugs for Secondary Prevention of Atherosclerosis 467
4.7 Phase II Trials in Children 467
5 Informed Consent 467
6 Lipoprotein Measurements 468
6.1 Determining which Lipoprotein Parameters to Measure 468
6.2 Acceptable Methods of Lipoprotein Measurements 468
6.3 Cholesterol Absorption Studies 469
6.4 Standardization for Lipid Research Laboratories 469
7 Diet Constancy Monitoring 469
7.1 Goals of Diet Monitoring 469
7.2 Methods of Monitoring Food Intake 470
8 Selection of Efficacy Endpoints 471
9 Selection of Safety Endpoints 471
10 Pharmacokinetic, Pharmacodynamic Studies in Phase II Trials 472
References 472

1 INTRODUCTION

Phase II clinical trials are of crucial, strategic importance in the development of lipid-active compounds and can supply the earliest and possibly most accurate data on short-term safety and efficacy and dose-related therapeutic and toxic effects of a new compound. Potential interactions with commonly used drugs such as analgesics, hormones, or other drugs frequently administered to dyslipidemic patients may also be detected in late phase II trials.

Phase II studies are usually conducted in 75-500 patients and may take 2-5 years to complete. The length of drug exposure is relatively short — 2-6 months — depending on the mechanism of action and known or predicted onset of the therapeutic effects. The safety profile determined in phase I may suggest or dictate the size of the sample and lengths of exposure in early phase II studies.[1]

We have proposed that studies in late phase I and early phase II hypolipidemic drugs are possible in dyslipidemic patients. Patients who are completely healthy except for documented dyslipidemia could well substitute for healthy volunteer subjects without dyslipidemia to do studies of late phase I or early phase II with lipid-acting drugs; there are many advantages to this approach as follows: (1) earlier evidence can be gathered regarding the efficacy of the lipid-acting compound on correction of abnormal serum lipid levels, (2) dose-efficacy relationships can be elicited, (3) evaluation of a new lipid-acting drug in later phase I or early phase II in subjects with elevated serum lipoprotein levels may reveal the new drug to have pharmacokinetic parameters different from those previously obtained in normal subjects.

0-8493-9230-6/97/$0.00+$.50
© 1997 by CRC Press, Inc.

2 STUDY DESIGNS

Controlled double-blind, placebo vs. drug studies in parallel treated groups have been considered ideal designs and are favored by statistitians as well as governments' drug approval agencies such as the U.S. Federal Drug Administration (FDA). However, use of placebo-treated controls is becoming more difficult in trials longer than 3-6 months, as the benefits of correcting dyslipidemia are now well documented in terms of reduction of morbidity and mortality (see Section 4.6). It is conceivable that in the very near future ethical considerations may make it necessary to utilize positive treatment controls with a dose of a drug for which short-term side effects have been identical to placebo and the therapeutic potency has been clearly established, e.g., 10-20 mg/day of lovastatin.[2]

Cross-over designs (where each patient is his/her own control) are not as well accepted as parallel designs by statisticians and the FDA, yet they have advantages in documenting efficacy when interindividual dose-responses are largely variable such as is often the case in dyslipidemic patients. Thus cross-over designs are likely to obviate a need for a larger number of patients to detect statistically significant differences.[3,4]

Cross-over designs are also useful when studying effects on parameters with a wide range of intraindividual abnormality such as serum triglyceride levels.[5]

3 PROFESSIONAL STAFF REQUIREMENTS

The professional competence of the staff is important since the performance of a clinical trial requires specialized skills, thoroughness, and attention to detail. Thus, the training and adequacy of the personnel available to implement a protocol at the individual clinic site are crucial ingredients for success. The primary components of a model for phase II dyslipidemic drug evaluation are depicted in the scheme shown in Figure 1. This model depicts the essential interactions among all kinds of operations and/or staff possibly to be involved in the implementation of a clinical trial.

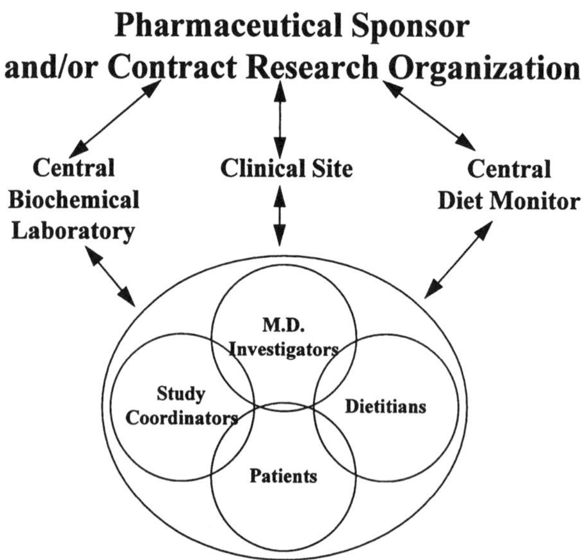

Figure 1 Essential interactions among operations and staff of a clinical trial.

The availability of a registered dietitian (RD) can become an issue in some sites; in certain studies, a dietitian may not need to be an essential part of the model if other diet instruction and monitoring sources are available. A centralized, preferably computer-assisted, diet analysis service can be very helpful (see details on diet monitoring below). In addition, a thorough and well-done videotape of basic dietary instruction is an alternative to a dietitian's in-person instruction (copies of such videos are available from the authors). Nurses or physician's assistants (PAs) who act as study coordinators can be trained to offer the subsequent supplementary dietary advice and coaching throughout the trial as required by the protocol.

The presence of other personnel in addition to those included in the basic model such as a recruiter, phlebotomist, and secretary can be very helpful and may be essential if a clinic site has a large number of subjects to enroll in a trial.

The question of what kind of healthcare provider should be the phase II study coordinator is important to consider. In our view, an RN is the ideal choice because nurses have a more holistic and versatile educational background than other medical professionals and are relatively easier to find and train. Furthermore, the first exposure of patients to a new drug may require refined clinical skills to detect subtle side effects. An option for a large clinic implementing late phase II clinical trials is to have study coordinators that come from various disciplines (i.e., RDs) who are supervised by a well-trained RN, PA, or MD.

4 SELECTION OF PATIENTS

4.1 Dyslipidemias

The knowledge from experimental and phase I studies on the effects of the new drug on lipoprotein regulation will determine the type of lipoprotein abnormalities to be studied. In most instances the new drug will be targeted toward correction of dyslipidemias which are of frequent occurrence and also known to result in significant atherosclerotic morbidity.

Most drugs are intended to lower blood levels of low density lipoprotein cholesterol (LDLC) or triglycerides, to raise blood levels of high density lipoprotein cholesterol (HDLC), or a combination of these effects. Changes in corresponding apoproteins are often also documented. In terms of Fredrickson phenotypes, the patients most frequently studied have types IIa, II, or IV. Types I, III, and V are relatively rare and/or complicated, and few drugs have been specifically developed for these patients. Patients with familial hypercholesterolemia are usually not mixed in with those described above who have more polygenic dyslipidemias. This applies to heterozygotes, and especially, homozygotes.

4.2 Concomitant Medications

It is ideal to test experimental drugs in the absence of all other medications to ensure that the effects on the therapeutic endpoints and/or side effects are from the new drug; however, it is also realistic to consider that the new lipid-acting drug will be used in populations taking other commonly used drugs such as analgesics, contraceptive hormones, postmenopausal replacement hormones, anti-allergic medications, thyroid replacement, and/or multiple vitamin preparations.

Antidepressant drugs (i.e., fluoxetine hydrochloride, Prozac™) and postmenopausal hormone replacements (estrogen with or without progesterone) are now quite commonly given to otherwise healthy people. The investigator as well as the sponsor must decide whether patients taking these compounds should be included in the trial. In general very early studies should exclude them, but late phase II studies may include such patients since they are likely to be eligible for later therapeutic trials. Since women at gestational age are often an exclusion, most other women in a phase II trial will be postmenopausal due to the expanding number of women on postmenopausal hormone replacement; excluding women on these drugs may make it difficult if not impossible to find female patients for the phase II trial. Anticoagulant use is a contraindication as well as drugs with potential effects on lipoprotein regulation mechanisms,[6] i.e., thiazide, diuretics, steroids, etc.

4.3 Concurrent Illnesses

The presence of illnesses that may affect lipid levels or lipoprotein regulation mechanisms should be ruled out, i.e., diabetes, hypothyroidism, renal, pancreatic or liver disease, severe obesity, etc. Some diseases that can be well controlled such as hypothyroidism could be accepted in phase II trials if the level of control is uniform and the hormone replacement is constant throughout the trial. Use of diabetic patients is usually avoided because of the likely possibility of serum lipoprotein level fluctuations secondary to variable diabetes control during the trial.

4.4 Clinical-Biochemical Laboratory Baselines

Routine biochemical tests, i.e., liver and renal function, should be normal except for the allowance of minor elevations in some biochemical tests occasionally present in patients with dyslipidemia. These include:

- Borderline low thyroid function tests
- Mild elevations of serum creatine phosphokinase (SCPK)[7,8] levels (see details below)

- Mild elevations in serum bilirubin levels, as seen in as many as 10% of the population with Gilbert's syndrome
- Mild elevation of serum creatinine due to some degree of renal atherosclerosis

SCPK is quite commonly elevated in dyslipidemics as previously described.[4,9,10] Therefore, moderate — up to twofold elevations — of SCPK should not preclude participation in phase II trials.

Abnormal "liver function tests" are not uncommonly seen in dyslipidemics with fatty infiltration of the liver. However, monitoring levels for abnormalities in these tests are crucial to rule out hepatotoxic effects of drugs. Therefore, it is necessary that in the very early phase II trials the liver function tests be normal before drug administration. This would include primarily the results of alanine aminotransferase levels (ALT). Minor elevations in serum aminotransferase levels (AST) can be tolerated only if ALT levels are normal; elevations of AST may often follow SCPK when SCPK elevations are secondary to the dyslipidemic condition as explained above or to strenuous physical exercise.

Serum bilirubin elevations are permitted only if due to Gilbert's syndrome (fasting hyperbilirubinemia) which is present in as many as 10% of the normal population and manifested by hyperbilirubinemia which is exacerbated by prolonged fasting. Patients with Gilbert's syndrome can be accepted in trials if there are no other abnormalities in liver function or indications of other causes of abnormal bilirubin metabolism. Alkaline phosphotase levels are to be normal or not larger than twice the upper limit of normal at baseline. Normal gallbladder sonograms may be required if the new drug is suspected of affecting gallstone formation.

Fasting blood glucose levels should be normal, but levels up to 140 mg/dl are usually accepted, provided there is no other evidence of diabetes.

4.5 Other Considerations in the Selection of Subjects-Patients

When the specific inclusion and exclusion criteria of the protocol have been considered, other considerations of lifestyle and/or personality need to be applied to the selection process.

Types of patients who may need special consideration before inclusion as subjects of phase II protocols:

1. Patients who regularly take many prescription drugs. The concerns are possible interference with measurements of endpoints, drug interactions, and possibly multiple other illnesses, complaints, or even hypochondria.
2. Persons who take an excessive number of food supplements or herbal remedies. Autoprescription and arbitrary compliance to the protocol regimens can be an obstacle. The possibility of drug interactions must also be considered.
3. Individuals seemingly unable to follow simple instructions. The concern is their capacity to keep appointment times, fasting the required number of hours before laboratory specimens, and taking medicines properly.
4. Patients with very complicated medical histories. This could be an indication of poor overall health, poor health maintenance, or even hypochondria.
5. Individuals with a history of rapid weight gain or loss. This could signal a history of "yo-yo" dieting or serious and chronic eating disorders.
6. Traveling sales people. Questions arise about the stability of lifestyle habits, ability to keep regular appointments, and eat uniform diets.
7. Persons with variable geographic stability. This includes seasonal workers and individuals whose work involves frequent travel. They may not be able to keep visits required or complete the study.
8. Patients failing to disclose concomitant medications, lifestyle habits. or past medical history. Implies unreliability.
9. Subjects of extremely low socioeconomic status if associated with a disregard for preventive health, unstable domiciles, and unstable nutritional status.
10. Persons on extremely high or low fat diets. This could adversely affect studies with certain types of drugs, e.g., fat-cholesterol absorption inhibitors or drugs whose solubility characteristics may be affected by extreme dietary fat levels; i.e., a vegetarian would be an inappropriate subject in whom to study a drug that affects fat absorption.
11. Patients with a current or past history of debilitating neurological disease, severe depression, or a past/present history of mental illness. These individuals are likely to have unstable lifestyle habits and/or noncompliance. True informed consent may be impossible to obtain in such individuals. Other examples include Alzheimer's disease or dementia.

12. Women of childbearing potential who indicate a poor compliance in the use of a birth control method. A common characteristic is an inability to recall the date of their last menstrual period and showing no concern for the risk of a pregnancy.
13. Subjects with epilepsy. Even if under control, unexpected symptoms can occur which can compromise the study drug. In addition, antiepileptic drugs can produce hematological abnormalities and a variety of drug interactions.
14. Subjects who had recent (last 6 months) or unstable cardiovascular disease with consequent unpredictable risk of illness during the study.
15. Subjects with any recent or recurrent symptomatic illness.

Good study candidates often have the following behavior patterns:

- Subjects who indicate interest in the dietary and drug benefits of a study or who indicate a commitment to a healthy lifestyle.
- Subjects that display a moderate degree of compulsiveness are usually excellent for research studies. Examples are the individual who comes to the clinic with cholesterol profile results of the past 5 years.
- Subjects who ask questions during a reading of the informed consent. This can indicate that they are processing the information presented.
- Subjects who bring in detailed previous medical records. Individuals that do this usually have a high degree of concern for their health.

4.6 Ethical Issues in Testing Drugs for Secondary Prevention of Atherosclerosis

It is now consensus that patients who had angioplasties, coronary bypass surgery, myocardial infarctions, or documented morbidity from arteriosclerotic vascular disease should be given pharmacotherapy as soon as lifestyle intervention is shown to be insufficient to bring serum LDLC levels below 100 mg/dl or at the minimum, below 130 mg/dl. It is therefore becoming difficult to approve the use of placebo control trials in such patients, more so if placebos are to be administered for longer than the 3 months of the preceding lifestyle intervention period.

4.7 Phase II Trials in Children

Dyslipidemia-induced atherosclerotic cardiovascular disease takes many years to be of health consequence in dyslipidemic children. It is then unlikely that new drugs will be tested in children before phase III or even phase IV studies have ensured absolute safety of the new compound.

5 INFORMED CONSENT

It is most important that the consent be written in a level of language that anyone with at least an eighth grade education can comprehend. For example, a word like "abdominal" could be replaced by "stomach"; the word "randomized" could be replaced by "assigned by lottery."

Sponsor or institutional review board (IRB) may mandate statements on the consent instrument which deals with liability issues. Insofar as is possible, lengthy and complicated legal terms and phrases should be avoided as these increase the likelihood of patient comprehension. Layman's terms should always be used.

The consent instrument should be carefully reviewed with the patient, paragraph by paragraph, after the patient has had an opportunity to read it. Encourage the patient to interrupt to ask questions. The interaction between study personnel and patients is an essential ingredient because in this way an assessment of a patient's comprehension can be made. Truly informed patients help ensure better study results by maximizing compliance, cooperation, and interest of subjects.

Consent instruments should contain a clear description of the treatments patients may receive on a research protocol. If the study contains the possibility of several treatment options, these should be clearly stated with a percentage chance specified for randomization to each option.

An excellent way to achieve informed consent that is also conservative of staff and patient's time is with group enrollment sessions. This method of patient enrollment has shown itself to be very efficient at our clinic and the group process can enhance patient comprehension and cooperation. Qualified patients can be enrolled at the same time the study coordinator reviews the consent and dietary instruction can be given either by a dietitian or by video. Sufficient phlebotomists should be available for obtaining the required lab work on these patients, before or after such a session.

6 LIPOPROTEIN MEASUREMENTS

6.1 Determining which Lipoprotein Parameters to Measure

The goal of therapy with most dyslipidemic drugs is either to lower LDLC or total triglyceride, or raise HDLC levels. Whatever the drug, it is critical to measure as accurately as possible the parameter expected to be affected. The decision about how many variables to measure depends upon several considerations: the expected mechanism of action of the drug, the research question being asked (i.e., safety vs. efficacy vs. mechanism), and the funds available. One of the four levels of laboratory lipoprotein determinations below can be chosen depending on the specific study requirements:

Level 1: Basic lipid profile containing total cholesterol, triglycerides, HDLC, and an estimated LDLC (for triglyceride and/or HDLC targeted drugs).

Level 2: Above plus directly measured LDLC (for LDLC targeted drugs) or for studies allowing serum triglyceride levels above 400 mg/dl.

Level 3: Above plus apolipoproteins A-1 and B-100, Lp(a), and LDLC/HDLC subfraction analyses (for more extensive investigations on effects and/or mechanisms of any dyslipidemic drugs).

Level 4: Above plus apolipoprotein E (apoE) genotype (for drug with possible interaction with intestinal absorption mechanisms), other apolipoproteins with variable roles in pro- or anti-atherogenic processes (C, E, A-IV, B-48, etc.), and LDLC oxidation susceptibility (for drugs with potential antioxidant properties). Measurement of lipoprotein a [Lp(a)] which is a newly discovered pro-atherogenic and pro-thrombotic risk factor. Measurement of intestinal cholesterol and/or fat absorption for drugs acting on these parameters.

6.2 Acceptable Methods of Lipoprotein Measurements

1. Total serum cholesterol is usually measured enzymatically.[11] The total cholesterol value is the sum of all the cholesterol in all the lipoproteins in the blood: LDL, HDL, and very low density lipoproteins (VLDL; containing about 70, 20, and 10%, of the total cholesterol, respectively). About 70% of the cholesterol is esterified and 30% is unesterified (free). In any clinical trial of a hypolipidemic agent, it is never sufficient to simply measure the total cholesterol level; the three lipoproteins noted above should always be determined (see below).
2. Triglycerides are also measured by enzymatic methods.[11] When triglyceride levels are the primary target for therapy, glycerol-blanking is essential.[12] Glycerol-blanking refers to the mathematical removal of background serum glycerol levels. (Glycerol falsely elevates serum triglyceride levels because most enzymatic assays measure the amount of glycerol liberated from serum triglycerides after treatment with lipase.) Free glycerol already present in the serum is measured before addition of lipase and then subtracted from the total "triglyceride" measured after incubation with lipase. Failure to glycerol-blank triglyceride measurements may lead to errors if the treatment under investigation alters serum free glycerol levels as well as triglyceride levels themselves.
3. For determination of LDLC, there are two common approaches: one is to measure the total cholesterol, the HDLC, and the triglyceride level, and then <u>estimate</u> the LDLC level using the Friedewald equation:[13]

   $$\text{LDLC} = \text{Total C} - (\text{HDLC}) - (\text{Triglycerides}/5)$$

   This method is adequate for estimating LDLC in routine patient care, but in trials of new drugs which target LDL specifically, it is more appropriate to measure LDLC directly. This has been done traditionally with the ultracentrifuge by a method known as "beta-quantification."[14] In this procedure, the plasma is spun to float the VLDL particles which are then removed. The cholesterol content of the infranatant (containing only LDL and HDL) is determined enzymatically, and the HDLC value subtracted giving the LDLC value. This method is relatively labor-intensive, but with newer ultracentrifuges (e.g., Beckman TL-100) the spin can be accomplished in 2 h (instead of the usual 18) and the analysis finished in 3 h.

   A newer method of directly measuring LDL is by an immunoseparation kit[15] (Sigma Diagnostics, St. Louis, MO). In this technique, whole serum is mixed with a reagent containing microbeads to which all non-LDL lipoproteins bind. After centrifugation the only cholesterol-containing lipoproteins remaining in solution are LDL, thus measurement of the cholesterol content gives LDLC directly.
4. This parameter is rarely of primary interest in clinical trials. It is a reflection of the number of VLDL particles in circulation which the total triglyceride level adequately estimates. VLDLC is either estimated by the Friedewald equation (above) or by difference in the beta-quantification procedure.

5. HDLC[16] is almost always measured directly in serum or plasma after precipitation of all apolipoprotein B-containing lipoproteins with a divalent cation (Ca^{+2}, Mg^{+2}, Mn^{+2}) and a polyanion (dextran sulfate, heparin). This method is adequate for nearly all clinical trials unless HDL subfractions are under study in which case either ultracentrifugal or dual-precipitation methods can be used.
6. Measurement of the primary protein conponents of lipoproteins (the apolipoproteins) has recently gained popularity. Apolipoprotein A-1 (apo A-1) and apo B-100[17] are the major proteins of HDL and LDL/VLDL, respectively. Measuring apo A-1 levels is a surrogate of HDLC. Apo B-100 estimates the total number of LDL and VLDL particles in circulation because there is only one apo B-100 molecule per particle. There continues to be controversy about the relative clinical significance of apoprotein vs. lipoprotein cholesterol measurements in clinical practice.[18-20] Although these are often measured in clinical trials (usually by radioimmunoassay or immunoturbidometric assays), they are usually considered secondary or confirmatory to the primary tests of lipoprotein cholesterol levels.
7. This lipoprotein (Lp "little a")[21] is basically an LDL particle which contains an extra, carbohydrate-rich protein called apo (a) attached covalently to apo B-100. Elevated levels of Lp(a) appear to confer increased risk of coronary heart disease (CHD), the mechanism proposed is related to the experimental demonstration in that Lp(a) cholesterol is accumulated in atherosclerotic arteries and in addition it interferes with fibrinalysis (a normal antithrombotic mechanism). Lp(a) levels appear to be largely genetically determined. Neither low-fat diets nor most current drugs will lower Lp(a) levels. Niacin is the most well-known exception to this rule.[22] At present it has not yet been proven that lowering Lp(a) levels will reduce CHD risk. However, there is ample experimental and epidemiological data to support such a possibility. It is often measured in clinical trials of new drugs but not as a primary variable.
8. Since there is growing evidence that oxidized LDL may be atherogenic, it is becoming more common to test lipid-acting drugs and antioxidative vitamins[23] for their ability to reduce the susceptibility of LDL to *in vitro* oxidation. Although there are several methods used,[24] the most common is to measure the lag time after incubation of isolated LDL with copper ions. Whether this (or any other test) accurately reflects the *in vivo* susceptibility to oxidation is not clear.

6.3 Cholesterol Absorption Studies

New drugs are often designed in an attempt to lower serum LDL levels by inhibiting the absorption of dietary and biliary cholesterol from the intestine. Among these are ACAT inhibitors[25] and synthetic saponins.[26] Documenting this mechanism of action requires specialized dual-isotopic procedures which measure either cholesterol excreted in stools[27] or plasma isotope ratios.[14]

6.4 Standardization for Lipid Research Laboratories

Laboratories utilized in phase II trials with dyslipidemic drugs must be standardized.[28] The CDC-NHLBI Lipid Standardization Program is primarily designed for lipid research laboratories. Accuracy and precision is evaluated quarterly for total cholesterol, triglycerides, and HDLC. Clinical laboratories and manufacturers may utilize the services of the Cholesterol Reference Method Laboratory Network which was recently established by the CDC.

7 DIET CONSTANCY MONITORING

7.1 Goals of Diet Monitoring

There are several goals of diet monitoring in clinical trials with lipid-acting drugs:

1. To detect differences in diet compliance between or among treatment groups or within a single drug treatment group at different doses. This is important because changes in dietary fat may have similar effects on LDL levels as pharmaceutical agents. Saturated fat and cholesterol downregulate the LDL receptor retarding hepatic removal of LDL from the plasma, thus resulting in increased plasma LDL. For overweight individuals, excessive caloric intake may enhance LDL synthesis by stimulating VLDL production. Weight loss and fish oil derived omega-3 fatty acids decrease the synthesis of VLDL reducing triglyceride levels. Thus dietary factors can influence the same lipoprotein parameters as lipid-lowering drugs. Because diets are difficult to control in outpatient settings, they should be monitored to detect dietary changes that could influence lipid endpoints.
2. To facilitate feedback to the patient and increase patient understanding of how diet influences their own lipid profile. In this way structured diet monitoring may enhance compliance not just to diet but to other lifestyle habits and even medications. Dyslipidemic patients who are randomized to placebo

treatment will receive the benefit of diet education if nothing else. This encourages patient participation and should increase the likelihood of the protocol meeting ethical standards of the IRB.

3. In the U.S., the third goal of diet monitoring is to meet all requirements and recommendations of the FDA recommendations regarding diet monitoring in lipid trials as follows:

- Relevant dietary composition and caloric intake as well as physical activity level should be assessed for each treatment group at baseline and during active therapy. Compliance with diet and medication should be quantified
- All patients should receive a standard diet
- Dietary regimens should be controlled and defined
- Data on dietary compliance and composition should be obtained at least every two months
- An analysis (of the final data) by degree of dietary and drug compliance should be performed

(Excerpts from the 1990 FDA draft "Guidelines for the Clinical Evaluation of Lipid-Altering Agents in Adults and Children").

4. By systematically requiring diet monitoring, which includes standardized diet counseling, investigators attain another goal which is to document compliance to the National Cholesterol Education Program (NCEP) treatment guidelines which require diet education before initiating pharmacologic intervention.

7.2 Methods of Monitoring Food Intake

Diet record is a self-documented record of foods (and quantities) consumed during a specified time interval, commonly 3-7 days. Training the subject in record keeping is essential and will involve the patient estimating portion size or actually weighing portions for improved accuracy. Once the record is completed, it should be reviewed and analyzed. One method of analyzing the diet record is to assign scores to all the foods consumed based on their predicted hypercholesterolemic effect. An example of this is the Food Record Rating designed for use in the MRFIT trial.[29] This method requires a highly trained nutritionist and does not yield specific nutrient data. It therefore does not meet the FDA requirement for quantifying dietary composition and caloric intake. A computer-assisted analysis of the diet record using a complete and up-to-date database is currently the preferred method of monitoring diets in phase II and III clinical trials. This method, when implemented by knowledgeable dietitians, should meet all FDA guidelines.

The duplicate plate method involves preparing weighed meals for the subject who, after eating, weighs and records the amounts of food not eaten. Duplicate meals are retained and the appropriate amounts (after subtracting the uneaten portion) can be analyzed in a laboratory for nutrient composition or calculated using a computer-assisted analysis. This method is much more accurate but is time-consuming, expensive and may alter eating habits; application is usually limited to metabolic studies.

The recall method is similar to the food record but relies on the patient remembering what they have eaten over a specified interval of time such as the past 24 h. It is generally limited to 48 h and is less able to describe the individual's usual pattern.[30] It may be analyzed by scoring or computer-assisted analysis.

The diet history method involves repeated food records or recall records to be obtained over a period of time to identify food intake patterns. It is useful for food habit and epidemiological studies as well as education programs. Diet History records may be analyzed to yield estimated but not absolute nutrient intake data and therefore does not meet the FDA guidelines.

The food frequency method employs food lists from which the patient selects not only the foods usually eaten but also the frequency of consumption and usual portion sizes. Because this method provides descriptive data only, absolute calorie and nutrient calculations cannot be obtained. Semi-quantitative food frequency forms have been developed to improve the accuracy of the data but none are as good or as well-implemented as diet records.

The **RISCC rating** shows that once a quantitative assessment has been obtained by one of the above-described methods, it is necessary to express the nutrient composition in a manner which is both easy to understand and analyze statistically. Since current dietary guidelines from the NCEP are almost universally used in clinical trials of dyslipidemic drugs, comparison to these guidelines will be essential for documentation of compliance or dietary constancy. Unfortunately there are many nutrients for which recommendations exist (cholesterol; saturated, monounsaturated, and polyunsaturated fatty acids; carbohydrate; etc.), and determining if patient diets meet all of these criteria for all of the nutrients can be cumbersome. There is thus a need for a simplified method for comparing patient diets to national guidelines.

The RISCC rating system was devised by investigators at our clinic for this purpose. RISCC stands for "ratio of ingested saturated fat and cholesterol to calories" and is calculated by determining (from an analysis of a diet record) the amount of saturated fat (g), cholesterol (mg), and kcalories consumed on average per day. These are then combined in the equation below to arrive at the RISCC score for the patient's diet.

$$\text{RISCC} = [(1.01 \times \text{saturated fatty acids}) + (0.05 \times \text{cholesterol})]/(\text{kcalories}/1{,}000)$$

The RISCC equation is the cholesterol saturated fat index of Connor et al.[31] calculated for the entire diet and adjusted for total kcalories. Once determined, the RISCC score can be compared to the RISCC scores of the NCEP step 1 and 2 diets. The RISCC score of the typical American diet is >20; that of the step 1 diet is 14-20; and that of the step 2 diet is ≤13.

The RISCC equation allows the major hyperlipidemic factors in the diet to be combined in one number and normalized to total energy intake (as a surrogate of body size). It also facilitates statistical evaluation of the change in diet compliance over a study. If mean RISCC scores do not change from baseline to the end of the study, then overall dietary stability has been documented. In addition, diet constancy *between* treatment groups can readily be compared to show that any changes in plasma lipid levels were not due to dietary changes. The RISCC system has been used successfully in a number of recently published[32-35] clinical trials.

8 SELECTION OF EFFICACY ENDPOINTS

Until a few years ago the FDA had arbitrarily established requirements that any new hypolipidemic drug should lower cholesterol levels by a mean of at least 15% in a dyslipidemic population. More recent advancements in knowledge of atherogenicity related to lipoprotein levels have made this concept antiquated. The National Cholesterol and Triglycerides guidelines set by NIH panels are more likely used as the current standards. Requirements for efficacy are now based on reaching a certain lower level for the abnormal lipid or lipoprotein. The goal level depends on the clinical type of patients and whether treatment is as described in detail in recent publications.[36,37]

In summary, it is now desirable to have treatments which lower LDL cholesterol down to 160, 130, or even 100 mg/dl (depending on the patient), lower triglyceride levels below 200 mg/dl and/or raise HDLC to the highest possible extent, ideally over 45 mg/dl.

9 SELECTION OF SAFETY ENDPOINTS

Phase II studies are concerned primarily with short-term safety and efficacy of the new drug. Because of the potentially life long need for dyslipidemic drug therapy, a period of 1 or even 2 years of treatment is a relatively short-term documentation of safety.

The major short-term safety concerns are related to the following organs:

Eyes — due to the potentially irreversible nature of the side effects and the role of lipids in the metabolism of the lens tissue. Target: rule out cataract formation or other ocular dysfunction.

Hepatobiliary — due to the pivotal role of the liver in lipoprotein regulation mechanisms and the first-pass effect and/or hepatic metabolism and/or biliary excretion/recirculation of many drugs. Target: rule out hepatotoxicity and/or other pathogenicity effects. Bile lithogenicity studies to discard the drug enhancing formation of gallstones.

Muscle — due to the antecedent frequency of muscle-related disorders in dyslipidemia with or without associated drug therapy. Target: rule out myopathies or associated myotoxicity.

Endocrine-gonadal function — due to active participation of cholesterol in normal endocrine and other homeostatic mechanisms. Goal: rule out effects on gonadal function.

Neuropsychiatric — due to the major lipid component of organs in this system and the differences in lipid/water partition coefficient among drugs. Goal: rule out sleep or behavioral changes.

10 PHARMACOKINETIC, PHARMACODYNAMIC STUDIES IN PHASE II TRIALS

Phase II studies may be ideal to initiate in-depth studies of pharmacokinetics as well as pharmacodynamics of the new compound. Pharmacokinetic data obtained from phase II studies may facilitate the planning of studies for future clinical development of a new drug by eliciting (1) important kinetic changes among populations of different age, sex, and ethnic characteristics, (2) potential kinetic changes in reference to different lipoprotein abnormality patterns, (3) pharmacokinetic behaviors that may suggest the best time of drug administration that will render the best efficacy or safety, (4) inappropriate dosages or dosage schedules, (5) the importance of active or inactive metabolites, (6) changes in efficacy and/or safety at different ages, (7) abnormal efficacy or safety in people of different age, sex, or other interindividual variables, and (8) drug interactions that could be clinically relevant to future clinical use of the drug.

We therefore advocate that pharmaceutical manufacturers use phase II trials to expand the gathering of pharmacokinetic and pharmacodynamic data to further the knowledge of drug disposition and to possibly correlate this data with efficacy — safety outcome of the trials.

REFERENCES

1. Spilker, B., *Inside the Drug Industry,* Prous Science Publishers, Barcelona, Spain, 1990, chap. 5.
2. Bradford, R. H., Shear, C. L., Chremos, A. N., Dujovne, C. A., Downton, M., Franklin, F. A., Gould, L., Hesney, M., Higgins, J., Hurley, D. P., Langendorfer, A., Nash, D. T., Pool, J. L. and Schnaper, H., Expanded clinical evaluation of lovastatin (EXCEL) Study Results. 1. Efficacy in modifying plasma lipoproteins and adverse event profile in 8245 patients with moderate hypercholesterolemia, *Arch. Intern. Med.,* 151, 43, 1991.
3. Dujovne, C. A. and Krehbiel, P., Considerations for controlled clinical testing of safety and efficacy of new hypolipidemic drugs, *Proc. of the IX International Symposium on Drugs Affecting Lipid Metabolism,* Florence, Italy, Paoletti, R., Ed., Springer-Verlag, Berlin, 1987, pp. 136-141.
4. Dujovne, C. A ., Weiss, P. and Bianchine, J. R., Comparative clinical therapeutic trial with two hypolipidemic drugs: clofibrate and nafenopin (SU-13437), *Clin. Pharmacol. Ther.,* 12, 117, 1971.
5. Dujovne, C. A., Azarnoff, D. L., Pentikainen, P., Manion, C. and Hurwitz, A., A comparative trial of clofibrate and nicotinyl alcohol tartrate in hyperlipoproteinemic patients, *Am. J. Med. Sci.,* 277, 255, 1979.
6. Dujovne, C. A., The lipid-hypertension treatment connection, *Perspec. Lipid Disord.,* 6, 20, 1989.
7. Dujovne, C. A., Findings and interpretation of changes in serum alkaline phosphatase, creatine phosphokinase, bilirubin and liver scanning in patients receiving hypolipidemic drugs, in *Drugs Affecting Lipid Metabolism,* Fumagalli, R., Kritchevsky, D. and Paoletti, R., Ed., Elsevier/North-Holland Biomedical Press, 1980, pp. 293-300.
8. Dujovne, C. A., Differentiation of toxic from spurious abnormalities after drug administration in man in drug effect on laboratory test results, in *Developments in Clinical Biochemistry,* Vol. 2, Siest, B., Ed., Martinus Nijhoff Publishers, The Hague, Netherlands, 1980, pp. 214-220.
9. Dujovne, C. A., Azarnoff, D. L., Huffman, D. H., Pentikäinen, P., Hurwitz, A. and Shoeman, D. W., One-year trials with halofenate clofibrate, and placebo, *Clin. Pharmacol. Ther.,* 19, 352, 1976.
10. Dujovne, C. A., Pitfalls in the adequate control of hypolipidemic drug trials, in *Proc. Interamerican Congr. Clin. Pharmacol. Ther., Caracas, Venezuela,* pp. 93, 1982.
11. Warnick, G. R., Enzymatic methods for quantitation of lipoprotein lipids, *Methods Enzymol.,* 129, 101, 1986.
12. Cole, T., Glycerol blanking in triglyceride assays: Is it necessary?, *Clin. Chem.,* 36, 1267, 1990.
13. Friedewald, W. T., Levy, R. I. and Fredrickson, D. S., Estimation of the concentration of LDL-cholesterol in plasma without the use of the ultracentrifuge. *Clin. Chem.,* 18, 449, 1972.
14. Belcher, J. D., McNamara, J. R., Grinstead, G. F., Rifai, N., Warnick, G. R. and Bachorik, P., Measurement of low-density lipoprotein cholesterol concentration, in *Laboratory Measurement of Lipids, Lipoproteins and Apolipoproteins,* Rifai, N., Warnick and G. R., Eds., American Association for Clinical Chemistry Press, Washington, D.C., 1994, pp. 107-124.
15. Singh, J., Kulig, K. and Lucco, L, Determination of direct LDL cholesterol in human serum with triglycerides ≤400 mg/dl by Genzyme Immunoseparation reagent (Gen-LDL) kit, *Clin. Chem.,* 40, 1099, 1994.
16. Wiebe, D. A. and Warnick, G. R., Measurement of high density lipoprotein cholesterol concentration, in *Laboratory Measurement of Lipids, Lipoproteins and Apolipoproteins,* Rifai, N. and Warnick, G. R., Eds., American Association for Clinical Chemistry Press, Washington, D.C., 1994, pp. 91-106.
17. Stein, E. A., Clinical significance and measurement of apolipoproteins A1 and B, in *Laboratory Measurement of Lipids, Lipoproteins and Apolipoproteins,* Rifai, N. and Warnick, G. R., Eds., American Association for Clinical Chemistry Press, Washington, D.C., 1994, pp. 141-154.
18. Vega, G. L. and Grundy, S. M., Does measurement of apoB have a place in cholesterol management? *Arteriosclerosis,* 10, 668, 1990.
19. Sniderman, A. D. and Silberberg, J., Is it time to measure apolipoprotein B? *Arteriosclerosis,* 10, 665, 1990.
20. Naito, H. K., The clinical significance of apolipoprotein measurements. *J. Clin. Immunoassay,* 9, 11, 1986.

21. Markovina, S. M., Levine, D. M. and Lippi, G., Lp(a): Structure, measurement and clinical significance, in *Laboratory Measurement of Lipids, Lipoproteins and Apolipoproteins,* Rifai, N. and Warnick, G. R., Eds., American Association for Clinical Chemistry Press, Washington, D.C., 1994, pp. 235-263.
22. Illingworth, D. R., Stein, E. A., Mitchell, Y. B., Dujovne, C. A., Frost, P. H., Knopp, R. H., Tun, P., Zupkis, R. V. and Greguski, R. A., Comparative effects of lovastatin and niacin in primary hypercholesterolemia: A prospective trial, *Arch. Intern. Med.*, 154, 1586, 1994.
23. Dujovne, C. A., Harris, W. S., Gerrond, L. L., Fan, J. and Muzio, F., Comparison of effects of probucol versus vitamin E on *ex vivo* oxidation susceptibility of lipoproteins in hyperlipoproteinemia, *Am. J. Cardiol.*, 74, 38, 1994.
24. Jialal, I. and Scaccini, C., Laboratory assessment of lipoprotein oxidation, in *Laboratory Measurement of Lipids, Lipoproteins and Apolipoproteins,* Rifai, N. and Warnick, G. R., Eds., American Association for Clinical Chemistry Press, Washington, D.C., 1994, pp. 307-321.
25. Harris, W. S., Dujovne, C. A., von Bergmann, K., Neal, J., Akester, J., Windsor, S. L., Greene, D. and Look, Z., Effects of the ACAT inhibitor CL 277,082 on cholesterol metabolism in humans, *Clin. Pharmacol. Ther.,* 48, 189, 1990.
26. Harwood, H. J. J., Chandler, C. E., Pellarin, L. D., Bangerter, F. W., Wilkins, R. W., Long, C. A., Cosgrove, P. G., Malinow, M. R., Marzetta, C. A., Pettini, J. L., Savoy, Y. E. and Mayne, J. T. Pharmacologic consequences of cholesterol absorption inhibition: alteration in cholesterol metabolism and reduction in plasma cholesterol concentration induced by the synthetic saponin b-tigogenin cellobioside (CP-88818; tiqueside), *J. Lipid Res.,* 34, 377, 1993.
27. Crouse, J. R. and Grundy, S. M., Evaluation of a continuous isotope feeding method for measurement of cholesterol absorption in man, *J. Lipid. Res.,* 19, 967, 1978.
28. Meyers, G. L., Cooper, G. L., Henderson, L. O., Hassamer, D. J. and Kimberly, M. M., Standardization of lipid and lipoprotein measurements, in *Laboratory Measurement of Lipids, Lipoproteins and Apolipoproteins*, Rifai, N. and Warnick, G. R., Eds., American Association for Clinical Chemistry Press, Washington, D.C., 1994, pp. 177-205.
29. Multiple Risk Factor Intervention Trial Research Group, Risk factor changes and mortality results, *JAMA*, 248, 1465, 1982.
30. Jackson, B., Dujovne, C. A., DeCoursey, S., Beyer, P., Brown, E. F. and Hassanein, K., Methods to assess relative reliability of diet records: Minimum records for monitoring lipid and caloric intake, *J. Am. Diet. Assoc.*, 86, 1531, 1986.
31. Connor, S. L., Gustafson, J. R., Artaud-Wild, S., M., Classick-Kohn, C. J. and Connor, W. E., The cholesterol-saturated fat index for coronary prevention: Background, use and a comprehensive table of foods, *J. Am. Diet. Assoc.*, 89, 807, 1989.
32. Hunninghake, D. B., Stein, E. A., Dujovne, C. A., Harris, W. S., Feldman, E. B., Miller, V. T., Tobert, J. A., Laskarzewski, P. M., Quiter, E., Held, J., Taylor, A. M., Hopper, S., Leonard, S. B. and Brewer, B. K., The efficacy of intensive dietary therapy alone or combined with lovastatin in outpatients with hypercholesterolemia, *N. Engl. J. Med.*, 328, 1213, 1993.
33. Dujovne, C. A., Eff, J., Ferraro, L., Goldstein, R. J., Gotto, A. M., Hall, W. D., Harris, W. S., Held, S. J., Herd, A., Hunninghake, D. B., Johnson, B. F. and Sztern, M. I., Comparative effects of atenolol vs. celiprolol on serum lipids and blood pressure in hyperlipidemic and hypertensive subjects, *Am. J. Cardiol.,* 72, 1131, 1993.
34. Harris, W. S., Windsor, S. L. and Dujovne, C. A., Effects of four doses of n-3 fatty acids given to hyperlipidemic patients for six months, *J. Am. Coll. Nutr.*, 10, 220, 1991.
35. Locker, P. K., Jungbluth, G. L., Francom, S. F. and Hughes, G. S., for the Lifibrol Study Group, Lifibrol: A novel lipid-lowering drug for the therapy of hypercholesterolemia, *Clin. Pharmacol. Ther.,* 57, 75, 1995.
36. Bay, H. E., Dujovne, C. A. and Lansing, A. M., Drug treatment of dyslipidemias: Practical Guidelines for the primary care physician, *Heart Dis. Stroke*, 1, 357, 1992.
37. Bays, H. E. and Dujovne, C. A., Drugs for treatment of patients with high cholesterol blood levels and other dyslipidemias, in *Progress in Drug Research,* Vol. 43, Jucker, E., Ed., Birkhäuser Verlag, Basel, Switzerland, 1994, pp. 9-41.

Chapter 35

Development of Antidiabetic Therapy Phases I and II

J. Raymond Bratty and Finian Kelly

CONTENTS

1 Introduction 475
2 Biochemistry and Pathology 476
3 Goals of Drug Development 476
4 Preclinical Pharmacology 477
5 Clinical Development of Antidiabetic Drugs 477
5.1 Phase I 477
5.1.1 First Human Exposure 477
5.1.2 Duration of Action Following a Single Dose 478
5.1.3 Interaction with Food 478
5.1.4 Mass Balance Study 478
5.1.5 Initial Repeat-Dose Tolerability Trial 478
5.2 Phase II 478
5.2.1 Dose-Ranging 479
5.2.2 24-h Profile 479
5.2.3 Special Populations (Renal, Hepatic, Elderly) 479
5.2.4 Mode of Action Studies 479
6 Conclusion 480
References 480

1 INTRODUCTION

Diabetes mellitus (Gr. diabetes: siphon, mellitus sweet, original diagnosis polyurea and sweet tasting urine) is a prevalent biochemical derangement where insulin-sensitive cells are relatively deficient in glucose despite a paradoxical abundance of glucose in the plasma. Hyperglycemia is diagnostic[1-4] for the two main forms, namely, insulin-dependent diabetes mellitus (IDDM) and non-insulin-dependent diabetes mellitus (NIDDM). (Table 1) Hyperglycemia is currently the primary target of drug treatment, quantified in risk (for insulin-dependent diabetics, IDDM) by the Diabetes Control and Complication Trial.[5] In this trial 1441 patients with IDDM were randomized to either intensive or conventional insulin treatment. The intensive treatment reduced the adjusted mean risk of retinopathy by 76% in the primary prevention cohort (no baseline retinopathy n = 726) and reduced the average risk of progression by 54% in the secondary intervention cohort (retinopathy at baseline, n = 715), over a mean 6.5 years. Microalbuminuria and clinical neuropathy were also reduced by intensive treatment, which carried a two- to threefold increase in severe hypoglycemia. Intensive treatment reduced glycated hemoglobin by approximately 2% absolute compared to conventional treatment and the mean values for a seven-point blood glucose profile from 12.8 mmol/l to 8.6 mmol/l. There is no reason to believe these results would not apply to patients with noninsulin-dependent diabetes mellitus (NIDDM).[6]

The glucose levels diagnostic of diabetes are expected to give rise to complications[5,7] and the area represented by impaired glucose tolerance (IGT) may carry increased risk of complication or diabetes, though not all subjects with IGT progress to diabetes mellitus.[8-10] Plasma (or blood) glucose conventionally estimated over time by measurement of glycated hemoglobin, usually HbA_{1c}, is therefore the cardinal endpoint for the treatment and prevention of complications in diabetes mellitus.[5]

0-8493-9230-6/97/$0.00+$.50
© 1997 by CRC Press, Inc.

Table 1 Venous Plasma Concentration Diagnostic of Diabetes Mellitus or Impaired Glucose Tolerance (IGT), Fasted or 2 h after a 75-g Glucose Load

	Fasted Glucose		2-h Post Glucose Load
Diabetic	≥7.8 mmol/l	or	≥11.1 mmol/l
IGT	<7.8 mmol/l	and	7.8 to 11.1 mmol/l
"Normal"	<7.8 mmol/l		<7.8 mmol/l

Based on WHO criteria.

2 BIOCHEMISTRY AND PATHOLOGY

Diabetes mellitus is a familial disease with both a genetic component and environmental influence, mainly through diet and exercise. A high incidence of NIDDM on the island of Nauru and among the Pima Indians has provided much of the understanding of the pathogenesis of NIDDM and the literature on it. It is agreed that the evolution of NIDDM requires a deficiency in both insulin secretion and resistance,[11] though there is currently debate about which defect comes first.[11-13]

In animal models of NIDDM there is increased gluconeogenesis from amino acids, decreased conversion of glucose into fatty acids, and preferential use of fat as a substrate rather than glucose, especially by the liver. In man the hepatic glucose output is elevated in NIDDM compared to normals and correlates to the degree of fasting hyperglycemia ($r = 0.847$),[11] though recent advances in estimation of hepatic glucose output suggest a more modest elevation than previously thought.[14] Furthermore, glucose oxidation and storage (as glycogen) are impaired in NIDDM.[11] Nonesterified fatty acids are elevated and contribute toward insulin resistance as measured by the glucose clamp. These derangements and the ensuing complications are or have been targets of (mainly oral) drug development programs.

3 GOALS OF DRUG DEVELOPMENT

Diagnosis of NIDDM is often by chance and 50% of patients already have complications at diagnosis[15] and must therefore have been diabetic for some years previously.

Therapeutic targets therefore include:

1. Earlier diagnosis — random screens or screening of first degree relatives of diabetics.
2. Prevention — measures include treatment of IGT (controversial), treatment of the obese, as obesity is a risk factor for diabetes, or intervention to prevent ß-cell loss in IDDM, e.g., immunosuppressants.
3. Control of glucose metabolism.
   - Insulin-releasing agents, e.g., sulfonylureas, amino acid derivatives, insulinotropin, and "non-sulfonylurea" agents. Most agents will cause hypoglycemia in a proportion of patients but some newer agents such as L-686 398 have the promise of glucose-dependent release of insulin.[16]
   - Insulin sensitizers, e.g., the thiazolidinediones of which troglitazone (CS045) is the most advanced. Some agents in this class have been associated with hematotoxicity and cardiac hypertrophy in animal species.
   - Alpha glucosidase inhibitors, designed to delay postprandial absorption of carbohydrate. Adverse events are mainly gastrointestinal including flatulence.
   - Drugs acting mainly or partly on the liver to reduce hepatic glucose output, e.g., biguanides. The biguanides have been associated with rare but serious lactic acidosis.
   - Drugs which increase energy expenditure, e.g., the $ß_3$-agonists, though inadequate adrenoceptor selectivity with some molecules has led to tremor and heart rate changes.
4. Control of lipid metabolism. Free fatty acids, if elevated, cause increased fatty acid oxidation in the liver and lead to inappropriately elevated hepatic glucose output. Therapeutic maneuvers include attempting to reduce the concentration of plasma free fatty acids or to inhibit hepatic fatty acid oxidation.
5. Prevention of complications:
   - Neuropathy. Aldose reductase inhibitors have been developed to test the hypothesis that the nerve damage is caused by formation of sorbitol from glucose, catalyzed by the enzyme aldose reductase.
   - Aminoguanidine is under investigation to test the hypothesis that retinopathy and nephropathy can be reduced by inhibiting the formation of advanced glycosylation end products, by means other than glucose reduction.

The challenge for the healthcare industry is to effect earlier diagnosis and better treatment of diabetes mellitus before complications become established by screening and improved lowering of blood glucose.

No regulatory guidelines on diabetes currently exist; however, it is clearly worth achieving any reduction in HbA_{1c},[5] but the magnitude required will depend on the adverse event profile of any given agent. One clinically relevant change for a glucose-lowering agent was suggested as 1% HbA_{1c} relative to placebo,[17] though some regulatory agencies currently accept a reduction relative to placebo of 10% baseline HbA_{1c} and Acarbose has just been recommended for U.S. approval with a smaller decrease in glycated hemoglobin. Commercial advantage may be derived from a greater treatment induced reduction in HbA_{1c} than either the regulatory hurdle or established therapy such as sulfonylurea. The DCCT showed that the relationship between the rate of progression of retinopathy and glycated hemoglobin level was a continuum[5] and therefore the use of polypharmacy may be justified to bring glycated hemoglobin as close to normal as possible.

The minimum safety exposure is set down in the ICH guidelines[18] as 1500 patients exposed, 3-600 for 6 months and 100 for 1 year. As this is a chronic treatment, however, some regulatory agencies may ask for considerably more patient exposure to assess safety; early dialog is advisable. As the principal endpoint for a glucose-lowering drug is HbA_{1c}, it follows that dose-ranging studies of minimum 2-3 months duration (to reach the asymptote using this slowly changing endpoint) are required and efficacy trials are currently expected to be of 6 months duration in most territories. Requirements are constantly evolving and historically have usually become more difficult, though placebo-controlled trials of less than 6 months duration may be acceptable.

4 PRECLINICAL PHARMACOLOGY

Many models of diabetes have been investigated, none thus far appears entirely predictive of man and the choice of model is often based on availability and possession of historical in-house data. There are models of NIDDM with various degrees of obesity, hyperinsulinemia and glycemia.[19] In some test models a nonstatistically significant elevation in insulin may masquerade as apparent extrapancreatic activity.

Toxicological class-effects may be evident, e.g., anemia and cardiac hypertrophy with certain thiazolidinediodes,[20,21] liver toxicity, implantation losses in fertility studies with hypoglycemics, or rat thyroid effects with some sulfonylureas.[22] As with any NCE potential target organs must be identified and appropriate clinical measures incorporated into the phase I/II protocols.

The half-life of biosynthetic agents may be greatly reduced in foreign toxicological species if an immune response is mounted, rendering the toxicological data less predictive of man.

5 CLINICAL DEVELOPMENT OF ANTIDIABETIC DRUGS

With such a diversity of mechanisms of action and pathological targets it is only possible to outline a general plan of development with a few personal observations.

5.1 Phase I

The objective is to provide preliminary tolerability, metabolism, and kinetic data in order to set reasonably safe parameters for phase II. If possible, estimations of dose-range, regimen, interaction with food, and theoretical drug interactions should be provided in order to focus the expensive, and necessarily cautious, phase II studies.

5.1.1 First Human Exposure

This is customarily conducted in healthy volunteers but a more difficult decision must be made when developing biosynthetic agents (especially where a host vs. agent reaction is expected) or in the case of immunosuppressives. Adequate toxicological cover is required (in the U.K. this is outside the Medicines Act but ethically the standard required for patients should apply). An ascending-dose, cross-over design in two alternating parallel groups has the advantage of speed and limited individual drug exposure. This may not be a good choice if the dose-response is steep or metabolism variable, as there is then potentially a relatively large within-subject increment in effect. Incorporation of randomized placebo is recommended and preferably blinding of subject and investigator, if different from the study director who may be unblinded for the purpose of safety review.

This design accommodates, say, 8 dose levels allowing a low starting dose, e.g., 1/100 or 1/64 of the no-effect level in the most sensitive species and a conservative incremental regimen.

The upper dose should be set on a case-by-case basis taking into account the animal pharmacology and the no-effect level from the toxicology studies. The design can incorporate an oral glucose tolerance test 2-3 h post-dose when an effect from a single dose might be evident and blood may be collected for glucose and hormones of interest. If the drug produces glucose lowering in healthy volunteers, a dose-response curve should emerge which identifies appropriate doses for further study. Preliminary kinetic profiles will help with selection of regimen and design of future kinetic studies.

5.1.2 Duration of Action Following a Single Dose

If the drug is glucose lowering acutely in volunteers a good indication of duration of effect together with kinetic proportionality may be obtained using doses within the range identified in the first study. This may be fully randomized and properly designed based on the kinetic knowledge obtained in the first study, assuming no safety concern. Subjects may be fasted overnight then for a further 8 or 10 h post-dose. Proportional doses to cover the dose range and placebo are administered and the effect followed. Dynamic-kinetic modeling[23] should confirm the optimal dose-range/regimen (admittedly based on single dose work), may reveal the presence of active metabolite(s) by virtue of an exaggerated anticlockwise hysteresis in a time-sequential plot of parent drug concentration against response, and should help in the interpretation of any unusual kinetic findings.

5.1.3 Interaction with Food

This standard study can be quickly conducted in healthy volunteers but in addition to the effects of food on the pharmaceutical preparation, which usually necessitates a two-way cross-over study, it may be useful to incorporate a placebo (three-way cross-over) to allow dynamic effects on postprandial glucose to be detected. A kinetic interaction or suggestion of a dynamic interaction may indicate further testing in diabetic patients[24-26] where it is probably impractical to administer the drug more than 30 min predose.

5.1.4 Mass Balance Study

Conventionally this is conducted using drug labeled with ^{14}C at a metabolically stable part of the molecule. Information from this study will allow the identification of metabolites, routes of excretion, and appropriateness of the species used in toxicological studies.

Structure-activity relationships may allow the activity of putative metabolites to be estimated prior to synthesis and testing. In the U.K. approval for the administration of radiolabeled material to humans, in addition to ethical and any other approval, is required from ARSAC.[27]

5.1.5 Initial Repeat-Dose Tolerability Trial

It is desirable to establish repeat-dose tolerability in man as early as possible, and this may be conducted in patients or healthy volunteers. The upper doses may be curtailed in a volunteer study due to hypoglycemia, a limited degree being ethically acceptable, and furthermore treatment-related changes in glucose and insulin may paradoxically imply insulin resistance if exogenous insulin or certain insulinotropic drugs are administered to healthy volunteers.[28]

The recruitment of diabetic patients to such a study poses a longer time scale but allows preliminary dose-finding. Patients may be exposed, for example, to several 5-day or 7-day exposures to different treatments on the basis of adequate toxicology under careful assessment. Two or more parallel groups afford a good range of doses/regimens.

This study may incorporate challenge meals or OGTT's and may even include 24-h profiling, but blood volume to be drawn off is likely to be limiting and this relatively simple tolerability study should not be over complicated. In the absence of sample size calculation 6–10 subjects and two on placebo may be adequate on each leg where assessment of tolerability is the main objective.

5.2 Phase II

The program director should now have an understanding of the likely dose range over which his drug will be effective, hopefully has not seen evidence of toxicity, is aware of the half-life, EC_{50}, dynamic/kinetic relationship, and knows whether or not there is a kinetic (and possibly dynamic) food interaction. He will be reassured that the metabolite profile is covered by the toxicological species or is being investigated and will have an inkling about the activity of the human metabolites. In order to rationally develop this drug the minimum effective dose and most suitable regimen will need to be identified. Many drugs have been developed at too high a dose or too optimistic a regimen.[29] Based on the duration of action study, dynamic-kinetic model and kinetic half-life and the patient tolerability study, one or two regimens can be chosen for the formal dose-ranging studies.

Theoretical drug interactions can be identified based on a knowledge of the pharmacology and metabolism. Protein displacement occurs when protein binding is high, the volume of distribution low, and usually is not clinically important if the drug is a base.[30] High renal clearance may indicate the possibility of drug competition for one of the renal excreter systems and interactions at the hepatic level may be investigated by *in vitro* cytochrome P450 work, identification of the P450 subtype involved, and a knowledge of other substrates/inhibitors, e.g., tolbutamide, CYP2C9.

It is well to proceed cautiously at this stage and patients should be as devoid of concomitant disease and drugs as possible, even though this will adversely impact on the recruitment rate.

5.2.1 Dose-Ranging

The relative advantages and disadvantages of titration and parallel group designs are well known;[31,32] a parallel group study is probably best as a baseline run-in and 2-3 months' treatment duration (to estimate HbA_{1c}) are required. The longer the treatment duration and the more severe the patients are on entry, the more difficult will be justification to include placebo. At present, placebo-controlled dose-range studies are possible. If no placebo is incorporated the dose response can be analyzed by Williams' test.[17]

5.2.2 24-h Profile

When an estimate of likely dose and regimen is available a 24-h profile study can be conducted in patients randomized to drug or placebo in a cross-over design. Useful data on 24-h cover will evolve, including hormone data and postprandial effects. Unfortunately, while 24-h glucose AUC is related to HbA_{1c} the 95% confidence intervals are large and formal dose-range studies ideally require HbA_{1c} measurements.

5.2.3 Special Populations (Renal, Hepatic, and Elderly)

Based on metabolic route, appropriate investigation in renally or hepatically impaired subjects should be undertaken. Diabetics have a high prevalence of renal impairment and it will be useful to know the dosing schedule in renally impaired subjects before phase III in order to include as many of these patients as possible in the regulatory submission.

In addition, as NIDDM is a significant disease of the elderly, the ICH guidelines for geriatrics will apply.[33] These guidelines also make comment on the scope and nature of interaction studies and usefulness of kinetic data from young and elderly volunteers.

5.2.4 Mode of Action Studies

In order to understand the new drug and its potential in the market, mode of action studies should commence in phase I/II with the objective of confirming animal pharmacology and developing clinical advantage.

1. Whole body insulin sensitivity — The hyperinsulinemic euglycemic clamp technique[34] is useful in estimating the change in insulin sensitivity following treatment with a pharmaceutical agent. An insulin releaser may induce, despite the high prevailing insulin level, endogenous release of insulin which will flaw the study. This may be detected by measurement of C-peptide and overcome by the addition of a somatostatin infusion. One difficulty is that the degree of insulin resistance is affected by changes in the ambient glucose level,[35,36] and indirect effects may be measured where plasma glucose reduction has occurred. One approach for an insulin releaser is to conduct the trial in C-peptide negative (following a test glucagon or meal stimulus) IDDM patients. In patients responding to drug the clamped glucose values should preferably be isoglycemic within subject, obtained if necessary by overnight equilibration or by "gating." Other less direct methods of assessing insulin sensitivity are available.[37]
2. Pancreatic response to glucose — The hyperglycemic clamp technique[34] demonstrates first and second phase insulin response to glucose *in vivo*. First and second phase responses are characteristically diminished in NIDDM but may be restored by drugs or an improvement in the glucose milieu.[38,39]
3. Liver metabolism — New data indicates that earlier studies overestimated suppression of hepatic glucose production due to tracer nonsteady state.[14,40] The assumptions for tracer studies and implication of the position of the label on tracer recycling should be considered.[41] Real time correction for enrichment appears highly desirable, but necessitates use of a radioactive method and appropriate ethical consideration and license (in U.K. by ARSAC[27]). Gluconeogenesis may be followed by using labeled precursors e.g., alanine or glycerol. Adequate time (e.g., 10 h) must be allowed to achieve steady state.[41]

4. Muscle metabolism — If the clamp studies indicate an improvement in glucose disposal, muscle biopsy or nuclear magnetic resonance may be used to investigate glycogen synthesis[42,43] or GLUT4 transporter activity. Cannulation of forearm artery and vein allows estimation of metabolite flux and extraction through forearm skeletal muscle.[44]
5. Fat metabolism — Metabolite flux across human subcutaneous adipose tissue may be investigated by cannulation of a superficial vein on the arterior abdominal wall and venous sampling, for example, during exercise[45] or periprandially.[46]

6 CONCLUSION

At the end of phase II it is possible, if development is straightforward, to establish efficacy to the satisfaction of the program director, choose a dose-range and regimen, have most of the kinetics available, and possibly define the clinical/marketing advantage.

NOTE ADDED IN PROOF

For a review of new agents to combat hyperglycemia, see Bailey CJ, Flatt PR, Development of Anti-diabetic Drugs, in *Drugs, Diet and Disease,* Vol. 2, Eds., Ioannides C, Flatt PR, Prentice Hall, Hemel Hempstead, 1996, pp. 281-326.

REFERENCES

1. National Diabetes Data Group. Classification and diagnosis of diabetes mellitus and other categories of glucose intolerance. *Diabetes* 1979;28:1039-57.
2. World Health Organisation Study Group. Diabetes Mellitus. Technical Report series 727 Geneva WHO 1985.
3. Harris MI, Hadden WC, Knowler WC, Bennett PH. International Criteria for the diagnosis of diabetes and impaired glucose tolerance. *Diabetes Care* 1985;8:562-7.
4. Modan M, Harris MI, Halkin H. Evaluation of World Health Organisation and National Diabetes Data Group Criteria for impaired glucose tolerance: results from two national samples. *Diabetes* 1989;38:1630-5.
5. DCCT Research Group. The effect of intensive treatment of diabetes on the development and progression of long-term complications in insulin-dependent diabetes mellitus. *N. Engl. J. Med.* 1993;329:977-86.
6. American Diabetes Association. Implications of the diabetes control and complications trial. *Diabetes Care* 1993; 16:1517-1520.
7. Jarrett RJ, Keen H. Hyperglycaemia and diabetes mellitus. *Lancet* 1976;1009-12.
8. Pettitt DJ, Knowler, WC, Lisse JR, Bennett, PH. Development of retinopathy and proteinuria in relation to plasma glucose concentration in Pima Indians. *Lancet* 1980;1050-1052.
9. Eriksson KF, Lindgarde F. Impaired glucose tolerance in a middle-aged male urban population: a new approach for identifying high-risk cases. *Diabetologia* 1990;33:526-31.
10. Jarrett RJ, Keen H, Fuller JH, McCartney M. Worsening to diabetes in men with impaired glucose tolerance ("borderline diabetes"). *Diabetologia* 1979;16:25-30.
11. De Fronzo RA, Bonadonna RC, Ferrannini E. Pathogenesis of NIDDM: A balanced overview. *Diabetes Care* 1992;15:318-368.
12. Vaag A, Henriksen JE, Beck-Nielsen H. Decreased insulin activation of glycogen synthase in skeletal muscles in young non-obese Caucasian first-degree relatives of patients with noninsulin-dependent diabetes mellitus. *J. Clin. Invest.* 1992;89:782-788.
13. O'Rahilly S, Hattersley A, Vaag A, Gray H. Insulin resistance as the major cause of impaired glucose tolerance: a self-fulfilling prophesy? *Lancet* 1994;344:585-589.
14. Jeng C-Y, Sheu WH-H, Fuh M M-T, Chen Y-D I, Reaven GM. Relationship between hepatic glucose production and fasting plasma glucose concentration in patients with NIDDM. *Diabetes* 1994;43:1440-1444.
15. United Kingdom Prospective Diabetes Study VI. Complications in newly diagnosed Type 2 diabetic patients and their association with different clinical and biochemical risk factors. *Diabetes Res.* 1990;13:1-11.
16. Leibowitz et al. A novel insulin secretagogue is a phosphodiesterase inhibitor. *Diabetes* 1995;44:67-74.
17. Gueriguian JL. (Executive Secretary) September 23-24 1991. Meeting of the Endocrinologic and Metabolic Drugs Advisory Committee, FDA, Rockville, MD.
18. The extent of population exposure to assess clinical safety, ICH Guideline III/5084/94.
19. Bailey CJ, Flatt PR. Models for testing new hypoglycaemic drugs, in *New Antidiabetic Drugs,* Eds. Bailey and Flatt (1990), Smith-Gordon and Company Ltd IBSN 1-85463-017-2.
20. Deldar A, Williams G, Stevens, C. Pathogenesis of thiazolidinedione induced haematotoxicity in the dog. *Diabetes* (1993); 42 (Suppl.1):A179, P57A.

21. Williams GD, Deldar A, Jordan WH, Gries C, Long GG, Dimarchi RD. Subchronic toxicity of the thiazolidinedione, Tanabe-174, in rat and dog. *Diabetes* (1993); 42 (Suppl. 1):A186, P59A.
22. Atterwill CK, Jones C and Brown CG. Thyroid gland II — Mechanisms of species-dependent thyroid toxicity, hyperplasia and neoplasia induced by xenobiotics. In *Endocrine Toxicology,* Eds Atterwill CK, Flack JD, P137-182, Cambridge University Press, New York, 1992, ISBN: 0 521 40225 5.
23. Byron WD, Rotherham NE, Bratty JR. Relationship between hypoglycemia response and plasma concentration of BTS 67 582 in healthy volunteers. *Br. J. Clin. Pharmacol.* 1994;38:433-439.
24. Sartor G, Lundquist I, Melander A, Schersten B, Wahlin-Boll E. Improved effect of glibenclamide on administration before breakfast. *Eur. J. Clin. Pharmacol.* 1982;21:403-408.
25. Wahlin-Boll E, Melander A, Sartor G, Schersten B. Influence of food intake on the absorption and effect of glipizide in diabetics and in healthy subjects. *Eur. J. Clin. Pharmacol.* 1980;18:279-283.
26. Samanta A, Jones GR, Burden AC, Shakir I. Improved effect of tolbutamide when given before food in patients on long-term therapy. *Br. J. Clin. Pharmacol.* 1984;18:647-8.
27. Administration of Radioactive Substances Advisory Committee (ARSAC). Notes for guidance on the administration of radioactive substances to persons for purposes of diagnosis, treatment or research, 1993 ARSAC Secretariat, Department of Health 80-94 Eileen House, Newington Causeway, London SE1 6EF.
28. Godfried MH, Romijn JA, Endert E, Sauerwein HP. Metabolic effects of hypoglycaemic counterregulation during sustained mild hyperinsulinaemia and constant glucose availability in healthy men. *Nutrition* 1994;10:5-10.
29. Shah RR. Clinical pharmacokinetics: current requirements and future perspectives from a regulatory point of view. *Xenobiotica* 1993;23:1159-1193.
30. Stockley IH. *Drug Interactions: A Source Book of Adverse Interactions, Their Mechanisms, Clinical Importance and Management.* Blackwell Scientific Publications, Oxford, ISBN 0-632-03721-0.
31. Dose-response information to support drug registration, ICH Guideline III/3376/93.
32. Sheiner LB, Beal SL, Sambol NC. Study designs for dose-ranging. *Clin. Pharmacol. Ther.* (1989); 46:63-77.
33. Studies in support of special populations: *Geriatrics,* ICH Guideline III/3388/93.
34. De Fronzo RA, Tobin JD, Andres R. Glucose clamp technique, a method for quantifying insulin secretion and resistance. *Am. J. Physiol.* 1979;237:E214-223.
35. Andrews WJ, Vasquez B, Nagulesparen M, Klimes I, Foley J, Unger R, Reaven GM. Insulin therapy in obese, noninsulin-dependent diabetes induces improvements in insulin action and secretion that are maintained for 2 weeks after insulin withdrawal. *Diabetes* (1984); 33:634-642.
36. Firth RG, Bell PM, Rizza RA. Effects of tolazamide and exogenous insulin on insulin action in patients with noninsulin-dependent diabetes mellitus. *N. Engl. J. Med.* 1986; 314:1280-6.
37. Fulcher GR, Walker M, Alberti KGMM. The assessment of insulin action *in vivo. International Textbook of Diabetes Mellitus,* Eds. Alberti KGMM, De Fronzo RA, Keen H, Zinimet P., John Wiley & Sons, New York, 1992.
38. Henry RR, Wallace P, Olefsky JM. Effects of weight loss on mechanisms of hyperglycaemia in obese noninsulin-dependent diabetes mellitus. *Diabetes* 1986; 35:990-98.
39. Ferner RE, Rawlins MD, Alberti KGMM. Impaired beta-cell responses improve when fasting blood glucose concentration is reduced in noninsulin-dependent diabetes. *Q. J. Med.* (1988); 66:137-146.
40. Hother-Neilsen O, Hendriksen JE. Insulin dose-response effect on glucose turnover rates in man. Re-evaluation using labeled glucose infusates for constant plasma specific activity. *Diabetes* 1994; 43 (Suppl) A158, P50A.
41. Wolfe RR. *Glucose Metabolism in Radioactive and Stable Isotope Tracers in Biomedicine: Principles and Practice of Kinetic Analysis.* Wiley-Liss, New York, 1992.
42. Rothman DL, Shulman RG, Shulman GI. NMR studies of muscle glycogen synthesis in normal and noninsulin dependent diabetic subjects. *Biochem. Soc. Trans.* 1991;19:992-994.
43. Rothman DL, Shulman RG, Shulman GI. ^{31}P Nuclear magnetic resonance measurements of muscle glucose–6–phosphate. *J. Clin. Invest.* 1992;89:1069-1075.
44. Walker M, Fulcher GR, Catalano C, Petranyl G, Orskov H, Alberti KGMM. Physiological levels of plasma non-esterified fatty acids impair forearm glucose uptake in normal man. *Clin. Sci.* 1990;79:167-174.
45. Hodgetts V, Coppack SW, Frayn KN, Hockaday TDR. Factors controlling fat mobilisation from human subcutaneous adipose tissue during exercise. *J. Appl. Physiol.* (1991); 71: 445-451.
46. Frayn KN, Coppack SW, Humphreys SM, Clark ML, Evans RD. Periprandial regulations of lipid metabolism in insulin treated diabetes mellitus. *Metabolism* (1993); 42:504-10.

Part XII. Assessment of the Effects of Chemotherapeutic Agents

Chapter 36

Antibiotic Development

André Bryskier

CONTENTS

1 Introduction 486
2 Preselection 486
3 Essential Documentation 487
3.1 Use of the Compound 488
3.2 Data Required to Begin Phase I and II Trials 490
3.2.1 Microbiological Assays — HPLC 490
3.2.2 Regression Lines 490
3.2.3 Reference Strains 491
4 "Core" Dossier 491
4.1 Common Pathogens 492
4.1.1 Gram-Positive Cocci 492
4.1.1.1 *Staphylococcus aureus* 492
4.1.1.2 Coagulase-Negative Staphylococci 493
4.1.1.3 *Streptococcus pneumoniae* 493
4.1.1.4 *Streptococcus* spp. 493
4.1.1.5 *Enterococcus* spp. 493
4.1.1.6 Other Gram-Positive Cocci 493
4.1.2 Gram-Positive Bacilli 493
4.1.3 Gram-Negative Cocci 494
4.1.3.1 *Neisseria meningitidis* 494
4.1.3.2 *Neisseria gonorrhoeae* 494
4.1.4 Gram-Negative Bacilli 494
4.1.4.1 Enterobacteriaceae 494
4.1.4.2 *Pseudomonas aeruginosa* and Other Species 494
4.1.4.3 Other Gram-Negative Bacilli 495
4.1.5 Anaerobes 497
4.2 Other Microorganisms 497
4.2.1 *Helicobacter pylori* 497
4.2.2 *Campylobacter* spp. 497
4.2.3 *Borrelia* spp. 497
4.2.4 *Treponema pallidum* 498
4.2.5 *Mycoplasma* spp. and *Ureaplasma* spp. 498
4.2.6 *Nocardia* spp. 498
4.2.7 *Leptospira* spp. 498
4.3 Intracellular Pathogens 499
4.4 Mycobacteria 499
4.4.1 *Mycobacterium tuberculosis* 499
4.4.2 Atypical Mycobacteria 499
4.4.3 *Mycobacterium leprae* 499
5 Animal Models 500
5.1 Nondiscriminatory Models 500
5.2 Discriminative Models 500
6 Specific Indications 500
7 Mechanisms of Action and Resistance 500
8 Interaction with Fecal and Oral Flora 501

0-8493-9230-6/97/$0.00+$.50
© 1997 by CRC Press, Inc.

9 Clinical Microbiology and Phases I and II: Determining the Dose 501
9.1 Phase II Trials 501
9.2 CSF Activity 501
9.3 Pharmacodynamics 501
9.3.1 Concentration-Dependent Drugs 502
9.3.1.1 Fluoroquinolones 502
9.3.1.2 Aminoglycosides 502
9.3.2 Time-Dependent Drugs 502
9.3.3. Pharmacodynamic Models Simulating Human Pharmacokinetics 502
10 Place of Clinical Microbiology During Phase II and II Trials 503
10.1 Pathological Specimens 503
10.2 Determination of Antibacterial Activity 503
10.3 Antibiophenotype 504
10.4 Centralizing the Test 504
10.5 Inhibition Zone Diameter/MIC Correlations 504
11 Epidemiology of Resistance — A Survey 504
12 Automated System 506
13 Conclusion 506
References 507

1 INTRODUCTION

The life of an antibiotic is made up of a complex series of events which begin with its design and continue well after its release onto the market.

The design of an antibiotic is the first important event; it results from the chemist's wish to create a new chemical entity from a known series of compounds or to detect and isolate antibacterial activity in the fermentation broth of selected bacterial or fungal strains, and finally to modify the molecular structure. A further possibility is full synthesis of a new chemical entity based on state-of-the-art scientific know-how and creativity. Among the more recent examples are the penems, which were conceived in 1976 by Woodward and which are chemical hybrids between penams and cephems. Preselected compounds must pass the essential hurdle of toxicological testing. If the results are compatible with clinical development, microbiological studies will determine suitability for phase I then phase II trials. In parallel with clinical development, experimental work is undertaken to establish the specific pharmacology dossier which will be the new compound's microbiological "identity card." Further experimental studies will be necessary to determine the optimal conditions of use, e.g., adaptation to automats for determining antimicrobial susceptibility. Research on antibacterial activity must not stop after the license application has been filed, and much importance must be given to post-marketing epidemiological surveys and the search for new indications. The latter may arise with the onset of new epidemiological situations; one example is the demonstration of the differential activity of 2-amino-5-thiazolyl cephalosporins on strains of *Streptococcus pneumoniae* resistant to penicillin G (Table 1).

Antibiotic development remains a complex process. Antibiotics are drugs which help in restoring the equilibrium between invading bacteria and the host defense system. Unlike the situation in other therapeutic fields, drugs used to combat infectious diseases are directed against an external agent, i.e., the bacterial pathogen. As a result, the preselection step will be based on antibacterial performance *in vitro* and *in vivo*. Determining antibacterial activity is the cornerstone of development. Guidelines can aid clinical development (Beam et al., 1992, 1993), but, with the exception of specific prerequisites for the different pathological settings, there are no guidelines for the microbiological development of an antibacterial agent.

2 PRESELECTION

A future antibacterial agent is simply one compound in a series of compounds prepared by chemists. Preselection is a crucial step in the life of a new drug. Once a compound has been synthesized, its activity *in vitro* is determined on a panel of strains containing selected bacterial genera and species. The choice of this panel is a complex affair. It is the result of a compromise between the design requirements established for the new research project and a systematic analysis of the activity of all new antibacterial

Table 1 *In Vitro* Activities of Cephems Against *Streptococcus pneumoniae*

	Pen-S (MIC < 0.12 mg/l)		Pen-I (MIC 0.12-≤ 1.0 mg/l)		Pen-R (MIC > 1.0 mg/l)	
	MIC_{50}	MIC_{90}	MIC_{50}	MIC_{90}	MIC_{50}	MIC_{90}
Cefotaxime	0.03	0.03	0.25	1.0	1.0	2.0
Ceftriaxone	0.03	0.03	0.25	1.0	1.0	2.0
Cefpirome	0.01	0.03	0.12	0.5	0.5	1.0
Ceftazidime	0.25	0.25	2.0	16.0	16.0	16.0
Cefodizime	0.03	0.03	0.5	2.0	2.0	4.0
Cefclidin	0.25	0.5	1	4	8	8
Cefozopran	0.03	0.06	0.25	1	2	2
Cefluprenam	0.03	0.03	0.25	1	1	1
Cefepime	0.03	0.03	0.25	1	1	2
Cefoselis*	0.03	0.125	0.125	0.5	1	1
Ceftizoxime	0.06	0.06	0.5	8.0	16.0	16.0

Data taken from Frémaux A et al., 1992, 1995 and Spangler et al., 1994.

entities against common pathogens. The panel can be particularly difficult to establish when the aim is to extend the "natural" activity of a chemical family to other bacterial genera. The classical example is the macrolides. Currently, the aim of research on new macrolides is to increase antibacterial activity for naturally susceptible species, but also to counter cross-resistance to erythromycin and to extend the activity to strains resistant to erythromycin such as *S. pneumoniae.* The ketolides are one example of the results of this research (Agouridas et al., 1994).

The panel is also difficult to establish when testing a new chemical entity. A recent example is daptomycin, a lipopeptide, the antibacterial spectrum of which essentially covers Gram-positive cocci and bacilli.

The choice of strains with different antibiophenotypes, and that of comparator compounds, is also critical, as it will determine the early life of the new compound.

Activity *in vivo* determines the next step, which consists of testing the efficacy of preselected compounds in nonspecific experimental models of infection when administered by the parenteral (subcutaneous or intraperitoneal) or oral route (Table 2).

Table 2 *In Vitro* and *In Vivo* Comparative Activities of Erythromycin and Roxithromycin

	Compounds	MIC (mg/l)	PD_{50} (mg/kg)	PD_{50}ery/ PD_{50} roxi
S. aureus Giorgio	Erythromycin	0.3	120	3.2
	Roxithromycin	0.6	37	
S. pneumoniae I	Erythromycin	0.02	375	5.6
	Roxithromycin	0.04	67	

From Chantol J-F, Bryskier A, Gasc J-C, *J. Antibiotics* 1986, 39, 660-668. With permission.

The work done during the preselection phase will lead to the selection of candidates for clinical development. This is mainly based on *in vitro* and *in vivo* activity, but also on the toxicology of the different compounds. Certain preselected compounds more active than the final selected candidate may not be chosen because of their toxicity. The selection process is aimed at choosing the compound with the best and most well-balanced antibacterial spectrum and the best safety profile in animals (Table 3). After the selection phase, the third step is microbiological development, a prerequisite for clinical development.

3 ESSENTIAL DOCUMENTATION

The documentation process is composed of two parts: the first consists of gathering the information required for microbiological tests and the second enables clinical studies to begin.

Table 3 *In Vivo* Activities of Roxithromycin Derivatives

	MIC (mg/l)	ED_{50} (mg/kg) *S. aureus* infection	ED_{50} (mg/kg) Streptococcus infection
Roxithromycin	0.296	3.84	2.3
RU 29065	0.126	2.36	20
RU 29702	0.118	1.55	12
Erythromycin	0.151	1	1

From Gasc J-C, Gouin d'Ambrière S, Lutz A, Chantol J-F, *J. Antibiotics* 1991, 44, 651-668. With permission.

3.1 Use of the Compound

The data acquired during this phase are essential for beginning experimental work and for establishing the microbiological part of the license application dossier.

The following physical and chemical properties are essential.

Physical and chemical properties:

- Solubility of the compound in water and the different solvents used in microbiology
- If the compound is poorly soluble or insoluble in water, the mode of dissolution must be mentioned on the instruction form for the experimenters
- Interactions with calcium, zinc, and magnesium
- Need for certain growth factors in the culture medium

The *in vitro* activity of cephalosporins containing a catechol moiety differs according to whether or not the culture medium contains excess iron. The compounds will be tested on a medium containing 2,2′-dipyrridyl, which depletes the medium of iron (≤50 g/l), and on iron-rich medium (600-2400 μg/l instead of 250-300 μg/l). The activity of mupirocine can be modified by the addition of blood when the medium contains isoleucine. Fosfomycin MICs are determined on Mueller Hinton medium containing 25 mg/l of glucose-6-phosphate. The antibiotic disks are loaded with 25 μg of glucose-6-phosphate (5 μg of fosfomycin) (Andrews et al., 1983). Sulfonamides and benzylpyrimidines (trimethoprim and brodimoprime) must be tested on a medium poor in thymidine. It is possible to use thymidine-phosphorylase (0.025-0.1 U/ml of medium) or simply to add 5% of lysed horse erythrocytes to Mueller Hinton medium. MICs of cefuroxime, ceftizoxime, cefotaxime, cefmenoxime, and ceftriaxone varied markedly with both commercial brand and blood content of the broth used to culture *Enteroccocus faecalis*. The use of Mueller Hinton broths supplemented with 5% lysed sheep blood frequently resulted in MICs that are ≥16 times lower than the MICs obtained with these same broths without blood (Sahm et al., 1984).

- Influence of the culture medium on minimal inhibitory concentrations. Mueller Hinton medium obtained from the same manufacturer (batch) or different manufacturers can give rise to different bacterial growth, leading to false results; hence the need to follow the M-23 recommendations of the NCCLS committee of the American Society for Microbiology (1993). The quality of Iso-Sensitest medium has been called into doubt for the determination of aminoglycoside activity, owing to a lack of standardization (King et al., 1993). Carbapenem susceptibility of *Pseudomonas aeruginosa* has been shown to increase in low basic amino acid media (Fukuoka et al., 1991). Basis amino acids such as L-lysine competitively inhibit carbapenem permeation through the OrpD channel to the periplasm in *P. aeruginosa* by binding to a site in the OrpD channel (Trias et al., 1990).
- Stability of the compound in culture medium with time and at different temperatures and pH values. For example, ansamycin activity on *Mycobacterium tuberculosis* diminishes with time in PBS and medium 7 H9 (Table 4).

It is thus best to test antibiotic stability in the culture medium before determining antibacterial activity.

The factors influencing bacterial growth must also be determined. This is not essential during the first phase of development, but is required information in the license dossier. The effect of different inocula on MIC values must also be tested. The best example is the cephalosporins (Eng et al., 1985). The increase in the MIC value reflects stability to hydrolysis by ß-lactamases (Table 5).

Similarly, certain compounds become less bactericidal as the inoculum increases. The bactericidal activity of the fluoroquinolones falls at bacterial inoculum above 10^8 CFU/ml and they become bacteriostatic above an inoculum of 10^{10} CFU/ml (Smith et al., 1988). A certain number of microorganisms require an atmosphere enriched in CO_2 for growth, but CO_2 influences antibacterial activity by modifying

Table 4 Ansamycin Stability in 7 H9 Broth Medium with and without Tween 80 (0.05% v/v-37°C, Solution 1mg/l)

		Ansamycin Concentrations in Broth Medium (mg/l)		
		Day 0	Day 2	Day 7
	Tween 80 +	0.8	0.88	0.22
Rifampicin	Tween 80 –	0.8	0.70	0.44
	PBS	0.8	0.82	0.42
	Tween 80 +	0.68	0.03	0
FCE 22807	Tween 80 –	0.69	0.35	0.16
	PBS	0.85	0.34	0.21
	Tween 80 +	0.80	0.06	0
FCE 22250	Tween 80 –	0.84	0.40	0.18
	PBS	0.94	0.61	0.19
	Tween 80 +	0.70	0	0
SPA-S-565	Tween 80 –	0.90	0.46	0.13
	PBS	0.80	0.45	0.07

From Dickinson JM, Mitchison DA, *Tubercle* 1990, 71, 109-115. With permission.

Table 5 Parenteral Cephems: *In Vitro* Inculum Effects

	E. coli		S. typhimurium		K. pneumoniae	
(CFU/ml)	5×10^5	5×10^7	5×10^5	5×10^7	5×10^5	5×10^7
Cefotaxime	0.06	0.5	0.06	0.5	0.06	0.5
Ceftriaxone	0.06	1.0	0.5	4.0	0.25	4.0
Ceftazidime	0.12	8.0	0.5	16.0	0.12	8.0
Cefoperazone	0.25	8.0	1.0	32	0.12	8.0

From Eng RHK, Cherubin C, Smith SM, Buccini F, *Antimicrob. Agents Chemother.* 1985, 28, 601-606. With permission.

the pH of the culture medium. The best example is the macrolides (Felmingham et al., 1987; Siebor et al., 1993). The pH of the medium can also directly modify the activity of a compound. Fluoroquinolones which possess a piperazine ring in position 7 are less active in acid medium than in alkaline medium. In contrast, compounds which do not have substituents in position 7 are more active in acid than alkaline medium (anionic compounds; Bryskier et al., 1994).

The presence of horse serum in the culture medium is often necessary for bacterial growth. It is essential to check that the MIC values do not vary. Klugman et al. (1994) have shown that the addition of horse serum to Mueller Hinton medium does not significantly modify the activity of 2-amino-5-thiazolyl cephalosporins on *S. pneumoniae* (Table 6). It is possible to use these enriched media to determine the MICs of the different cephalosporins, regardless of the strain of *S. pneumoniae*. The effect of human serum on the activity of a new agent could be evaluated employing pooled normal human serum combined with Mueller Hinton medium to yield 50% final concentration.

The problem of activity in the presence of serum has been studied in detail with daptomycin (Lee et al., 1991). Indeed, this compound is very active *in vitro* on *E. faecalis*, but in therapeutic use at the recommended doses it is only moderately active, owing to strong binding to plasma proteins. It is not essential to test antibacterial activity in the presence of human serum for the licensing dossier, or for a knowledge of the basic characteristics of the compound. Indeed, the level of specific proteins (antibodies, complement, etc.) and nonspecific proteins (serum albumin, α_1-glycoprotein, etc.) varies from one individual to the next. In addition, the reactivity of serum, even when pooled, is difficult to standardize. As a result, the analysis of experimental results is complex. As for the fluoroquinolones, their stability and antibacterial activity must be determined in urine (Table 7), and is generally reduced in function of the urinary pH.

Table 6 Effect of Addition in the Growth Medium of 50% Horse Serum on ß-Lactams Activities

	MIC_{50} (mg/l)	
	Medium Without Serum	**Medium + 50% Horse Serum**
Penicillin G	0.015	0.03
Cefpirome	0.03	0.03
Cefotaxime	0.015	0.03
Ceftriaxone	0.015	0.03
Ceftazidime	0.03	0.5
Cefodizime	0.06	0.12
Cefepime	0.03	0.015

From Klugman KP, Saunders J, 6th Int. Congr. Infect. Dis. Prague, 1994. With permission.

Table 7

	MIC (mg/l) Geometric Means		
	Urine pH 5.8	**Urine pH 6.8**	**Mueller Hinton Broth pH 7.4**
Norfloxacin	5.2	3.9	0.083
Ofloxacin	2.9	0.9	0.69

From Chantot JF, Bryskier A, *J. Antimicrob. Chemother.*, 1985, 16, 475-484. With permission.

3.2 Data Required to Begin Phase I and II Trials

3.2.1 Microbiological Assays — HPLC

The choice of culture medium, pH, and test strain is crucial for the future development of the compound. The method must be sufficiently sensitive (large inhibition zone relative to the standard curves) and reproducible. The test strain must belong to a reference collection or, in the case of a new strain, be registered with a national collection for easy access. A chemical assay method, such as HPLC, must also be developed, and a good correlation must be obtained between microbiological and chemical methods.

3.2.2 Regression Lines

Before beginning phase II clinical trials it is essential to supply clinical microbiology laboratories with *in vitro* recommendations. In practice, this means determining the antimicrobial susceptibility of the strain responsible for the infection with an agar diffusion method (antibiogram). This is done in the majority of hospital laboratories by means of a qualitative method based on inhibition zone diameters around a disk loaded with a known amount of antibacterial agent. However, difficulties arise because the diameter of the paper disk can vary according to the country, e.g., 6 mm in Europe and 9 mm in Japan. The amount of active substance contained on the disk can also vary from one country to another. For example, in the majority of European countries and the U.S., disks of the new oral cephalosporins such as cefpodoxime are loaded with 10 µg, whereas in Germany they are loaded with 30 µg. This makes it difficult to interpret German epidemiological data.

The regression line is different in France (SFM; Soussy et al., 1994), Germany (DIN, 1984), the U.K. (BSAC, 1991), Sweden (Ericsson et al., 1971; Swedish reference group, 1981), The Netherlands (WRG, 1981), the U.S. (NCCLS, 1993) and Japan (1984). In general the BSAC and DIN systems recommend lower breakpoints than those of the SFM and NCCLS committees. However, this is not always true, particularly for the fluoroquinolones, for which the SFM breakpoints are 1-4 mg/l and those of the BSAC 2-8 mg/l. In Europe there have been attempts at harmonization, which have given rise to consensus breakpoints (TCB; Baquero, 1990; Williams, 1990).

In the U.K., microbiologists use the method of Joan Stokes (1954, 1993), which compares the inhibition zones between the edge of the paper disk and the edge of the growth zone of a reference strain and the clinical isolate on the same plate. The radius is the difference between these two zones and, depending on its size, it is possible to determine if an antibiotic is active, moderately active, or inactive (Table 8).

Table 8 Levofloxacin Radius, J. Stokes Method

	Radius (mm)	
	S. aureus NCTC 6571	*E. coli* NCTC 10418
Susceptible	≥7	≥9
Intermediately-S	>3 – <7	>3 – <9
Resistant	≤3	≤3

From Felmingham D, Grüneberg RN, Personal communication, 1994.

3.2.3 Reference Strains

It is essential to test the antibiotic against reference strains for reasons of quality control. Currently, there is a "nomenclature jungle," with ATCC (U.S.) and NCTC (U.K.) often covering the same strains. In the U.S., quality assurance is well standardized. The inhibition zone diameters and MIC values for reference strains are submitted to the NCCLS committee of the American Society for Microbiology. After acceptatance, they are officially published by the committee.

The "classical" strains of *Escherichia coli, P. aeruginosa,* or *S. aureus* pose no problem, but the interpretation of values for *Haemophilus influenzae, S. pneumoniae,* or *Neisseria gonorrhoeae* is more delicate. As regards anaerobes, there is currently no consensus within the NCCLS committee, but discussions are ongoing. According to the recommendations of document M-23 of the NCCLS committee, the activity of the new antibacterial agent must be tested with five batches of culture medium from two manufacturers, and a reference batch of Mueller Hinton medium. The activity on each reference strain must be tested 20 times. Two batches of disks must be tested, and a minimun of five laboratories must participate.

4 "CORE" DOSSIER

These microbiological data are an important part of the European toxicology-pharmacology expert report in the license application dossier for the new antibacterial agent. It involves determining the antibacterial spectrum and activity of the compound. Whatever the compound, a knowledge of its intrinsic activity is required, in terms of bacteriostatic (MIC) and bactericidal (MBC) activities. Against common pathogens, the compound must be tested on a sufficient number of strains (about 100) to determine the MIC_{50} and MIC_{90} values.

In addition, several centers in different regions must be involved. Three types of strain can be tested: reference strains to identify possible resistance mechanisms, collection strains from a laboratory having participated in other studies and serving as a reference, and freshly isolated clinical strains.

All authors publishing MIC data have to define their method of calculating MIC_{50}. MIC_{50} can be calculated in at least two different ways. The first method is to assemble all data into an "orderly" array and to select the median value as MIC_{50}. The second method is to accumulate data and then determine MIC_{50} by interpolation from graph of accumulated percent strains inhibited vs. MIC (Reed et al., 1938, Hamilton-Miller, 1977; Finland et al., 1976). Davies (1990), in a theoretical model, has shown that traditional MIC_{50}, MIC_{75}, and MIC_{90} values have poor discrimination. He stressed that in comparative clinical trials, geometric mean MIC values are a better parameter for assessing whether one agent performed better than another. The MIC_{50} reflects the intrinsic activity of the compound and it is this which establishes the spectrum and activity of the compound, whereas the MIC_{90} only reflects the different resistance mechanisms and depends on the center and the way in which the strains are collected.

To determine the intrinsic value of a compound, it is essential that it is tested on the different bacterial species composing a genus, and also on a panel of isolates with resistance antibiophenotypes. King et al. (1995) pointed out that partial MICs reports such as ≤ or > designations should be discouraged for new agents, because this leaves us ignorant of the true activity of a new compound.

It is also essential to determine the antibacterial activity of the potential metabolites of the antibacterial agent. When a metabolite is active and accounts for an important part of the drug kinetics, the parent compound and its metabolite must be tested together to ensure that there is no antagonism (e.g., clarithromycin and 14-OH clarithromycin).

4.1 Common Pathogens

The bacterial species and genera are divided into four groups depending on their morphology and Gram staining.

4.1.1 Gram-Positive Cocci

4.1.1.1 Staphylococcus aureus

A distinction is generally made between *S. aureus* strains which produce penicillinases and those which are resistant to methicillin. Staphylococcal ß-lactamases have been classified immunologically into types A, B, C, and D (Rosdahl, 1973). Type A and C are commonly found in hospital isolates while strains producing the type B enzyme, with less hydrolytic activity toward penicillin G, are isolated less frequently. The type D enzyme seems to be rare (Kernodle et al., 1990).

Strains which produce a penicillinase account for more than 80% of isolates in some areas. When testing a new antibacterial agent on these phenotypes, it is important to have a panel of strains possessing the four enzymes A, B, C, and D. Cephalothin is more stable to penicillinase A hydrolysis than cefazolin. Other antistaphylococcal agents must be tested in comparison, such as fusidic acid, which is a good marker of type D penicillinase.

When seeking to demonstrate the activity of a new chemical entity on strains resistant to methicillin, one must use strains belonging to the four classes described by Tomasz et al. (1991) and strains with the MODSA phenotype. The results which lead to BORSA phenotype remain unclear.

Jabès et al. (1993) clearly showed the differential activity of penems and carbapenems depending on the class of staphylococcal strain (Table 9). These compounds are apparently active on classes 1 and 2, but totally inactive on classes 3 and 4. Moreover, it is recommended to test the *in vitro* activity of the compounds with agar trypicase-soy medium containing 2% NaCl. The inoculum must be 10^4 CFU/spot and the incubation temperature 30°C. When the inoculum is small with classes 1 and 2, there is a major risk of failing to detect heterogeneous hyperresistant strains (Table 9). It is also necessary to test the compound on multiresistant strains, taking into account resistance to aminoglycosides (gentamicin and amikacin), macrolides, fluoroquinolones, and cyclines.

Table 9 Penems In Vitro Activities Against MRSA

	MIC (mg/l)				
	Clinical Isolates	Class 1 CDC-1	Class 2 SN-7	Class 3 SN-43	Class 4 COL
Methicillin	100	3.12	6.25	>100	>100
Ritipenem	0.39	0.19	0.39	100	100
Imipenem	1.56	0.09	0.19	25	25
Meropenem	12.5	0.19	1.56	25	100
Ciprofloxacin	0.19	0.39	0.78	25	6.25

From Jabès D et al. *Bioorg. Med. Chem. Lett.* 1993, 3, 2165-2170. With permission.

One should test macrolides, lincosamides, and streptogramins on strains whose genetic resistance mechanism is known (inducible or constitutive). Recently, this type of study was done to analyze the activity of RP 59500 (Table 10).

Table 10 *In Vitro* Activities of RP 59500 Against *S. aureus*

	MIC (mg/l)		
	RP 57669	RP 54476	RP 59500
M(S) MLS_B (S)	1	2	0.1
M(R) MLS_B (I)	2	2	0.12
M(R) MLS_B (R)	30	4	0.5

From Barrière JC, Bouanchaud DH, Desnottes JF, Paris, JM, *Expert Opin. Invest. Drugs* 1994, 32, 115-131. With permission.

4.1.1.2 Coagulase-Negative Staphylococci

The coagulase-negative staphylococci include several species. Again, it is necessary to test antibacterial activity on strains both susceptible and resistant to methicillin. The species most frequently involved in infections are *S. epidermidis, S. saprophyticus,* and *S. haemolyticus.* As regards other species, about 30 strains are sufficient to gain an idea of the new compound's potential activity.

4.1.1.3 Streptococcus pneumoniae

The emergence of strains resistant to penicillin G, and multiresistant strains, necessitates a good deal of work to determine the antipneumococcal profile of a new compound. The most simple method is to determine the comparative *in vitro* activity of the compound on strains which are susceptible (MIC < 0.12 mg/l), intermediately susceptible (MIC 0.12-1 mg/l), or resistant to penicillin G (MIC >1 mg/l). One must now add to this panel strains resistant to cefotaxime (MIC ≥2 mg/l) and also those with diminished susceptibility (MIC 0.5-1 mg/l) and multiresistant strains, particularly those resistant to erythromycin (MIC > 1 mg/l), tetracycline, chloramphenicol, and co-trimoxazole. It is compulsory to detect erythromycin-resistant strains, but also to differentiate inducible and constitutive mechanism of resistance. The best 16-membered ring macrolide against erythromycin-resistant isolates seems to be rokitamycin (Leclercq, personal data). If rokitamycin MIC values are ≤8-16 mg/l or >16 mg/l, it is concluded that strains harbor respectively, an inducible or a constitutive mechanism of erythromycin resistance. It is preferable to determine MIC in agar rather than broth media (even Schaedler's medium), as the results are more variable in the latter. However, these tests are inadequate, as bactericidal activity must be tested on strains with different resistance phenotypes to ß-lactams with different inocula. With ß-lactams and fluoroquinolones, bactericidal activity falls as the inoculum increases above 10^6 CFU/ml. This modification can be identified by the killing curves method (Baquero, personal communication, 1994).

4.1.1.4 Streptococcus spp.

Antibacterial activity on group Lancefield A, B, C, G, and F streptococci must be determined using a classical method. The panel must include strains resistant to erythromycin, particularly *S. pyogenes.*

It is more difficult to determine activity on viridans streptococci. Bacteriostatic and bactericidal activity must be determined on penicillin G tolerant strains. Bactericidal activity is determined by the killing curves method. The *in vitro* activity has to be determined against the main species which composed the viridans streptococci group.

4.1.1.5 Enterococcus spp.

The susceptibility of the different species of enterococci is determined on a panel of strains susceptible or resistant to vancomycin and gentamicin; in the latter case the strains must have a high level of resistance to aminoglycosides (MIC > 1000 mg/l). In the future it will no doubt be necessary to add ß-lactamase-producing strains. The bactericidal activity of the compound is determined by the killing curves method, as with daptomycin.

4.1.1.6 Other Gram-Positive Cocci

As a prerequisite for the evaluation of clinical efficacy in endocarditis, *in vitro* studies have to be carried out on *Gemella* spp., *Stomatococcus, Micrococcus,* and *Aerococcus* spp. (Eiffel et al., 1994).

4.1.2 Gram-Positive Bacilli

Antibacterial activity must be determined on *Listeria monocytogenes, Erysipelothrix rhusopathiae, Bacillus anthracis,* and *Bacillus* spp., *Lactobacillus* spp., *Pediococcus* spp., *Leuconostoc* spp., *Rhodococcus equi,* and *Corynebacterium diphtheriae* and *Corynebacterium* spp. (*C. jeikeium, C. urealyticum,* etc.).

Activity on *C. jeikeium* must always be determined, as there are few active drugs. Activity on *Arcanobacterium (Corynebacterium) haemolyticum* and *Actinomycetes (Corynebacterium) pyogenes* should also be tested (Martinez-Martinez et al., 1994). There is increasing interest in *C. diphtheriae* because of the diphtheria outbreak in Russia and the Ukraine (CDR, 1994). Against *C. diphtheriae,* MIC value determinations have to be done against the two biotypes: *mitis* and *gravis* and against toxigenic and nontoxigenic isolates. The toxigenic strain *C. diphtheriae* var. *gravis* NCTC 10648, the non toxigenic strain *C. diphtheriae* var. *gravis* NCTC 10356, and the nontoxigenic strain *C. diphtheriae* var. *mitis* NCTC 11397 have to be included as controls (Maple et al., 1994).

4.1.3 Gram-Negative Cocci

Whether for *N. gonorrhoeae* or *N. meningitidis*, it is necessary to test strains with different resistance phenotypes to antibacterial agents.

4.1.3.1 *Neisseria meningitidis*

A fall in the activity of penicillin G (Saez-Nieto et al., 1990) has been observed in certain regions. The resistance mechanism is similar to that of *S. pneumoniae*. Susceptibility to penicillin G varies according to the region and serogroup in Spain. It has recently been shown that strains belonging to serogroup C have diminished susceptibility to penicillin G. The intensive use of rifampicin prophylaxis accounts for the emergence of strains resistant to this antibiotic. The test panel must thus include strains susceptible to antibacterial agents, strains with diminished susceptibility to penicillin G, and strains resistant to rifampicin and macrolides (spiramycin and erythromycin). The strains should belong to the serogroups most frequently isolated, i.e., B, C, and A. Killing curves must be constructed for the different strains of *N. meningitidis*. Some chloramphenicol-resistant isolates have also been described.

4.1.3.2 *Neisseria gonorrhoeae*

The emergence of strains of *N. gonorrhoeae* resistant to penicillin G, tetracyclines, spectinomycin, and, more recently, with diminished susceptibility to fluoroquinolones (Knapp et al., 1994; Puttman et al., 1992) means that the compound must be tested on strains with different resistance phenotypes. It is probable that strains resistant to 2-amino-5-thiazolyl cephalosporins and fluoroquinolones will have to be added in the near future.

4.1.4 Gram-Negative Bacilli

4.1.4.1 Enterobacteriaceae

The Enterobacteriaceae form a vast family, but a few simple rules could be sufficient to obtain the antibacterial profile of a new compound. It must be borne in mind that Enterobacteriaceae produce enzymes which hydrolyze ß-lactams (Philipon et al., 1994) and inactivate aminoglycosides to varying degrees (Miller, 1994), or become resistant to the fluoroquinolones by chromosomal mechanisms (Bryskier, 1993). The new compound must be tested on:

- Isogenic strains, such as *E. coli* 600, which possess different enzymes capable of hydrolyzing ß-lactams or inactivating aminoglycosides.
- Strains resistant to fluoroquinolones by known mechanisms.
- Reference strains which produce the different ß-lactamases (class 1, extended-spectrum, broad-spectrum, etc.) or enzymes which inactivate aminoglycosides (use strains producing the most frequent enzymes in each bacterial species).

Initially, studies will be limited to species frequently involved in infectious diseases. Activity on less frequent species has to be determined as a second step.

In practice the *in vitro* activity of new compound must be determined on *E. coli, Klebsiella pneumoniae, K. oxytoca, Citrobacter diversus, C. freundii, Serratia marcescens, Enterobacter cloacae, E. aerogenes, Morganella morganii, Providencia* spp., *Proteus* spp., *Shigella* spp., *Salmonella* spp. and *Yersinia enterocolitica, Hafnia* spp.

Salmonellae and shigellae occupy a special place among the Enterobacteriaceae. The new antibacterial agent must be tested on strains resistant to antibiotics recommended in the therapy of these diseases, i.e., ampicillin, chloramphenicol, and co-trimoxazole for salmonellae, and additionally tetracyclines and nalidixic acid for shigellae. Strains resistant to fluoroquinolones are still rare, and are not to be included in a standard panel.

A minimum of the following *Salmonella enterica* serovars must be tested: Typhi, Enteritidis, and Typhimurium, with strains presenting different antibiophenotypes; other serovars can be tested depending on the local epidemiology. As regards shigellae, activity must be tested on the four serogroups, *Shigella sonnei, S. flexneri, S. dysenteriae,* and *S. bodyi*. The number of clinical isolates will be large with the first two species, which account for most infections. Again, it is necessary to use a panel composed of susceptible strains and strains resistant to co-trimoxazole, tetracyclines, and nalidixic acid. Strains resistant to fluoroquinolones remain rare.

4.1.4.2 *Pseudomonas aeruginosa and Other Species*

The activity of the new antibacterial agent must be tested on wild strains (clinical isolates and collections) and strains with known resistance phenotypes, i.e., ß-lactamase producers (carbenicillinases, oxacillinases, and cephalosporinases), and strains resistant to fluoroquinolones, aminoglycosides (gentamicin, tobramycin, amikacin, and netilmicin), C-3'-quaternary ammonium cephems, and imipenem (outermembrane permeability mutants, OprD, OrpJ, OprM, and OprN mutants).

Bactericidal activity must be determined alone and in combination with other antibacterial agents (checkerboard and killing curve methods). A sufficient number of strains of species other than *P. aeruginosa* must be included in the determination of antibacterial activity so as to complete the antibacterial spectrum.

4.1.4.3 Other Gram-Negative Bacilli

The following bacterial genera must be included in the characterization of the antibacterial spectrum: *Aeromonas hydrophila* and five other species (Janda et al., 1991), *Stenotrophomonas (Xanthomonas) maltophilia, Burkholderia cepacia, Vibrio* spp., *Alcaligenes* spp., *Acinetobacter* spp., *Bordetella bronchiseptica, Flavobacterium* spp., *Alteromonas, Comamonas,* and *Vibrio cholerae.*

Acinetobacter spp.

Antibacterial activity must be tested on about 100 strains of *A. baumannii* with different resistance phenotypes to antibiotics (five phenotypes), particularly to N-acyl penicillins (piperacillin), α-carboxy penicillins (ticarcillin), alone or combined with a ß-lactamase inhibitor (clavulanic acid or tazobactam) and aminoglycosides (Joly-Guillou et al., 1988).

The other species of *Acinetobacter* should also be included in the panel, but a much smaller sample of strains is required.

Vibrio cholerae

The susceptibility profile differs between *V. cholerae* O1 (responsible for the 7th pandemic; classic biotype or El Tor) and the new strain of Sub-Indian continent (Bangladesh) origin which is responsible of the 8th pandemic (*Vibrio cholerae* O 139) and which is resistant to co-trimoxazole and furans. Certain strains of *V. cholerae* non-O_1 have been isolated from patients who do not have a choleriform syndrome but rather bacteriemia often of gastrointestinal origin and which are usually nonsusceptible to colistin.

The new agent must be tested on the three types of *V. cholerae* and strains with phenotypic resistance to ampicillin, tetracyclines, and sulfonamides.

Haemophilus spp.

The susceptibility of *H. influenzae* should be studied on a panel of strains comprising ß-lactamases producers and nonproducers, and strains resistant to ampicillin through a nonenzymatic mechanism. Cephalosporins have diminished activity on these latter strains, and oral and parenteral cephalosporins must be included among the comparators. The most controversial question is the nature of the medium used to determine the MIC (Erwin et al., 1993; Jones et al., 1994). There should be equal numbers of type b and non-b *H. influenzae*. The other species such as *H. parainfluenzae, H. haemolyticus, H. parahaemolyticus, H. paraphrohaemolyticus* and *H. aegyptius* will be studied later. Certain species are responsible for liver abscesses, endocarditis, and purulent meningitis.

Moraxella spp.

The genus Moraxella includes the following species: *M. lacunata, M. bovis, M. nonliquefaciens, M. phenylpyruvica, M. otlantae*, and *O. osloensis, M. lacunata* and *M. nonliquefaciens* cause conjunctivitis and purulent meningitis in humans.

M. catarrhalis

This upper-airway commensal can cause superinfections in patients with chronic bronchitis and ENT infections such as otitis media. Some strains of *M. catarrhalis* produce ROB-1 and ROB-2 ß-lactamases and the three antibiotypes must be tested.

Bordetella pertussis

The causative agent of whooping cough is generally susceptible to macrolides, which are the drugs of choice. Susceptibility testing is done on strains of *B. pertussis* and *B. parapertussis*. The culture medium and growth conditions are specific for *B. pertussis*.

HACEK

This acronym covers Gram-negative bacteria which are infrequent human pathogens but can cause severe endocarditis. The members comprise *Haemophilus aphrophilus, Actinobacillus actinomycetemcomitans, Cardiobacterium hominis, Eikenella corrodens,* and *Kingella* spp.

The activity of new compounds must be tested against this group as a prerequisite if clinical trials are planned to be conducted in patients suffering from endocarditis.

Pasteurella spp.

P. multocida is responsible for skin infections following dog and cat bites and scratches. In the panel of strains tested, ROB-1 ß-lactamase producing strains have to be included.

Haemophilus ducreyi

This is a fastidious organism. Special culture medium must be made up no more than three days before use. The strains tested should have different resistance phenotypes, i.e., ß-lactamase (TEM-1, ROB-1) producers and nonproducers, and strains resistant and susceptible to tetracyclines, sulfonamides, and kanamycin. Strains resistant to erythromycin and 2-amino-5-thiazolyl cephalosporins remain rare.

Capnocytophaga

The genus *Capnocytophaga* comprises three species of Gram-negative bacilli: *C. ochracea, C. sputigena,* and *C. gingivalis*. This opportunistic pathogen can cause suppurative oral infections, ENT and bone tissue infections, and a few cases of endocarditis have been reported. Strains of *Capnocytophaga* are classically resistant to 5-nitroimidazoles and aminoglycosides. The *in vitro* activity of the new antibacterial agent must be determined as a prerequisite if endocarditis trial are scheduled.

Stenotrophomonas (Xanthomonas) maltophilia

S. maltophilia is an opportunistic pathogen usually involved in nosocomial infections, particularly in intensive care units. Susceptibility testing of *S. maltophilia* remains to be standardized. In particular, it has been shown that the disk diffusion method is unreliable and that the inhibition zone diameters depend on the medium and its zinc content. *S. maltophilia* produces at least two enzymes: carbapenemase resistant to clavulanic acid and a cephalosporinase susceptible to clavulanic acid. Strains producing small amounts of imipenemase are more susceptible to the ticarcillin-clavulanic acid combination than to combinations containing sulbactam or tazobactam (piperacillin-tazobactam). The new compound should be tested on strains susceptible and resistant to the ticarcillin-clavulanic acid combination.

Burkholderia spp.

Group II of *Pseudomonas pseudomallei* has recently been rebaptized *Burkholderia* spp. (Yabuuchi et al., 1992). This group comprises *B. pseudomallei, B. mallei, B. cepacia, P. gladioli, B. picketti, B. carophylli,* and *B. solonacearum*.

B. cepacia has become an important opportunistic pathogen, but is also increasingly isolated from patients with cystic fibrosis. Clinical isolates are often multiresistant. Classically, *B. cepacia* is susceptible to ceftazidime, piperacillin, and co-trimoxazole, but its susceptibility to carbapenems and fluoroquinolones is variable. Most strains are resistant to aminoglycosides and chloramphenicol.

Antibacterial activity must be tested on strains resistant to one or several of the following antibiotics: imipemen, ceftazidime, co-trimoxazole, piperacillin, and ciprofloxacin. Many isolates from bronchial secretions of patients with cystic fibrosis produce carbapenemases (Simpson et al., 1993).

4.1.5 *Anaerobes*

Antibacterial activity against anaerobes must be tested in a specialized laboratory. The Gram-negative bacilli (*Bacteroides* spp., *Porphyromonas* spp., *Prevotella* spp., *Fusobacterium* spp.) to be tested include strains resistant to clindamycin and cephamycins (cefoxitin and cefotetan). Strains resistant to 5-nitroimidazoles (metronidazole and derivatives) are infrequent (Dublanchet et al., 1986).

Activity must be determined on two different culture media (Wilkins-Chalgren, NCCLS 11 A norms; and Brucella medium). Combination activities with metronidazole and clindamycin have to be tested with the new antibacterials especially against pathogens involved in intra-abdominal sepsis or in dental infections.

Antibacterial activity against non-spore-forming Gram-positive bacteria has to be determined (*Peptococcus* spp., *Peptostreptococcus* spp., *Eubacterium* spp., *Bifidobacterium* spp., and *Propionibacterium* spp.) and against Gram-negative cocci such as *Veillonella* spp. Activity on *Clostridium difficile* is determined separately from the other clostridia.

4.2 Other Microorganisms

The antibacterial activity of a new compound is tested in special conditions against the following species: *Treponema pallidum, Borrelia* spp., *H. pylori, Campylobacter* spp., *Mycobacterium* spp., *Mycoplasma* spp., *Leptospira* spp., and *Ureaplasma urealyticum.*

4.2.1 *Helicobacter pylori*

It is now recognized that *H. pylori* is involved in duodenal ulcers and chronic gastritis type B. Antibacterial activity *in vitro* will be determined at gastric pH if the compounds are acid-stable. It is necessary to determine antibacterial activity in combination with Hep-2 cells, although they dislike excessively acidic media (pH < 6). As anti-ulcer drugs such as H_2-blockers and proton pump inhibitors (omeprazole, lanzoprazole) are often used therapeutically in this setting, the activity of the antibacterial agent must be tested in their presence; indeed, some such compounds have intrinsic antibacterial activity (e.g., lanzoprazole; Mégraud et al., 1991).

The incidence of *H. pylori* resistance to metronidazole varies from 7-49% according to the center. However, there is no standard method for assessing susceptibility to metronidazole, and this also accounts for the wide variability of resistance. De Cross et al. (1993) have developed a method for determining the susceptibility of *H. pylori* to metronidazole by a disk diffusion method, using a modified version of the Kirby- Bauer method. It is moderately reliable, with a difference of 10.7% between the agar dilution and disk diffusion method. Xia et al. (1994) have proposed the following break points (Table 11). Currently there are no reference strains for quality control.

Table 11 Metronidazole Break Points on *Helicobacter pylori*

	Inhibition Zone Diameters (mm)	MIC (mg/l)
Susceptible	≥26	<4
Intermediately-S	20-26	4-8
Resistant	≤20	>8

4.2.2 *Campylobacter* spp.

C. jejuni and *C. coli* are the most frequent pathogens in this genus. *C. jejuni* is more susceptible to antibiotics than *C. coli*. The panel should include strains resistant to macrolides and fluoroquinolones. Reina et al. (1995) have shown a progressive increase in the percentage of *Campylobacter* resistant to fluoroquinolones. In Spain a slight increase in erythromycin rates has been observed as well as an increase in the number of strains with simulutaneous resistance to erythromycin an fluoroquinolones. All erythromycin-resistant strains were also resistant to other available macrolides. When new chemical entities are tested on *C. jejuni*, it is compulsory to include strains resistant to erythromycin and fluoroquinolones.

4.2.3 *Borrelia* spp.

Borrelia spp. are responsible for Lyme disease, which is endemic in the northern hemisphere. Genetic studies have identified several species of *Borrelia*: *B. burgdorferi, B. garanii, B. afzelii,* and B. VS 461

(Péter et al., 1993), which cause different clinical manifestations. *B. burgdorferi* is often associated with rheumatic symptoms, while *B. garinii* and *B. afzelii*, respectively, are associated with neurological disease and cutaneous manifestations (*acrodermatitis chronica atrophicans*). It is necessary to test a new agent against all the different species. BSK II medium is used and the number of spirochetes is determined by using a Petroff-Hausser counting chamber.

The *in vitro* activity of the new agent will be determined against wild strains as well as strains from stock collection which grow more rapidly after multiple subculture than the former. Care must be taken to avoid false results. Above all, the culture pellet must be reseeded in antibiotic-free medium to detect the presence of the spirochete, taking care to read the results after a sufficient time (several days) to allow for regrowth. The discrepancy between the *in vitro* results obtained from different teams is partially due to the lack of standardization, and it was recently clearly shown that the different species of *Borrelia* do not have the same susceptibility to antibacterial agents (Péter et al., 1994; Table 12).

Table 12 Antibacterial Susceptibility of *Borrelia* spp.

	B. burgdorferi BE 1	*B. garinii* VS 102	*B. afzelii* ACA1
Doxycycline	0.25	0.125	0.25
Amoxicillin	0.25	0.125	0.25
Roxithromycin	0.062	0.015	0.125
Ceftriaxone	0.031	0.031	0.031
Cefodizime	0.125	0.125	0.25
Cefpirome	0.25	0.25	0.125
Cefpodoxime	4.0	1.0	1.0

From Péter O, Bretz AG, *Recent Adv. lyme Borreliosis Dis.*, 1994, 167-174. With permission.

4.2.4 *Treponema pallidum*

T. pallidum is the etiologic agent of syphilis. Its treatment is based on benzylpenicillin. However, a therapeutic alternative is necessary when the patient has delayed-type hypersensitivity reactions to penicillin G. There are no *in vitro* culture models, but Stamm et al. (1988) developed a model which combines bacterial extraction from infected rabbit testis and inhibition of [^{35}S]-methionine incorporation into trichloroacetic acid precipitable protein of *T. pallidum* freshly extracted from infected rabbit testis 4 h after a 4-h contact between the organism and the antibiotic. A comparative rabbit model with penicillin G (Lukehart et al., 1990) can be used to quantify the potential activity of the new antibacterial agent in the treatment of syphilis. This experimental work must be confirmed by clinical studies (Verdon et al., 1994).

4.2.5 *Mycoplasma* spp. and *Ureaplasma* spp.

Few compounds (macrolides, fluoroquinolones, and cyclines) are active on these bacterial species. Methods are poorly standardized and interpretation of the results is often delicate. It is difficult to compare results between different laboratories. The following species should be tested: *M. pneumoniae, M. hominis,* and *M. genitalium.* The human pathogenicity of the other mycoplasmas is more controversial, and for the time-being it is not necessary for licensing purposes to test the activity of the new compound. The *in vitro* activity of the new agent has to be tested against selected *U. urealyticum* strains susceptible and resistant to tetracyclines (Kenny et al., 1986, 1993).

4.2.6 *Nocardia* spp.

Nocardia spp. rarely cause infections in immunocompetent hosts. The genus *Nocardia* includes the following species: *N. asteroides, N. brasilensis,* and *N. farcinica. N. asteroides* is susceptible to aminoglycosides, 2-amino-5-thiazolyl cephalosporins, sulfonamides, and tetracyclines (Wallace et al., 1988).

4.2.7 *Leptospira* spp.

Leptospirosis is a endemozoonosis due to *Leptospira* spp., which comprises several serogroups and serovars. The serogroups are *L. icterohemmorrhagiae, L. canicola, L. grippothyphosa,* and *L. australis.* The determination of the antibacterial activity against these pathogens is fastidious and has to be carried out in highly specialized laboratories.

4.3 Intracellular Pathogens

Few antibiotics are able to penetrate into phagocytic cells, but the following do show intracellular bioactivity: macrolides, fluoroquinolones, tetracyclines, ansamycins, streptogramins, and lincosamides. The first step in the investigation of intracellular bioactivity is to determine the kinetics of penetration and efflux, as well as the precise subcellular site of accumulation. This work must be comparative in the same class of antibacterials. As the methodology varies from one laboratory to another, it is preferable, if possible, to have the results from two different teams.

The second step consists of testing the intracellular activity of the antibacterials on intracellular pathogens. This type of study is usually conducted with *Mycobacterium tuberculosis* and *M. avium complex* (Rastogi et al., 1995), but will probably soon be extended to other intracellular genera and species.

Certain intracellular bacteria such as *Brucella* spp. grow readily on agar and broth medium. MIC and MBC values give some indication as to the compound's activity, but they must be compared with intracellular concentrations and the site of antibiotic accumulation in the cell as well as the *Brucella* cellular location.

The determination of activity on *Chlamydia* spp. will vary according to the species. In the case of *C. trachomatis*, activity must be tested on cell cultures (the McCoy or HeLa cell lines) and on animal models (e.g., fertility of mice infected by *C. trachomatis* and treated with the antibiotic relative to a control). With *C. psittaci*, activity is tested *in vitro* on cell cultures and in a mouse model of pneumonia. As regards *C. pneumoniae*, only *in vitro* models have been validated thus far. Activity on *Rickettsia* and related organisms is determined on cell cultures. The results vary from one laboratory to another, owing to the use of different methods. Activity must be tested on the principal species, including *R. conorii, R. rickettsii, R. prowazeki, R. tsutsugamuchi, R. typhi,* and *Coxiella burnettii.*

Activity on *Rochalimaea* spp. (*Bartonella*) is determined on Vero cells; note that *R. hanselae* is becoming an important opportunistic pathogen with the onset of the AIDS epidemic; activity on the different species of *Ehrlichia*, as well as *A. felis*, must also be determined. *In vitro* activity on *Legionella* spp. is determined on two media with a reference strain. However, overall activity must be tested in the presence of macrophages and also in guinea pig experimental pneumonia.

4.4 Mycobacteria

According to the pathogenicity of the different *Mycobacteria* species, it is important to distinguish the antibacterial activity of a new agent against *M. tuberculosis, M. leprae,* and "atypical" mycobacteria.

4.4.1 *Mycobacterium tuberculosis*

The antibacterial activity of the new agent has to be tested on the reference strain H_{37RV} and H_{37RV} strains with different resistance phenotypes (streptomycin, INH, rifampicin, ethambutol, etc.).

If the new agent is active on these different H_{37RV} strains, it will be tested on a panel of clinical isolates, including strains of *M. africanum, M. bovis*, and *M. bovis* BCG.

The second step consists of assessing combinations with established antitubercular drugs *in vitro* and in animal models.

Antibacterial activity *in vitro* is classically determined on Löwenstein-Jensen agar containing the antibiotic. However, Middlebrook agar is now preferred (7 H10 or 7 H11 plus 10% oleic acid-albumin-dextrose-catalase, and with or without Tween 80, at pH 6.6). Pyrazinamine activity is tested on the same medium but at pH 5.8, or on Bactec at two different pH values (6.8 and 7.4).

4.4.2 *Atypical Mycobacteria*

The new antibacterial agent will be tested alone and in combination against different strains of *M. avium complex* isolated from HIV-seropositive and seronegative patients. The drug will be tested in the presence of macrophages and various antibiotics. Depending on the results, studies in Beige mice will be conducted. Activity should also be determined on other atypical mycobacteria such as *M. chelonei, M. fortuitum,* and *M. kansasii* (Rastogi et al., 1993).

4.4.3 *Mycobacterium leprae*

The need for new drugs effective against leprosy means that all candidate compounds (mainly fluoroquinolones and macrolides) must be tested alone and in combination.

5 ANIMAL MODELS

Two types of animal models must be used: nondiscriminatory models and specific models of experimental infections (Zak et al., 1990).

5.1 Nondiscriminatory Models

These models belong to the preselection phase. After determining *in vitro* activity, it is essential to assess *in vivo* activity after parenteral and oral dosing. Indeed, *in vitro* activity does not necessarily correlate with *in vivo* activity (poor absorption, marked metabolism, or toxicity). These models of systemic infections are used to test activity on Gram-positive cocci (*S. aureus, S. pyogenes, S. pneumoniae,* and *Enterococcus faecalis*), Enterobacteriaceae and *P. aeruginosa*, using comparators belonging to the same chemical class (if available).

The panel must include strains with different antibiophenotypes, e.g., *P. aeruginosa* strains with different susceptibility to imipenem and ceftazidime. However, it is sometimes difficult to test these strains *in vivo* as they are not always sufficiently virulent in mice.

5.2 Discriminatory Models

Two types of experimental infections can be used, and these studies could be prerequisite for further clinical development. Target infections include lower respiratory tract infection (e.g., *K. pneumoniae*), experimental pyelonephritis, endocarditis, experimental abscesses due to *Bacteroides fragilis*, experimental osteomyelitis due to *S. aureus* or *P. aeruginosa*, and experimental diarrhea in the piglet.

Mice immunodepressed with steroids or cyclophosphamide, or neutropenic mice, are used to predict activity in immunodepressed and neutropenic patients. Activity in otitis media due to *H. influenzae* is tested in the gerbil or in the chinchilla, although this latter model is controversial.

The second type of infection is more specific for the microorganism. These models are prerequisites for clinical testing in respiratory tract infections by *Legionella pneumophila* (guinea pig) and genital tract infections by *Chlamydia trachomatis* (mice). The Syrian hamster model for respiratory tract infections due to *M. pneumoniae* is not yet validated.

6 SPECIFIC INDICATIONS

If a precise clinical indication is sought, then detailed pharmacologic studies must be done. One example is pneumococcal infections. The emergence of strains with decreased susceptibility (resistant to penicillin G or multiresistant) necessitates microbiological validation of this indication.

The first step is to determine *in vitro* activity (MIC and MBC) on a panel of strains with variable susceptibility to penicillin G and cefotaxime. Multiresistant strains (including erythromycin, tetracyclines, cotrimoxazole, and kanamycin) are also tested. If the activity of a fluoroquinolone is to be determined, strains of variable susceptibility (e.g., with ofloxacin MICs of ≤ 2 mg/l and >2 mg/l) should also be tested. The second step involves determining bactericidal activity by the killing curves method with different inocula (10^5 and 10^7 CFU/ml). The third type of study is more complex, as it involves determining the selective potential of the compound, and the frequency and rate of mutations (particularly with fluoroquinolones). These experiments have to be carried out *in vitro* and *in vivo*, the latter model has to be defined (Drugeon et al., 1994). Comparative, experimental models of systemic infection (respiratory and meningeal) are used to determine potential therapeutic activity and will guide the choice of doses for Phase II trials. The same approach is used for other pathogens such as *S. aureus* and *P. aeruginosa*.

7 MECHANISMS OF ACTION AND RESISTANCE

The licensing authorities will wish to know the mechanism of action and the mechanisms of resistance (determined using state-of-the-art techniques, which are rapidly evolving). Our understanding of these mechanisms varies with the chemical class. The best-known are those of the ß-lactams, fluoroquinolones, mupirocine, and fosfomycin. In the case of ß-lactams, studies involve outermembrane penetration, interaction with peptidoglycan synthesis, inhibition of PBP of the different bacterial species, hydrolytic susceptibility to different crude ß-lactamases, and *in vitro* susceptibility of the new compound to whole bacterial cell producing ß-lactamases, induction of cephalosporinases, and the inhibitory activity of ß-lactamases (e.g., cephamycins, penems). With fluoroquinolones, it is necessary to study outermembrane uptake, affinity for DNA gyrase, and the DNA-gyrase-DNA complex, topoisomerase IV and the Nor A efflux system of *S. aureus*. The activity of new fluoroquinolones must be tested on the different mutants.

8 INTERACTION WITH FECAL AND ORAL FLORA

Administration of antibacterial agents is the most common and significant cause of ecological disturbance in the normal oral and intestinal microflora (Nord et al., 1990). The impact of a new antibacterial agent on the human fecal and oral flora has to be carried out when phase II had been completed (daily dose determination and administration rhythm).

The aim of these studies is threefold: (1) to determine the amount of product eliminated in the feces over 24 h or longer, together with the duration of this elimination after administration of single or repeated doses; (2) to quantify changes in the anaerobic flora and Enterobacteriaceae, together with the time required for the flora to return to normal after completion of the treatment; and (3) to detect emergence of *C. difficile* and the level of *C. difficile* toxins (Edlund et al., 1993). If studying a ß-lactam antibiotic, a fourth target could be the determination of selected strains producing a high level of ß-lactamases (Bellido et al.).

9 CLINICAL MICROBIOLOGY AND PHASES I AND II: DETERMINING THE DOSE

The dose and dosing schedule is crucial in the development of a new antibacterial agent. Studies conducted *in vitro* and *in vivo* will contribute to the proposed daily dose, which has to be validated during Phase II trials.

9.1 Phase II Trials

One example is the daily dose of oral roxithromycin. Roxithromycin has similar antibacterial activity to erythromycin A but is three to ten times more active *in vivo* in nondiscriminative models of experimental infections, mainly owing to its favorable pharmacokinetics (Chantot et al., 1986). The first roxithromycin Phase II trials were done with one third of the erythromycin A recommended dose, i.e., 600 mg/day (Roussel Uclaf, data on file, 1984). Dose-finding studies in fact showed that the optimal daily dose was 300 mg (Akoun et al., 1986).

Microbiological studies help in the choice of dose for phase II trials, as do pharmacodynamic models. In the second phase, a certain number of models can be used to validate the chosen dosage, such as the indexes proposed by Schentag (1991) and Ellner et al. (1981), serum, or CSF bactericidal activity.

9.2 CSF Activity

The CSF concentration must be at least ten times the MIC for the pathogen if bactericidal activity is to be obtained (Täuber et al., 1984, 1989). CSF levels depend on the phase of meningitis. After a cefotaxime dose of 200 mg/kg/day by the intravenous route, concentrations are higher during the acute phase of the infection (1.7-7 mg/l) and fall slightly during the attenuation phase (1.2-4 mg/l); during the resolutive phase the concentrations are about 1 mg/l (0.7-1.3 mg/l; Periti et al., 1984). When antibacterial activity falls, as for example with penicillin G in strains of *S. pneumoniae*, the administered dose must be increased to maintain this minimum ratio of CSF/MIC values of 10:1, and CSF bactericidal activity titer of 1:8 (Täuber et al., 1989).

9.3 Pharmacodynamics

Antibacterial agents can be divided into three categories. The first is composed of compounds such as aminoglycosides and fluoroquinolones which possess concentration-dependent bactericidal activity. The second is ß-lactams and glycopeptides, the bactericidal activity of which is time-dependent. The third group comprises compounds whose activity is mainly bacteriostatic, such as the macrolides and tetracyclines. Pharmacokinetic parameters and *in vitro* activity (MIC and MBC) are used to assess or predict therapeutic efficacy.

Currently, the following parameters are studied: area under the curve (AUC) above the MIC, the peak serum concentration/MIC ratio, the time during which serum concentrations are above the MIC (T > MIC), AUIC (the AUC/MIC ratio; Schentag, 1991). The concentration of the drug in the fluid surrounding the microorganism is what drives it into the bacterial cell and delivers it to the binding site. Because the majority of microorganisms live in the interstitial fluid, drug concentrations and kinetics have to be known in the extravascular fluid.

9.3.1 Concentration-Dependent Drugs

Forrest et al. (1993) were the first to determine a clinical breakpoint by evaluating the integration of a drug's pharmacokinetic and pharmacodynamic properties and relating this to the patient's response to treatment. Study results clearly demonstrated that the AUIC value was the best predictor of clinical response (Forrest et al., 1993). It has been applied to parenteral cephalosporins, fluoroquinolones, aminoglycosides, metronidazole, and daptomycin, but could be used for other antibiotic families. The AUIC must be at least 125.

9.3.1.1 Fluoroquinolones

In the case of the fluoroquinolones, which are more rapidly bactericidal, an index of 250 has been proposed by Schentag as the threshold for strong bactericidal activity. At AUIC <125 ($\log_{10}$ ~2.25), the overall cure rate was 42%, whereas at AUICs >125, the probability of clinical cure was 80%. In terms of time to bacterial eradication, the median time to eradication was >32 days at an AUIC <125, 6.6 days at an AUIC of 125-250, and 1.9 days at an AUIC >250 ($p < 0.005$).

A general rule for 4-quinolones that exhibit concentration-dependent killing kinetics, serum concentrations approximately 10 times greater than the MIC are needed to kill Gram-negative organisms, while concentrations one to four times the MICs are adequate to kill Gram-positive organisms (Forster et al., 1986). When concentration-dependent antibacterials cannot achieve Cp/MIC ratios of 8 to 10, the time element of the product (AUC) cannot be ignored. This especially applied for bacteria moderately susceptible *in vitro* to 4-quinolones.

The ratio AUIC is determined with MIC_{90} values, but it seems reasonable to determine $AUIC_{50}$ (MIC_{50} values), $AUIC_{90}$ (MIC_{90} values), and $AUIC_{GM}$ (MIC geometric mean), which will give a better idea of the activity of a 4-quinolone in an average clinical isolates (e.g., *S. pneumoniae*).

9.3.1.2 Aminoglycosides

The killing rate is stronger with aminoglycosides when serum concentrations are markedly higher than the MIC. Optimal activity is reached when the plasma concentration is 10-12 times the MIC (Moore et al., 1984a,b). Antibacterial activity will depend on the duration and intensity of exposure. Bolus administration provides an early, intense bactericidal effect but low bactericidal activity at later times. This phenomenon can lead to the selection of bacteria with a low level of resistance. When the Cmax/MIC ratio is at least 8, there is a high probability of bacterial eradication. In animal models, a single dose of an aminoglycoside is associated with less lesions of the Corti organ and renal cells than multiple daily dosing.

9.3.2 Time-Dependent Drugs

The killing rate of ß-lactams is time-dependent and concentration-independent. The time during which serum concentrations are above the MIC is the best predictor of therapeutic activity. The bactericidal activity of ß-lactams is saturable (depending on the concentration) and seems to be optimal when the serum concentration is 4 to 8 times higher than the relevant MBC. Above this concentration bactericidal activity no longer increases but may decrease (Eagle's effect, 1950). Given this saturation phenomenon, it is the time during which the concentration is saturating (T>MIC) which must be optimized rather than the intensity of exposure (dose increment). Efficacy is optimum if T>MIC, is respectively, 100 and 50% for Gram-negative bacteria and Gram-positive cocci. This means that serum concentrations must be above the MIC between two drug intakes for Gram-negative bacilli and only for 50% of the time in the case of Gram-positive cocci, given the absence of a post-antibiotic effect (Vogelman et al., 1985). However, these predictive factors can be erroneous. For example, ceftriaxone has excellent bactericidal activity on *Shigella* spp. with a CMI_{90} of 0.06 mg/l (Peloux et al., 1994). A single dose of ceftriaxone gives a plasma concentration which remains above the MIC beyond 48 h. In a comparative, double-blind study of the efficacy of ceftriaxone after a single dose in adults with shigellosis, a clinical response was obtained but fecal elimination of shigellae was the same as after ampicillin or a placebo (Kabir et al., 1986; Loleka et al., 1991).

9.3.3 Pharmacodynamics Models Simulating Human Pharmacokinetics

In conventional *in vitro* tests, bacteria are exposed to a constant concentration of antibiotic throughout the period of test. This does not reflect the situation in humans, where the concentration of antibiotic in the serum and tissues is constantly changing, according to absorption and elimination rates and any metabolism of compounds. *In vitro* kinetic models can be used to simulate the concentrations of antibiotics measured in the serum and extravascular fluid of man following conventional dosage and to assess their antibacterial activities (Grasso et al., 1978).

This model may be used to study direct comparative activity, effect of different dosage regimens to predict breakpoints values more accurately, and interaction studies looking for either synergy or antagonism at concentrations likely to be achieved in man.

10 PLACE OF CLINICAL MICROBIOLOGY DURING PHASE II AND III TRIALS

The clinical dossier for antibacterial agents includes a microbiological section. The aim is to achieve harmonious clinical development, and this involves a program of quality control assurance which, for the moment, is still in its infancy (or nonexistent).

Microbiological development covers several aspects:

1. Collection and transport of pathological specimens
2. Isolation and identification of pathogen(s)
3. Determination of the antibacterial activity of the test compound and comparators
4. Phenotyping of the strain
5. Correlation of *in vitro* activity with clinical efficacy for the determination of breakpoints

During clinical trials, MIC values and zone diameter inhibition have to be determined for each clinical isolate. The quality control strains have to be used and MIC values and zone diameters determined. A full report with all the microbiological data has to be written. These results will be compulsory to validate the quality control strains and the breakpoints.

10.1 Pathological Specimens

Pathological specimens include blood, urine, stools, bronchial secretions, bronchoalveolar lavage fluid, CSF, pleural fluid, pericardial fluid, ascites, joint fluid, pharyngotonsillar samples, and various pus.

The sampling conditions and the way in which the specimen is transported to the clinical laboratory (transport medium, time required, etc.), must be stated and standardized. Norms must be established for cytological examination, direct microscopic examinations after staining (Gram, May Grünwald Giemsa, etc.), and for bacterial isolation and identification.

Quantification may be necessary for certain pathological samples such as urine and bronchial brushing specimens. The results of cytobacteriological examinations must be provided together with biochemical results in certain infections like purulent meningitis. Bacterial identification must be thorough. For example, "*Salmonella* spp." is not acceptable. Indeed, the predicted activity of a parenteral cephalosporin will differ between *S. enterica* serovar Enteritidis and Typhimurium. This latter is located intracellularly, and ß-lactams are inactive as this are concentrated into cells. The same is true for streptococci, which must be identified by their Lancefield group and, in cases of therapeutic failure, other features. Pneumococcal serogroups and serotypes must be known with precision, and this information can only be obtained in specialized laboratories. In the case of *H. influenzae*, not only the serotype has to be obtained (type b and non-type b) but also biotype which can be useful if bacterial eradication is not obtained, and this is used to check the identity of the strains isolated at the beginning of the infection and during treatment (Kilian, 1976).

When the same bacterial species is isolated after completion of the treatment or during treatment (clinical and/or microbiological signs of failure), it must be checked that the strain present at the outset of the infection is the same as that responsible for the treatment failure. Certain bacterial species can be subjected to fine analysis by means of gel-pulsed-field electrophoresis. This method gives good results with most Enterobacteriaceae, except for *Salmonella* spp. and *E. coli*. It can also be used for *S. pyogenes* and *S. aureus*.

10.2 Determination of Antibacterial Activity

The susceptibility of the clinical isolate thought to be responsible for the infection should be tested in the clinical microbiology laboratory belonging to the participating center. The minimun requested is the antibiotic susceptibility testing by mean of an antibiogram. In the microbiological section of the study book the detailed identity of the pathogen should be clearly mentioned together with the type of the pathological sample and the inhibition zone diameters and MIC values. The MIC and inhibition zone diameters for the appropriate quality control strain must be noted precisely. To facilitate later analysis of the clinical results, particularly in case of therapeutic failure, this test should include other antibiotics in order to define the antibiophenotype of the strain responsible for the infection.

The method for antibiotic susceptibility testing must be noted on the record form for microbiology; the different possibilities include the method of Kirby-Bauer (Bauer *et al.*, 1966), the flooded method (Chabbert, 1982), and the methods of Joan Stokes (1993) in the U.K. with particular reference strains (*S. aureus* NCTC 6571, *E. coli* NCTC 10418, *S. pneumoniae* NCTC 12140; Snell et al., 1988; BSAC, 1991). It is essential to know the type of agar medium, with the manufacturer's name, the batch number, and the expiry date for ready-to-use preparations. When the media are made up from dehydrated powder, it is necessary to add a reproducibility test with a reference strain. The use of additives such as blood (horse, sheep, rabbit, etc.) must be mentioned, together with growth factors, CO_2 concentration, etc.

The origin of the test disks (manufacturers), batch number, quality controls, and details of storage must also be given, together with the way in which the diameter of the inhibition zone is measured (caliper, ruler, optical device, etc.).

10.3 Antibiophenotype

Certain tests are done routinely. For example, with *S. pneumoniae*, disks loaded with 1 μg of oxacillin can be used to predict if the strain is resistant to penicillin G. It is wise to add a ceftizoxime disk, as if the diameter is ≤15 mm there is a strong probability that the strain is resistant to cefotaxime and ceftriaxone (MIC ≥2 mg/l). This test appears to be less reliable if the strains have diminished susceptibility to cefotaxime (MIC: 1 mg/l). All these data can be confirmed by determining the MIC value. Another example is the determination of the activity of a new ß-lactam on Enterobacteriaceae. Cefotaxime, ceftazidime, and, if possible, aztreonam must be tested in association with co-amoxyclav to detect extended spectrum ß-lactamases (double-test technic; Jarlier et al., 1988).

In the case of the aminoglycosides, it also possible to determine the enzymatic profile of a bacterial strain for different enzymes and membrane permeability abnormalities depending on the inhibition zone diameters (Table 13; Miller, 1992).

10.4 Centralizing the Tests

All isolates must be stored in good conditions (storage media, temperature, lyophilization, etc.). A single laboratory should centralize all strains isolated during the clinical trial. All the strains must be reidentified precisely, including serogroups or serotypes, and ß-lactamases or enzymes inactivating aminoglycosides must be detected. The MIC must be routinely redetermined if the results are to be analyzable. In the case of bacterial species whose growth is reputed to be difficult, e.g., *S. pneumoniae, S. pyogenes, M. catarrhalis,* and *H. influenzae*, it is useful to run an antibacterial susceptibility test (antibiogram) and to determine the MIC value of antibiotics tested in parallel. This provides information on the vitality of the strain and avoids underestimating the MIC because of poor growth. For a given bacterial species, the culture medium and its additives must be of the same batch and from the same manufacturer. It must be routinely validated with a reference strain.

Other tests, e.g., killing curves, can be done on a given strain if the microbiological response occurs slower than expected in comparison with the majority of isolates for a given bacterial species.

Certain bacterial species must be tested for tolerance phenomena, as for example, with benzylpenicillin and viridans streptococci or 2-amino-5-thiazolyl cephalosporins and *H. influenzae*. The simplest test consists of determining the MIC and MBC (Allen et al., 1978; Goessens, 1993).

10.5 Inhibition Zone Diameter/MIC Correlations

The correlation between the disk method and MIC technique must be established in certain countries, such as the U.S. This involves multicenter studies, based on fresh clinical isolates collected over a given period and including the major bacterial species growing aerobically or in anaero-aerobic conditions such as Enterobacteriaceae and commonly responsible for clinical infections.

11 EPIDEMIOLOGY OF RESISTANCE — A SURVEY

It is exceedingly difficult to predict the epidemiology of resistance at the time when a new compound will be released, as 5 to 10 years will elapse between its synthesis, the beginning of development and its release, and the situation can evolve rapidly. The first signs of changes in the activity of an antibacterial agent on one or several species must be detected as early as possible. The best example of such signs is the decrease in the susceptibility of *N. gonorrhoeae* to fluoroquinolones (Knapp et al., 1994; Putnam

Table 13 Inhibition Zone for 50% of the Clinical Isolates (Aminoglycoside Resistant (1989-1991).

	Test Disc Load (μg)	Diameter (mm)	Gram-Negative Bacilli							Gram-Positive Cocci	
			AAC(3)-IV	AAC(3)-I	AAC(2')	AAC(3)-VI	ANT(2") + AAC(3)-III	ANT(4')-II	APH(3')-VI	APH(2") + AAC(6)	ANT(4') -I
Gentamicin	10	22 ± 4	12	13	14	6	8	20	24	6	20
Tobramycin	10	21 ± 5	6	21	13	17	9	14	26	6	7
Netilmicin	30	25 ± 5	15	25	24	21	22	20	27	18	36
Amikacin	30	22 ± 6	23	23	24	21	22	18	8	16	22
Isepamicin	30	24 ± 6	25	25	24	23	23	18	8	16	21

Adapted from Miller GH., 1992.

et al., 1992). Previous studies had shown a slight decrease in the *in vitro* activity of fluoroquinolones on ß-lactamase-producing strains.

A decrease in the activity of cefuroxime and other cephalosporins (Table 14) has recently been reported on *H. influenzae* ß-lactamase-producing strains resistant to ampicillin (James et al., 1993).

There is a major risk of emergence of strains resistant to fluoroquinolones among Enterobacteriaceae producing extended spectrum ß-lactamases (TEM-3, etc.), as a change in the killing rate of ciprofloxacin has been observed; this occurred at the sixth hour instead of the second hour as seen with strains that do not produce this enzyme. Recently, strains of *S. pneumoniae* resistant to sparfloxacin (MIC: 8 mg/l) have been detected during clinical studies (Garau et al., 1994) with a potential risk of dissemination.

Table 14 ß-Lactams Activities on *H. Influenzae* Isolates Resistant to Ampicillin and Nonproducing ß-Lactamases

	MIC$_{90}$ (mg/l)		
	Strains with Decrease Susceptibility	Susceptible Strains	*H. influenzae* NCTC 11931 (MIC)
Ampicillin	5.16	0.52	0.5
Amoxicillin	11.9	0.92	1.0
Coamoxyclav	6.20	0.64	1.0
Imipenem	6.19	4.14	1.0
Cefazolin	>55.4	30.0	16.0
Cefadroxil	>118.7	35.6	16.0
Cefaclor	>59.1	5.29	4.0
Cefuroxime	5.9	0.69	1.0
Cefotaxime	0.24	<0.06	0.03
Cefepime	1.48	0.11	0.1
Cefpirome	0.70	<0.06	0.06
Cefpodoxime	0.93	0.086	0.1
Cefixime	0.62	0.05	0.06

From James PA, Hossain FK, Lewis DA, White DG, *J. Antimicrob. Chemother.* 1993, 32, 239-246. With permission.

Regular monitoring of cephalosporin activity will enable a gradual increase in MIC to be detected, even if values remain within the therapeutic range. This epidemiological surveillance is difficult in practice, as it requires a colossal effort. A certain number of epidemiological survey could be initiated, but the most realistic approach is to analyze the relevant scientific publications and studies done by scientific societies such as the European Society of Clinical Microbiology.

12 AUTOMATED SYSTEM

The used of automated microdilution system for MIC determinations has become increasingly popular during the last decade. Comparative testing of the new drug to an accepted reference method (e.g., NCCLS) has to be carried out to determine clinical efficacy, reproductibility, efficacy with challenge strains from the reference centers, stability, and quality control ranges.

Examples are Autobac®, Vitek®, and API® test strips. The latter two methods are unsatisfactory, as they are inflexible and cannot be used to test a new compound. Other techniques such as E-test strips have been started to be used for routine MIC determinations, but their use necessitates a certain degree of experience, particularly for difficult species such as *S. pneumoniae*.

All this work must start during the late development phase and the results must be available when the new drug is marketed.

13 CONCLUSION

Clinical pharmacology plays several roles in the field of antimicrobial chemotherapy. The first is to determine the intrinsic activity of the new compound and its antibacterial spectrum. The second is to determine the activity of the new agent relative to compounds used in a given infection. The third is to determine activity in a given epidemiological setting, such as pneumococcal infections due to strains resistant to penicillin G, *Shigella* resistant to ampicillin and tetracyclines, staphylococcal infections resistant to oxacillin, enterococcal strains resistant to vancomycin, Enterobacteriaceae producing extended-spectrum ß-lactamases, and multiresistant tuberculous bacilli. Finally, it has a prospective role for new opportunistic agents such as *Rhodococcus equi* and *Leuconostoc* and *Pediococcus* spp. One of the crucial duties is to pay attention to the evolution of bacterial resistance.

REFERENCES

Agouridas C, Bonnefoy A, Chantot JF, Ketolides, a new distinct semi-synthetic class of macrolides : *in vitro* and *in vivo* antibacterial activity, 34th Intersci. Conf. Antimicrob. Agents Chemother., Orlando, FL, 1994, F-168.

Akoun G, Bertrand A, Cambarrère I, Constans P, Dumont R, Guibout P, Kamarec J, Marsac J, Robillard M, Sauvaget J, Thibault P, Voisin C, Safran C, Clinical evaluation of roxithromycin (RU 28965) in the treatment of hospitalized patients with lower respiratory tract infections, In Butzler JP, Kobayashi H, *Macrolides: a Review with an Outlook on Future Development,* Excerpta Medica, Amsterdam, 1986, 95-99.

Allen JL, Sprunt K, Discrepancy between minimum inhibitory and minimum bactericidal concentrations of penicillin for group A and group B ß-hemolytic streptococci, *J. Pediatr.* 1978, 93, 69-71.

Andrews JM, Baquero F, Beltran JM, Carton E, Crockaert F, Golernado M et al., International collaborative study on standardization of bacterial sensitivity to fosfomycin *J. Antimicrob. Chemother.* 1983, 12, 357-361.

Baquero F, European standards for antibiotic susceptibility testing : towards a theoretical consensus, *Eur. J. Clin. Microbiol. Infect. Dis.* 1990, 9, 492-495.

Barrière JC, Bouanchaud DH, Desnottes JF, Paris JM, Streptogramins analogues *Expert Opin. Invest. Drugs* 1994, 32, 115-131.

Bauer AW, Kirby WMM, Sherris JC, Turck M, Antibiotic susceptibility testing by a standardized single disc method, *Am. J. Clin. Pathol.,* 1966, 45, 493-496.

Beam TR Jr, Gilbert DN, Kunin C, European guidelines for the clinical evaluation of anti-infectives drug products, *Eur. Soc. Micobiol. Clin. Infect. Dis.,* 1993.

Beam TR Jr, Gilbert DN, Kunin C, Guidelines for the evaluation of anti-infective drug products, *Clin. Infect. Dis.* 1992, 15, Suppl. 1.

British Society for Antimicrobial Chemotherapy, A guide to sensitivity testing, *J. Antimicrob. Chemother.* 1991, 27, Suppl. D 1-47.

Bryskier A, Fluoroquinolones: mechanisms of action and resistance, *Int. J. Antimicrob. Agents* 1993, 2, 151-184.

Bryskier A, Veyssier P, Kazmierczak A, Fluoroquinolones, propriétés physicochimiques et microbiologiques, *Encyclopédie Médico-Chirurgicales-Maladies Infectieuses*, 1994, 8-004-B-10.

Chabbert YA, Sensibilité bactérienne aux antibiotiques In Le Minor L, Veron M, *Bactériologie Médicale,* Flammarion, Paris, 1982 p. 204-212.

Chantot J-F, Bryskier A, Gasc J-C, Antibacterial activity of roxithromycin: a laboratory evaluation, *J. Antibiotics* 1986, 39, 660-668.

Chantot J-F, Bryskier A, Antibacterial activity of ofloxacin and other 4-quinolone derivatives: *in vitro* and *in vivo* comparison, *J. Antimicrob. Chemother.* 1985, 16, 475-484.

Communicable Disease Report, Diphteria in Ukraine, CDR weekly 1994, 4, (38).

Cooper GL, Louie A, Baltch AL, Chu RC, Smith RP, Ritz WJ, Michelsen P, Influence of zinc on *Pseudomonas aeruginosa* susceptibilities to imipenem *J. Clin. Microbiol.* 1993, 31, 2366-2370.

Davies BI, The importance of the geometric MIC, *J. Antimicrob. Chemother.* 1990, 25, 471-472.

DeCross AJ, Marschall BJ, Mc Callum RW, Hoffman SR, Barrett LJ, Guerrant RL, Metronidazole susceptibility testing for *Helicobacter pylori*: comparison of disk, broth and agar dilution methods and their clinical relevance, *J. Clin. Microbiol.* 1993, 31, 1971-1974.

Deutsche Institut für Normung, Methoden zur Empfindlichkeitsprüfung von Bakteriellen Krankenheitseregern (außer Mycobacterien) gegen chemotherapeutika 1984, DIN 58940.

Dickinson JM, Mitchison DA, *In vitro* activities against mycobacteria of two-long-acting rifamycins, FCE 22807 and CGP 40/469 A (SPA-S-565), *Tubercle* 1990, 71, 109-115.

Doern GV, *In vitro* susceptibility testing of *Haemophilus influenzae*: review of new national committee for clinical laboratory standards recommendations, *J. Clin. Microb.* 1992, 3035-3038.

Drugeon HB, Drocourt V, Garrafo R, *Streptococcus pneumoniae*: conditions d'apparition des mutants résistants vis a vis de la sparfloxacine et de la ciprofloxacine dans un modèle expérimental animal, *Réunion Soc. Franc. Microbiol.* 1994.

Dublanchet A, Caillou J, Emond JP, Chardon H, Drugeon HB, Isolation of *Bacteroides* strains with reduced sensibility to 5-nitro-imidazoles, *Eur. J. Clin. Microbiol.* 1986, 5, 346-347.

Eagle H, Fleishman R, Musselman AD, Effect of schedule of administration on the therapeutic efficacy of penicillin, *Am. J. Med.* 1950, 9, 280-289.

Edlund C, Nord CE, Ecological impact of antimicrobial agents on human intestinal microflora, *Alpe Adria Microbiol. J.* 1993, 3, 137-164.

Ellner PD, Neu HC, The inhibitory quotient: a method for interpreting minimum inhibitory concentration data, *J. Am. Med. Assoc.* 1981, 246, 1575-1578.

Eng RHK, Cherubin C, Smith SM, Buccini F, Inoculum effect of ß-lactam antibiotics on Enterobacteriaceae, *Antimicrob. Agents Chemother.* 1985, 28, 601-606.

Ericsson HM, Sherris JC, Antibiotic sensitivity testing — Report of an international collaborative study, *Acta. Pathol. Microbiol. Immunol. Scand.* 1971, section B, suppl 217, 1-90.

Erwin ME, Jones RN, Roxithromycin *in vitro* susceptibility testing of *Heamophilus influenzae* by NCCLS methods, *J. Antimicrob. Chemother.* 1993, 32, 652-654.

Felmingham D, Grüneberg RN, personal communication, 1994.

Felmingham D, Robbins MJ, Marais R, Ridgway GL, Grüneberg RN, The effect of carbon dioxide on the *in vitro* activity of erythromycin and RU 28965 against anaerobic bacteria, *Drugs Exp. Clin. Res.* 1987, 13, 195-199.

Finland M, Garner C, Wilcox C, Sabath LD, Susceptibility of recently isolated bacteria to amikacin *in vitro*: comparison with other aminoglycoside antibiotics, *J. Infect. Dis.* 1976, 134, Suppl. S-297-307.

Forrest A, Nix DE, Ballow CH, Goss TF, Birmingham MC, Schentag JJ, Pharmacodynamics of intravenous ciprofloxacin in seriously ill patients, *Antimicrob. Agents Chemother.* 1993, 37, 1073-1081.

Forster JK, Lentino JR, Strodtman R, Divicenzo C, Comparison of *in vitro* activity of quinolone antibiotics and vancomycin against gentamicin and methicillin-resistant *S. aureus* by time kill kinetic studies, *Antimicrob. Agents Chemother.* 1986, 30, 823-827.

Frémaux A, Sissia G, Rosembaum M, Geslin P, *In vitro* activity of cefpirome (HR 810) a new parenteral cephalosporin against penicillin-susceptible and resistant pneumococci, 32nd Intersci. Conf. Antimicrob. Agents Chemother. Anaheim, 1992, 102.

Fukuoka T, Masuda N, Takenouchi T, Sekina N, Iijima M, Ohya S, Increase in susceptibility of *Pseudomonas aeruginosa* to carbapenem antibiotics in low aminoacid media, *Antimicrob. Agents Chemother.* 1991, 35, 529-532.

Garau J, Vercken JB, Efficacy of sparfloxacin in the treatment of 312 cases of pneumococcal community-acquired pneumonia: a pool data analysis, 5th Int. Symp. New Quinolones, Singapore, 1994.

Gasc J-C, Gouin d'Ambrière S, Lutz A, Chantot J-F, New ether oxime derivative of erythromycin A. A structure activity relationship study, *J. Antibiotics* 1991, 44, 651-668.

Goessens WHF, Basic mechanisms of bacterial tolerance of antimicrobial agents, *Eur. J. Clin. Microbiol. Infect. Dis.* 1990, 9, 9-12.

Graig W, Pharmacodynamics of antimicrobial agents as a basis for determining dosage regimens, *Eur. J. Clin. Microbiol. Infect. Dis.* 1990, 9, 6-8.

Grasso S, Meinardi G, De Carneci I, Tamassia V, New, *in vitro* model to study the effect of antibiotic concentration and rate of elimination on antibacterial activity, *Antimicrob. Agents Chemother.* 1978, 13, 570-576.

Hamilton-Miller JMT, Calculating MIC_{50}, *J. Antimicrob. Chemother.* 1991, 27, 863-864.

Hamilton-Miller JMT, Towards greater uniformity in sensitivity testing, *J. Antimicrob. Chemother.* 1977, 3, 385-392.

Hammerschlag MR, Antimicrobial susceptibility and therapy of infections caused by *Chlamydia pneumoniae, Antimicrob. Agents Chemother.* 1994, 38, 1873-1878.

Jabès D, Rossi R, Della Bruna C, Perrone E, Alpegiani M, Andreini BP, Visenti G, Zarini F, Francheschi G, Activity of new penems against defined MRSA strains, *Bioorg. Med. Chem. Lett.* 1993, 3, 2165-2170.

James PA, Hossain FK, Lewis DA, White DG, ß-lactam susceptibility of *Haemophilus influenzae* strains showing reduced susceptibility to cefuroxime, *J. Antimicrob. Chemother.* 1993, 32, 239-246.

Janda JM, Recent advances in the study of the taxomnomy, pathogenicity, and infectious syndromes associated with the genus *Aeromonas, Clin. Microb. Rev.* 1991, 4, 397-410.

Jarlier V, Nicolas MH, Fournier G, Phillipon A, Extended broad-spectrum ß-lactamases conferring transferable resistance to newer ß-lactam antibiotics in Enterobacteriaceae: hospital prevalence and susceptibility pattern, *Rev. Infect. Dis.* 1988, 10, 867-878.

Joly-Guillou ML, Vallée E, Bergogne-Bérézin E, Phillipon A, Distribution of ß-lactamases and phenotype analysis in clinical strains of *Acinetobacter calcoaceticus, J. Antimicrob. Chemother.* 1988, 22, 597-604.

Jones RN, Doern GV, Gerlach HE, Hindler J, Erwin ME, Validation of NCCSL macrolide (azithromycin, clarithromycin, and erythromycin) interpretive criteria for *Haemophilus influenzae* tested with the *Haemophilus* test medium, *Diagn. Microbiol. Infect. Dis.* 1994, 18, 243-249.

Kabir I, Butler T, Khanam A, Comparative efficacies of single intravenous dose of ceftriaxone ans ampicillin for shigellosis in a placebo-control trial, *Antimicrob. Agents Chemother.* 1986, 29, 645-648.

Kenny GE, Cartwright FD, Effect of pH, inoculum size, and incubation time on the susceptibility of *Ureaplasma urealyticum* to erythromycin *in vitro, Clin. Infect. Dis.* 1993, 17, Suppl. 1, S-215-218.

Kenny GE, Cartwright FD, Roberts MC, Agar dilution method for determination of antibiotic susceptibility of *Ureaplasma urealyticum, Ped. Infect. Dis. J.* 1986, 6, Suppl. 5, S-332-334.

Kernodle DS, Mc Graw PA, Stratton CW, Kaiser AB, Use of extracts versus whole-cell bacterial suspensions in the identification of *Staphylococcus aureus* ß-lactamase variants, *Antimicrob. Agents Chemother.* 1990, 34, 420-425.

Kilian M, A taxonomic study of the genus *Haemophilus*, with the proposal of a new species, *J. Gen. Microbiol.* 1976, 93, 9-62.

King A, Phillips I, Standardization of Iso-Sensitest, *Agar. J. Antimicrob. Chemother.* 1993, 32, 339.

King A, Philips I, Reporting *in vitro* activity of new antimicrobial agents, *J. Antimicrob. Chemother.* 1995, 35, 227.

Klugman KP, Saunders J, *In vitro* susceptibility of penicillin-susceptible and penicillin-resistant pneumococci to parenteral third and fourth generation cephalosporins, *6th Int. Cong. Infect. Dis.* Prague, 1994.

Knapp JS, Washington JA, Doyle LJ, Neal SW, Parekh MC, Rice RJ, Persistence of *Neisseria gonorrhoeae* strains with decreased susceptibilities to ciprofloxacin and ofloxacin in Cleveland, Ohio, from 1992 through 1993, *Antimicrob. Agents Chemother.* 1994, 38, 2194-2196.

Lee BL, Sachdeva M, Chambers HF, Effect of protein binding of daptomycin on MIC and antibacterial activity, *Antimicrob. Agents Chemother.* 1991, 35, 2505-2508.

Loleka S, Vibulbandhikit S, Poonyarit P, Response to antimicrobial therapy for shigellosis in Thailand, *Rev. Infect. Dis.* 1991, 13 Suppl. 4, S-42-6.

Lukehart SA, Fohn MJ, Baker-Zander SA, Efficacy of azithromycin for therapy of active syphilis in the rabbit model, *J. Antimicrob. Chemother.* 1990, 25, Suppl. A, 91-99.

Maple PCA, Efstratiou A, Tsevena G, Rikushin Y, Deshevoi S, Jahkola M, Vuopia-Varkila J, George RC, The *in vitro* susceptibilities of toxigenic strains of *Corynebacterium diphtheriae* isolated in northwestern Russia and surrounding areas to ten antibiotics, *J. Antimicrob. Chemother.* 1994, 34, 1037-1040.

Martinez-Martinez L, Suarez AI, Ortega MC, Perea EJ, Comparative *in vitro* activities of new quinolones against coryneform bacteria, *Antimicrob. Agents Chemother.* 1994, 38, 1439-1441.

Mégraud F, Boyanova L, Lamoulliate H, Activity of lanzoprazole against *Helicobacter pylori, Lancet* 1991, 337, 1486.

Miller GH, and Aminoglycoside resistance study group, Resistance to aminoglycosides in *Pseudomonas, Trends Microbiol.*, 1994, 2, 347-352.

Moore RD, Smith CR, Lietman PS, Association of aminoglycoside plasma levels with therapeutic outcome in gram-negative pneumonia, *Am. J. Med.* 1984a, 77, 657-662.

Moore RD, Smith CR, Lietman PS, The association of aminoglycoside plasma levels with mortality in patients with Gram-negative bacteria, *J. Infect. Dis.* 1984b, 149, 443-448.

National Committee for Clinical Laboratory Standards, Development of *in vitro* susceptibility testing criteria and quality control parameters — tentative guideline — Document M 23-T NCCLS, Villanova PA, 1993.

Nickolai DJ, Lammel CJ, Byford BA, Morris JH, Kaplan EB, Hadley WK, Brooks GF, Effects of storage temperature and pH on the stability of eleven ß-lactam antibiotics in MIC trays, *J. Clin. Microbiol.* 1985, 21, 366-370.

Nord CE, Edlund C, Impact of antimicrobial agents on human intestinal microflora, *J. Chemother.* 1990, 2, 218-237.

Peloux I, Le Noc P, Bryskier A, Le Noc D, *In vitro* activity of cefpirome and five other cephems against enteric pathogens, 34th Intersci. Conf. Antimicrob. Agents Chemother., Orlando, FL, 1994, E-28.

Periti P, Sueri L, Tosi M, Ciammarughi R, Cadco P, Milanesi B, Cefotaxime in the cerebral fluid and serum in patients with purulent meningitis, *J. Antimicrob. Chemother.* 1984, 14, Suppl. B, 117-123.

Péter O, Bretz AG, *In vitro* susceptibility of *Borrelia burgdorferi, Borrelia garinii* and *Borrelia afzelii* to 7 antimicrobial agents, *Advances in Lyme Borreliosis Research,* Cevenini R, Sambri V, La Placa M, 1994 p. 167-170.

Péter O, Bretz AG, Polymorphism of outer surface proteins of *Borrelia burgdorferi* as a tool for classification, *Zentralbl. Bakteriol.* 1992, 277, 28-33.

Philipon A, Arlet G, Lagrange PH, Origin and impact of plasmid-mediated extended-spectrum beta-lactamases, *Eur. J. Clin. Microbiol. Infect. Dis.* 1994, 13, Suppl. 1, 17-29.

Putnam SD, Lavin BS, Stone JR, Oldfield III EC, Hoper DG, Evaluation of the standardized disk diffusion and agar dilution antibiotic susceptibility test methods by using strains of *Neisseria gonorrhoeae* from the United States and Southeast Asia, *J. Clin. Microbiol.* 1992, 30, 974-980.

Rastogi N, Labrousse V, Bryskier A, Intracellular activities of roxithromycin used alone and in association with other drugs against *Mycobacterium avium* complex in human macrophages, *Antimicrob. Agents Chemother.* 1995, 39.

Rastogi N, Goh KS, Bryskier A, *In vitro* activity of roxithromycin against 16 species of atypical mycobacteria and effect of pH on its radiometric MICs, *Antimicrob. Agents Chemother.* 1993, 37, 1560-1562.

Reed LJ, Muench H, A simple method for estimating fifty percent endpoints, *Am. J. Hygiene* 1938, 27, 493-497.

Reina J, Ros MJ, Fernandez-Baca V, Resistance to erythromycin in fluoroquinolone-resistant *Campylobacter jejuni* strains isolated from human feces, *J. Antimicrob. Chemother.* 1995, 35, 351-352.

Rosdahl VT, Naturally occuring constitutive ß-lactamase of novel serotype in *Staphylococcus aureus, J. Gen. Microbiol.* 1973, 77, 229-231.

Saez-Nieto JA, Vazquez JA, Marcos C, Meningococci moderately resistant to penicillin, *Lancet* 1990, 54.

Sahm DF, Baker CN, Jones RN, Thornsberry C, Influence of growth medium on the *in vitro* activities of second- and third-generation cephalosporins against *Streptococcus faecalis, Antimicrob. Agents Chemother.* 1984, 20, 561-567.

Schentag J, Correlation of pharmacokinetic parameters to efficacy of antibiotics: relationships between serum concentrations, MIC values, and bacterial eradication in patients with Gram-negative pneumonia, *Scand. J. Infect. Dis.* 1991, Suppl. 74, 218-234.

Siebor E, Kazmierczak A, Factors influencing the activity of macrolide antibiotics *in vitro* In *Macrolides, Chemistry, Pharmacology and Clinical Use*, Bryskier AJ, Butzler J-P, Neu HC, Tulkens PM, Blackwell-Arnette, Paris 1993, 197-203.

Simpson IN, Hunter R, Govan JRW, Nelson JW, Do all *Pseudomonas cepacia* produce carbapenemases? *J. Antimicrob. Chemother.* 1993, 32, 339-341.

Smith JT, Lewin CS, Chemistry and mechanisms of action of the quinolone antibacterials, *The Quinolones,* Andriole VT (ed). Academic Press, New York, 1988, p. 23-82.

Snell JJS, George RC, Perry SF, Erdman YG, Antimicrobial susceptibility testing of *Streptococcus pneumoniae* quality assessment results, *J. Clin. Pathol.* 1988, 41, 384-387.

Soussy CJ, Cluzel R, Courvalin P et le Comité de l'antibiogramme de la société française de microbiologie, Definition and determination of *in vitro* antibiotic suscptibility breakpoints for bacteria in France, *Eur. J. Clin. Microbiol. Infect. Dis.* 1994, 13, 238-246.

Stamm LV, Stapleton JT, Bassford PJ, *In vitro* assay to demonstrate high-level erythromycin resistance of a clinical isolate of *Treponema pallidum, Antimicrob. Agents Chemother.* 1988, 32, 164-169.

Stokes EJ, Ridgway GL, Wren MWD, *Clinical Microbiology,* 7th edition, Edward Arnold, London 1993, pp. 234-278.

Stokes EJ, Antibacterial drugs, In *Clinical Bacteriology,* Edward Arnold, London 1955, pp. 157-192.

Täuber MG, Zak O, Scheld WM, Hengstler B, Sande MA, The postantibiotic effect in the treatment of experimental meningitis caused by *Streptococcus pneumoniae* in rabbits, *J. Infect. Dis.* 1984, 149, 575-583.

Täuber MG, Kunz S, Zak O, Sande MA, Influence of antibiotic dose, dosing interval, and duration of therapy on outcome in experimental pneumococcal meningitis in rabbits, *Antimicrob. Agents Chemother.* 1989, 33, 418-423.

The Swedish reference group for antibiotics, A revised system for antibiotic sensitivity testing, *Scand. J. Infect. Dis.* 1981, 13, 148-152.

Tomasz A, Nachman S, Leaf H, Stable classes of phenotypic expression in methicillin-resistant clinical isolates of staphylococci, *Antimicrob. Agents Chemother.* 1991, 35, 124-129.

Trias J, Nikaido H, Protein D_2 channel of *Pseudomonas aeruginosa* outermembrane has binding site for basic aminoacids and peptides, *J. Biol. Chem.* 1990, 265, 15680-15684.

Verdon MS, Handsfield HH, Johnson RB, Pilot study of azithromycin for treatment of primary and secondary syphilis, *Clin. Infect. Dis.* 1994, 19, 486-488.

Vogelman BS, Craig WA, Postantibiotic effects, *J. Antimicrob. Chemother.* 1985, 15, Suppl. A, 37-46.

Wallace RJ, Steele LC, Susceptibility testing of *Nocardia* species for the clinical laboratory, *Diagn. Microbiol. Infect. Dis.* 1988, 9, 155-166.

Werkgroep Richtlijnen Govoeligheidsbepalingen report, Standaardisatie van govoeligheidsbepalingen, WRG Bilthoven 1981.

White RL, Kays MB, Friederich LV, Brown EW, Koonce JR, Pseudoresistance of *Pseudomonas aeruginosa* resulting from degradation of imipenem in an automated susceptibility testing system with predried panels, *J. Clin. Microbiol.* 1991, 29, 398-400.

Wilkins TD, Chalgren S, Medium for use in antibiotic susceptibility testing of anaerobic bacteria, *Antimicrob. Agents Chemother.* 1976, 10, 926-928.

Williams JD, Prospects for standardisation of methods and guidelines for disc susceptibility testing, *Eur. J. Clin. Microbiol. Infect. Dis.* 1990, 9, 496-501.

Xia H, Keane CT, Beattie S, O'Morain CA, Standardization of disk diffusion and its clinical significance for susceptibility testing of metronidazole against *Helicobacter pylori, Antimicrob. Agents Chemother.* 1994, 38, 2357-2361.

Yabuuchi E, Kosako Y, Oyaizu H, Yano I, Hotta H, Hashimoto Y et al., Proposal of *Burkholderia* gen nov and transfer of seven species of the genus *Pseudomonas* homology group II to the new genus with the type species *Burkholderia cepacia* (Pallrini and Holmes, 1981) comb nov 1992, *Microbiol. Immunol.* 1992, 36, 1251-1275.

Zak O, O'Reilly T, Animal models as predictors of the safety and efficacy of antibiotics, *Eur. J. Clin. Microbiol. Infect. Dis.* 1990, 9, 472-478.

Chapter 37

Antiviral Drugs

Whaijen Soo

CONTENTS

1 Introduction 511
2 Drug Classes 512
3 Prophylaxis 512
  3.1 Aims of Therapy 512
  3.2 Study Design 513
  3.3 Clinical Assessments 513
  3.4 Laboratory Assessments 513
4 Acute Infections and Recurrent Episodes 513
  4.1 Study Design 514
  4.2 Clinical Assessments 514
    4.2.1 Clinical Signs and Symptoms 514
    4.2.2 Quality of Life 514
    4.2.3 Resolution of Viral Lesions 515
    4.2.4 Prevention of Complications 515
  4.3. Laboratory Assessments 515
5 Chronic Infection 515
  5.1 Study Design 515
    5.1.1 The Use of Surrogate Markers 515
    5.1.2 Other Design Issues 516
  5.2 Clinical Assessments 516
    5.2.1 Death or Life-Threatening Events 516
    5.2.2 Quality of Life Measurements 516
    5.2.3 Other Assessments 516
  5.3 Laboratory Assessments 517
    5.3.1 Virological Measurements 517
    5.3.2 Immunological Measurements 517
    5.3.3 Other Assessments 517
6 Combination Therapy 517
7 Drug Resistance 518
8 Safety Evaluation 518
9 Conclusions 518
References 519

1 INTRODUCTION

Viral infections lead to a spectrum of diseases of varying severity and duration. Infections caused by many respiratory and enteric viruses, for example, usually lead to acute illnesses without much chronicity. Antiviral therapy for these acute infections should provide early resolution of signs and symptoms associated with the disease, reduce viral shedding, and prevent secondary complications. These treatment goals can also be applied to therapy for recurrent episodes of acute illness caused by some of the herpes virus infections such as herpes simplex (HSV) and varicella zoster (VZV). Most agents for acute viral illnesses are only effective when given early in the manifestation of disease symptoms and signs. To maximize the clinical benefits of these drugs, use during a prodromal phase or even for postexposure prophylaxis should be considered, if the safety and tolerance of a particular drug have been well established.

0-8493-9230-6/97/$0.00+$.50
© 1997 by CRC Press, Inc.

Infections by papillomaviruses (HPV), cytomegalovirus (CMV), hepatitis viruses B and C (HBV and HCV), and immunodeficiency viruses (HIV), on the other hand, might not cause obvious acute illnesses but can cause chronic diseases leading to serious clinical sequelae. Antiviral therapy for these chronic viral infections, therefore, should aim to arrest the progression of the disease and reduce the chance of late adverse consequences. Since drugs for chronic viral illnesses will have to be used for an extended period of time, long-term tolerance becomes a key consideration in the risk-to-benefit assessment for each drug with regard to the viral illness to be treated.

Immunization should remain the primary approach to the prevention of viral infections. When effective vaccines are not available for use in a particular target population, chemoprophylaxis should be considered. These circumstances include use in immunodeficient individuals and individuals with hypersensitivity to existing vaccines, as well as in conjunction with late vaccination. For seasonal chemoprophylaxis against diseases such as influenza, drug therapy should be initiated as soon as an outbreak is recognized. For other prophylactic use, the duration and the timing of initiation of prophylaxis will depend on knowledge of the natural history of the disease.

2 DRUG CLASSES

Attempts to develop antiviral therapy in the past 50 years have met with only limited success, largely due to our lack of knowledge about virus-specific functions as target sites. Most antiviral drugs, such as idoxuridine, vidarabine, zidovudine, didanosine, and zalcitabine, are nucleoside analogs that interfere with viral nucleic acid synthesis by inhibiting viral DNA polymerases.[1,2] This inhibition of viral enzyme, however, is not selective enough, and all these drugs cause significant toxicities due to their inhibitory actions on host enzymes. One notable exception is acyclovir, which is relatively nontoxic since its activation can only be achieved by a virus-specific process.[3] Other drugs, such as amantadine and rimantadine, interfere with the entry of the influenza virus.[4] Recent advances in molecular virology and recombinant technology, however, have enabled us to better understand the virus life cycle, and thus recognize additional virus-specific functions to be targeted for therapeutic intervention. One excellent example of these new targets is HIV proteinase.[5,6] Based on the transitional state of this enzyme, a number of potent inhibitors of HIV replication have been designed and some have shown promise in early phase clinical trials.[7] Other new target sites include virus-specific integrase and regulatory enzymes responsible for amplification of viral replication.[8] Rational drug design based on structure analysis, and simple screening procedures suitable for high-flux random screening can now be used to identify drug candidates which inhibit these target sites.

A different approach to antiviral therapy is the use of immunomodulators. This is a relatively new class of compounds, many of which have nonspecific immunomodulatory effects. The primary objective for the use of an immunomodulator is to enhance the cytotoxic killing of infected cells which serve as reservoirs for further spread of the virus. One particular immunomodulator, alpha-interferon, has been extensively studied. Alpha-interferon, however, has independent immunomodulatory and antiviral effects, probably through different mechanisms of action.[9] It is possible that the efficacy of alpha-interferon against viral hepatitis and papilloma viral infection, for example, is due to both the antiviral and the immunomodulatory effects of this compound. Other immunomodulators such as gamma-interferon, interleukin-2, and interleukin-12 have also been studied for their potential use against various viral diseases.[10,11] These immunomodulators clearly do not have a direct antiviral effect. Although there is preliminary evidence suggesting that these immunomodulators can indeed enhance immune functions in patients with viral illnesses,[12] it is too early to predict whether the observed immunomodulatory effects can be translated into clinical efficacy.

3 PROPHYLAXIS

3.1 Aims of Therapy

The aim of chemoprophylaxis is to prevent the infection and/or clinical manifestation of disease caused by a particular virus. For viral infections leading to significant chronic sequelae, prevention of infection is critical. For viral infections causing only acute illnesses, prevention of clinical disease should be adequate. In the latter case, the development of an immune response to subclinical infection could be a potentially desirable feature of prophylaxis, since immunity may be established against reinfection.

3.2 Study Design

To demonstrate efficacy of chemoprophylaxis in a natural setting usually requires a large number of patients, because of low infection rates. This problem can be circumvented in early phase evaluation by the selection of a subpopulation with higher infection rates, such as prison inmates, nursing home residents, and other institutionalized populations,[13] as well as individuals who are less immunocompetent because of medications, transplantations, or lack of vaccination. If such a subpopulation is not available, the use of an artificial challenge model can be considered.[14] The extrapolation of data from challenge to natural studies, however, is not always successful. This is because the viral load, the infection rate, and the strains of virus used in a challenge study might be very different from those occurring in the natural setting.

Owing to the unpredictability of the outbreak and the variability of the immune status of each individual against a particular viral infection, efficacy data from uncontrolled, open studies are not reliable. Phase II pilot efficacy studies, therefore, should be double-blind and controlled, while Phase I single and multiple ascending-dose pharmacokinetic and tolerance studies can remain open and uncontrolled.

Study of the efficacy of chemoprophylaxis in the prevention of chronic viral infections, such as HIV, is generally difficult due to the low attack rate, even in the postexposure setting.[15] Very large sample size will be required for drugs with high efficacy. Early phase studies can only be used to primarily establish safety profiles.

Because of high rate of perinatal transmission of HIV, the efficacy of chemoprophylaxis can be demonstrated with a reasonable number of patients.[16] Large controlled trials can be planned based on efficacy and safety data from early phase studies in pregnant women.[17-19]

3.3 Clinical Assessments

The primary efficacy endpoint is prevention of laboratory-documented viral illness during chemoprophylaxis. Laboratory documentation is especially critical in respiratory viral infections, because many different respiratory viruses cause diseases with similar signs and symptoms. For example, in a prophylaxis study comparing rimantadine with placebo in young volunteers, 14% of those who took drug had a clinical diagnosis of influenza A illness, yet only 3% had true influenza A illness documented by the laboratory.[20] On the other hand, laboratory documentation might not be required for study of suppression of recurrence, since in this case patients are usually familiar with the specific clinical signs and symptoms associated with the disease, so that accurate diagnosis can be made clinically.

The severity of viral illness that develops during chemoprophylaxis should also be monitored. Illness developing during chemoprophylaxis could be less severe or with fewer complications, which supports further the activity of the drug.

3.4 Laboratory Assessments

Many methods are now available to confirm virus infection. Antibody tests are available for the detection of either seroconversion or increases in antibody titers.[21] Other tests such as antigen-capture assays detect the presence of the virus or its components in the infected individuals. Viral culture, if positive, is a useful indication for the infectivity of the patients. Negative culture results, however, may not always indicate the absence of the virus, and could be due to the difficulty in standardizing the culture technology itself, especially if virus is sensitive to exposure outside the host or is present in very low titers. Recent availability of diagnostic tests based on amplification technologies such as polymerase chain reaction (PCR)[22-24] and branched-DNA[25-27] assays will no doubt simplify and facilitate the confirmation of viral infection.

4 ACUTE INFECTIONS AND RECURRENT EPISODES

The aims of treatment for acute infection include some or all of the following: relief of signs and symptoms of acute viral illnesses, early resolution of viral lesions, reduction in viral shedding, and prevention of secondary complications. Usually similar study designs and efficacy parameters can be used for initial infection as well as recurrent episodes of illness. In some viral diseases, however, the signs and symptoms may be different between initial infection and subsequent recurrences.

4.1 Study Design

The timing of initiation of therapy and the frequency of efficacy measurements are two elements critical to a successful treatment study of acute viral infections. The earlier drug treatment can be started, the more likely benefits of the drug can be shown. Results from studies on influenza A and herpes simplex showed that, to have significant efficacy against these acute illnesses, drugs must be given within 48 to 72 h after signs and symptoms of diseases are first noted. Ideally, drug therapy should not be initiated until laboratory diagnosis is made. However, when a rapid diagnostic test is not available, treatment may be started without laboratory diagnosis if the disease is life-threatening or the drug under study is relatively nontoxic. Under these circumstances, a retrospective laboratory diagnosis should be made. Drug therapy can be commenced even earlier with self-initiation of therapy by patients, provided that pretherapy baseline information can be accurately recorded by patients themselves or through other types of arrangements. Earlier initiation of therapy might also be needed for efficacy in the treatment of acute viral illnesses in children.[28-30]

Many acute infections are self-limited and patients usually recover without therapy in a few days. Therefore, efficacy of a drug can be demonstrated only during a narrow window of time. Demonstration of more rapid improvement with therapy might require that patients be monitored frequently with more than one observation per day. This close monitoring may require housing patients with diseases that otherwise would not require hospitalization, a procedure bound to increase the cost of a study and present additional management problems.

Because there is much variation in the clinical course of acute disease among infected individuals, drug efficacy for symptomatic relief can only be evaluated in double-blind, controlled studies.[31] A randomized trial of vidarabine vs. foscarnet in patients with acyclovir-resistant HSV was terminated early due to clear evidence of the superiority of foscarnet in terms of time to healing, resolution of pain, and cessation of viral shedding.[32] At the time of closure only 14 of a projected 26 patients had been enrolled, indicating the potential power of a controlled trial to rapidly detect large differences in efficacy between treatments.

Although early phase tolerance studies can still be open and uncontrolled, it should be emphasized that toxicities of a drug can sometimes be confused with symptoms and signs of the disease to be treated. In this case, further clarification of drug toxicity can only be obtained from a controlled study.

4.2 Clinical Assessments

4.2.1 Clinical Signs and Symptoms

The most important efficacy parameters in clinical assessments are measurements of signs and symptoms. Because clinical manifestations of an acute infection include many signs and symptoms, analysis of change in each sign and symptom individually can be cumbersome and often uninterpretable. One approach to simplify this analytical nightmare is to establish a simple scoring system for signs and symptoms, as was used in studies with rimantadine for the treatment of influenza A illness.[33] Another approach is to select only key symptoms as primary parameters for analysis. For example, only pain and itching were evaluated in most studies with acyclovir and interferons for the treatment of herpes simplex,[34] while both acute pain and postherpetic neuralgia have been used as key efficacy parameters for herpes zoster.[35,36] A third approach employs "transformed" parameters that provide general measurement of the rate of recovery from illness. Examples of transformed parameters include "time to 50% improvement" and "time to last fever," which were effectively used in data analysis of rimantadine studies.[37] These parameters help to eliminate repeated analysis at each time-point.

4.2.2 Quality of Life

Improvement of quality of life in acute viral illnesses can provide supportive evidence for the activity of the drug. Simple evaluation of productivity such as return to work, class attendance, etc. can sometimes provide useful evidence for practical benefits of the drug. For example, in a study in college students who had acute influenza illness, those who were treated with rimantadine were able to return to classes earlier than those who were treated with placebo.[38] Treatment of immunocompetent zoster patients >50 years old with valaciclovir resulted in a reduction both in days lost from work and in the need for help at home, as compared to treatment with acyclovir.[39]

More sophisticated instruments are now available to help evaluate changes in overall behavior or perceptions such as psychosocial functioning and general well-being. These methods will be discussed later in this chapter.

4.2.3 *Resolution of Viral Lesions*

This clinical assessment is primarily restricted to herpetic lesions. Resolution of viral lesions is usually measured by time to healing, time to crusting, and duration of vesicle/ulcer. Some of these parameters are more appropriate than others for a particular type of herpetic lesion, depending on the natural course of the disease. For example, time to crusting is probably more reliable than time to healing for herpes zoster lesions.[40] It should be emphasized that a precise definition of these parameters might not be as critical as a simple one that is strictly followed, especially among different study centers in a multicenter trial. In addition, consistent observations of lesions by one or only a very limited number of observers are required, since the assessment of lesions can be subjective.

4.2.4 *Prevention of Complications*

The particular viral disease under study determines the difficulty with which this parameter can be adequately assessed. Prevention of dissemination of lesions in herpes zoster in immunocompromised patients, for example, is easy to demonstrate, since dissemination can be clearly defined and the incidence of dissemination without drug therapy is high. In a study to evaluate alpha-interferon for the treatment of zoster in immunosuppressed patients with cancer, dissemination of zoster occurred in 58% of patients who received placebo, but only in 17% of those who received interferon.[35] On the other hand, to demonstrate prevention of secondary complications such as pneumonia or death from influenza infection requires a large number of patients, since the incidence of complications is low. In some viral diseases, a clear-cut causal relationship between the primary infection and secondary complications can be difficult to establish.

4.3 Laboratory Assessments

Viral culture data provide key measurements of an antiviral effect. Presence of viruses from either herpetic lesions or nasal wash of patients with influenza illness, for example, can be identified by culture. The sensitivity of culture techniques depends on the particular viral disease under study. For influenza virus, quantitative techniques for viral isolation have been well established, and data on viral shedding are fairly reliable. These culture assays were effectively used to demonstrate that significantly fewer patients with influenza illness were shedding virus after two-day therapy with rimantadine as compared with those who received placebo. In addition, those who continued to shed virus despite rimantadine therapy had significantly lower viral titers as compared with placebo recipients.[38] On the other hand, interpretation of viral culture data from studies with herpes simplex is not as straightforward. Positive culture cannot be obtained from herpetic lesions in up to 50% of recurrent episodes, so that culture-negative and -positive lesions might have to be evaluated separately.[34] It is hoped that the availability of PCR assays will significantly increase the sensitivity in the identification of viral lesions.[41]

5 CHRONIC INFECTION

The primary aims of therapy for chronic viral illnesses should be to arrest disease progression and reduce the chance of the late adverse sequelae of infection. The ultimate goal is to completely eliminate pre-existing viral infection, but this is probably not realistic at the present time. Owing to viral-gene integration and the development of latency, active viral replication does not take place in many infected cells. Phenotypically and functionally, these cells closely resemble their noninfected counterparts, leaving few targeting opportunities for drug discovery.

5.1 Study Design

5.1.1 *The Use of Surrogate Markers*

The evaluation of antiviral agents for chronic viral illness frequently follows a two-step process. Virological or immunological surrogate markers are usually used as endpoints for drug activity during early phase studies so that a long study period can be avoided. Once drug activity is demonstrated and therapeutic index determined, long-term studies will be needed to evaluate efficacy on the basis of clinical endpoints which can be rare and might require months or even years to reach.

Although the use of surrogate markers to evaluate drug activity in early phase trials is universally accepted, registration approval based on surrogate marker data is still controversial. Response in CD_4 cell counts has been used as the basis for approval for didanosine, zalcitabine, and stavudine for the treatment of advanced HIV disease. CD_4 cell counts, however, have been shown to partially satisfy the criteria for a valid surrogate marker as defined by The Institute of Medicine.[42] In addition, the treatment effect on CD_4 cell counts can only explain less than half of the eventual clinical benefit with therapy.[43,44] Other immunologic and virologic endpoints, including ß-$_2$-microglobulin, HIV p24 antigen, and neopterin have also been tested as surrogate markers in early trials. Unfortunately, these parameters have proven to be of only very limited, if any, prognostic value.

Recent data on viral load measurement based on amplification technology suggest that these parameters might be alternative surrogate markers in addition to CD_4 cell counts[45-47] for evaluation of drug therapy against HIV disease, as well as supportive markers for efficacy of drug therapy against hepatitis C.[48]

In designing early phase studies using surrogate markers as endpoints, sample size and frequency of measurement must be specified to address both selection and regression-to-the-mean biases, as well as intra- and intersubject variabilities. These biases can best be minimized through the use of a randomized control group.

5.1.2 Other Design Issues

The response of patients with chronic viral illnesses to therapy frequently depends on the length of the disease at the time of therapy. In diseases such as chronic active hepatitis B and HPV infection, it has been shown that the longer patients have had the disease the less likely it is that they will respond. To ensure a balanced study population, stratification of patients based on the length of their disease should be considered.

Dose-range and the frequency of dosing to be used in early phase studies should be determined on the basis of effective *in vitro* antiviral concentrations and single-dose pharmacokinetics of the drug in humans.

5.2 Clinical Assessments

5.2.1 Death or Life-Threatening Events

When possible, death or life-threatening events should be used as clinical endpoints. These parameters provide the most impressive and often dramatic results for the efficacy of a drug. For example, in a placebo-controlled phase II study on zidovudine in patients with acquired immunodeficiency syndrome (AIDS) or advanced AIDS-related complex (ARC), only 1 of 145 patients taking the drug but 16 of 137 patients taking placebo died after 3-6 months of treatment.[49] This convincing evidence for efficacy resulted in an early termination of the study, leading to the registration approval of the drug. Much larger sample size and longer study duration, however, were required to allow enough clinical events for efficacy evaluation in patients with less advanced HIV disease. Death or life-threatening events due to other chronic viral illnesses could take a lifetime to develop or occur with very low incidence. In these diseases, primary efficacy endpoints will be laboratory parameters.

5.2.2 Quality of Life Measurements

Methodology to measure quality of life has been developed over the past decade. Some of these methods, such as the General Health Rating Index[50] and the Sickness Impact Profile,[51] have been developed to assess sense of well-being and satisfaction with life, intellectual functioning, overall physical condition, overall emotional state, and ability to perform in social roles. Other more specific instruments, such as the Psychological General Well-being Schedule,[52] have been designed primarily to measure general psychological status. Clinically relevant comparative measures of health status and function in patients with advanced HIV disease undergoing treatment with various antiretroviral agents have been obtained through use of the HIV-PARSE. This is a self-administered instrument designed to assess symptom impact, disability, health status, and function.[53] In pediatric trials, patients can be tested for social behavior, language skills, attention span, memory and learning, motor speed, problem solving, and visual acuity.[54] It should be emphasized that there is no single method that is sensitive, specific, and yet able to cover the breadth of all aspects of quality of life. A composite index, based on all available instruments, should be developed for each chronic viral illness under study.

5.2.3 Other Assessments

Depending on the disease, other assessments may be appropriate. For example, patients with HIV infection also develop neurological abnormalities and cognitive function impairment. Thus, demonstration of improvement in neurological and cognitive functions can be supportive evidence for efficacy.[55] For efficacy evaluation in children, neuropsychologic testing can include age-appropriate tests of general intelligence such as the Bayley Scales of Infant Development (ages <2$^1/_2$ years), the McCarthy Scales of Children's Abilities ($2^1/_2$ to $5^1/_2$ years), and the Wechsler Intelligence Scales for Children ($>5^1/_2$ years).[54] In patients with chronic hepatitides, specific measurements are also available for the evaluation of signs and symptoms associated with compromised liver functions.

5.3 Laboratory Assessments

5.3.1 Virological Measurements

Commercial assays are available for quantitative measurements of components associated with various viruses such as HBV, HCV, and HIV. In HBV infection, the plasma levels of both HBV-DNA and HBV-DNA polymerase seem to correlate well with the amount of viral particles. A significant decrease in these parameters with therapy should therefore reflect antiviral activity of the drug. Moreover, continuous suppression of these HBV viral markers has been associated with reversion of serological status of patients and improvement in liver histology.[56] Hepatitis B surface antigen is an accepted marker for HBV, however, no such antigen has yet been observed for HCV. Preliminary results suggest that HCV RNA levels parallel the course of ALT values, indicating the possible utility of the viral marker as a surrogate. In HIV infection, reduction of viral load as measured by amplification strategy such as RNA-PCR seems to correlate with better clinical outcome.

Viral cultures in the past have not been reliable efficacy parameters for chronic viral illnesses due to problems with reproducibility. Recent establishment of microculture titering of plasma HIV viral load helped establish another valid viral load measurement. This assay methodology, however, is time-consuming and labor-intensive.

Antibodies against specific viral antigens represent another important class of markers for virological assessments. The presence of these antibodies is commonly correlated with a less active phase of viral replication. Appearance of these antibodies during drug therapy, therefore, strongly suggests that the activity of the disease has been slowed down or arrested. For example, appearances of antibodies to HBV core antigen and surface antigen have been established as major milestones for efficacy in the therapy of chronic active hepatitis B.[57]

5.3.2 Immunological Measurements

When the immune system serves as the direct target of a virus, as with HIV infection, normalization or improvement of immune function can be used as key evidence for efficacy. In other viral illnesses improvement in immune function can also be used as supportive evidence for efficacy.

Several immunological tests have been widely used for the evaluation of various immune functions. Routine cell counts of total various subtypes of white blood cells provide a quick glimpse of overall status of the immune system. Specific measurements of subsets of T lymphocytes, such as helper population (CD_4) and suppressor population (CD_8), are useful as surrogate markers for efficacy evaluation of HIV therapy, but are not generally useful for other viral illnesses. Other measurements of immune functions are now possible for testing both *in vitro* and *in vivo*. The most commonly used *in vitro* assay is the lymphocytic response to mitogenic and antigenic stimulation, a general assay to assess the overall function status of cellular immunity.[58] More specific assays such as antibody-dependent, cell-mediated cytotoxicity should be used only when infected cells can serve directly as target cells for cytotoxic killing in the *in vitro* assay.[12] Cutaneous delayed-type hypersensitivity (DTH) tests have been widely used to evaluate the T-cell functionality *in vivo*.[59] However, the DTH test has not been standardized thus far, and cannot be considered a validated efficacy parameter at the present time.

5.3.3 Other Assessments

Additional efficacy parameters may be used when their association with the disease under study is clearly established. For example, improvement in liver function tests during therapy is supportive evidence for the efficacy of drugs for chronic hepatitis B and C, while improvement in liver histology is considered key evidence for efficacy for both chronic hepatitides. Any new parameter being explored as a potential efficacy endpoint should preferably be tested first with an established drug.

6 COMBINATION THERAPY

For chronic viral diseases, such as HIV, the use of available drugs is limited due to insufficient potency with poor long-term efficacy, toxicities, and emergence of drug resistance. The goals for combination therapy will depend on the patient populations under consideration. For patients with advanced or terminal diseases, combination therapy should provide maximal potency[60,61] and reduce the incidence of viral resistance. For relatively asymptomatic patients with earlier stage disease, on the other hand, good tolerance can be a primary concern for any regimen to be of practical value.

Selection of combination regimens for early phase testing should be based on *in vitro* data on synergy, and lack of cross resistance, overlapping toxicities, and drug-drug interactions. Doses of each drug to be used in the combination regimen shoud be carefully considered, with the goal to maximize the antiviral effect through use of the highest dose of each drug that a patient can tolerate in monotherapy trials. Pharmacokinetic studies of combination drug use should be done as early as possible to help ensure correct dose selection for efficacy studies.

7 DRUG RESISTANCE

The emergence of drug-resistant strains of poliovirus was reported in laboratories as early as 1961,[62] but the clinical significance of drug resistance has not been adequately evaluated until recently.[63] Drug-resistant strains of various viruses have now been isolated from man. These resistant strains may have either existed in the environment before drug therapy and were selected during drug treatment, or have arisen by mutation from sensitive progenitor strains during therapy.

Early detection of resistant strains depends on the availability of sensitive laboratory methods and the careful study design of clinical trials. In studies on acute infections, for example, symptoms and signs of the illness as well as viral shedding should be followed during the entire length of the study, so that any rebound in illness and/or viral shedding late in drug therapy can be recognized and potential emergence of resistant strains of virus evaluated. Short-term clinical trials may be sufficient to identify rapid development of viral resistance, such as that seen with the non-nucleoside HIV reverse transcriptase inhibitor L-697,661.[64]

Virulence and infectivity of drug-resistant strains of virus can best be studied in a postcontact study. In chronic infections the emergence of resistant strains should always be considered a possible cause for the loss of response to drug therapy.

8 SAFETY EVALUATION

Standard evaluations of adverse reactions are discussed elsewhere in this book. However, it is important to emphasize that in early phase studies when a control arm is not used, the toxicities of a drug may be exaggerated because of difficulty in separating toxicities associated with the drug from symptoms and signs of the illness. For example, the gastrointestinal toxicities seen in patients who received rimantadine or amantadine for acute influenza illness could be due to either drug or the illness.[33] Similarly, hematological and neurological toxicities from HIV infection have made evaluation of toxicities of zidovudine[65] and dideoxycytidine[66] difficult. When no control arm is included in a trial for comparison, careful attention should be given to the temporal relationship of the observed toxicity and drug therapy, as well as the reversibility of side effects after termination of therapy. If possible, rechallenge with drug should be considered to provide direct evidence for the causal relationship. In life-threatening diseases such as AIDS, one should use caution not to drop the development of a drug candidate until it is clearly demonstrated that the limiting toxicity is due to the agent under study.

The recent experience of five deaths due to FIAU therapy in patients with chronic active hepatitis disease brought attention to safety monitoring in early phase studies, emphasizing the need for an adequate follow-up period after the conclusion of a study, especially when there is a possibility that drug toxicity could mimic either the underlying disease or the toxicity associated with concomitant medications.[67]

9 CONCLUSIONS

The search for new antiviral drugs has shifted in recent years from limited nucleoside research and opportunism to rational drug design, including the establishment of target sites such as viral proteinase, integrase, or DNA polymerase, and development of rapid screening procedures to identify lead compounds targeted at these sites. Antiviral research has been accelerated tremendously by the mobilization of the scientific research community to discover treatments for AIDS. It is expected that, through this research effort, many new classes of drugs will be developed in the next few decades, not only for HIV infection but for other viral illnesses as well.

Methodologies for the evaluation of antiviral drugs have been developed for many viral illnesses. For prophylaxis, a small early phase study with the artificial challenge model should provide useful information on activity of the drug, but a large study in a natural setting is ultimately required to establish efficacy of the drug. For acute infections, drug therapy should be initiated early, and the signs and symptoms of illness should be monitored frequently during drug therapy to demonstrate early improvement. Reduction of viral shedding should be demonstrated, and the potential development of resistant strains should be followed closely. For chronic viral infections, viral load measurements, immunological markers, and, if appropriate, quality of life measurements should be evaluated for drug activity in early phase trials. Since correlation between reduction in viral markers, improvement in immune function, and efficacy in clinical endpoints, such as survival or prevention of disease progression, has not been established, efficacy demonstrated with laboratory surrogate markers has to be followed by long-term trials using clinical events as endpoints.

For many viral illnesses, treatments are either available or under development for control of the disease, but no cure is on the horizon. With the availability of new biotechnologies such as antisense, gene therapy, humanized monoclonal antibody, and therapeutic vaccines, however, there could be no boundary for future antiviral therapy. For the first time, these technologies can provide us with opportunities to consider cure instead of control of the disease. The development of these new technologies as antiviral therapies, however, might require the establishment of new paradigms in laboratory assessments and clinical evaluation for the cure of diseases. More sensitive diagnostic tests, such as PCR and nucleic acid probes, will be required to verify eradication of infection in various tissues. Different laboratory markers specific to the mechanisms of action of these therapies have to be developed as possible surrogate markers. Lastly, more creative and efficient clinical trial methodologies will be needed which allow use of a reasonable sample size and study duration for demonstration of efficacy in patients with earlier stages of disease.

REFERENCES

1. Herdewijn, P. A. M. M., Mini-Review, Novel nucleoside strategies for anti-HIV and anti-HSV therapy, *Antiviral Res.*, 19, 1, 1992.
2. Keating, M. R., Antiviral agents, Symposium on Antimicrobial Agents, Part VI, *Mayo Clin. Proc.*, 67, 160, 1992.
3. Balfour, H. H. Jr., Acyclovir and other chemotherapy for herpes group viral infections, *Annu. Rev. Med.*, 35, 279, 1984.
4. Koff, W. C. and Knight, V., Effect of rimantadine on influenza virus replication, *Proc. Soc. Exp. Biol. Med.*, 160, 246, 1979.
5. Roberts, N. A., Martin, J. A., Kinchinton, D., Broadhurst, J., Craig, J. C., Duncan, I. B., Galpin, S. A., Handa, B. K., Kay, J., Krohn, A., Lambert, R. W., Merrett, J. H., Mills, J. S., Parkes, K. E. B., Redshaw, S., Ritchie, A. J., Taylor, D. L., Thomas, G. J., and Machin, P. J., Rational design of peptide-based HIV proteinase inhibitors, *Science*, 248, 358, 1990.
6. Vacca, J. P., Dorsey, B.D., Schleif, W.A., Levin, R. B., McDaniel, S. L., Darke, P. L., Zugay, J., Quintero, J.C., Blahy, O. M., Roth, E., Sardana, V. V., Schlabach, A. J., Graham, P. I., Condra, J. H., Gotlib, L., Holloway, M. K., Lin, J., Chen, I.-W., Vastag, K., Ostovic, D., Anderson, P. S., Emini, E. A., and Huff, J. R., L-735,524: An orally bioavailable human immunodeficiency virus type 1 protease inhibitor, *Proc. Natl. Acad. Sci. U.S.A.*, 91, 4096, 1994.
7. Vella, S., Update on antiretroviral therapy, presented at the Tenth International Conference on AIDS, Yokohama, Japan, August 7-12, 1994.
8. Mitsuya, H. and Broder, S., Strategies for antiviral therapy in AIDS, *Nature*, 325, 773, 1987.
9. Clemens, M. J. and McNurlan, M. A., Regulation of cell proliferation and differentiation by interferons, *Biochem. J.*, 226, 345, 1985.
10. Scott, P., IL-12: Initiation cytokine for cell-mediated immunity, *Science*, 260, 496, 1993.
11. Sneller, M., Cytokine therapy of HIV infection, presented at the Fourth Triennial Symposium, New Directions in Antiviral Chemotherapy, San Francisco, California, November 10-12, 1994.
12. Weinhold, K. J., Lyerly, H. K., Matthews, T. J., Tyler, D. S., Ahearne, P. M., Stine, K. C., Langlois, A. J., Durack, D. T., and Bolognesi, D. P., Cellular anti-gp120 cytolytic reactivities in HIV-1 seropositive individuals, *Lancet*, i, 902, 1988.
13. Atkinson, W. L., Arden, A. H., Patiarca, P. A., Leslie, N., Lui, K.-J., and Gohd, R., Amantadine prophylaxis during an institutional outbreak of type A (H1N1) Influenza, *Arch. Int. Med.*, 146, 1751, 1986.
14. Dawkins, A. T., Gallager, L. R., Togo, Y., Hornick, R. B., and Harris, B. A, Studies on induced influenza in man, *J. Am. Med. Assoc.*, 203, 1095, 1968.
15. Henderson, D. K. and Gerberding, J. L., Prophylactic zidovudine after occupational exposure to the human immunodeficiency virus: an interim analysis, *J. Infect. Dis.*, 160(2), 321, Aug., 1989.

16. Connor, E. M., Sperling, R. S., Gelber, R., Kiseley, P., Scott, G., O'Sullivan, M. J., VanDyke, R., Bey, M., Shearer, W., Jacobson, R. L., Jimenez, E., O'Neill, E., Bazin, B., Delfraissy, J. F., Culnane, M., Coombs, R., Elkins, M., Moye, J., Stratton, P., and Balsley, J., Reduction of maternal-infant transmission of Human Immunodeficiency Virus Type I with zidovudine treatment, *N. Engl. J. Med.,* 331 (18), 1173, 1994.
17. O'Sullivan, M. J., Boyer, P. J., Scott, G. B., Parks, W. P., et al., The pharmacokinetics and safety of zidovudine in the third trimester of pregnancy for women infected with human immunodeficiency virus and their infants: phase I acquired immunodeficiency syndrome clinical trials group study (Protocol 082), *Am. J. Obstet. Gynecol.*, May, 168(5), 1510, 1993.
18. Sperling, R. S., Roboz, J., Dische, R., Silides, D. et al., Zidovudine pharmacokinetics during pregnancy, *Am. J. Perinatol.*, 9(4), 247, 1992.
19. Watts, D. H., Brown, Z. A., Tartaglione, T., Burchett, S. K. et al., Pharmacokinetic disposition of zidovudine during pregnancy, *J. Infect. Dis.*, Feb., 163(2), 226, 1991.
20. Dolin, R., Reichman, R. C., Madore, H. P., Maynard, R., Linton, P. N. and Weber-Jones, J., A controlled trial of amantadine and rimantadine in the prophylaxis of influenza A infection, *N. Engl. J. Med.*, 307, 580, 1982.
21. Van Voris, L. P., Betts, R. F., Menegus, M. A., Murphy, B. R., Roth, F. K., and Douglas, G., Jr., Serological diagnosis of influenza A/USSR/77 H1N1 infection; value of ELISA compared to other antibody techniques. *J. Med. Virol.*, 16, 315, 1985.
22. Kwok, S., Chang, S.-Y., Sninsky, J. J., and Wang, A, A guide to the design and use of mismatched and degenerate primers, *PRC Methods and Applications*, Manual Supplement, 3, S39, 1994.
23. Mulder, J., McKinney, N., Christopherson, C., Sninsky, L., Greenfield, L., and Kwok, S., Rapid and simple PCR assay for quantitation of Human Immunodeficiency Virus Type 1 RNA in plasma: application to acute retroviral infection, *J. Clin. Microbiol.*, 32(2), 292, 1994.
24. Sninsky, J. J., In Application of the polymerase chain reaction to the detection of viruses,*Viral Hepatitis and Liver Disease*, Williams & Wilkins, Baltimore, MD, pp. 799, 1991.
25. Martinot-Peignoux, M., Marcellin, P., Gournay, J., Gabriel F. et al., Detection and quantitation of serum HCV-RNA by branched DNA amplification in anti-HCV positive blood donors, *J. Hepatol*, 20(5), 676, 1994.
26. Urdea, M. S., Horn, T., Fultz, T. J., Anderson, M. et al., Branched DNA amplification multimers for the sensitive, direct detection of human hepatitis viruses, *Nucleic Acids Symp. Ser.,* (24), 197, 1991.
27. Urdea, M. S., Wilber, J. C., Yeghiazarian, T., Todd, J. A. et al., Direct and quantitative detection of HIV-1 RNA in human plasma with a branched DNA signal amplification assay, *AIDS*, 7 Suppl. 2, S11, 1993.
28. Balfour, H. H., Jr., Kelly, J. M., Suarez, C. S., Heussner, R. C., Englund, J. A., Crane, D. D., McGuirt, P. V., Clemmer, A. F., and Aeppli, D. M., Acyclovir treatment of varicella in otherwise healthy children, *J. Pediatr.*, 116, 633, 1990.
29. Balfour, H. H., Jr., Rotbart, H. A., Feldman, S., Dunkle, L. M., Feder, H. M. Jr., Prober, C. G., Hayden, G. F., Steinberg, S., Whitley, R. J., Goldberg, L., Mcguirt, P. V., and the Collaborative Acyclovir Varicella Study Group, Acyclovir treatment of varicella in otherwise healthy adolescents, *J. Pediatr.*, 120, 627, 1992.
30. Dunkle, L. M., Arvin, A. M., Whitley, R. J., Rotbart, H. A., Feder, H. M., Feldman, S., Gershon, A. A., Levy, M. L., Hayden, G. F., McGuirt, P. V., Harris, J., and Balfour, H. H., A controlled trial of acyclovir for chickenpox in normal children, *N. Engl. J. Med.*, 325, 1539, 1991.
31. Straus, S., Corey, L., Burke, R. L., Savarese, B., Barnum, G., Krause, P. R., Kost, R. G., Meier, J. L., Sekulovich, R., Adair, S. F., and Dekker, C. L., Placebo-controlled trial of vaccination with recombinant glycoprotein D of herpes simplex virus type 2 for immunotherapy of genital herpes, *Lancet,* 343, 1460-63, 1994.
32. Safrin, S., Crumpacker, C., Chatis, P., Davis, R., Rush, J., Kessler, H. A., Landry, B., Mills, J., and other members of the AIDS Clinical Trials Group, A controlled trial comparing foscarnet with vidarabine for acyclovir-resistant mucocutaneous herpes simplex in the acquired immunodeficiency syndrome, *N. Engl. J. Med.*, 325, 551, 1991.
33. Hall, C. B., Dolin, R., Gala, C. L., Markovitz, D. M., Zhang, Y. Q., Madore, P. H., Disney, F. A., Talpey, W. B., Green, J. L., Francis, A. B., and Pichichero, M. E., Children with influenza A infection: treatment with rimantadine, *Pediatrics*, 80, 275, 1987.
34. Sacks, S. L., Treatment of genital herpes, In DeClercq, E. (Ed.), *Clinical Use of Antiviral Drugs*, Martinus Nijhoff, Boston, pp. 87, 1988.
35. Winston, D. J., Eron, L. J., Ho, M., Pazin, G. Kessler, H., Pottage, J. C., Jr., Gallagher, J., Sartiano, G., Ho, W. G., Champlin, R. E. and the Hoffmann-La Roche Zoster Study Group Recombinant interferon alpha-2a for treatment of herpes zoster in immunosuppressed patients with cancer, *Am. J. Med.*, 85, 147-51, 1988.
36. Gilden, D. H., Herpes zoster with postherpetic neuralgia - persisting pain and frustration, *N. Engl. J. Med.,* 330(13), 932, 1994.
37. Wingfield, W. L., Pollack, D., and Grunert, R. R., Therapeutic efficacy of amantadine HC1 and rimantadine HC1 in naturally occurring influenza A2 respiratory illness in man, *N. Engl. J. Med.*, 281, 579, 1969.
38. Van Voris, L. P., Betts, R. F., Hayden, F. G., Christmas, W. A., and Douglas G., Jr., Successful treatment of naturally occurring influenza A/USSR/77 H1N1, *J. Am. Med. Assoc.*, 245, 1128, 1981.
39. Smiley, M. L., Valaciclovir for VZV infections, presented at the Fourth Triennial Symposium, New Directions in Antiviral Chemotherapy, San Francisco, California, November 10-12, 1994.
40. Degreef, H., Famciclovir Herpes Zoster Clinical Study Group, Famciclovir, a new oral antiherpes drug: results of the first controlled clinical study demonstrating its efficacy and safety in the treatment of uncomplicated herpes zoster in immunocompetent patients, *Antimicrob. Agents*, 4, 241, 1994.

41. Cone, R. W., Hobson, A. C., Brown, Z., Ashley, R., Berry, S., Winter, C., and Corey, L., Frequent detection of genital herpes simplex virus DNA by polymerase chain reaction among pregnant women, *JAMA*, 272(10), 792, 1994.
42. Weiss, R., Mazade, L., eds. Institute of Medicine, Surrogate endpoints in evaluating the effectiveness of drugs against HIV infection and AIDS: September 11-12, 1989 Conference Summary, Washington, D.C.: National Academy Press, 1990.
43. DeGruttola, V., Wulfsohn, M., Fischl, M., and Tsiatis, A., Modeling the relationship between survival and CD_4 lymphocytes in patients with AIDS and AIDS-Related Complex, *J. AIDS*, 6, 359, 1993.
44. Lagakos, S., Immunologic and virologic endpoints, presented at the Inter-Company Collaboration for AIDS Drug Development Surrogate Marker Workshop, Washington, D.C., September 21, 1994.
45. Mellors J., Detection of plasma HIV RNA by branched DNA signal amplification predicts outcome after seroconversion, presented at the Inter-Company Collaboration for AIDS Drug Development Surrogate Marker Workshop, Washington, D.C., September 21, 1994.
46. Hartigan, P., PCR as a surrogate marker for clinical endpoint, presented at the Inter-Company Collaboration for AIDS Drug Development Surrogate Marker Workshop, Washington, D.C., September 21, 1994.
47. Welles, S., Prognostic capacity of plasma RNA copy number in patients enrolled in ACTG Protocol 116B/117, presented at the Inter-Company Collaboration for AIDS Drug Development Surrogate Marker Workshop, Washington, D.C., September 21, 1994.
48. Osada, T., Iwabuchi, S., Takatori, M., Murayama, M., and Iino, S., Serum levels of HCV-RNA determined by branched DNA (bDNA) probe assay in chronic hepatitis C: method and clinical significance on interferon (IFN) therapy, *Nippon Rinsho,* 52(7), 1747-53, 1994.
49. Fischl, M. A. D. A., Richman, D. D., Grieco, M. H., Gottlieb, M. S., Volberding, P. A., Laskin, O. L., Leedom, J. M., Groopman, J. E., Mildvan, D., Schooley, R. T., Jackson, G. G., Durack, D. T., King, D., and the AZT Collaborative Working Group, The efficacy of azidothymidine (AZT) in the treatment of patients with AIDS and AIDS-related complex, *N. Engl. J. Med.*, 317, 185, 1987.
50. Ware, J., General health rating index. In Wenger, N. K., Mattson, M. E., Furberg, C. D., and Elinson, J. (Eds.), *Assessment of Quality of Life in Clinical Trials of Cardiovascular Therapies*, Le Jacq Publishing, New York, pp. 184, 1984.
51. Bergner, M., The sickness impact scale. In Wenger, N. K., Mattson, M. E., Furgerg, C. D., and Elinson, J., (Eds.), *Assessment of Quality of Life in Clinical Trials of Cardiovascular Therapies*, Le Jacq Publishing, New York, pp. 152, 1984.
52. Dupuy, H. J., The psychological general well-being index, In Wenger, N. K., Mattson, M. E., Furberg, C. D., and Elinson, J. (Eds.), *Assessment of Quality of Life in Clinical Trials of Cardiovascular Therapies*, Le Jacq Publishing, New York, pp. 170, 1984.
53. Bozzette, S. A., Kanouse, D., Berry, S., Duan, N., Downes-LeGuin, T., Hays, R., Petinnelli, C., Richmann, D. D., Gocke, D., and Kahn, J., with the 3300 Investigators and ACTG, Relative effects of ddC or ddI vs ZDV on health status, function and disability in N3300 (ACTG 114) and ACTG 116b/117, presented at the VIII International Conference on AIDS/III STD World Congress, Amsterdam, The Netherlands, July 19-24, 1992.
54. Pizzo, P. A., Butler, K., Balis, F., Brouwers, E., Hawkins, M., Eddy, J., Einloth, M., Falloon, J., Husson, R., Jarosinski, P., Meer, J., Moss, H., Poplack, D. G., Santacroce, S., Wiener, L., and Walters, P., Dideoxycytidine alone and in an alternating schedule with zidovudine in children with symptomatic human immunodeficiency virus infection, *J. Pediatr.,* 117(5), 799, 1990.
55. Schmitt, F. A., Bigley, J. B., McKinnis, R., Logue, P. E., Evans, R. W., Drucker, J. L., and the AZT Collaborative Working Group, Neurophysiological outcome of zidovudine treatment of patients with AIDS and AIDS-related complex, *N. Engl. J. Med.*, 319, 1573, 1988.
56. Alexander, G. J. M., Brahm, J., Fagan, E. A., Smith, H. M., Daniels, H. M., Eddleston, A. L. W. F., and Williams, R., Loss of HBsAg with interferon therapy in chronic hepatitis B virus infection, *Lancet*, ii, 66, 1987.
57. Perrillo, R. P., Regenstein, F. G., Peter, M. G., DeeSchryver-Kecskemeti, K., Bodicky, C. J., Campbell, C. R., and Kuhns, M. C., Prednisone withdrawal followed by recombinant alpha interferon in the treatment of chronic type B hepatitis, *Annu. Int. Med.*, 108, 95, 1988.
58. Yarchoan, R. and Nelson, D. L., A study of the functional capabilities of human neonatal lymphocytes for *in vitro* specific antibody production, *J. Immunol.*, 131, 1222, 1983.
59. Yarchoan, R., Klecker, R. W., Weinhold, K. J., Markham, P. D., Lyerly, H. K., Durack, D. T., Gelmann, E., Nusinoff-Lehrman, S., Blum, R. M., Barry, D. W., Shearer, G. M., Fischl, M. A., Mitsuya, H., Gallo, R. C., Collins, J. M., Bolognesi, D. P., Myers, C. E., and Broder, S., Administration of 3′-azido-3′-deoxythymidine, an inhibitor of HTLV-III/LAV replication, to patients with AIDS or AIDS-related complex, *Lancet*, i, 575, 1986.
60. Meng, T. C., Fischl, M. A., Boota, A. H., Spector, S. A., Bennett, D., Bassiakos, Y., Lai, S., Wright, B., and Richman, D. D., Combination therapy with zidovudine and dideoxycytidine in patients with advanced human immunodeficiency virus infection, A phase I/II Study, *Ann. Intern. Med.,* 116, 13-20, 1992.
61. Schooley, R., Combination antiretroviral therapy in previously untreated individuals, presented at the Tenth International Conference on AIDS, Yokohama, Japan, August 7-12, 1994.
62. Melnick, J. L., Crowther, D., and Barrera-Oro, J., Rapid development of drug-resistant mutants of poliovirus, *Science, N.Y.*, 134, 551,1961.

63. Erice, A., Balfour, H. H., Jr., Resistance of human immunodeficiency virus, type 1 to antiretroviral agents: a review, *Clin. Infect. Dis.,* 18, 149, 1994.
64. Saag, M. S., Emini, E. A., Laskin, O.L., Douglas, J., Lapidus, W. I., Schleif, W. A., Whitley, R. J., Hilderbrand, C., Byrnes, V. W., Kappes, J. C., Anderson, K. W., Massari, F. E., Shaw, G. M., and the L-697,661 Working Group, Short-term clinical evaluation of L-697, 661 a non-nucleoside inhibitor of HIV-1 reverse transcriptase, *N. Engl. J. Med.*, 329(15), 1065, 1993.
65. Richman, D. D., Fischl, M. A., Grieco, M. H., Gottlieb, M. S., Volberding, P. L., Laskin, O. L., Leedom, J. M., Groopman, J. E., Mildvan, D., Hirsch, M. S., Jackson, G. G., Durack, D. T., Nusinoff-Lehrman, S., and the AZT Collaborative Working Group, The toxicity of azidothymidine in the treatment of patients with AIDS and AIDS-related complex, *N. Engl. J. Med.*, 317, 192, 1987.
66. Yarchoan, R., Perno, C. F., Thomas, R. V., Klecker, R. W., Allain, J.-P., Wills, R. J., McAtee, N., Fischl, M. A., Dubinsky, R., McNeely, M. C., Mitsuya, H., Pluda, J. M., Lawley, T. J., Leuther, M., Safai, B., Collins, J. M., Myers, C. E., and Broder, S., Phase I studies of 2',3'-dideoxycytidine in severe human immunodeficiency virus infection as a single agent and alternating with zidovudine (AZT), *Lancet*, i, 76, 1988.
67. Marsh, E., Drug trial deaths deemed unavoidable, *Science,* 264, 1530, 1994.

Chapter 38

Anticancer Drugs

Lee Schacter, Martin Birkhofer, Stephen Carter, Renzo Canetta, Susan Hellmann, Nicole Onetto, Catherine Weil, Benjamin Winograd, and Marcel Rozencweig

CONTENTS

1 Introduction 523
2 Healthy Volunteers 525
3 Patient Studies — General Considerations 525
3.1 Suitability 525
3.2 Risk: Benefit 525
3.3 Controls 526
4 Patient Studies — Phase I 526
4.1 Selection Criteria 526
4.2 Safety Considerations 527
4.2.1 Dose Calculation 528
4.3 Methods 528
4.3.1 Dose Escalation 528
4.3.2 Retreatment Interval 528
4.3.3 Endpoint of Phase I Trials for Cytotoxics 529
4.3.4 Determination of Route and Schedule 529
4.3.5 Pharmacokinetics 529
4.4 Size and Duration of Trials 530
4.4.1 Number of Patients at Each Dose Level 530
5 Patient Studies — Phase II 530
5.1 Selection Criteria 530
5.2 Safety Considerations 530
5.3 Methods 531
5.3.1 Response and Survival 531
5.3.2 Response Criteria 531
5.3.3 Spectrum of Activity 531
5.3.4 Patient Selection 531
5.3.5 Duration of Treatment 531
5.3.6 Statistical Considerations 532
5.3.7 Surrogate Markers 532
6 Decision Making 532
7 Conclusions 533
References 533

1 INTRODUCTION

Cancer represents a heterogeneous group of diseases characterized by the uncontrolled proliferation of phenotypically abnormal cells. This proliferation appears to arise from one or more changes in the genome of mature cell (somatic cell mutation) leading to the loss of normal growth regulation. In some cases (cancer families) a hereditable genomic variation may underlie the disease. To a variable extent, malignant tumors phenotypically resemble the cell type from which they derive and are classified by the cell of origin, e.g., adenocarcinomas arise from secretory cells, squamous cell tumors from epithelial cells, sarcomas from mesodermal cells, etc. The natural history of each tumor type demonstrates a wide variation of behavior within a tumor type. Therapy is dependent on the type of tumor, location, stage (extent) at diagnosis, and patient factors (willingness and ability to undergo treatment). Primary treatment

0-8493-9230-6/97/$0.00+$.50
© 1997 by CRC Press, Inc.

for most tumors is surgical which can be curative if all disease can be resected or may be diagnostic or palliative (relief of symptoms due to tumor bulk and/or location). It is an absolute rule that no patient may be treated for cancer until a malignancy is confirmed by pathological examination. Radiotherapy is used to treat localized or regional disease with curative or palliative intent. Radiotherapy may be preferable to surgery for localized disease if resection is more likely to cause significant morbidity than radiation.

A variety of drugs are available for the treatment of malignant diseases. Therapeutic agents can be divided into two broad groups, biologicals and cytotoxic agents. Relatively few biological agents are currently in standard use. These include the enzyme L-asparaginase used to deplete the serum levels of asparagine, an amino acid required for the growth of some leukemia cells but not normal cells; the antiviral agent interferon α used to treat some leukemias, melanoma, Kaposi's sarcoma, and other cancers;[1] and interleukin-2 (IL-2), a mediator of inflammation active in the treatment of kidney cancer and melanoma.[2] In addition, hematopoietic growth factors for granulocytes, granulocytes and macrophages, and erythrocytes are commonly used to reduce or modify the myelosuppression caused by many cytotoxic drugs.

More than 45 drugs are currently approved for cancer treatment in the U.S.[3] These can be classified into a variety of ways, one of which is shown (Table 1).

Table 1 Classes of Anticancer Compounds

Class Examples		
Alkylating Agents		
Azathioprine	Cyclophosphamide	Melphalan
Busulfan	Estramustine	Mitomycin C
Carmustine	Ifosfamide	Nitrogen Mustard
Chlorambucil	Lomustine	Procarbazine
		Thiotepa
Nucleoside Analogs/Metabolic Inhibitors		
Cladribine (2CDA)	Fludarabine	Pentostatin
Cytosine arabinoside	5-Fluorouracil	Streptozocin
Dacarbazine (DTIC)	Methotrexate	6-Thioguanine
Floxuridine	op'-DDD	
DNA Intercalators/Crosslinkers		
Actinomycin D	Cisplatin	Mitoxantrone
Bleomycin	Daunorubicin	Mithramycin
Carboplatin	Doxorubicin	
Topoisomerase Inhibitors		
Etoposide	Teniposide	
Microtubule Active Agents		
Paclitaxel	Vinblastine	Vincristine
Biologicals		
Asparaginase	Interferon α	Interleukin-2
Hormones/Hormone Antagonists		
Aminoglutethimide	Leuprolide	Octreotide
Diethylstilbestrol	Megestrol acetate	Tamoxifen
Flutamide	Medroxyprogesterone	
Mechanism of Action Uncertain		
Altretamine	Hydroxyurea	

Tumor cells are derived from normal ones, often as a result of relatively "minor" genomic changes and are biochemically similar to them. Critical differences between normal and malignant cells have not been found which would allow selective killing of malignant cells. As a result, the cytotoxic drugs used to treat cancers have a very small therapeutic index. Although the safety profile of each drug is unique, most cytotoxics have one or more of the following unwanted side effects: myelosuppression, immune suppression, nausea and vomiting, anorexia, alopecia, and mucositis. The safety profile of biologicals is generally related to their natural biological function. Those which are foreign proteins can cause serum sickness while inflammatory mediators cause inflammatory symptoms. Because of their toxicity anticancer drugs require careful phase I evaluation. However, because many are used only for relatively short periods of time and with palliative intent, long-term dosing and toxicities may not initially be a primary concern. Chronic toxicity becomes an issue when agents are used over longer periods as in the adjuvant setting.

A number of tumors can be cured with chemotherapy. These include Hodgkin's disease, some non-Hodgkin's lymphomas, testicular cancer, gestational trophoblastic tumors, acute lymphoblastic leukemia, and limited small cell cancer of the lung. Adjuvant chemotherapy may result in cure or significantly improved disease-free survival in Wilm's tumors, osteogenic sarcoma, rhabdomyosarcoma, breast cancer, and colorectal cancer. However, for most patients palliation is the goal when drugs are used in the treatment of cancer. Endpoints must therefore focus on real, albeit transient, benefits to the patient such as symptomatic improvement, delayed time to tumor recurrence, prolonged survival, or improved quality of life.

2 HEALTHY VOLUNTEERS

Because of their small therapeutic index, serious side effects, and significant potential for damage to DNA, anticancer drugs are not tested in normal subjects. Although some biological agents might be considered safe enough to test in healthy volunteers, unknown risks makes such testing unlikely.

3 PATIENT STUDIES — GENERAL CONSIDERATIONS

3.1 Suitability

The initial studies (phase I) of cancer drugs are carried out in patients with malignant diseases which have proved unresponsive to treatment with established modalities or for which there are no accepted therapies. Patients with a variety of malignancies may be entered in phase I trials while for phase II studies, patients are selected by tumor type. Most patients treated in phase I have had prior surgery and/or radiotherapy and usually one or more chemotherapy regimes. Phase I patients typically have relatively advanced cancers and may die of progressive disease during the course of a study.

The ethical construct on which cancer patients are treated with compounds of unknown efficacy in phase I and II trials is the possibility of clinical benefit to the patient being treated. Antineoplastic agents selected for testing in man must have shown evidence of activity against tumors in one or more animal models. However, the predictive value of preclinical models for cancer treatment is unknown. Drugs which do not have activity in such models are not tested in man; thereby making the true negative rate unknown and precluding a calculation of predictive value. In general, only one of every ten anticancer compounds brought to the clinic will have significant activity in man. Trials are therefore designed to expose as few patients as possible to ineffective agents while at the same time gathering the data required to determine optimal drug dosing (phase I) and efficacy (phase II).

Unless specifically selected for activity in pediatric tumors, antineoplastic drugs are first tested in adult subjects with normal cognitive function. If the drug is found to be active in adults its study will then be extended to children. As in adults, testing in pediatric patients is warranted only in patients without other, better therapeutic options.

3.2 Risk: Benefit

Although the drugs and combinations now used and being studied may carry with them a significant risk of adverse events, this is considered acceptable because of the rapidly fatal nature of many cancers and the lack of less toxic, effective alternatives. The acceptable level of toxicity is directly proportional to the morbidity and mortality of the malignancy being treated and the potential for benefit. Treatments with significant potential for side effects are more acceptable for rapidly growing quickly, lethal malignancies which may be cured, such as acute leukemia, than for more slow growing cancers, such as carcinoid. In addition, during phase I patients treated at lower doses are less likely to experience side effects or have a beneficial response to treatment than those treated at higher doses. With most cytotoxic agents the probability of benefit increases in parallel to the risk of side effects.

Patients treated in phase I and II trials must understand that their disease has reached a point at which there are no known effective therapies and that they are being offered treatment with an experimental agent whose toxicity and efficacy are unknown (phase I) or whose toxicity is known but efficacy remains to be proven (phase II). This is significantly different from phase III in which a control and experimental arms of presumably equivalent efficacy are being compared.

Participation in phase I and II trials of cancer drugs offers patients the hope that the agent being tested will be beneficial to them. Many patients also derive satisfaction from the knowledge that they are helping to find more effective cancer treatments even if they do not directly benefit.

3.3 Controls

Phase I and II studies of cancer drugs are usually uncontrolled trials. In some disease settings, such as advanced nonsmall cell lung cancer, where no effective therapy exists, a best supportive care control arm without specific anticancer treatment may be appropriate in phase II or III. Blinding is usually impractical and could put patients at risk. Randomized phase II studies may be an attractive design in situations where it is important to avoid selection bias in comparing response rates of a new agent to one of proven activity. Such trials can be designed to allow expansion into pivotal phase III investigations if preliminary data warrant such a change.

4 PATIENT STUDIES — PHASE I

4.1 Selection Criteria

Cancer patients selected for phase I trials must meet two types of criteria: the first designed to protect them from unnecessary risks while maximizing the chance of benefit, and the second to allow adequate testing of the agent (Table 2). To protect the patient, only individuals for whom no effective treatment of their malignancy is available are eligible for phase I trials. This usually means that the patient has disease spread beyond surgical control or relapsing following surgery, radiation therapy and/or chemotherapy. To maximize the possibility of benefit to the patient, those treated should not have very advanced, preterminal disease. Subjects should be selected who can be followed long enough for any response or delayed toxicity to be documented. Patients must, therefore, have a life expectancy of at least 8-12 weeks following drug administration. In addition, most cytotoxics affect the bone marrow. Patients receiving these agents in phase I studies must have adequate marrow function as demonstrated by normal numbers of circulating white blood cells and platelets. Because the toxicity of the new agent is uncertain, it is important that patients receiving the drug are able to metabolize and excrete it normally. Subjects must therefore have adequate hepatic and renal function. Informed consent consistent with the declaration of Helsinki[4] and national requirements must be obtained.

Table 2 Commonly Used Inclusion and Exclusion Criteria for Phase I Trials

Inclusion	Exclusion
Histologically confirmed cancer	Pregnancy or lactation
Age >18 and <75 physiologic	Brain metastases
Performance status ECOG ≤3	Active infection
Life expectancy >9 weeks	Major organ dysfunction
No prior cytotoxics within 4 weeks (6 weeks for nitrosureas)	Any medical or psychiatric condition which would put patient at risk
Prior radiotherapy restricted to ≤ 30% of marrow bearing bone	
WBC >4000/mm^3, platelets >100,000/mm^3	
Serum creatinine ≤1.5 mg/dl	
Normal hepatic function	
Ability to give informed consent	

The type of patient entered when higher doses are used may differ from those treated at the lowest dose of drug. At the beginning of the phase I trial, heavily pretreated patients with a poor performance status are usually entered. Since no toxicity is expected at the starting dose, such patients can be safely treated. As experience with the drug accumulates, better-risk individuals are given the drug as the possibility of a therapeutic benefit may increase.

It is important to determine the maximum tolerated dose (MTD) of a new drug in patients with both good and poor prognostic factors. For instance, it is important to know whether patients with impaired marrow function can be treated at the same dose as those with normal hematopoietic capability or if patients previously treated with radiation and/or cytotoxic agents can tolerate the same dose as those without such prior therapy. The MTD is that dose which if exceeded would put patients at unacceptable risk. It is a dose which causes predictable and reversible toxicity usually in one third or more of patients. Unacceptable toxicities might include reduction in granulocyte numbers to <1000/cmm, platelets to <50,000/cmm, elevations in liver enzymes by more than 2.5-fold or increases in serum creatinine of a similar magnitude. Hair loss is not considered a serious toxicity while intractable vomiting is. If adverse effects are first observed among high risk patients additional subjects with fewer risk factors for toxicity, such as prior therapy or poor performance status, should be treated at the same dose. The advent of growth factors such as granulocyte colony-stimulating factor (G-CSF) has added a new dimension to the determination of the MTD. Routine use of such factors may allow treatment at significantly higher doses of drug without dose limiting myelosuppression. Other agents which prevent what otherwise might be dose limiting toxicity are also available such as mesna which protects patients from bladder toxicity caused by ifosfamide. Phase I trials may therefore include an initial stage in which the MTD is determined without a protector such as G-CSF and a second stage in which the MTD is determined using the protecting agent.

A well-designed phase I study will identify a dose at which patients can safely be treated and one which can benefit the patient.

4.2 Safety Considerations

Adverse events can reasonably be expected to occur in at least some patients treated with any anticancer drug. Trials with these compounds should only be conducted by experienced investigators and at institutions with the facilities to provide adequate care regardless of the toxicity encountered.

Cytotoxic agents have a variety of toxicities some of which can be life-threatening (Table 3).

Table 3 Common Toxicities of Cytotoxic Agents

Myelosuppression	Renal dysfunction
Immune suppression	Hepatic dysfunction
Nausea, vomiting	Pulmonary dysfunction
Anorexia	Mucositis
Alopecia	Peripheral nervous system

In addition to identifying an appropriate dose for later phase trials and demonstrating biological activity, phase I trials are designed to identify all significant short-term side effects of a new compound. Although valuable information about side effects can be obtained from animal toxicology studies and prior experience with other compounds in the same class, unexpected toxicities can be observed in the phase I testing of anticancer drugs. Intensive patient monitoring is therefore vital. Antitumor drugs may have short-term, delayed, and late toxicities. Side effects occurring within 3 to 6 weeks of dosing are generally considered acute or short-term, those observed after several months are considered delayed, and those observed after 6 or more months can be called late. Examples of common acute effects include emesis, mucositis, myelosuppression, transient decreases in renal function, or transient hepatic abnormalities. Renal failure, peripheral neuropathy, pulmonary fibrosis, and cardiomyopathy are examples of toxicities which may occur after months of treatment while secondary leukemia occurring in long-term survivors would be a late side effect.

Phase I trials are best suited to the identification of acute toxicities since patients in these trials frequently have advanced malignancies and are treated for a relatively short period. The identification of delayed and late toxicities may not occur until phase II or III trials are conducted. Acute changes in hepatic, renal, and marrow function require frequent laboratory assessment. Blood samples are generally collected twice a week following dosing for 3 to 6 weeks or until any toxicity has resolved, whichever is longer. Intensive monitoring allows for more rapid increases in dose, minimizing the number of patients treated. For cytotoxic drugs this is generally 4 to 6 weeks after treatment. In addition to frequent laboratory testing, patients must be interviewed and undergo a physical examination to detect other toxicities such as appetite change, nausea and vomiting, diarrhea or constipation, confusion or neuropathy, pulmonary, or other symptoms. If an unexpected toxicity is identified during a trial, the protocol may need to be modified to protect patients, minimize the toxicity, and fully evaluate the side effect. Protocol changes in dosing, routes and schedule of administration, or concomitant treatment such as antiemetics or hydration may be needed to minimize toxicity.

A critical safety issue is the determination of the starting dose for a new compound. The first human subjects should be exposed to doses which can reasonably be expected to cause little or no toxicity. On the other hand, the starting dose should not be too remote from efficacious levels.

The starting dose in man is based on data from animals. Retrospective analyses of the relationship between dosing and toxicity in animals and in humans provide the rationale for predicting a safe starting dose for a new agent in humans from animal studies.[5-7] A safe starting dose in man for the vast majority of cytotoxic drugs has been empirically found to be either one tenth of the LD_{10} in rodents or one third of the lowest dose causing toxicity (toxic dose low: TDL) in a larger mammal such as the dog. If there is a discrepancy between one tenth of the LD_{10} in rodents and one third of the TDL in dogs, the lower starting dose should be chosen to reduce the risk to patients.

4.2.1 Dose Calculation

Many drugs are dosed on a mg/kg basis or a fixed dose regardless of the patient's size. Because of the narrow margin between therapeutic and toxic doses of cytotoxic drugs, the amount administered must be more carefully determined. A number of studies[8-10] have demonstrated that dosing based on body surface area is the most accurate method for administering appropriate doses of cytotoxic drugs to patients. In addition, comparison of toxic and therapeutic effects between species is most accurate when body surface area is used as the denominator. Nomograms have been developed to convert height and weight into surface area (m^2) for both adults and children as well as conversion factors from mg/kg to mg/m^2 for various species.[10] Doses of almost all cytotoxic drugs are determined using body surface area whether in early clinical trials or routine clinical use.

4.3 Methods

4.3.1 Dose Escalation

Traditional cytotoxic drugs rarely exhibit activity at doses completely devoid of side effects. Because the starting dose in phase I is targeted to be below the MTD and usually nontoxic, it is important to make the transition from an inactive nontoxic starting dose to an active dose as rapidly as possible, to minimize the number of patients treated at inactive levels.

Two general approaches to dose escalation have been used. An empiric approach can be employed in which doses are increased according to a predetermined numerical formula. One such formula is the Fibonacci escalation, named for an Italian mathematician who described this type of numerical sequence.[11] The pattern described by Fibonacci is 1,1,2,3,5.... in which each number is the sum of the two preceding values. In practice various modifications of the Fibonacci progression are used. Other formulas can be used such as doubling the dose until the first signs of toxicity are observed and then increasing it at a slower rate (e.g., 50% or 33%) until the MTD has been identified. As the MTD is approached, the dose may have to be increased *or* decreased to clearly define optimum dosing.

The second general approach to dose escalation is based on drug pharmacokinetics. The human MTD for many cytotoxics occurs when the area under the plasma drug concentration-time curve (AUC or $C \times T$) is the same as the AUC in mice at the mouse LD_{10}.[12,13] Although it may be possible to use the AUC to more efficiently determine dosing by reducing the number of dose escalations required, this approach has not been widely adopted.

4.3.2 Retreatment Interval

The time between treatments with a new agent is determined by: the time required for recovery from acute toxic effects as observed in animals, other toxicology data from animals, the nature of the agent being studied, and preliminary observations in treated patients. For example, a new chemotype demonstrating delayed hepatotoxicity in animals will require prolonged careful monitoring of liver function prior to retreatment, while an analog of an existing drug such as doxorubicin, which is known to cause early cytopenia as the first manifestation of its toxicity, may be dosed more frequently in phase I.

In many trials a patient starting treatment at a particular dose level can be retreated at the next higher dose level *if* he/she has shown no toxicity at the initial level *and* if other patients administered the drug at the higher level have been followed for a period adequate to determine the safety of the higher dose level. However, dose escalation of individual patients may confound the evaluation of the dose effect relationship.

4.3.3 Endpoint of Phase I Trials for Cytotoxics

The objectives of phase I trials for cytotoxic agents are to: (1) identify the most common toxicities and (2) define the dose (MTD) at which these toxicities become a significant risk to the patient. Achievement of these goals allows the design of phase II efficacy trials.

Cytotoxic agents can cause a wide variety of toxicities. Prominent targets of these drugs are the bone marrow, oral mucosa, hair follicles, and gastrointestinal mucosa. These organs must be monitored closely for toxic effects. Toxicities are generally rated by use of the scales promulgated by the World Health Organization (WHO publication No. 48, WHO Publications Center U.S., 49 Sheridan Ave., Albany, N.Y. 12210). A number of cooperative research groups have begun to use "common toxicity criteria" (CTC) which differs only slightly from the WHO system. The CTC have yet to appear as a publication.

4.3.4 Determination of Route and Schedule

Cytotoxic drugs can be given by various routes and schedules. Preclinical studies often provide some information on whether or not the new agent's activity is route- or schedule-dependent. Unless preclinical trials unambiguously indicate superior activity via a particular route or schedule, most drugs are tested by intravenous administration using more than one schedule. Patient and physician convenience are an important factor in determining schedules.

Most cytotoxics are given intravenously in phase I, but if oral absorption in animals has been good and GI toxicity mild, the oral route might be chosen.

For cytotoxic drugs the interval between dosing is a function of the time it takes to recover from drug-induced toxicity. The higher the dose, the longer recovery usually takes. For most new cytotoxic agents the MTD and dose limiting toxicities (DLT) are determined using three different schedules: a single dose given at intervals determined by the time to full recovery (usually every 3 or 4 weeks); daily doses for 5 days, with retreatment when there is full recovery; and once weekly for 3 to 4 weeks, again with retreatment when there is full recovery. Testing of prolonged daily treatment is not routinely performed until the toxicity of the drug in man has been evaluated and the possibility of a cumulative effect determined.

4.3.5 Pharmacokinetics

The traditional, dose-dependent approach to the development of anticancer drugs has not incorporated pharmacokinetics (pK) or pharmacodynamics in the decision-making process for selection of starting dose in phase I clinical trials, the establishment of dose escalation criteria for phase I, or for the selection of dose and/or schedule of administration for the later stages of clinical trials. Generally, for a new chemotherapeutic agent, pharmacokinetic data are collected from a limited number of patients in order to describe pK parameters. Indeed, the incorporation of pharmacokinetic data into current oncologic practice has usually occurred *post hoc*, with compounds that have already completed advanced phases of development, as for example, the use of methotrexate levels to adjust folinic acid dosage in patients receiving high dose methotrexate with leucovorin rescue, or the individualization of carboplatin dosage targeted to AUC and platelet count.

More recently, alternative approaches to early stage development of anticancer compounds have attempted to prospectively incorporate pharmacokinetic data into decision-making processes with regard to selection of starting doses for phase I and into defining new criteria for dose escalation for phase I trials based on drug exposure (AUC) rather than on dose. Pharmacologically guided dose escalation schemes[12,13] have evolved from a recognition of the need to provide a better rationale in the design of these trials.

For some chemotherapeutic agents, clearance and exposure can vary by as much as three- to tenfold between patients administered identical doses of a drug. In addition, there is evidence that total exposure to certain agents correlates with toxicity and/or efficacy.[14] Thus, rather than empiric dose escalation in phase I, several investigators have proposed dose escalation schemes based on AUC. This approach has been applied retrospectively, to agents which had already completed phase I clinical trials where pharmacokinetic data were available for analysis[13] as well as prospectively, in a limited number of clinical trials of new chemotherapeutic agents.[15-18] Additional prospective data are needed before the impact of this approach on trial methodology can be evaluated.

Pharmacologically guided selection of starting dose and dose escalation for phase I necessitates early development of validated analytic methods for use in animal toxicology as well as in phase I clinical trials. In addition, toxicology should optimally be carried out using clinical material administered via the same route and on a schedule similar to that proposed for clinical study.[11] Alternatively, pharmacokinetic data from several animal species may be considered to attempt to prospectively define optimal scheduling for man. While useful data can be derived from animals, differences in drug disposition and metabolism between man and other species make extrapolation from other species to humans less than certain.

Another potentially important role for detailed pharmacokinetic evaluation would be the development of orally active chemotherapeutic agents, where issues such as bioavailability, bioequivalence, and drug disposition under different conditions (i.e., fed vs. fasted) and in different populations (e.g., good vs. poor performance status) might need to be addressed. The effects of altered excretory function on the disposition of orally active agents might also require study.

With regard to development of biologic agents for cancer therapy, particularly monoclonal antibodies, recently issued draft guidelines indicate that pharmacokinetic data may play a central role in the selection of dose and schedule of administration for efficacy trials.[19]

4.4 Size and Duration of Trials

4.4.1 Number of Patients at Each Dose Level

In the vast majority of phase I trials of cytotoxic agents, at least three patients are entered at each dose level. The number of patients at each dose level is kept small, to allow the most rapid possible increase in dose from a nontoxic inactive level to an active, albeit toxic, one. *Assuming* that there is a probability of achieving toxicity in 50% of the patients at a given dose level, the probability of missing toxicity in three consecutive patients is $0.5 \times 0.5 \times 0.5 = 0.125$. This number of patients gives an 87.5% confidence (1.0 to 0.125) that the dose is nontoxic if no adverse events are seen. If four patients are entered, the confidence becomes 93.75% and with five patients it becomes 96.875%.[11] Many, if not most, trials enter additional patients if one or more of three patients at any given dose level exhibit toxicity, to ensure the validity of the observation and to be able to give a better assessment of the frequency of the event. At the suspected MTD, experience is expanded in a larger number of patients to more clearly identify the optimal dose and the toxicities which may be expected in phase II trials enrolling patients with various risk factors.

5 PATIENT STUDIES — PHASE II

5.1 Selection Criteria

Early phase II trials are designed to identify ineffective drugs through testing in a minimum number of patients. Meaningful results in small numbers of patients require a homogeneous population. Therefore, in addition the criteria used to select patients for phase I, those treated in phase II trials must have a specific tumor type and measurable disease. Prior treatment becomes more important in phase II studies. Responses are more likely to occur with initial drug treatments than with therapies which follow an initial failure to respond or relapse. The use of an experimental phase II agent as first line treatment may be appropriate in a number of malignancies. This is especially true if responses in one or more tumor types have been observed during phase I. The tumor types in which chemotherapy has not been proven to extend survival or improve quality of life in patients are controversial and changes as new drugs and combinations are tried and found to be effective or ineffective. Nonsmall lung cancer, metastatic colon cancer, metastatic melanoma, gastric cancer, pancreatic cancer, hepatoma, metastatic cervical cancer, and soft tissue sarcomas are still considered by many as unresponsive to available chemotherapeutics and therefore appropriate settings for the testing of new drugs in previously untreated patients.[20]

The ability to evaluate response to therapy is critical for inclusion of patients in phase II trials. The most commonly used endpoint is reduction in tumor size. Patients treated in phase II trials must have tumor masses which can be measured in two dimensions perpendicular to each other, either by physical palpation or an imaging procedure. Tumor markers such as chorioembryonic antigen (CEA) or prostate specific antigen (PSA) may also be helpful in evaluating response of a tumor to treatment, but the reduction in measurable tumor mass remains a prerequisite for the demonstration of drug activity.

5.2 Safety Considerations

Phase II studies focus on efficacy. Data on toxicity are collected and because of the longer duration of treatment, delayed effects may be more apparent than in the phase I setting. Laboratory tests are performed prior to each course of treatment and at least once between courses, usually at the time maximum renal, hepatic, or hematopoietic toxicity is expected. Patients are evaluated clinically prior to each course for adverse events which have occurred since the prior dose. As with phase I trials, if unexpected toxicities become manifest during phase II, protocols may need to be amended to protect patients and/or gather more information about the toxicity.

5.3 Methods

In phase I the critical issue addressed is the determination of the MTD of the new agent and the identification of the toxic effects of the compound. In phase II the emphasis is evaluation of antitumor activity.

The elucidation of activity has two restraints: first is the need to avoid treating large numbers of patients with ineffective agents and second, the need to avoid false-negative results. It is more important not to mistakenly label as inactive an agent which has activity than to label as active one which is not. An error in identifying as active an agent which is not will be corrected as trials continue. If an active agent is erroneously labeled as ineffective, its development may be abandoned.

5.3.1 Response and Survival

While the ultimate goal of cancer chemotherapy is cure, few cytotoxic drugs have had an obvious and dramatic impact on survival in phase II studies which are designed to detect tumor shrinkage and not improved survival. Trials designed to detect increased survival require large numbers of patients, prolonged followup, and are carried out in phase III.

It is generally accepted that tumor shrinkage is required for improved survival, and that the higher the response rate, the more likely it is that these responses will result in prolonged life. Therefore, response is used in phase II as a surrogate endpoint. Even if not associated with improved survival, reducing tumor burden can relieve symptoms and improve quality of life.

5.3.2 Response Criteria

For the purpose of phase II trials, activity is defined as the ability to induce complete and/or partial responses. A complete response is defined as the complete disappearance of all signs and symptoms of the disease for at least 4 weeks. A partial response is the reduction by 50% or more in the volume of all measurable disease for 4 weeks or more. Other types of responses have been defined (mixed, less than partial, and stabilization), but these are generally considered of little clinical or biological significance. Measurable is generally defined as any mass which can be palpated or seen by an imaging technique and whose size can be determined. Pleural effusions or leptomeningeal disease would not be considered measurable. To measure a tumor mass, the two largest perpendicular diameters are multiplied. If more than one measurable mass is present, the size of each is determined and summed. An overall response rate, the sum of the complete and partial rates, is usually reported. In addition, duration of response, time to progression, and survival are determined.

5.3.3 Spectrum of Activity

New agents are usually tested in malignancies which are common and/or have lesions which can be followed for response. Typically, phase II studies will be conducted in a number of tumor types including breast cancer, nonsmall cell lung cancer, small cell lung cancer, colorectal cancer, ovarian cancer, hypernephroma, melanoma, and squamous cell carcinoma of the head and neck. In addition, preclinical or phase I trial results can suggest tumors which should be evaluated in phase II. The demonstration of activity in one tumor type does not predict for activity in others. Each tumor type of interest must be studied to determine a drug's activity in that malignancy.

5.3.4 Patient Selection

As described previously (Section 5.1), selection of phase II patients is determined by the tumor types to be studied, prior threatment of the patients, and the need to test the new agent in patients with the best possible chance of responding. Therefore, patients must have measurable disease and a defined tumor type. Prior treatment should be minimal. In some settings, where chemotherapy is of marginal benefit (Table 4), the patients may have had no prior drug treatment.

5.3.5 Duration of Treatment

Few tumors respond to a single cycle of any chemotherapeutic agent. Unless there is clear-cut progression, two cycles of therapy are given before response is assessed. Often, individual patients are allowed to continue treatment if, in the investigator's opinion, they are benefiting from therapy.

Table 4 Response of Cancer to Existing Chemotherapy

Unresponsive to Existing Chemotherapy	Minor Response to Existing Chemotherapy	Response to Chemotherapy
Melanoma	Colorectal cancer	Breast cancer
Hypernephroma (renal cell carcinoma)	Hepatoma	Small cell lung cancer
Pancreatic carcinoma	Squamous cell carcinoma of the head and neck	Lymphoma (Hodgkin's and non-Hodgkin's)
	Nonsmall cell lung cancer	Leukemia (all forms)
		Ovarian carcinoma
		Germ cell tumors

5.3.6 Statistical Considerations

The initial (early) goal of phase II trials is to reject ineffective agents while treating the smallest number of patients possible. If no responses are seen in 14 consecutive patients, there is 95% probability that the response rate is <20%. If 19 consecutive patients show no response, it is possible to be 95% sure that the response rate is <15%.[11] If no responses are seen in 14 or 19 patients, the drug is generally considered to be of little value as a single agent in that disease.

If responses are seen treatment of more patients increases the accuracy with which the response rate can be predicted. To estimate the response to within ±15% of its true value with 95% confidence, 45 patients must be entered. Most trial designs call for the entry of a fixed number of *evaluable* patients, usually 24 or 30.[21] Once activity has been observed, expanded phase II trials allow for more careful definition of activity in a specific patient population.

Response data should be based on evaluable patients. Evaluable patients are all individuals entered into the study who met the entry criteria and for whom sufficient data are available to allow evaluation of response. Very sick patients are not entered into such studies. Patients must be expected to live long enough to receive two courses of treatment allowing time for an effective agent to exert its antitumor activity.

The endpoint of the early phase II trial of a new cytotoxic is the identification of sufficient activity to warrant further development. The endpoint of late phase II trials is the more accurate definition of the degree and spectrum of activity, as well as further quantitative determination of acute and chronic side effects.

5.3.7 Surrogate Markers

Surrogate markers, parameters which are more easily measured than the ultimate endpoint of prolonged survival are the basis of phase II trials. These studies use tumor shrinkage as a surrogate endpoint for clinical benefit (survival). The implicit assumption is that to affect survival an anticancer drug must cause objective decrease in tumor mass.

In contrast, the primary endpoints for phase I trials are toxicity for cytotoxic agents and appropriate biological effects for compounds designed to affect immunity, inflammation, or other biologic functions.

6 DECISION MAKING

Data from phase I trials should provide the information needed to treat patients in phase II using optimal doses and schedules. In addition, data on the type and severity of adverse events will be accumulated which will be important in the drug profile evaluation. Since phase I trials of anticancer drugs are not designed to demonstrate activity, decisions about further development of a compound are not usually made based on the results of such trials. However, severe, unexpected, or uncontrollable toxicities could lead to a decision to discontinue the development of a compound. In contrast, if significant activity (tumor shrinkage) is seen during phase I it may be possible to accelerate development of a compound.

The Go/No Go decision for anticancer compounds is usually made following phase II. The percent of patients responding, the quality of these responses, and tumor types in which responses, are observed are all factors when considering whether or not to continue development of a new agent. In general a compound active in a relatively rare tumor type will be of less interest than one active in a common tumor. A drug with a high response rate will probably have more appeal than one with less activity. Drugs which can cause responses in previously treated patients may be more attractive than those which work well only in previously untreated patients. In addition the spectrum of activity and response rate in each tumor type will be compared to other available compounds. Finally each pharmaceutical company will set its own criteria for the selection of compounds. Some companies may welcome a drug likely to have a relatively narrow indication while others will require significant activity in common tumors such as breast, colon and/or lung cancer (Table 5).

Table 5 Factors Considered in Go/No Go Decision Making after Phase II Evaluation of Anticancer Compounds

Types of tumors responding to the new agent
Antitumor efficacy in each tumor type
Toxicity of the compound
Potential for incorporation into multidrug regimes and combined modality treatment programs
Availability of other drugs to treat the tumors in which the new agent is active
Ability to devise a strategy leading to rapid registration for important indications
Probability of successful registration

Data from phase II trials are essential in designing phase III studies. These data should be adequate to allow the development of a registrational strategy which will minimize the time to registration and result in the widest possible indications. However, they are not usually critical components of a registrational dossier in the U.S. Approval of anticancer drugs by the FDA as well as other regulatory agencies has traditionally required demonstration of improved survival or quality of life in two well controlled randomized trials. This usually requires comparison of the new drug alone or in combination to the best currently available treatment for each cancer for which approval is sought. Depending on the new drug's activity and the tumor type being treated, the trials may seek to show superiority, altered toxicity, or equivalence. Of note, in order to gain regulatory approval, a new drug does not have to be proven superior to existing treatment but only documented to be safe and effective.

In situations where the new drug is novel and unusually active, phase II data may suffice for registration. Such a setting could be one in which there is no conventional therapy available and phase II data show a reproducible significant response rate with prolongation of survival or significant palliation compared to historical experience. The regulatory environment for anticancer compounds is in flux in North America, Europe, and Japan. Activity in phase II has sufficed for registration in Europe and Japan in the past and continues to do so in Japan. Europe, however, is moving rapidly toward requirements similar to those in the U.S. at a time when the FDA is showing some flexibility in its standards. In addition, discussions among North American, Japanese, and European regulatory agencies have taken place aimed at "harmonizing" registrational requirements. At this time, however, a unique registrational strategy must be designed for each new anticancer drug based on phase I and II data and regulatory requirements.

7 CONCLUSIONS

Phase I and II trials of anticancer drugs have unique characteristics when compared to trials of most other agents. Because life-threatening conditions are being treated and with a dearth of effective agents, compounds with significant toxicity and small therapeutic indexes are routinely developed. This precludes testing in normal volunteers, requires exceptional care in determining doses and schedules, reduces the importance of pharmacokinetics, and results in special ethical considerations which impact on trial design.

REFERENCES

1. Hansen, R. M. and Borden, E. C., Current status of interferons in the treatment of cancer, *Oncology*, 6, 19-24, 1992.
2. Whittington, R. and Faulds, D., Interleukin-2. A review of its pharmacological properties and therapeutic use patients with cancer, *Drugs*, 46, 446-514, 1993.
3. Schacter, L. P., Anderson, C., Canetta, R. M., Kelley, S., Nicaise, C., Onetto, N., Rozencweig, M., Smaldone, L. and Winograd, B., Drug discovery and development in the pharmaceutical industry, *Semin. Oncol.*, 19, 613-621, 1992.
4. Code of Federal Regulations, Vol. 52, No. 53, Page 8845, 1987.

5. Penta, J. S., Rozencweig, M., Guarino, A. M. and Muggia, F. M., Mouse and large-animal toxicology studies of twelve antitumor agents: Relevance to starting dose for phase I clinical trials, *Cancer Chemother. Pharmacol.* 3, 97-101, 1979.
6. Rozencweig, M., Dodion, P., Nicaise, C., Piccart, M. and Kenis, Y., Approach to phase I trials in cancer patients, in *New Approaches in Cancer Therapy,* Cortes-Funes, J. H. and Rozencweig, M., Eds, Raven Press, New York, 1982, 1-13.
7. Rozencweig, M., VonHoff, D. D., Staquet, M. J., Schein, P. S., Penta, J. S., Goldin, A., Muggia, F. M., Freireich, E. J. and DeVita, V. T. Jr., Animal toxicology for early clinical trials with anticancer agents, *Cancer Clin. Trials*, 4, 21-28, 1981.
8. Crawford, J.D., Terry, M.E. and Rourke, G.M., Simplification of drug dosage calculation by application of the surface area principle, *Pediatrics*, 5, 783-790, 1950.
9. Pinkel, D., The use of body surface area as a criterion of drug dosage in cancer chemotherapy. *Cancer Res.*, 18, 853-856, 1958.
10. Freireich, E. J., Gehan, E. A., Rall, D. P., Schmidt, L. H. and Sipeer, H. E., Quantitative comparison of toxicity of anticancer agents in mouse, rat, hamster, dog, monkey and man, *Cancer Chemother. Rep.*, 50, 219-244, 1966.
11. Geller, N. L., Design of phase I and II clinical trials in cancer: A statistician's view, *Cancer Invest.*, 2, 483-491, 1984.
12. EORTC Pharmacokinetics and Metabolism Group, Pharmacokinetically guided dose escalation in phase I clinical trials. Commentary and proposed guidelines. *Eur. J. Cancer Clin. Oncol.*, 23, 1083-1087, 1987.
13. Collins J.M., Zaharko D.S., Dedrick R.L. and Chabner B.A., Potential roles for preclinical pharmacology in phase I clinical trial. *Cancer Treat Rep.*, 70, 1, 73-80, 1986.
14. Evans, W.E. and Relling, M.V., Clinical pharmacokinetics-pharmacodynamics of anticancer drugs. *Clin. Pharmacokin.*, 16, 327-336, 1989.
15. Collins J.M., Grieshaber C.K. and Chabner B.A., Pharmacologically guided phase I clinical trials based upon preclinical drug development. *J. Natl. Cancer Inst.*, 82, 1321-1326, 1990.
16. Foster B.J., Graham M.J., Newell D.R., Gumbrell, L.A. and Calvert, A.H., Phase I study of the anthrapyrazole CI941 with pharmacokinetically guided dose escalation. *Proc. ASCO*, 7, 64, 1988.
17. Gianni L., Vigano L., Surbone A. et al., Pharmacology and clinical toxicity of 4′-iodo-4′-deoxydoxorubicin: An example of successful application of pharmacokinetics to dose escalation in phase I trials. *J. Natl. Cancer Inst.* 82: 469-477, 1990.
18. Politi P., Setser A., Bastian H., Ford, H., Xie, F., Kelley, J., Jordan, E., Dahut, B., Allegra, C., Hamilton, J.M., Arbuck, S., Chen, A., Agbaria, R. and Grem, J., Pharmacologically guided phase I trial of cyclopentenyl cytosine (CPC) with biochemical monitoring. *Proc. ASCO*, 12, 142, 1993.
19. Center for Biologics Evaluation and Research, FDA: Draft points to consider in the manufacture and testing of monoclonal antibody products for human use, 1994.
20. Krakoff, I.H., Cancer chemotherapeutic and biologic agents, *CA-A J. Clin.*, 41, 264-278, 1991.
21. Gehan, E. A. and Schniederman, M. A., Experimental design of clinical trials, in *Cancer Medicine,* Holland, J. F. and Frei, E., Eds, Lea & Febiger, Philadelphia, 1973, 531.

Part XIII. Assessment of Drugs Affecting the Inflammatory Process and Pain

Chapter 39

Analgesics

R. L. Holland

CONTENTS

1 Introduction ... 537
2 Studies of Efficacy in Volunteers ... 537
 2.1 Volunteer Pain Models ... 537
 2.2 Pain Measurement in These Models ... 538
  2.2.1 Visual Analog Scales ... 538
  2.2.2 Category Judgments ... 538
  2.2.3 Physiological Variables ... 538
   2.2.3.1 Cerebral Event Related Potentials ... 538
   2.2.3.2 The Nociception Flexion Reflex ... 539
   2.2.3.3 Other Measures ... 539
 2.3 Which Measures, in which Volunteer Models, Respond to which Drugs? ... 539
 2.4 Recommendations ... 539
3 Early Studies of Efficacy in Patients ... 539
 3.1 Introduction ... 540
 3.2 Useful Paradigms for Investigating the Clinical Efficacy of Novel Analgesics ... 540
  3.2.1 Acute Pain ... 540
   3.2.1.1 Postoperative Pain ... 540
   3.2.1.2 Other Acutely Painful Conditions ... 541
  3.2.2 Chronic Pain ... 541
   3.2.2.1 Pain Due to Cancer ... 541
   3.2.2.2 Chronic Arthritic Conditions ... 541
   3.2.2.3 Other Chronic Pains ... 541
 3.3 Discussion and Recommendations ... 542
4 Other Studies Usefully Performed at an Early Stage of Analgesic Development ... 542
 4.1 Volunteer Studies ... 542
  4.1.1 Opioids ... 542
  4.1.2 Other Analgesics ... 542
 4.2 Patient Studies ... 542
 4.3 Later Clinical Pharmacological Studies ... 542
5 Conclusion ... 542
References ... 542

1 INTRODUCTION

Kinetics and tolerance studies are common to all novel drugs and are addressed elsewhere in this volume. Therefore this chapter will concentrate on methods to evaluate efficacy and then touch upon other pharmacodynamic properties of analgesics which can sometimes be explored. In this chapter some methods for studying new drugs in volunteers and patients will be described. It will be shown that although the methods may lack scientific validity, they can generate valuable information.

2 STUDIES OF EFFICACY IN VOLUNTEERS

2.1 Volunteer Pain Models

Many methods of causing pain in volunteers have been investigated. Examples include:

0-8493-9230-6/97/$0.00+$.50
© 1997 by CRC Press, Inc.

1. Electrical shocks to the finger (Seki, 1978; Bromm et al., 1986); to the forearm (Buchsbaum et al., 1981a,b); to the tooth pulp (Gracely et al., 1982); to the earlobe (Stacher et al., 1982); and directly onto or into a nerve (Schady and Torebjork, 1984; Willier, 1985).
2. Mechanical pressure on the finger (Bromm and Scharein, 1982a,b) or the interdigital web (Forster et al., 1988).
3. Hand immersion in cold water (De Jalon et al., 1985).
4. Ischemia (Smith and Beecher, 1969; Posner, 1984; Segerdahl et al., 1994).
5. Heat on the skin (Hougs and Skoulby, 1957; Gracely et al., 1988).
6. Jets of gas into the nostril (Kobal et al., 1994).

2.2 Pain Measurement in These Models

There are rather few methods available. They consist of either asking the volunteer to quantify subjectively pain intensity or attempting to measure some physiological correlate of the pain. Usually an attempt is made to relate the pain intensity to the magnitude of the stimulus causing the pain. Typical parameters analyzed are the stimulus intensity at which pain is just perceived (threshold) and the maximum stimulus tolerated by the subjects (tolerance).

Two methods for quantifying self-reported pain have been developed.

2.2.1 Visual Analog Scales

Visual analog scales are lines, usually horizontal, anchored at both ends by terms such as "no pain" and "worst possible pain." Pain intensity can be indicated by placing a mark on the line (see Sriwatanakui et al., 1983, for review) or by moving a cursor along a computer-generated scale (Posner, 1984). The score is usually taken as the distance from the "no pain" end.

2.2.2 Category Judgments

This is the more common technique. At its simplest, this devolves to asking whether a particular stimulus intensity is painful or not. Usually, however, several categories of painfulness are used (see, e.g., Buchsbaum et al., 1981a,b; De Jalon et al., 1985). Perhaps surprisingly, this methodology lends itself to some fairly sophisticated psychophysics. It is possible, for example, using the technique of cross-modality matching, to give certain categories of painfulness absolute scores which are consistent between subjects as well as within a subject (Gracely et al., 1982; Gracely and Dubner, 1987).

Most research into category judgments of pain intensity has focused upon the pain threshold and upon delineating accurately the stimulus intensity at that boundary. Typically, but least accurately, the threshold is sought by use of a steadily rising stimulus intensity (see, e.g., Wolff et al., 1976; Stacher et al., 1982). A better technique is to use the method of limits, in which ascending and descending stimulus intensities are used. This can be improved still further with the use of random double staircases (see Gracely et al., 1988). Although these techniques are usually used to delineate the prepain-pain category boundary, in principle they can be applied to any category boundary, e.g., moderate to severe pain.

Another approach to category judgment uses sensory decision theory (SDT). Statistical techniques are used to examine subject categorizations of a large number of brief, variable-intensity stimuli (usually electrical pulses). Two parameters are derived. One is an index of discrimination ability, often called sensitivity, which is obtained from accuracy and error rates. The other, often called response bias, is a measure of the conservatism with which the subject makes a judgment during that experiment (Buchsbaum et al., 1981a,b).

2.2.3 Physiological Variables

Several physiological variables have been quantified in an attempt to obtain more objective data.

2.2.3.1 Cerebral Event Related Potentials

There have been many attempts to relate changes in the electroencephalogram with the presence or absence, and intensity of pain (see, e.g., Buchsbaum et al., 1981b; Bromm and Scharein, 1982a; Fernandes de Lima et al., 1982; Bromm et al., 1986). The usual technique has been to present many brief painful stimuli, usually electrical, and then to average the cerebral potentials over the next 300 ms or so — "evoked potentials." A negative potential is usually evident about 120-150 ms after the stimulation, and this is followed by a positive component about 100 ms later. The amplitudes of these waves are typically related to the intensity of the stimulation and sometimes correlate with the self-reported pain intensity (Kobal et al., 1994). However, it is by no means clear that these waves represent "pain", as they can be evoked at low amplitude by non-noxious A delta fiber stimulation (Chudler and Dong, 1983).

2.2.3.2 The Nociception Flexion Reflex

A painful stimulus to a limb produces a spinal reflex withdrawal of that limb from that stimulus. Willer (1985) stimulated the peroneal nerve of volunteers at the ankle and recorded electrical activity in the ipsilateral biceps femoris. This electromyogram response was quantitatively linearly related to the stimulus intensity and to the self-reported pain intensity. However, again, an EMG response can be produced by low-amplitude (subpain threshold) electrical stimuli.

2.2.3.3 Other Measures

Autonomic functions have frequently been measured during volunteer pain studies. However, these measures typically relate more to the anxiety of the subjects and to the physical procedures (e.g., cold pressor), than to the intensity of the pain experience (Chapman et al., 1985).

2.3 Which Measures, in which Volunteer Models, Respond to which Drugs?

In essence this question can be answered as follows: in double-blind, placebo-controlled, crossover, single-dose studies (1) a reasonable dose of an opioid will reduce the intensity of subjectively assessed pain, using practically any measure in practically any volunteer model; and (2) it is very difficult to detect effects with other types of analgesics.

Thus, therapeutic doses of opioids provide pain relief in: (1) electrically induced pain (Wolff, 1976; Buchsbaum et al., 1981a,b; Gracely et al., 1982; Bromm et al., 1986; Stacher et al., 1986, 1987); (2) cold-induced pain (Wolff et al., 1976; De Jalon et al., 1985; Holland et al., 1988); (3) ischemic pain (Posner, 1984; Segerdahl et al., 1994); and (4) thermal pain (Stacher et al., 1982).

The most clear-cut effects are on tolerance and pain intensity after a constant stimulus rather than on threshold. One possible explanation for this is that the opioid effect is proportional to the pain intensity. However, a more interesting possibility is that moderate to severe pain, especially if it is increasing, more reliably represents the clinical situation with its associated anxiety and stress (Chapman et al., 1985).

Evidence for pain relief by nonopioid analgesics is much more difficult to obtain.

1. Electrically induced pain. Some studies have found high doses of a nonsteroidal anti-inflammatory drug (NSAID) to have effects on pain threshold (Wolff et al., 1976; Stacher et al., 1982, 1986). Occasionally, other parameters have also been affected: e.g., aspirin, on all categories of painfulness (Seki, 1978) and zomepirac, on pain intensity to constant stimulus (Schady and Torebjork, 1984).
2. Cold-induced pain. NSAIDs produce little if any effect (Wolff et al., 1976; De Jalon et al., 1985; Telekes et al., 1987).
3. Ischemic pain. Aspirin 600 mg produced some effects (Smith and Beecher, 1969) but not paracetamol (Telekes, A., personal communication). Adenosine had some effects especially in combination with other analgesics (Segerdahl et al., 1994).
4. Thermal threshold. Diclofenac 75 mg and 150 mg affected this (Stacher et al., 1986).
5. Mechanical pressure. Aspirin 1.5 mg affected category judgments (Forster et al., 1988).
6. Jets of Gas into Nostril. Ibuprofen was not effective (Kobal et al., 1994).

With the well-known bias in favor of publishing positive results, it is probable that many negative studies of nonopioids remain unpublished. It might be, therefore, that the few positive published examples cited above represent chance findings. Two other points should also be noted. First, these studies often used very high doses of NSAIDs, which can have other (nonanalgesic) CNS effects (Telekes et al., 1987). Second, effects on pain threshold are the least reliable of analgesic measures (Beecher, 1957; Chapman et al., 1985), as thresholds are particularly affected by placebo and instructional set.

2.4 Recommendations

If a new drug is an opioid, it is worth investigating its efficacy in a volunteer model. Electrical stimulation and cold-induced pain are both reliable and convenient techniques. Both can predict therapeutic single doses and duration of action. However, neither has been properly explored for false-positives, i.e., drugs which might produce apparent pain relief but are not clinical analgesics. However, diazepam did not affect an electrical pain test (Gracely et al., 1982) and the vasodilator nifedipine did not affect the cold pain test (Holland et al., 1988).

For drugs which are not opioids there are no really appropriate volunteer models. Only the electrical pain test has consistently shown pain relief with nonopioids, and even then, this effect is typically on the least reliable measure (threshold) and only occurs with high doses. The occasional positive effects of antidepressant-like drugs in this model are also worrying. It is not clear that imipramine (Bromm et al., 1986) and RO15-8081 (Stacher et al., 1987) are clinically effective analgesics, whereas fluradoline (rejected in the Bromm et al., 1986, experiment) does seem to produce postoperative analgesia (Jones and McQuay, 1987).

3 EARLY STUDIES OF EFFICACY IN PATIENTS

3.1 Introduction

Testing analgesics in patients is in some ways easier than in volunteers. After all, if the patients find, on average, that the drug produces adequate relief of a diagnosed pain, then the drug is by definition an analgesic, provided that it is not acting to improve the underlying disease process.

3.2 Useful Paradigms for Investigating the Clinical Efficacy of Novel Analgesics

Any clinical situation in which pain features could, in theory, be used to assess analgesic efficacy. However, clearly: (1) it is easier to use paradigms in which the patient's physical condition is otherwise more or less stable and (2) it is better to use conditions in which the cause of the pain has been diagnosed. Most of the studies which follow have satisfied both of these criteria.

3.2.1 Acute Pain

3.2.1.1 Postoperative Pain

In many ways postoperative pain represents the "gold standard" clinical study of an analgesic, as efficacy can be reliably demonstrated in double-blind, placebo-controlled parallel group single-dose studies. Pain post dental surgery has become perhaps the best characterized patient model (e.g., Bakshi et al., 1994; Fricke et al., 1993; Kiersch et al., 1994; Nelson et al., 1994; Patel et al., 1991), though really any form of surgery can be satisfactory. A typical study is described below.

The patients are assessed for suitability and informed consent is obtained preoperatively. After operation the patients are monitored until they complain of moderate or severe pain. At this point they are randomized to receive a single dose of one of the several treatments (typically placebo, two or three doses of the active medication, and a positive control). They are then monitored frequently by a trained observer (often a nurse) for the expected duration of action of the analgesics. Observation times are usually pretreatment, then 1/2, 1, 2, 3, 4, 5, and 6 h post treatment. The patients are usually asked to rate their pain intensity on a four- (or sometimes five-) point scale — 0: none; 1: mild; 2: moderate; 3: severe (4: very severe). They usually also rate their pain intensity on a 100 mm visual analog line and their pain relief on a typical five- (or six-) point scale — (-1: worse); 0: no relief; 1: some relief; 2: good relief; 3: excellent relief; 4: complete relief. Additional parameters that can be analyzed include: the time at which pain is "half gone"; pain adjectives presented randomly; and the time at which escape analgesia is required (treatment failure). It is important that the same observer be used throughout for a particular patient, and preferably for the whole study, as the patient's responses to these self-evaluations will depend upon the instructional set. It is also desirable to use a trained and experienced observer, as this allows consistent behavior in the face of anxious, sedated, or nauseated patients.

Analysis of these different category scales and analog scales is relatively straightforward. For the pain intensity measures (category and analog), the pretreatment measure is used as a baseline and the analyzed value is usually the difference from baseline (i.e., pain intensity difference, PID; or pain analog intensity difference, PAID). Separate analyses are usually carried out at each time-point, and, in addition, a time-weighted average value is usually computed (SPID and SPAID). Patients who drop out are typically allocated their initial value for the remainder of the analyzed time-points — as though the treatment had been ineffective. The pain relief scores are usually analyzed directly, and once again a total time-weighted pain relief score (TOTPAR) is usually generated.

A great deal of literature has been published on the relative merits of different category and analog scales in this postoperative situation. However, when a large number of studies were reviewed (Liltman et al., 1985), it was clear that intensity difference ratings, visual analog scale (VAS) scores, and pain relief scores all correlated extremely highly. There was little difference in their abilities to detect drug effects, with perhaps the pain relief scales and VAS scales being slightly more sensitive than intensity scales. The fact that the different scales all gave the same answers is hardly surprising. Patients will attempt to describe whether the drug gives effective pain relief, whatever method is used to ask this question of them. It should also be noted that the data manipulations used to compute PID and PAID essentially convert scores of intensity to scores of pain relief. Importantly, it has been shown that patients prefer adjectival descriptions to VAS, with as many as 11% failing to understand and cope with the latter (Kremer et al., 1981; Jensen et al., 1986).

With appropriate stratification for operation site and patient age, and with sufficient patients per group (usually 30 per treatment dose), postoperative pain studies are highly effective at showing both opioid (see, e.g., Downing et al., 1981; Calimlin et al., 1982) and NSAID (see, e.g., McQuay et al., 1986; O'Hara et al., 1987) analgesia. This technique has even been extended to investigations of analgesia produced by corticosteroids (Olstad and Skjelbred, 1986) and antidepressants (Levine et al., 1986).

Another route to assessing pain relief is to analyze the numbers of patients who require additional analgesia (Sechzer, 1977). More elegantly, the total amount of additional analgesic requested can be quantified by use of a patient-controlled analgesia system (e.g., Harmer et al., 1983; Fredman et al., 1995). However, this technique may produce additional problems, given the extreme variation that occurs in analgesic demand postoperatively with such a system.

3.2.1.2 Other Acutely Painful Conditions

Techniques validated by frequent use in postoperative pain have been equally successfully applied to other acutely painful conditions. Obstetric pain is one such, with analgesia being demonstrated during labor (Frank et al., 1987), and in postpartum pain, e.g., episiotomy, uterine cramp, and cesarean section (Bloomfield et al., 1986; Sunshine et al., 1986). Similar studies have been performed equally successfully in acute renal and ureteric colic (Warren et al., 1985), acute trauma, acute back pain, and sciatica (Clissoid and Beresford, 1987).

3.2.2 Chronic Pain

The assessment of an analgesic in chronically painful conditions is problematic. Clearly, the diagnosis is of fundamental importance, and not all conditions are appropriate for analgesic intervention. It is rare for patients to suffer only one pain at a time. The interplay between mental state and perceived pain intensity is crucial. Outcome measures must include more than just pain relief, with assessments of quality of life being more relevant.

3.2.2.1 Pain Due to Cancer

Deschamps et al., (1988) reviewed the use of category scales and VAS in studies of pain due to cancer, noting that both types of scale tended to focus only on intensity. The authors advocated the use of the McGill Pain Questionnaire (MPQ; Melzack, 1975) as a more appropriate tool. However, there would be substantial problems in using the MPQ in a drug study. It is difficult and time-consuming to administer, and there is little consensus as to how to score it. Nonetheless, the philosophy of the MPQ is appropriate to cancer pain (e.g., Hays et al., 1994).

A particular problem with cancer pain is the ethical requirement for the physician to alleviate that pain. Pain control in such patients typically has two phases during maintenance treatment, a titration period during which increasing doses of an analgesic are administered, and a maintenance phase. The maintenance dose for longer term pain control can be highly variable between patients (40-400 mg of oral morphine daily; Hanks et al., 1987) and in this situation cross-over comparisons of different preparations can be the most relevant design for a clinical study (e.g., Bruera et al., 1995). Another approach is to regard an admission for cancer pain as equivalent to an acutely painful condition. For example, Stambaugh and McAdams (1987) performed a placebo-controlled single-dose study directly equivalent to postoperative pain studies. Alternatively, placebo can be avoided in the same situation by demonstrating a dose response (Chary et al., 1994).

3.2.2.2 Chronic Arthritic Conditions

Clinical trials in these conditions are extremely complex, with multiple outcome measures. Honig (1983) presented a good example of an appropriate study on the long-term pain relief provided by zomepirac in osteoarthritis. Four separate pains were scored, each on a four-point scale: pain at rest, pain on motion, pain at night, and joint tenderness (joint swelling was also scored on the same scale). Functional status was scored on at least 11 separate movements and activities related to daily living.

3.2.2.3 Other Chronic Pains

Simple studies can be performed but are usually confounded by diagnosis and previous treatment. Patients who present to chronic pain clinics usually have pains which will not respond to simple treatments. Moreover, chronic pain causes low mood, but chronic pain can also be a presentation (symptom) of depression.

3.3 Discussion and Recommendations

The early phase evaluation of novel analgesics in patients is relatively easily undertaken in acutely painful conditions. Postoperative pain, particularly after orthopedic or dental surgery, is a well-validated model sensitive to both major classes of analgesic. Although patient numbers need to be large (>30 per group), the conditions are common, patient recruitment can be rapid, and the studies are easy to analyze and have sensible outcome measures.

Chronically painful conditions are much more complex, and rarely suitable for the early phase investigation of new drugs.

4 OTHER STUDIES USEFULLY PERFORMED AT AN EARLY STAGE OF ANALGESIC DEVELOPMENT

4.1 Volunteer Studies

4.1.1 Opioids

Opioids have a large number of well-known side effects relating to their specificities for particular receptor subtypes. Estimates of opioid-induced sedation can be obtained from simple tests of psychomotor performance and validated visual analog scales (e.g., Telekes et al., 1987). Similarly, the likelihood of respiratory depression can be determined by looking for effects on the ventilatory response to rebreathing CO_2 (Keats, 1985; Telekes et al., 1987). Abuse liability can be addressed by giving the drug to opioid-experienced volunteers (usually ex-addicts) who can self-assess euphoria, dysphoria, and "drug liking." In the presence of trained observers, double-blind, placebo-controlled studies can give reliable and predictive results (Jasinsky and Preston, 1985; Preston et al., 1987). Other effects which can be sought in volunteers include hormonal responses and gastrointestinal effects (by use of techniques to measure delay in gastric emptying, such as the H_2 breath test, or simply measuring the time until the next stool).

4.1.2 Other Analgesics

It is not, in general, as profitable to seek effects of NSAIDs in volunteers as it is for opioids. However, occasionally CNS effects can be detected, such as self-assessed sedation and *increased* respiratory responsiveness to rebreathing CO_2 (Telekes et al., 1987).

4.2 Patient Studies

Before investigating dose response in a postoperative pain model, it is imperative to have information about possible kinetic and dynamic interactions with other drugs used in the postoperative period. These include: anesthetics (inhalational and induction agents, e.g., barbiturates); neuromuscular blocking drugs; drugs used to reverse neuromuscular blockade; and antiemetics. This sort of information can be obtained by performing a limited rising-dose tolerance study of the potential analgesic in postoperative patients.

4.3 Later Clinical Pharmacological Studies

The safe and therapeutic dose having been established, there are many further clinical pharmacological studies to be performed. For example, drug interaction studies will be required, and dynamic/kinetic studies in particular patient populations (the elderly, impaired renal or hepatic function). However, these studies are perhaps best deferred until the later phase of drug investigation.

5 CONCLUSION

While some of the methodologies described above may be criticized, they contribute to the development of a new analgesic. Kinetic and tolerance studies are as important as with any drug, and at least some of this work must be performed in the most likely experimental testbed for the analgesic — postoperative pain. Volunteer pharmacodynamic models have much to offer with regard to questions about tolerance, side effects, and abuse potential, but are probably only predictive of efficacy for opioids.

REFERENCES

Bakshi, R., Frenkel, G., Dietlein, G., Meurer-Witt, B. and Sinterhauf, U. (1994) A placebo controlled comparative evaluation of diclofenac dispersible versus ibuprofen in postoperative pain after third molar surgery. *J. Clin. Pharmacol.* 34, 225-230.

Beecher, H. K. (1957). The measurement of pain. *Pharm. Rev.*, 9, 59-209.

Bloomfield, S. S., Mitchell, J., Cissell, G. and Barden, T. P. (1986). Analgesic sensitivity of two post-partum pain models. *Pain*, 27, 171-9.

Bromm, B., Meier, W. and Scharein, E. (1986). Imipramine reduces experimental pain. *Pain*, 25, 245-57.

Bromm, B. and Scharein, E. (1982a). Response plasticity of pain evoked reactions in man. *Physiol. Behav.*, 28, 109-16.

Bromm, B. and Scharein, E. (1982b). Principal component analysis of pain related cerebral potentials to mechanical and electrical stimulation in man. *Electroenceph. Clin. Neurophysiol.*, 53, 94-103.

Bruera, E., Fainsinger, R., Spachynski, K., Babul, N., Harsanyi, Z. and Darke, A.C. (1995) Clinical efficacy and safety of a novel controlled-release morphine suppository and subcutaneous morphine in cancer pain: a randomized evaluation. *J. Clin. Oncol.*, 13 1520-7.

Buchsbaum, M. S., Davis, G. C., Coppola, R. and Naber, D. (1981a). Opiate pharmacology and individual differences. I. Psychophysical pain measurements. *Pain*, 10, 357-66.

Buchsbaum, M. S., Davis, G. C., Coppola, R. and Naber, D. (1981b). Opiate pharmacology and individual differences. I. Somatosensory evoked potentials. *Pain*, 10, 367-77.

Calimlin, J. F., Sriwatanakul, K., Wardell, W. M., Lasagna, L. and Cox, C. (1982). Analgesic efficacy of parenteral metkephamid acetate in the treatment of postoperative pain. *Lancet*, i, 1374-5.

Chapman, C. R., Casey, K. L., Dubnet, R., Foley, K. M., Gracely, R. H. and Reading, A. E. (1985). Pain measurement: an overview. *Pain*, 22, 1-31.

Chary, S., Goughnour, B. R., Moulin, D. E., Thorpe, W. R., Harsanyi, Z. and Darke, A. C. (1994) The dose response relationship of controlled release codeine (Codeine Contin) in chronic cancer pain. *J. Pain Symp. Manage.*, 9, 363-71.

Chudler, E. H. and Dong, W. K. (1983). The assessment of pain by cerebral evoked potentials. *Pain*, 16, 221-44.

Clissold, S. P. and Beresford, R. (1987). Proquazone. A review of its pharmacodynamic and pharmacokinetic properties and therapeutic efficacy in rheumatic diseases and pain states. *Drugs*, 33, 478-502.

De Jalon, P. D. G., Harrison, F. J. J., Johnson, K. I., Kozma, C. and Schnelle, K. (1985). A modified cold stimulation technique for the evaluation of analgesic activity in human volunteers. *Pain*, 22, 183-9.

Deschamps, K., Band, P. R. and Coldman, A. J. (1988). Assessment of adult cancer pain: shortcomings of current methods. *Pain*, 32, 133-9.

Downing, J. W., Brock-Utne, J. G., Barclay, A. and Schwegmann, I. L. (1981). WY16225 (Dezocine) a new synthetic opiate agonist-antagonist and potent analgesic: comparison with morphine for relief of pain after lower abdominal surgery. *Br. J. Anaesth.*, 53, 59-63.

Fernandes de Lima, V. M., Chatrian, G. E., Lettich, E., Canfield, R. C., Miller, R. C. and Soso, M. J. (1982). Electrical stimulation of toothpulp in humans. I. Relationships among physical stimulus intensities, psychological magnitude estimates, and cerebral evoked potentials. *Pain*, 14, 207-32.

Forster, C., Anton, F., Reeh, P. W., Weber, E. and Handwerker, H. O. (1988). Measurement of the analgesic effects of aspirin with a new experimental algesimetric procedure. *Pain*, 32, 215-22.

Frank, M., McAteer, E. J., Cattermole, R., Loughman, B., Stafford, L. B. and Hitchcock, A. M. (1987). Nalbuphine for obstetric analgesia. A comparison of nalbuphine with pethidine for pain relief in labor when administered by patient controlled analgesia (PCA). *Anaesthesia*, 42, 697-703.

Fredman, B., Olsfanger, D. and Jedeikin, R. (1995) A comparative study of ketorolac and diclofenac on post laparoscopic cholecysectomy pain. *Eur. J. Anaesthesiol.* 12, 501-4.

Fricke, J., Halladay, S.C., Bynum, L. and Francisco, C.A. (1993) Pain relief after dental impaction surgery using ketorolac, hydrocodone plus acetaminophen, or placebo. *Clin. Ther.* 15, 500-9.

Gracely, R. H. and Dubner, R. (1987). Reliability and validity of verbal descriptor scales of painfulness. *Pain*, 29, 175-85.

Gracely, R. H., Dubner, R. and McGrath, P. A. (1982). Fentanyl reduces the intensity of painful toothpulp sensations: controlling for detection of active drugs. *Anesth. Analg.*, 61, 751-5.

Gracely, R. H., Lota, L., Walter, D. J. and Dubner, R. (1988). A multiple random staircase method of psychophysical pain assessment. *Pain*, 32, 55-63.

Hanks, G. W., Twycross, R. G. and Bliss, J. M. (1987). Controlled release morphine tablets; a double blind trial in patients with advanced cancer. *Anaesthesia*, 42, 840-4.

Harmer, M., Slattery, P. J., Rosen, M. and Vickers, M.D. (1983). Intramuscular on demand analgesia: double blind controlled trial of pethidine, buprenorphine, morphine and meptazinol. *Br. Med. J.*, 286, 680-2.

Hays, H., Hagen, M., Thirlwell, M., Dhaliwal, H., Babul, N., Harsanyi, Z. and Darke, A.C. (1994) Comparative clinical efficacy and safety of immediate release and controlled release hydromorphone for chronic severe cancer pain. *Cancer*, 74, 1808-16.

Holland, R. L., Harkin, N. E., Coleshaw, S. R K., Jones, D. A., Peck. A. W. and Telekes, A. (1988). Dipipanone and nifedipine in cold induced pain: analgesia not due to skin warming. *Br. J. Clin. Pharmacol.*, 24, 823-6.

Honig, S. (1983). Long-term therapy for the pain of ostearthrifis: a comparison of zomepirac sodium and aspirin. *J. Clin. Pharmacol.*, 23, 494-504.

Hougs, W. and Skouby, A. P. (1957). The analgetic action of analgetics, antihistaminics and chlorpromazine on volunteers. *Acta Pharmacol. Toxicol.*, 13, 405-9.

Jasinsky, D. R. and Preston, K. K. (1985). Assessment of dezocine for morphine like subjective effects and miosis. *Clin. Pharmacol. Ther.*, 38, 544-8.

Jensen, M. P., Karoly, P. and Braver, S. (1986). The measurement of clinical pain intensity: a comparison of six methods. *Pain,* 27, 117-26.

Jones, S. F. and McQuay, H. J. (1987). Letter to Editor. *Pain,* 28, 265.

Keats, A. S. (1985). The effect of drugs on respiration in man. *Annu. Rev. Pharmacol. Toxicol.*, 25, 41-65.

Kiersch, T. A., Halladay, S. C. and Hormel, P. C. (1994) A single dose, double blind comparison of naproxen sodium, acetaminophen, and placebo in post operative dental pain. *Clin. Ther.* 16, 394-404.

Kobal, G., Hummel, C., Gruber, M., Geisslinger, G. and Hummel, T. (1994) Dose related effects of ibuprofen on pain-related potentials. *Br. J. Clin. Pharmacol.*, 37 445-52.

Kremer, F., Atkinson, J. H. and Ignelzi, R. J. (1981). Measurement of pain: patient preference does not confound pain measurement. *Pain,* 10, 241-8.

Levine, J. D., Gordon, N. C., Smith, R. and McBryde, R. (1986). Desipramine enhances opiate post operative analgesia. *Pain,* 27, 45-9.

Liltman, G. S., Walker, B. R. and Scheider, B. E. (1985). Reassessment of verbal and visual analog ratings in analgesic studies. *Clin. Pharmacol. Ther.*, 38, 16-23.

McQuay, H. J., Poppleton, P., Carroll, D., Summerfield, R. J., Bullingham, R. E. S. and Moore, R. A. (1986). Ketorolac and acetaminophen for orthopaedic post operative pain. *Clin. Pharmacol. Ther.*, 39, 89-93.

Melzack, R. (1975). The McGill Pain Questionnaire: major properties and scoring methods. *Pain,* 1, 277-99.

Nelson, S. L., Brahim, J. S., Korn, S. H., Greene, S. S. and Suchower, L. J. (1994) Comparison of single dose ibuprofen lysine, acetylsalicylic acid, and placebo for moderate to severe postoperative dental pain. *Clin. Ther.* 16, 458-65.

O'Hara, D. A., Fragen, R. J., Kinzer, M. and Pemberton, D. (1987). Ketorolac tromethamine as compared with morphine sulfate for treatment of post operative pain. *Clin. Pharm. Ther.*, 41, 556-61.

Olstad, O. A. and Skjelbred, P. (1986). Comparison of the analgesic effect of a corticosteroid and paracetamol in patients with pain after oral surgery. *Br. J. Clin. Pharmacol.*, 22, 437-42.

Patel, A., Skelly, A.M., Kohn, H. and Preiskel, H.W. (1991) Double blind placebo controlled comparison of the analgesic effects of single doses of lornoxicam and aspirin in patients with post operative dental pain. *Br. Dent. J.* 170, 295-9.

Posner, J. (1984). A modified submaximal effort tourniquet test for evaluation of analgesics in healthy volunteers. *Pain,* 19, 143-51.

Preston, K. L., Bigelow, G. E. and Liebson, I. A. (1987). Comparative evaluation of morphine, pentazocine, and ciramadol in post addicts. *J. Pharmacol. Exp. Ther.*, 240, 900-10.

Schady, W. and Torebjork, H. E. (1984). Central effects of zomepirac on pain evoked by intraneural stimulation in man. *J. Clin. Pharmacol.*, 24, 42-35.

Sechzer, P. H. (1977). Evaluation of fenoprofen as a post operative analgesic. *Curr. Ther. Res.*, 21, 137-48.

Segerdahl, M., Ekblom, A. and Sollevi, A. (1994) The influence of adenosine, ketamine, and morphine on experimentally induced ischaemic pain in healthy volunteers. *Anesth. Analg.*, 79, 787-91.

Seki, T. (1978). Evaluation of effect of acetyl-salicylic acid using electrical stimulation on the forefinger of healthy volunteers. *Br. J. Clin. Pharmacol.*, 6, 521-4.

Smith, G. M. and Beecher, H. K. (1969). Experimental production of pain in man: sensitivity of a new method to 600 mg of aspirin. *Clin. Pharmacol. Ther.*, 10, 213-16.

Sriwatanakul, K., Kelvie, W., Lasagna, L., Calimlim, J. F., Weis, O. F. and Mehta, G. (1983). Studies with different types of visual analog scales for measurement of pain. *Clin. Pharmacol. Ther.*, 34, 234-9.

Stacher, G., Bauer, P., Scheider, C., Winklehner, S. and Schmierer, S. (1982). Effects of a combination of oral naproxen sodium and codeine on experimentally induced pain. *Eur. J. Clin. Pharmacol.*, 21, 485-90.

Stacher, G., Steinringer, H., Schneider, S., Mittelbach, G., Gaupman, G., Abatzi, Th.-A. and Stacher-Janotta, G. (1987). Effects of graded doses of a new 5-hydroxytryptamine/noradrenaline uptake inhibitor (RO 15-8081) in comparison with 60 mg codeine and placebo on experimentally induced pain and side effect profile in man. *Br. J. Clin. Pharmacol.*, 24, 627-35.

Stacher, G., Steinringer, H., Schneider, S., Mittelbach, G., Winklehner, S. and Gaupman, G. (1986). Experimental pain induced by electrical and thermal stimulation of the skin in healthy man: sensitivity to 75 and 150 mg diclofenac sodium in comparison with 60 mg codeine and placebo. *Br. J. Clin. Pharmacol.*, 21, 3543.

Stambaugh, J. E. and McAdams, J. (1987). Comparison of intramuscular dezocine with butorphanol and placebo in chronic cancer pain: a method to evaluate analgesia after both single and repeated doses. *Clin. Pharmacol. Ther.*, 42, 210-19.

Sunshine, A., Zighelboim, I., Laska, E., Siegel, C., Olson, N. Z. and DeCastro, A. (1986). A double blind parallel comparison of ketoprofen, aspirin and placebo in patients with post partum pain. *J. Clin. Pharmacol.*, 26, 706-11.

Telekes, A., Holland, R. L. and Peck, A. W. (1987). Indomethacin: effects on cold induced pain and the nervous system in healthy volunteers. *Pain,* 30, 321-8.

Warren, M. M., Boyce, W. H., Evans, J. W. and Peters, P. C. (1985). A double blind comparison of dezocine and morphine in patients with acute renal and ureteral colic. *J. Urol.*, 134, 457-9.

Willer, J. C. (1985). Studies on pain. Effects of morphine on a spinal nociceptive flexion reflex and related pain sensation in man. *Brain Res.*, 331, 105-14.

Wolff, B. B., Kantor, T. G. and Cohen, P. (1976). Laboratory pain induction methods for human analgesic assays. *Adv. Pain Res. Ther.*, 1, 363-7.

Index

INDEX

A

ABPI (ankle/brachial pressure index), 259, 262
ABPI research ethics guidelines, 118–122
Absorption, 390–391
  artificial stomas and, 391
  buccal, 391
  gastrointestinal, 8–9, 10, 390–391
  measurements of, 390–391
    HF capsule, 390–391
    intubation techniques, 390
  preliminary considerations, 27–29
  principles of, 169–170
ACE inhibitors, 227–228, 239, 243
Acinetobacter spp., 495
Acne, 442
Acute toxicity, animal studies, 36–37
Administrative issues, 67–100, see also Organizational issues
Adrenoreceptor antagonists, 239
Adverse effects, 166–167
  of diuretics, 421–422
  drug-induced gastrointestinal injury, 391–394
  of NSAIDs, 174, 394–395, 428, 539
  in vitro investigation of, 57–58
Age
  in antihypertensive studies, 218
  in atherosclerosis studies, 252
  body sway and, 301
  depression and, 340
Age-associated memory impairment (AAMI), 355, see also Alzheimer's disease/dementia
Aggression Rating Scale, 301–302
Aging, animal studies, 47
Alcohol (ethanol), 301
Aldose reductase, 476
Alzheimer's Disease Assessment Scale, 364
Alzheimer's disease/dementia, 355–368
  decision making, 368
  diagnosis and staging, 364
  healthy volunteers, 356–362
    selection criteria, 357–358
    study design, 358–362
  key literature examples, 368–369
  measurement
    cognitive/memory testing, 359–360
    hypoxia, 360
    neuroendocrine testing, 361
    non-CNS pharmacological effects, 361–362
    physiologic brain testing, 360–361
    scopolamine model of dementia, 360
  patient studies, 362–368
  pharmacodynamics, 358–382
  pharmacokinetics, 357, 358
Ambulatory blood pressure monitoring, 190–191
Ambulatory tremor monitoring (tremor Holter), 378
Amine pressor tests, 331–332
Aminoguanidine, 476
Anaerobic bacteria, 497
Analgesics, 537–542
  for acute pain, 540–541
  for chronic pain, 541
  healthy volunteers, 537–540
  NSAIDs, 174, 394–395, 428, 539
  patient studies, 540–542
Angina, effort, 207–208, see also Antianginal drugs
Angiography, quantitative, 200–201
Animal studies, 35–49
  acute toxicity, 36–37
  aging studies, 47
  carcinogenicity, 39–40
  categorization, 42
  chronic toxicity, 37–39
  ethical and moral issues, 42–43
  four R's of, 45
  hypersensitivity/immune response, 40–41
  importance of, 23–25
  limitations, 236
  neurotoxicity, 41
  new strategies, 46–47
    fixed dose oral toxicity, 46
    limit test, 46
    sequential studies/decision tree, 46
  recommendations for improvement, 42
  refinement of animal experiments, 43–45
  reproductive/developmental toxicity, 41
  transgenic species, 95–96
Ankle/brachial pressure index (ABPI), 259, 262
Antacids, interactions, 78
Antianginal drugs
  as contraindications for test subjects, 262
  evaluation methods
    pharmacodynamic profiling, 199–204
      atrial pacing, 201–202
      coronary blood flow assessment, 202
      hemodynamic studies, 199–201
      quantitative coronary angiography, 201
      radionuclide procedures, 202–204
    stress tests
      exercise, 204–208
      pharmacological, 204
  study design, 208–210
    patient selection, 208–209
    protocol, 209–210

Antianxiety drugs, see Anxiolytics and hypnotics
Antiarrhythmic agents, 213–215
  supraventricular arrhythmias, 215
  ventricular arrhythmias, 213–215
Antiasthmatic drugs, 291
  data analysis, 291
  study design, 283–291
    bronchial challenge experiments, 283–284
    efficacy measurement, 288
    number of patients, 288–290
    statistical methods, 290–291
    therapeutic trials (short-term), 283–288
Antibiophenotype tests, 504
Antibiotics, 485–507
  animal models, 500
  automated microdilution systems, 506
  "core" dossier, 491–499
    anaerobes, 497
    Borrelia spp., 497–498
    Campylobacter spp., 497
    gram-negative bacilli, 494–496
    gram-negative cocci, 494
    gram-positive bacilli, 493
    gram-positive cocci, 492–493
    Helicobacter pylori, 401–402, 497
    intracellular pathogens, 498
    Leptospira spp., 498
    mycobacteria, 498
    Nocardia spp., 498
    Treponema pallidum, 498
  CSF activity, 501
  essential documentation, 487–491
    data required to begin trials, 489–491
    use of compound, 488–489
  general considerations, 486
  interactions with fecal and oral flora, 501
  mechanisms of action and resistance, 500–501
  pharmacodynamics, 501–503
  preselection, 486–487
  resistance epidemiology, 505–506
  specific indications, 500
  study design, 503–505
Anticancer drugs, 523–533
  classes of, 524
  decision making, 532–533
  general considerations, 523–525
  healthy volunteer studies contraindicated, 525
  patient studies, 525–532
    phase I, 526–530
    phase II, 530–532
  pharmacokinetics, 529–530
  safety considerations, 527–528
  study design, 529
  surrogate markers, 530
Antidepressants, 329–341
  alternative dose-finding approaches, 338–339
  compliance issues, 339
  of future, 340–341
  healthy volunteers, 330–334
  interactions, 333–334
  markers of depression, 337–338, see also Depression
  patient studies
    alternative dose-finding approaches, 338–339
    compliance issues, 339
    concentration-response relationships, 338
    cost-benefit analysis, 339
    markers of depression, 337–338, see also Depression
    overdose, 339
    safety considerations, 334
    special populations, 339–340
      elderly, 340
      gender, 339
      pregnancy, 339–340
    study design, 334–337
  pharmacodynamics, 331–333
    amine pressor tests, 331–332
    autonomic function tests, 332
    electroencephalography (EEG), 332
    imaging techniques, 333
    modeling studies, 333
    psychomotor performance, 332
  pharmacokinetics, 331
  safety considerations, 331
  serotonin reuptake inhibitors, 60
  special populations, 339–340
  stereoisomerism, 334
  tricyclic, 301
Antiepileptic drugs, 305–314
  healthy volunteers, 306–309
  monotherapy studies, 312–313
  patient studies, 310–312
Antigen-IGE response, 443
Antihistamines, 24
Antihypertensive drugs, see also Diuretics
  decision making, 231–232
  diuretics, 415–422
  general considerations, 217
  healthy volunteer studies, 218–230
    age, 218
    gender, 218
    race, 218
    safety considerations, 219–220
    selection criteria, 219
    study design, 220–224
  patient studies, 230–232
    safety considerations, 230
    selection criteria, 230
    study design, 230–231
    surrogate markers, 231
  pharmacodynamics, 226–230
  pharmacokinetics, 224–225

Antiinflammatory drugs, see also Analgesics
  NSAIDs, 174, 394–395, 428, 539
  in skin disorders, 442
Antimicrobials, see also Antibiotics; Antiviral drugs
  antibiotics, 465–507
  antiviral drugs, 511–522
Antiparasitic drugs, 498, see also Antibiotics
Antiparkinsonian agents, 373–380
  decision making, 380
  healthy volunteers, 374–375
  patient studies, 375–380
Antipsychotics, 347–353
  decision making, 352–353
  general considerations, 347–348
  healthy volunteers, 348–349
  patient studies, 349–352
Antiseizure drugs, 305–314, see also Antiepileptic drugs
Anti-ulcer drugs, 401–410
  decision making, 410
  general considerations, 401–410
  healthy volunteers, 412–406
  key literature, 410
  patient studies, 406–409
Antiviral drugs, 511–519
  acute and recurrent infections, 513–515
  chronic infection, 515–517
  combination therapy, 517–518
  drug classes, 512
  general considerations, 511–512
  laboratory assessment, 517
  prophylaxis, 512–513
  resistance to, 518, 519
  safety evaluation, 518
Anxiolytics and hypnotics
  decision making, 324–325
  general considerations, 317–318
  healthy volunteers, 318–323
  patient studies, 323–324
  pharmacodynamic, 319–324
  pharmacodynamics, 319–324
    elderly persons, 322
    electroencephalography (EEG), 321
    psychomotor function testing, 319–320
    sleep studies, 321–322
    tolerance, rebound, and withdrawal, 322, 323–324
  pharmacokinetics, 318–319
  safety considerations, 322
APA Task Force, 338
ApoE gene in dementias, 356
Arrhythmias
  Cardiac Arrhythmia Suspension Trial (CAST), 214–215
  as side effects, 24
  supraventricular, 215
  and terfenadine-ketoconazole interactions, 60
  ventricular, 213–215
Artificial stomas, 391
Asberg Depression Rating Scale, 335
Aspirin, 262, see also Analgesics; Antiinflammatory drugs
Association of British Pharmaceutical Industry, see ABPI; Legal liability
Asthma, see also Antiasthmatic drugs
  airflow limitation measurements, 282
  antiasthmatic drugs, 282–292
  epidemiology and pathogenesis, 281–282
Atherosclerosis, see also Peripheral arterial occlusive disease
  healthy volunteers
    safety considerations, 252–253
    selection criteria, 252
    study design, 253–261
  measurement, 253–261
    blood vessel tone, 256–257
    coagulation and hemorrheology, 255–256
    coagulation system, 257–258
    vasodilatation, 253–255
  pathogenesis, 250–252
Atrial pacing, 201–202
Automated microdilution systems, 506
Autonomic function tests, 332
Autonomic system, pharmacological preliminary considerations, 18, 19
Autonomy of volunteer subjects, 105–106
Autoradiography, whole-body, 29–30

B

Beat-by-beat pressure (volume clamp method) blood pressure measurement, 189–190
Beck Depression Inventory, 335
Behavioral toxicity, 297
Beneficence, 104
Benzodiazepines, 301, see also Sedatives
Beta blockers, 239
Bicarbonate secretion test, 392
Biliary system, 387–388, 390–391
Bioavailability (absolute absorption), 170, 296–297
Biological properties, preliminary considerations, 7–9
Biopsy, gastrointestinal, 394–395
Biotechnology, 93–100
  background, 93–94
  conclusions, 99–100
  gene therapy, 97–99
    antisense, 98–99
    sense, 97–98
  perspective, 97
  technical support systems, 95–97
    cell separation techniques, 96
    DNA/RNA probes, 97

immuno-adsorption techniques, 96
polymerase chain reaction (PCR), 96–97
transgenic animals, 95–96
Blood cell counts, 258–259
Blood pressure
in exercise testing, 207
measurement, 188–191
ambulatory monitoring, 190–191
beat-by-beat pressure (volume clamp method), 189–190
hemodynamic, 200
Blood vessels of skin, 440
Body sway/saccadic eye movement analysis, 296–297
Bordetella pertussis, 496
Borrelia spp., 497–498
Bronchial challenge experiments, 283–284, see also Antiasthmatic drugs
Bronchodilators, see Antiasthmatic drugs
Buccal absorption, 391
Buccal assay, 394
Burkholderia spp., 496

C

CAD (coronary artery disease), see Peripheral arterial occlusive disease
Caffeine and antihypertensive studies, 219
CAMCOG software, 364–365
Campylobacter spp., 497
Cancer chemotherapeutic agents, 523–533, see also Anticancer drugs
Carbamazepine, 306, see also Antiepileptic drugs
Carcinogenicity, animal studies, 39–40
Cardiac arrhythmias, see Antiarrhythmic agents; Arrhythmias
Cardiac Arrhythmia Suspension Trial (CAST), 214–215
Cardiac catheterization, 199–200
left heart, 200
right heart, 199–200
Cardiac failure, 237–247, see also Heart failure
Cardiac glycosides, 238
Cardiography
displacement, 188
Doppler, 184–185
echo, 184–185, 187–188
impedance, 183–184
Cardiovascular system, 179–278, see also specific drug types
antianginal drugs, 197–210
evaluation methods, 199–210
pathophysiological aspects, 198–199
antiarrhythmic agents, 213–215
supreventricular arrhythmias, 215
ventricular arrhythmias, 213–215
antihypertensive drugs, 217–231
decision making, 231–232
in healthy volunteers, 218–230
patient studies, 230–231
atherosclerosis, lipid-acting drugs, 463–473
diuretic effects on, 416, see also Diuretics
heart failure, 237–247
adrenoreceptor antagonists, 239
decision making, 247
diuretics, 239
endpoints, 239
healthy volunteer studies, 239–244
NYHA classification, 237–238
patient studies, 244–247
positive inotropic drugs, 238–239
safety issues, 239
vasodilators, 238
ketoconazole-terfenadine interactions, 24, 60
noninvasive measurement, 179–192
blood pressure, 188–191
ambulatory monitoring, 190–191
beat-by-beat pressure (volume clamp method), 189–190
cardiac output/inotropic state, 183–188
choice of method, 186–187
CO_2 rebreathing techniques, 185–186
displacement cardiography, 188
Doppler/echo-Doppler cardiography, 184–185
echocardiography, 187–188
impedance cardiography, 183–184
systolic time-intervals, 187, 242–243
general considerations, 180–182
repeatability, 180–181
sensitivity, 182
validity, 181–182
heart rate, 191–192
interpretation, 182–183
methods, 183–192
vasodilatation, 243, 254–255
peripheral arterial occlusive disease, 249–274
Good Clinical Practice considerations, 273–274
healthy volunteers, 252–261
pathogenesis of atherosclerosis, 249–252
patient studies
critical limb ischemia, 267–273
intermittent claudication, 261–267
pharmacological preliminary considerations, 18, 19
CAST (Cardiac Arrhythmia Suspension Trial), 214–215
Cell separation
fluorescence-activated cell sorting (FACS), 96
physical parameter selection, 96
Chemical purity, 6
Chemotherapeutic agents, 485–533, see also Analgesics; Anticancer drugs; Antimicrobials
anticancer drugs, 523–533

antimicrobials
antibiotics, 485–507
antiviral drugs, 511–522
Children as subjects, 69–70, 109
Chlorpromazine, 301
Cholesterol-lowering drugs, 463–473, see also Lipid-acting drugs
Cholinergic theory of Alzheimer's disease, 360
Chromatography, 26, 96
Chronic toxicity, animal studies, 37–39
Cigarette smoking, see Smoking
Clearance, renal, see also Metabolism
in cirrhosis, 78
[^{31}Cr] excretion, 393
prediction of *in vivo in vitro*, 55–57
in renal failure, 78
Clearance tests, 415
CNS effects, see also specific drug types
Alzheimer's disease/dementia, 355–368
decision making, 368
healthy volunteers, 356–362
key literature examples, 368–369
patient studies, 362–368
antidepressants, 329–341
of future, 340–341
phase I studies, 330–334
phase II studies, 334–340
antiepileptic drugs, 305–314
healthy volunteers, 306–309
monotherapy studies, 312–313
patient studies, 310–312
antiparkinsonian agents, 373–380
decision making, 380
healthy volunteers, 374–375
patient studies, 375–380
antipsychotics, 347–353
Decision making, 352–353
general considerations, 347–348
healthy volunteers, 348–349
patient studies, 349–352
anxiolytics and hypnotics, 317–326
decision making, 324–325
general considerations, 317–318
healthy volunteers, 318–323
patient studies, 323–324
pharmacodynamics, 319–323
pharmacokinetics, 318–319
measurement, 295–302
general considerations, 295–296
neurophysiological measurements, 296–297
psychometric testing, 297–301
saccadic eye movement/body sway analysis, 301
subjective feelings, 301–302
Coagulation measurements, 255–260
Coagulation system, 19, 257–261
Cognitive impairment, 347–353, 355–368, 373–380, see also CNS effects
Cognitive/memory testing, 359–360
Colonic transit time, 389, see also Gastrointestinal system
Colonoscopy, 391, 393
Column chromatography, 96
Compensation for injury, 140–142
Computer-based systems, 46, 47, see also Modeling
dementia diagnosis, 364–365
Congestive heart failure, see Heart failure
Conjugation (phase II) enzymes, 53
Consent
ABPI forms for, 138–139, 151–153
in children, 133
in dementia research, 363
and disclosure of risks and research, 135–138
informed, 113–114, 132–139, 351–352, 363, 467
in lipid-acting drug studies, 467
of mentally handicapped, 133–134, 351–352
and negligence, 134–135
of patients, 113–114
and randomization and placebo controls, 138
and respect for autonomy, 105–106
and trespass to person, 132
of volunteer subjects, 105–106
Consent forms, 138–139, 151–153
Controls, placebo and informed consent, 138
CO_2 rebreathing techniques, 185–186
Coronary angiography, 200–201
Coronary artery bypass grafting, 268
Coronary artery disease (CAD), see Peripheral arterial occlusive disease
Coronary blood flow measurement
continuous thermodilution, 202
Doppler techniques, 202
electromagnetic flow profiles, 202
gas clearance, 202
positron emission tomography (PET scan), 202–204
radionuclide methods, 202–204
Corticosteroids, vasoconstrictor assay for potency, 442, see also Antiinflammatory drugs
Costing and administration, 81–92
complexity of research and, 82
conclusions, 91–92
cost/time tradeoff, 82–83, 339
country-specific pricing, 91
general considerations, 81–82
hospital overhead management, 90–91
incremental pricing, 91
investigator fee setting and budgeting, 88–89
opinion leader grants, 90
PICAS/CROCAS database, 82
selection of institutions, 88
setting payment levels, 89–90
simplification of protocols, 83–88

CPMP Guidelines, 125–127, see also Legal liability
[^{31}Cr] excretion in urine, 393, see also Clearance, renal
Criminal liability, 130
Critical flicker fusion threshold test, 299
Critical limb ischemia, 267–273, see also Peripheral arterial occlusive disease
CRP isoforms, 52–55
CSF activity of antibiotics, 501
Cytochromes P-450, *in vitro* studies, 52–55

D

Decision points in human studies, 67–79
  additional Phase II studies, 77–78
  discontinuance, 78–79
  entry-into-man, 68–69
  first efficacy studies, 75–77
  general considerations, 67–68
  tolerability studies, 68–75
Declaration of Helsinki, 112, 127, see also Ethical/legal considerations
Dementia, 355–368, see also Alzheimer's disease/dementia
Dementia Rating Scale, 364
Depression
  age and, 340
  assessment of, 335
  epidemiology, 334
  gender and, 339
  markers of, 337–339
Dermatitis, 442, 447–456, see also Eczema/dermatitis
Diabetes mellitus, 263, 475–480, see also Antidiabetic therapy
Diagnostic modalities, see Measurement
Dialysis in distribution studies, 29
Diarrhea induction, 394
Diet
  and antihypertensive studies, 220
  monitoring of, 469–471
Digitalis glycosides, 238, see also Heart failure
Digit symbol substitution, 300
Discontinuance of trials, 78–79
Displacement cardiography, 188
Distribution, 29–30, see also Pharmacodynamics; Pharmacokinetics
Diuretics, 239
  adverse-effect studies, 421–422
  extrarenal activity of, 416
  pharmacodynamics, 417–420
  pharmacokinetics, 417
  renal physiology and, 415–417
  study design, 420–421
DNA content of cellular exfoliation, 392
DNA/RNA probes, 97
Doppler/echo-Doppler cardiography, 184–185
Doppler laser flowmetry, 254–255, 392–393
Dosage
  decision points for
    determination of maximum, 74
    dose/response and time curve determination, 72–73
    duration of administration, 74–75
    duration of followup, 75
    escalation of, 70–71
    fed versus fasting administration, 75
    initial (entry-into-man), 70
    measurement parameters for humans, 72
    safety parameters, 71–72
    single- versus multiple-, 74
  form of (route of administration), 6–7
Dose, minimal eczema, 443
Dose/plasma concentration, 76–77, 165–166, 170–173
Dosing regimen selection, 159–160
Driving tests, 300–301
Drug-induced gastrointestinal injury, 391–395
  bicarbonate secretion test, 392
  biopsy, 394–395
  buccal assay, 394
  colonoscopy, 393
  [^{31}Cr] excretion in urine, 393
  diarrhea induction, 394
  DNA content of cellular exfoliation, 392
  fecal blood loss, 393
  gastric electrical transmural potential difference test, 392
  gastrointestinal hormone assays, 395
  gastroscopy, 393
  measurement, 391–394
  mucosal blood flow-laser Doppler flowmetry, 392–393
  pepsinogen in blood, 394
  saliva collection, 394
Drug interactions, see also Adverse effects
  antibiotics with fecal and oral flora, 501
  antidepressants, 333–334, 335
  antidiabetic drugs with food, 48
  antiepileptic drugs, 308–309
  in antihypertensive studies, 219
  organizational issues, 77–78
  over-the-counter drugs, 335
  in vitro investigation of, 58–60
Dynamic nailfold capillary microscopy, 255
Dyslipidemia, 463–473, see also Lipid-acting drugs
Dysrhythmia, see Antiarrhythmic drugs; Arrhythmias

E

ECG (electrocardiography), in exercise testing, 206–207
Echocardiography, 187–188
Echo-Doppler cardiography, 184–185

Eczema/dermatitis
  drug targeting, 448
  erythema dose-response curves, 443
  general considerations and subtypes, 447–448
  healthy volunteers, 454–455
  immune reactions, 443–444
  minimal eczema dose, 443
  patient studies, 455
  study design, 448–456
  weal reactions, 443
Efficacy
  decision points, 75–77
  first, 75–77
  pharmacological effects versus clinical benefit, 76
Effort angina, 207–208
Eicosanoids, 256
EKG (electrocardiography), in exercise testing, 206, 207
Elderly persons
  antidepressants in, 340
  anxiolytics and hypnotics in, 322
  decision to use, 69–70
  depression in, 340
  pharmacokinetics in, 174
  as volunteer subjects, 109
Electrocardiography (ECG), in exercise stress testing, 206–207
Electroencephalography (EEG), 332
  anxiolytics and hypnotics, 321
  quantitative pharmaco-EEG, 296–297, 332, 361
Enalapril, 227
Endocrine disorders, 463–480, see also Antidiabetic drugs; Lipid-active compounds; Metabolic disorders
Endothelin, 256
Enterobacteriaceae, 494
Enterococcus spp., 493
Entry-into man, see also Decision points in human studies
Entry-into-man, 68–69, 75–77, 220–221, see Entry-into-man
Enzyme isoform identification, 56–57
Enzymes for *in vitro* studies, 52–57
Epilepsy, 305–314, see also Antiepileptic drugs
Erythema, 443–444
Erythrocytes (RBCs), blood flow effects, 258
Esophageal motility, 386
Ethical/legal considerations, 103–153
  ABPI guidelines, 118–122
  in animal studies, 42–43
  in cancer chemotherapy trials, 525–526
  fraud and misconduct, 115–117
  healthy-volunteer research, 103–110
    beneficence, 104
    children, 109
    elderly, 109
    general considerations, 103
    impoverished persons, 108–109
    justice, 103–104
    non-maleficence, 104–105
    payment, 106–107
    prisoners, 109
    recruitment, 107–108
    respect for autonomy/consent, see Consent
    staff, 108
    students, 108
    women of childbearing potential, 109
  legal liabilities in clinical trials, 123–153
    ABPI Clinical Trial Compensation Guidelines, 149–151
    ABPI/Department of Health Form of Indemnity, 151–153
    clinical trial defined, 124
    compensation for injury, 140–144
    ethics committees', 139–140
    investigators', 130–139
    law and medical ethics, 124–127
    manufacturers', 127–130
    proof of causation, 144–145
    regulation under general principles of law, 127
    regulatory authorities', 140
    researchers' indeminities, 145–146
  patients as subjects, 111–122
    confidentiality, 122
    general and historical background, 111–112
    Good Clinical (Research) Practice guidelines, 115
    informed consent, 113–114
    research ethics committees, 112–113, 120–121
    U.K. Department of Health guidelines, 114
  promotion and marketing, 117–118
Ethylene glycol elixir case, 111–112
Evoked potential tests, 361, 539
Excretion, 31–32
Exercise testing
  contraindications, 205
  ECG data evaluation, 206–207
  indications, 206
  interpretation, 206
  intervention/ischemia endpoints, 208
  methods available, 204–205
  protocols, 205–206
Exercise training, 266
Eye movement analysis in CNS studies, 296–297

F

Fasting versus fed administration, 75
Fat measurement, 439
FDA (U.S. Food and Drug Administration), 111–112
Fecal blood loss test, 393

Fibrinolysis, 259–260
Fixed dose oral toxicity, 46
Flavin-containing monoxygenases, 53
Fluorescence-activated cell sorting (FACS), 96
Food intake monitoring, 469–471
Food interactions, 78, 174, 308
Four R's of animal studies, 45
Fraud and misconduct, 115–117
  detection of, 116–117
  prosecution of, 117
  reasons for, 115–116

G

GABA inhibitors, 309, see also Antiepileptic drugs
Gastric acid secretion, 401–410, see also Anti-ulcer drugs
  continuous intragastric monitoring, 405–406
  cytoprotective agents, 406
  nasogastric intubation/aspiration, 403–405
Gastric electrical transmural potential difference test, 392
Gastric motility, 386–387
Gastrointestinal absorption, see under Absorption
Gastrointestinal system, 385–396
  anti-ulcer drugs, 401–410
    decision making, 410
    general considerations, 401–410
    healthy volunteers, 406–412
    key literature, 410
    patient studies, 406–409
  drug-induced injury, 391–395
    bicarbonate secretion test, 392
    biopsy, 394–395
    buccal assay, 394
    colonoscopy, 393
    [^{31}Cr] excretion in urine, 393
    diarrhea induction, 394
    DNA content of cellular exfoliation, 392
    fecal blood loss, 393
    gastric electrical transmural potential difference test, 392
    gastrointestinal hormone assays, 395
    gastroscopy, 393
    mucosal blood flow—laser Doppler flowmetry, 392–393
    pepsinogen in blood, 394
    saliva collection, 394
  inflammatory bowel diseases, 395–396
  measurements
    absorption, 390–391
    gastric pH/acid secretion, 403–406
    motility, 386–389
    secretion, 389–390
  pharmacological preliminary considerations, 18, 19
Gastroscopy, 392, 393
Gender
  in antihypertensive studies, 218
  depression and, 339
Genitourinary system, 414–431
  diuretics, 415–422
    adverse-effect studies, 421–422
    extrarenal activity of, 416
    pharmacodynamics, 417–420
    pharmacokinetics, 417
    renal physiology and, 415–417
    study design, 420–421
  pharmacological preliminary considerations, 19
  renal side effects, 425–431
    general considerations, 425–427
    measurement, 427–431
    nephrotoxicity, 427
Glomerular filtration rate (GFR), 417–418, 427
Glucose tolerance disorders, 475–480
Good Clinical (Research) Practice, 115, 273–274, see also Ethical/legal considerations
Gram-negative bacilli, 494–496
Gram-negative cocci, 494
Gram-positive bacilli, 493
Gram-positive cocci, 492–493

H

HACEK microorganisms, 496
Haemophilus ducreyi, 496
Haemophilus spp., 495
Hair, 440, see also Skin
Hamilton Rating Scale for Depression, 335
Harpenden skinfold caliper, 439
Healthy volunteer (phase I) studies
  antidepressants, 331–334
  antidiabetes drugs, 477–478
  antiepileptic drugs, 306–309
  antihypertensive drugs, 218–230
  antiparkinsonian agents, 374–375
  antipsychotics, 348–349
  anti-ulcer drugs, 406–412
  anxiolytics and hypnotics, 318–323
  biosynthetic agents, 477
  contraindicated for anticancer drugs, 525
  decision to use, 69–70
  ethical/legal considerations, 103–110
    beneficence, 104
    children, 109
    compensation, 143
    elderly, 109
    general considerations, 103
    impoverished persons, 108–109
    justice, 103–104
    non-maleficence, 104–105
    payment, 106–107
    prisoners, 109
    recruitment, 107–108

respect for autonomy/consent, 105–106
staff, 108
students, 108
women of childbearing potential, 109
heart failure, 239–244
heart failure drugs, 239–244
peripheral arterial occlusive disease, 252–261
pharmaco-EEG studies, 297
Heart failure, 237–247
adrenoreceptor antagonists, 239
decision making, 247
diuretics, 239
endpoints, 239
healthy volunteer studies, 239–244
NYHA classification, 237–238
patient studies, 244–247
positive inotropic drugs, 238–239
safety issues, 239
vasodilators, 238
Heart rate measurement, 191–192
atrial pacing, 201–202
cardiovascular reflexes, 191
continuous R-R interval, 191
in exercise testing, 207
Helicobacter pylori, 401–402, 497, See also Anti-ulcer drugs
Helsinki Declaration, 112, 127
Hematologic system, pharmacological preliminary considerations, 19
Hemodynamics, 199–201
antihypertensive drugs and, 227–230
catheterization, 199–200
left heart, 200
right heart, 199–200
in peripheral arterial occlusive disease, 257–261
pressure measurements, 200
quantitative angiography, 200–201
Hemorrheology, 255–260
Hepatocyte cell line studies, 55, see also *In vitro* studies
HF (high frequency) capsules, 390–391
Holter (ambulatory) blood pressure monitoring, 190–191
Holter (ambulatory) tremor monitoring, 378
Hormones
as depression markers, 338
gastrointestinal, 395
H_2 receptor blockers, 401–402, see also Anti-ulcer drugs
Hypersensitivity
animal studies, 40–41
in asthma, 283
skin reactions, 443–444
Hypertension, see Antihypertensive drugs; Diuretics
Hypnotics, 317–326, see also Anxiolytics and hypnotics
Hypokalemia, diuretic-induced, 421
Hypoxia in vascular dementia, 360, see also Alzheimer's disease/dementia

I

IDDM (insulin-dependent diabetes mellitus), 475–480
Immune adsorption ferromagnetic beads, 96
Immune system
animal studies, 40–41
pharmacological preliminary considerations, 19
skin reactions, 443–444
Immuno-adsorption techniques, 96–97
column chromatography, 96
immune adsorption ferromagnetic beads, 96
panning, 96
Impedance cardiography, 183–184
Impoverished persons as volunteer subjects, 108–109
Infectious disease, see also Antibiotics; Antiviral drugs
bacterial, 485–506
viral, 511–518
Inflammation, 19
Inflammatory bowel diseases, 395–396
Informed consent, see Consent; Legal liability
Injury compensation insurance, 140–142
Inotropic drugs, 238–239, see also Heart failure
Insulin-releasing agents, 476
Insulin sensitizers, 476
Insurance, injury compensation, 140–142
Integumentary system, 437–456, see also Skin
Interactions, see Drug interactions
Intermittent claudication, 261–267, see also Peripheral arterial occlusive disease
Intestinal motility, 388–389
Intestinal secretion, 389–390
Intracellular pathogens, 498
Intragastric continuous monitoring, 405–406
Intubation, absorption measurement by, 380–391
Investigator's legal liability, 130–145, see also Legal liability
In vitro-in vivo extrapolation, 59–60
In vitro studies, 51–63
advantages of, 51–62
enzymes used in, 52–54
conjugation (phase II) enzymes, 53–54
cytochromes P-450, 52–53
flavin-containing monooxygenases, 53
experimental systems, 54–55
heterologous expression systems, 55
human liver tissue, 54–55
molecular models, 55
relevant applications, 55–60
In vivo drug clearance prediction *in vitro*, 55–57

Ischemia
cardiac, see Peripheral arterial occlusive disease
critical limb, 267–273, see also Peripheral arterial occlusive disease
Itching, 441, see also Eczema/dermatitis; Skin

J

Justice in use of volunteers, 103–104

K

Ketoconazole-terfenadine interactions, 24, 60
Kidney, see Renal

L

Lamotrigine, 307, 308, see also Antiepileptic drugs
Laser Doppler flowmetry, 254–255, 392–393
Legal liability, 123–153, see also Ethical/legal considerations
ABPI Clinical Trial Compensation Guidelines, 149–151
ABPI/Department of Health Form of Indemnity, 151–153
clinical trial defined, 124
compensation for injury, 140–144
ethics committees', 139–140
investigators', 130–139
consent, 132–135, 138–139, see also Consent
disclosure of risks and research, 135–138
general principles, 130–132
randomization and placebo controls, 138
law and medical ethics, 124–127
manufacturers', 127–130
criminal, 130
to investigator, 127
to research subject, 128–130
strict, 129–130
proof of causation, 144–145
regulation under general principles of law, 127
regulatory authorities', 140
researchers' indemnities, 145–146
Leptospira spp., 498
Leukocytes, blood flow effects, 259
Levodopa, see Antiparkinsonian agents
Limit test in animal studies, 46
Lipid-acting drugs, 463–473
diet monitoring, 469–471
efficacy endpoints, 471
informed consent, 467
lipoprotein measurements, 468–469
patient selection, 465–467
pharmacodynamics, 472
pharmocokinetics, 472
professional staff requirements, 464–465
safety endpoints, 471
study design, 464
Liver tissue *in vitro* studies, 54–55
Loop diuretics, 416, 421, see also Diuretics
Losartan, 230
Low molecular weight proteins, 428–429
Lymphocyte-borne skin response, 443

M

Manufacturers' legal liability
criminal, 130
to investigator, 127
to research subject, 128–130
strict, 129–130
MAO inhibitors, 330, 333–334, see also Antidepressants
Marketing ethics, 117–118
Maximal work capacity, 207, 208
Measurements, 165–167
cardiovascular noninvasive, 179–192, see also under specific drug types
blood pressure, 188–191
ambulatory monitoring, 190–191
beat-by-beat pressure (volume clamp method), 189–190
cardiac output/inotropic state, 183–188
choice of method, 186–187
CO_2 rebreathing techniques, 185–186
displacement cardiography, 188
Doppler/echo-Doppler cardiography, 184–185
echocardiography, 187–188
impedance cardiography, 183–184
systolic time-intervals, 187, 242–243
general considerations, 180–182
repeatability, 180–181
sensitivity, 182
validity, 181–182
heart rate, 191–192
interpretation, 182–183
methods, 183–192
of vasodilatation, 243, 254–255
CNS effects, 295–302
general considerations, 295–296
neurophysiological measurements, 296–297
psychometric testing, 297–301
saccadic eye movement/body sway analysis, 301
subjective feelings, 301–302
drug-induced gastrointestinal damage, 391–394
gastrointestinal system
absorption, 390–391
motility, 386–389
secretion, 389–390
in humans generally, 157–175
pain, 538–539

pharmacokinetic, 169–175, see also Pharmacokinetics
psychometric tests for depression, 335
pulmonary function testing, 283–284, 286
renal function
glomerular filtration rate (GFR), 417–418, 427
tubular function, 418–421, 428–429
skinfold test of body fat, 439
study design, 157–167, see also Study design
unwanted drug effects, 166–167
wanted drug effects, 166
Memory tests, 300, 359–360
Metabolic disorders
antidiabetic therapy, 475–480
goals of therapy, 476–477
modeling, 477
pathogenesis of diabetes mellitus, 475
phase II studies, 478–480
phase I studies, 477–478
lipid-acting drugs, 463–473
diet monitoring, 469–471
efficacy endpoints, 471
informed consent, 467
lipoprotein measurements, 468–469
patient selection, 465–467
pharmacodynamics, 472
pharmocokinetics, 472
professional staff requirements, 464–465
safety endpoints, 471
study design, 464
Metabolic preliminary considerations, 23–33
absorption and pharmacokinetics, 27–29
analytical methodology, 26
distribution, 29–30
excretion, 31–32
general drug disposition, 23–25
guidelines for, 25–26
metabolism, 30–31
physicochemical properties, 27
Metabolism
human and pharmacokinetics, 173
in vivo studies, 31
preliminary considerations, 30–31
in vitro studies, 30–31
METs (metabolic equivalents; maximal exercise tolerance), 207, 208
Microbiological studies, 485–506, see also Antibiotics
Microsomes, 54–55
Mini-Mental State Examination (MMSE), 364
Modeling
antidepressants, 333
Modeling, pharmakokinetic/pharmacodynamic, 171–173
Molecular properties, 9
Monitoring
ambulatory blood pressure (Holter), 190–191
ambulatory tremor (tremor Holter), 378
diet, 469–471
intragastric continuous, 405–406
Moraxella spp., 495
Motility, gastrointestinal, 386–389
Mucosal blood flow/laser Doppler flowmetry, 392–393
Multiple system atrophy, 376, 377, see also Parkinson's disease
Mycobacteria, 498
Myocardial oxygen consumption testing (MVO2), see Cardiovascular system

N

Nails, 440–441, see also Skin
Nasogastric intubation/aspiration, 403–405
Negligence, 128–129, see also Ethical/legal considerations
Neisseria gonorrhoeae, 494
Neisseria meningitidis, 494
NeoR gene, 97
Neuroendocrine markers
of Alzheimer's disease/dementia, 361
of depression, 338
Neuroleptics, 347–353, see also Antipsychotics
Neurophysiological measurements, 296–297
Neurotoxicity, animal studies, 41
Neurotransmitters as depression markers, 337
NIDDM (noninsulin-dependent diabetes mellitus), 475–480
Nitric oxide, 256
NMR spectroscopy, renal, 430–431
Nocardia spp., 498
Nociception flexion index, 539
Nonmaleficence, 104–105
Nonsteroidal anti-inflammatory drugs (NSAIDs), adverse effects of, 174, 394–395, 428, 539
Nootropics, 356
NSAIDs (nonsteroidal anti-inflammatory drugs), adverse effects of, 174, 394–395, 428, 539
NYHA classification of heart failure, 237–238

O

Opioids, 540, 542, see also Analgesics
Organizational issues, 67–100, see also Study design
biotechnology, 93–100
background, 93–94
conclusions, 99–100
gene therapy: sense and antisense, 97–99
technical support systems, 95–97
costing and administration, 81–92
complexity of research and, 82
conclusions, 91–92

cost/time trandeoff, 82–83
country-specific pricing, 91
general considerations, 81–82
hospital overhead management, 90–91
incremental pricing, 91
investigator fee setting and budgeting, 88–89
opinion leader grants, 90
PICAS/CROCAS database, 82
selection of institutions, 88
setting payment levels, 89–90
simplification of protocols, 83–88
decision points in human studies, 67–79
additional Phase II studies, 77–78
discontinuance, 78–79
efficacy studies, 75–77
entry-into-man, 68–69
general considerations, 67–68
tolerability studies, 68–75
Orphan drugs, 113–114
Overdose, antidepressants, 339

P

Pain
management of, 537–542, see also Analgesics
measurement of, 538–539
category judgments, 538
cerebral event related potentials, 538–539
nociception flexion index, 539
Parkinson's disease, 373–380
classification of, 377
differential diagnosis, 377
surrogate markers, 378–379
U.K. Parkinson's Disease Society Brain Bank Clinical Diagnostic Criteria, 378
Parozetine, 60
Pasteurella spp., 496
Patient (phase II) studies
anti-asthmatic drugs, 282–292
anticancer drugs, 525–532
antidepressants, 333–3340
antidiabetes drugs, 478–480
antiepileptic drugs, 310–312
antihypertensive drugs, 230–232
antipsychotics, 349–352
anti-ulcer drugs, 406–409
anxiolytics and hypnotics, 323–324
heart failure drugs, 244–247
legal liability and compensation, 143–145
lipid-acting drugs, 463–473
Patients
as research subjects, 111–122, see also Consent; Ethical/legal considerations; Legal liability
Patient studies
peripheral arterial occlusive disease
critical limb ischemia, 267–273
intermittent claudication, 261–267
Payment of volunteer subjects, 106–107
Pepsinogen in blood, 394
Peripheral arterial occlusive disease, 249–274
diagnostic modalities, 253–261
blood vessel tone, 256–257
coagulation and hemorrheology, 255–256
coagulation system, 257–258
hematopoietic system, 258–261
vasodilatation, 253–255
Good Clinical Practice considerations, 273–274
healthy volunteer studies, 252–261
atherosclerosis
safety considerations, 252–253
selection criteria, 252
study design, 253–261
pathogenesis of atherosclerosis, 249–252
patient studies
critical limb ischemia, 267–273
intermittent claudication, 261–267
PET scan (positron emission tomography), 202–204, 309, 333, 349, 361
pH, gastrointestinal, 8, 403–406
Pharmaceutical preliminary considerations, 3–13
biological considerations, 7–9
dosage form, 6–7
general, 15–16
general considerations, 3–4
physicochemical considerations, 9–11
preformulation considerations, 4–8
primary, 16–17
secondary, 17–20
autonomic system, 18, 19
cardiovascular system, 18, 19
CNS, 17–18, 19
gastrointestinal system, 18, 19
genitourinary system, 19
hematologic system (coagulation effects), 19
immune system, 19
respiratory system, 18, 19
U.S., U.K., and Europe compared, 18
Pharmacodynamics
Alzheimer's disease/dementia, 358–382, 364–366
antianginal drugs, 199–204
antibiotics, 501–503
antidepressants, 331–333
antiepileptic drugs, 309
antihypertensive drugs, 226–230
antiparkinsonian agents, 375
antipsychotics, 349
anti-ulcer drugs, 403–406, 407–409
anxiolytics and hypnotics, 319–324
atherosclerosis studies, 253–254
CNS drugs, 296–297
diuretics, 417–420, see also Renal function tests
heart failure drugs, 241–243
lipid-acting drugs, 472

Pharmacokinetic/pharmacodynamic modeling, 171–173
Pharmacokinetics
- absorption, 169–170
- Alzheimer's disease/dementia, 357, 358, 364
- anticancer drugs, 529–530
- antidepressants, 331
- antiepileptic drugs, 307–309
- antihypertensive drugs, 224–226
- antiparkinsonian agents, 375, 378
- antipsychotics, 349, 350
- anti-ulcer drugs, 403, 407
- atherosclerosis studies, 253
- bioavailability, 170
- diuretics, 417
- food effects on, 174
- heart failure drugs, 241
- human metabolism and, 173
- lipid-acting drugs, 472
- peripheral arterial occlusive disease, 265, 271
- plasma dose concentration, 76–77, 165–166, 170–173
- plasma drug concentration, 76–77, 165–166, 170–172
- preliminary considerations, 27–29
- in special patient groups, 174
  - elderly, 174
  - renal disease, 174

Phase II studies, see Patient (phase II) studies
Phase I studies, see Healthy volunteer (phase I) studies
Phenylethylamine, 337
Phenytoin, 306, see also Antiepileptic drugs
Physicochemical properties, 9–11, 27, see also Pharmacokinetics
PICAS/CROCAS database, 82
Placebo controls
- in dementia studies, 366–367
- and informed consent, 138
- in Parkinson's disease, 379

Plasma concentration of antidepressants, 338
Plasma/dose concentration, 76–77, 165–166, 170–173, see also Pharmacodynamics; Pharmacokinetics
- pharmacokinetic/pharmacodynamic modeling, 171–173
- time-course, 170–171

Plasma fibrinolysis, 259–260
Plasma protein-binding, 29
Plasminogen activator inhibitor, 260
Platelet function, 19
Platelet markers of depression, 337
Platelet tests, 258
Polymerase chain reaction (PCR), 96–97
Positron emission tomography (PET scan), 202–204, 309, 333, 361
Positron-emission tomography (PET scan), 349
Potassium-sparing diuretics, 416, 421, see also Diuretics
Preclinical assessment, see Animal studies
Preformulation considerations, 4–8
Pregnancy, depression/antidepressants in, 339–340
Preliminary considerations, 3–82
- animal tests as predictors, 35–49, see also Animal studies
  - acute toxicity, 36–37
  - aging studies, 47
  - carcinogenicity, 39–40
  - categorization, 42
  - chronic toxicity, 37–39
  - ethical and moral issues, 42–43
  - four R's of, 45
  - hypersensitivity/immune response, 40–41
  - limitations, 236
  - neurotoxicity, 41
  - new strategies, 46–47
    - computer-based systems, 47
    - fixed dose oral toxicity, 46
    - limit test, 46
    - sequential studies/decision tree, 46
    - *in vitro* testing, 46–47
  - physiological parameters
  - recommendations for improvement, 42
  - refinement of animal experiments, 43–45
  - reproductive/developmental toxicity, 41
- *in vitro* studies, 51–63
  - advantages of, 51–62
  - enzymes used in, 52–54
    - conjugation (phase II) enzymes, 53–54
    - cytochromes P-450, 52–53
    - flavin-containing monooxygenases, 53
  - experimental systems, 54–55
    - heterologous expression systems, 55
    - human liver tissue, 54–55
    - molecular models, 55
  - relevant applications, 55–60
    - case examples, 60
    - identification of enzyme isoforms, 56–57
    - prediction of interactions, 56–60
    - prediction of *in vivo* drug clearance, 55–56
    - understanding of side effects, 57–56
- metabolic, 23–33
  - absorption and pharmacokinetics, 27–29
  - analytical methodology, 26
  - distribution, 29–30
  - excretion, 31–32
  - general drug disposition, 23–25
  - guidelines for, 25–26
  - metabolism, 30–31
  - physicochemical properties, 27
- pharmaceutical background, 3–13
  - biological considerations, 7–9
  - dosage form, 6–7
  - general considerations, 3–4

physicochemical considerations, 9–11
preformulation considerations, 4–8
pharmacological, 15–20
general, 15–16
primary, 16–17
secondary by system, 17–20
Premature ventricular contrations (PVCs), 214–215
Prisoners as volunteer subjects, 109
Product License Application
see Study design
Pruritus, 441, see also Eczema/dermatitis; Skin
Pseudomonas spp., 494–495
Psoriasis, 441–442
Psychometric testing, 297–301
cognition and memory, 359–360
critical flicker fusion threshold test, 299
for depression, 335
digit symbol substitution, 300
driving tests, 300–301
general considerations, 297
memory tests, 300, 359–360
reaction time tests, 300
study methodology, 298–299
subject selection, 298
vigilance tasks, 299–300
Psychomotor function testing, 319–320, 332, 365
Psychomotor performance tests, 332
Psychotropic drugs, see CNS effects and specific drug types
PTCA (percutaneous transluminal coronary angioplasty), 269
Pulmonary function tests, 283–284, 286

Q

Quality of life, 514, 525–526
Quantitative angiography, 200–201
Quantitative pharmaco-EEG, 296–297, 332, 361

R

Race of subjects, in antihypertensive studies, 218
Radionuclide angiography, 202–204
Radionuclide labeling studies, 26, 393, 395
absorption, 28
antiepileptic drugs, 308
Randomization and informed consent, 138
RBCs (red blood cells), blood flow effects, 258
Reaction time tests, 300
Recruitment of volunteer subjects, 107–108
Reflectance spectrophotometry, 440
Renal dysfunction, 78, 174, 324
Renal function tests
electrolyte analysis, 428
glomerular filtration rate (GFR), 417–418, 427
low molecular weight proteins, 428–429
proton NMR spectroscopy, 430–431
tubular function, 418–421, 428–429
Renal physiology, 415–417
Repeatability, 180–181
Reproductive/developmental toxicity, animal studies, 41
Research ethics committees, 112–113, 120–121, 139–140, see also Ethical/legal considerations
Resistance to antimicrobials, 500–501, 504–506, 519
Respiratory gas exchange, 207
Respiratory system, 281–282
airflow limitation measurements, 282
antiasthmatic drugs, 282–292
asthma defined, 281–282
pharmacological preliminary considerations, 18, 19
Rest pain, See Peripheral arterial occlusive disease
Route of administration, 6–7, 160

S

Saccadic eye movement/body sway analysis, 296–297
Safety considerations
Alzheimer's disease/dementia, 359
anticancer drugs, 527–528
antidepressants, 331, 334
antiepileptic drugs, 307
antihypertensive drugs, 219–220, 230
antiparkinsonian agents, 374
antipsychotics, 348, 350
anti-ulcer drugs, 402–403
antiviral drugs, 518
anxiolytics and hypnotics, 322
in atherosclerosis studies, 252–253
heart failure drugs, 239
lipid-acting drugs, 471
Saliva collection, 394
Schizophrenia, 347–348, see also Antipsychotics
Scintigraphy, 393, 395
Scopolamine model of dementia, 360
Screening, 3–4
for substance abuse, 219
Sebaceous glands, 441
Sedatives, 317–326, see also Anxiolytics and hypnotics
Seizures, 305–314, see also Antiepileptic drugs
Self-image and skin disease, 441
Seligiline, see Antiparkinsonian agents
Sensitivity, 182
Serotonin reuptake inhibitors, 60, 330, 333–334, 340, see also Antidepressants
Sex (of subjects), see Gender
Side effects, see Adverse effects
Single photon emission computed tomography (SPECT), 361

Skin disorders, 441–442
adolescent acne, 442
dermatitis and eczema, 442, 447–456, see also Eczema
eczema/dermatitis
drug targeting, 448
general considerations and subtypes, 447–448
healthy volunteers, 454–455
patient studies, 455
study design, 448–456
inflammatory responses to therapy, 442–444
psoriasis, 441–442
structures, functions, and constituents of, 438–440
Sleep markers of depression, 338
Sleep studies, 321–322
Small intestine, see Gastrointestinal system
Smoking
and antihypertensive studies, 219
peripheral arterial occlusive disease and, 263
Solubility, 5, 9–10, 10
Spectrophotometry, reflectance, 440
SSRIs (selective serotonin reuptake inhibitors), 330, 333–334, 340, see also Antidepressants
Stability, 11
Staff as volunteer subjects, 108
Staphylococcus aureus, 492
Staphylococcus pneumoniae, 493
State-Trait Anxiety Inventory, 298, 301–302
Steal pehnomenon, 251
Stenotrophomonas (Xanthomonas) maltophilia, 496
Stereoisomerism, 334
STIs (systolic time intervals), 187, 242–243
Streptococcus spp., 493
Stress tests
exercise, 204–208
pharmacological, 204
Strict liability, 129–130
Students as volunteer subjects, 108
Study design, 157–167, See also Good Clinical (Research) Practices
alternative add-on, 311
Alzheimer's disease/dementia, 359–362, 367–368
antianginal drugs, 208–210
antibiotics, 503–505
anticancer drugs, 529–529
antidepressants, 334–337, 335–337
antihypertensive drugs
diet and, 220
early phase, 221–223
entry-into-man, 220–221
healthy volunteer studies, 220–224
patient studies, 230–231
statistical considerations in hemodynamics, 223
antiparkinsonian agents, 375–375, 377–378
antipsychotics, 348–352
anti-ulcer drugs, 403, 407–408
CNS testing, 297–301
cross-over, 311
dosing regimens, 159–160
enriched parallel, 312
general considerations, 157–159
heart failure studies
healthy volunteers, 239–244
patient studies, 244–247
inclusion/exclusion criteria, 159
measurements, 165–167, see also Measurement
plasma drug concentrations, 76–77, 165–166, 170–172
unwanted drug effects, 167
wanted drug effects, 166
number of subjects, 160
objectives, 158
peripheral arterial occlusive disease
healthy volunteers (atherosclerosis), 252–261
patient studies
critical limb ischemia, 267–273
intermittent claudication, 261–267
phase I (general), 161–164
first administration—repeat dose, 163–164
first administration—single dose, 161–163
phase II (general), 164–165
preliminary considerations, 26
route of administration, 160
study restrictions, 159
Substance abuse and antihypertensive studies, 219
Supraventricular arrhythmias, 215
Surrogate markers
anticancer drugs, 530
gastric acid secretion, 407–408
in hypertension, 231
Parkinson's disease, 378–379
in peripheral arterial occlusive disease, 265–266, 271–272
for schizophrenia/psychosis, 350–351
Systolic time-interval measurement, 187, 242–243

T

Tacrine (THA), 356, see also Alzheimer's disease/dementia
Terfenadine-ketoconazole interactions, 24, 60
Thermography, 255
Thiazide diuretics, 416, 421, see also Diuretics
Thromboangiitis obliterans (Buerger's disease), 269
Thrombosis, see Peripheral arterial occlusive disease
Tolerability studies, decision points, 58–75
Tolerance, rebound, and withdrawal, anxiolytics and hypnotics, 322, 323–324
Total peripheral resistance (TPR) measurement, 243
Toxicity, acute, 36–37
Trace amines as depression markers, 337
Transgenic animals, 95–96
Treponema pallidum, 498

Tricyclic antidepressants, 60, 301, 330, see also Antidepressants
Tryptamine, 337
Tubular function tests, 418–421, 428–429
Tumor infiltrating lymphocytes (TILs), 97

U

U.K. Parkinson's Disease Society Brain Bank Clinical Diagnostic Criteria, 378
Ulceration in peripheral arterial occlusive disease, 272
Ulcers, 401–410, see also Anti-ulcer drugs
Ultrasonography
  Doppler/echo-Doppler cardiography, 184–185, 202
  Doppler laser flowmetry, 254–255, 392–393
  in peripheral arterial disease, 262
  skin thickness measurement, 439
Unified Parkinson Disease Rating Scale, 378
Ureaplasma spp., 496
U.S. Food and Drug Administration (FDA), 111–112

V

Validity, 181–182
Vascular dementia, 355–368, see also Alzheimer's disease/dementia
Vasoconstriction, 256–260, see also Peripheral arterial occlusive disease
Vasoconstrictor assay for potency of corticosteroids, 442
Vasodilatation measurement, 243, 254–255
  dynamic nailfold capillary microscopy, 255
  laser Doppler flowmetry, 254–255
Vasodilators, 238
Venous occlusion plethysmography, 228–230
Ventricular arrhythmias, 213–215
Vibrio cholerae, 495
Vigabatrin, 307, see also Antiepileptic drugs
Vigilance tasks, 299–300
Volunteers, healthy, see Healthy volunteer (phase I) studies
VO_2 max, 207

W

WBCs (white blood cells), blood flow effects, 259
Wheal responses, 443
Whole-body autoradiography, 29–30
Withdrawal, 322, 324–325
Women of childbearing potential as volunteer subjects, 109

X

Xanthomonas (Stenotrophomonas) maltophilia, 496

Y

Young subjects, see Children

Z

Zung Self-Rating Depression Scale, 335

3 5282 00411 0758